CRITICAL CARE REVIEW for NURSES

CRITICAL CARE REVIEW for NURSES

Sheryle L. Wills, R.N., B.S.N., J.D.
Sharyn F. Tremblay, R.N., B.S.N., M.S.
with nine contributors

JONES AND BARTLETT PUBLISHERS, INC.
BOSTON   MONTEREY

Copyright © 1986 by Jones and Bartlett Publishers, Inc. © 1984 by Wadsworth, Inc. All rights reserved. No part of this book may be reproduced, stored in a retrieval system, or transcribed, in any form or by any means—electronic, mechanical, photocopying, recording, or otherwise—without the prior written permission of the publisher.

Editorial Office: Jones and Bartlett Publishers, Inc., 23720 Spectacular Lane, Monterey, CA 93940

Sales and Customer Service Offices: Jones and Bartlett Publishers, Inc., 20 Park Plaza, Boston, MA 02116

Printed in the United States of America
10 9 8 7 6 5 4 3 2

Library of Congress Cataloging-in-Publication Data

Critical care review for nurses.

   Reprint. Originally published: Monterey, Calif.: Wadsworth Health Sciences Division, c1984.
     Bibliography: p.
     Includes index.
     1. Intensive care nursing. 2. Intensive care nursing—Examinations, questions, etc. I. Wills, Sheryle L. II. Tremblay, Sharyn A. [DNLM: 1. Critical Care—examination questions. 2. Critical Care—nurses' instruction. WY 154 C934 1984a]
RT120.I5C775 1986   610.73'61   86-7491

ISBN 0-86720-368-4

Sponsoring Editor: *James Keating*
Production Services Coordinator: *Marlene Thom*
Production: *Multi-Media Publishing, Inc.*
Manuscript Editor: *Barbara Jensen*
Interior Design: *Julianne Simmons*
Cover Design: *Jamie Sue Brooks*
Illustrations: *Julianne Simmons*
Typesetting: *Lesa Moore*
Printing and Binding: *The Maple-Vail Book Manufacturing Group*

To Jimmy (Johnny America) Lynn
and
to Andy F. Ferrara.
The warmth of your being lingers to comfort me,
and heaven is **alive** with song.

CCRN CONTRIBUTORS

Jo Bozza, RN, BSN, CCRN (Pulmonary Chapter)
Critical Care Clinician
Assistant Director of Nursing
Community Hospital of the Palm Beaches
West Palm Beach, Florida

Nancy Carlstedt, RN, BS (Overview Chapter)
Associate Executive Director-Nursing
Humana Bennett Hospital
Plantation, Florida

Annette Castenholz, RN, CCRN (Gastrointestinal Chapter)
Critical Care Clinician
Memorial Hospital
Hollywood, Florida

Marilyn Doughman, BS, RN, CCRN (Psychosocial Chapter)
Nursing Administration
Humana Bennett Hospital
Plantation, Florida

Aileen Goldstein, RN, BSN, CNRN, CCRN (Nervous System and
Assistant Director of Nursing   Endocrine Chapter)
Memorial Hospital
Hollywood, Florida

Margaret Guthaus, RN, CCRN (Renal Chapter)
I.C.U. Supervisor
Al Baha General Hospital
Al Baha, Saudi Arabia
(formerly Coronary Care Unit
Borges Medical Center
Kalamazoo, Michigan)

D. Katherine Jackson, RN, BSN, MA (Nursing Process)
Faculty: Department of Nursing Technology
Broward Community College
Ft. Lauderdale, Florida

Jane Lundgren, BA, RN, CCRN, CNRN (Hematopoietic Chapter)
Community Faculty
Metropolitan State University
Minneapolis, Minnesota

Barbara A. Perra, RN, MS, CCRN (Cardiovascular Chapter)
Critical Care Consultant
Past Corporate Regional Coordinator—A-O Med. Div.
Director of Education
Bennett Community Hospital
Plantation, Florida

Sharyn F. Tremblay, RN, BSN, MS
Critical Care Consultant
Chairperson: Department of Nursing Technology
Broward Community College
Ft. Lauderdale, Florida

Sheryle L. Wills, RN, BSN, JD
Critical Care Consultant
Adjunct Faculty: Department of Nursing Technology
Broward Community College
Ft. Lauderdale, Florida

PREFACE

The role of the critical care nurse has matured to the level of specialist. Certification as a critical care nurse has become a professional requirement for those who seek a specialized practice in critical care. Standards for certification have been developed and serve two purposes: to standardize nursing practice and to establish standards of patient care. Certification is achieved by successfully completing the American Association of Critical Care Nurses' examination. Preparation for this examination is facilitated by the AACN's Core Curriculum. The Core identifies and establishes the knowledge base required for certification. This is achieved by using behavioral objectives, combined with an extensive outline of content knowledge.

Many critical care nurses preparing for the certification examination find that reviewing an extensive body of scientific knowledge and making the appropriate clinical applications necessitates a very difficult research through numerous sources, which then must be synthesized to provide a reviewing base for the examination. The purpose of this publication is to provide a succinct, yet comprehensive, review of the core material. It has been our purpose to develop this book to serve as the primary mechanism to prepare critical care nurses for their registry examination. To achieve this goal, the textual material reflects the principles and the practice of adult education within the framework of the Core Curriculum. **Critical Care Review for Nurses** incorporates in one book the resource material needed to master the Core Curriculum. By integrating the sciences, nursing process and systems approach to patient care, this text is applicable to any facet of critical care nursing.

Each chapter uses a format that incorporates a variety of learning techniques.

(1) **Behavioral objectives** are listed at the beginning of each chapter.

(2) **Topical outlines** provide an overview of textual material and can be used for conceptualizing the subject matter as a whole.

(3) The **body of the text** succinctly clarifies the vast amount of material required for a complete review.

(4) **Key concepts,** which are placed throughout the body of the text, are set in bold type. They are identified by the following symbol:

Key concepts are brief statements of significant material that must be understood by the reviewer for mastery of the Core Curriculum.

(5) **Key point recognition** is an evaluation tool using a true-false format so the reader can obtain immediate feedback on the material within a chapter. Correct answers for all false statements provide additional content reinforcement.

(6) The acronym **PASS** stands for **Program Assessment: Science and Situation.** It is a multiple-choice, self-evaluation tool at the end of each chapter. This instrument provides immediate self-assessment on the mastery of chapter content.

(7) A **practice examination,** utilizing a modified form of clinical simulation, concludes the text. It gives the reviewer practical experience with the new examination methodology introduced with the examinations administered for the first time in the summer of 1982. Use of this practice examination should be made under simulated testing conditions. Upon completion of the examination, the reviewer should immediately identify those weak areas requiring additional study and refer to the appropriate sections in the text. After mastery of these content areas has been achieved, the examination should be repeated.

It may be advantageous for the reviewer to wait several days before retaking the examination. Repeating the examination several days prior to the certifying examination is also recommended.

(8) Each content chapter in the book also contains a **survey summary.** These are provided in outline form so the reader may make a rapid preview, or a subsequent review, of material. The reviewer can use the survey summaries to identify the areas that may be most appropriate for concentrating study time or areas where it is desirable to refer to additional source material. For some, the surveys may provide a good way to integrate the content of each chapter after it has been carefully studied.

Critical Care Review for Nurses may be used in the following ways:

- As a self-paced, individualized study program
- In conjunction with a structured course
- As a reference source for periodic review following successful passage of the certification examination
- For self-evaluation throughout one's career in critical care nursing

Helping others is what critical care and **Critical Care Review for Nurses** are all about. We hope this text helps the critical care nurse by providing a time-saving, economical way to prepare for the CCRN examination.

ACKNOWLEDGMENTS

The editors extend their appreciation to all the contributors for their continued support, dedicated work, and high standards of care and teaching. Their numerous revisions and suggestions are responsible for the integration of massive amounts of material into a succinct, workable review text.

We would like to acknowledge the physicians who reviewed each chapter for medical accuracy. Special thanks to Richard Sandler, M.D., Plantation, Florida, for close scrutiny of the renal chapter and to David Weissberger, M.D., Medical Director Respiratory Therapy, Community Hospital of the Palm Beaches, Palm Beach, Florida, for reviewing the respiratory chapter.

We wish to thank the publisher's reviewers for their helpful comments and recommendations: Dr. Michael Carter, R.N., Ph.D.; Jo Ann Niemeyer, R.N., C.C.R.N.; Lynne Phillips, R.N., M.S.N.; Anna Seroka, R.N., C.C.R.N.; Nancy Townsend, R.N., M.N., C.C.R.N.

A very special acknowledgment to Karen Craparo, M.D., Director of Emergency Medical Services, Hollywood Medical Center, Hollywood, Florida, for her continued support, valued friendship and intimate chats. Special thanks for suggestions and final review of the cardiovascular chapter.

G.I. photographs are courtesy of R.H. Castenholz II, R.R.T., B.A. We are appreciative of his time taken from medical school to enhance the G.I. chapter.

And to Pam Cantello, the lady who typed by candlelight, we sincerely thank you and promise never to say "by tomorrow" again! We appreciate all those deadlines you met!

To all at Multi-Media Publishing in Denver who labored with us in the early development of this book which really belongs to all of us—we thank you.

And to Norman Dinerman, M.D., Denver, Colorado, we say thanks, "Storm," for your kind words, continued support and sense of humor.

We must acknowledge our families and their continued patience as we secluded ourselves in the writer's lair night after night to write. Thank you Michael, Michele, Ashley and Angela for not moving away while the door was closed.

Sheryle Lynn Wills
Sharyn Ferrara Tremblay

CONTENTS

Chapter One—Introduction 1

  I. Critical Care Nursing: An Overview 3
     Critical care: yesterday 3
     Attributes of the critical care nurse 4
     Professional relationships 4
     Multiple systems approach 5
     Cost containment in the critical care unit 6
     Legal responsibilities of the critical care nurse 6
 II. The Nursing Process 8
     Overview 8
       Assessment 8
       Planning 9
       Implementation 10
       Evaluation 10
     Case study 10
       Case history 10
     Summary 12

Chapter Two—Psychosocial Aspects of Critical Care 15

    I. Psychosocial Nursing 19
   II. Basic Human Needs 19
  III. Mental Attitudes 20
   IV. Stress 21
    V. Common Emotional States of the Critical Care Patient 22
       Anxiety 22
       Denial 23
       Depression 24
   VI. Aggressive Sexual Behavior 24
  VII. Inappropriate Responses to Stress: Addiction/Suicide 25
 VIII. Crisis 26
   IX. The Stresses of Critical Care 27
       The patient's viewpoint 27
         Pain 28
       The nurse's viewpoint 29
       The family's viewpoint 29
    X. Death and Dying 30
       Program Assessment: Science and Situation 33
       Key Point Recognition Answers 39
       PASS Answer Sheet 41
       Survey Summary 43

Chapter Three—Nervous System 45

   I. The Nervous System: Overview 51
  II. Anatomy and Physiology 51
      Skull 51
      Spinal column 53

Nervous tissue: cells of the nervous system 55
Transmission of nerve impulses 56
Reflex action 59
Cerebral metabolism 60
Divisions of cerebral tissue 60
Cerebral blood supply 63
The ventricular system 66
The spinal cord 67
Autonomic nervous system 70

III. Assessment of the Neurological System 73
Cranial nerve testing 73
Cerebellar function testing 75
Sensory system testing 76
Motor system testing 76
Reflex testing 76
Level of consciousness 77
Pupillary response 77
Motor strength and equality 77
Evaluation of vital signs 78
Laboratory and radiologic studies 78

IV. Pathological States and Nursing Management 79
Cerebral vascular accidents (CVA) 79
Pathophysiology 79
Clinical presentation 80
Diagnostic data 80
Nursing care 80
Cerebral aneurysm 81
Pathophysiology 81
Clinical presentation 81
Diagnostic data 81
Nursing care 81
Meningitis 82
Pathophysiology 82
Clinical presentation 82
Diagnostic data 82
Nursing care 83
Guillain-Barre syndrome (acute polyneuritis) 83
Pathophysiology 83
Clinical presentation 83
Diagnostic data 83
Nursing care 84
Head injury 84
Pathophysiology 84
Clinical presentation 85
Diagnostic data 85
Nursing care 86
Spinal cord injury 86
Pathophysiology 86
Clinical presentation 87

Diagnostic data 88
Nursing care 88
Myasthenia gravis 89
Pathophysiology 89
Clinical presentation 89
Diagnostic data 89
Nursing care 90
Tetanus 90
Pathophysiology 90
Clinical presentation 90
Diagnostic data 90
Nursing care 90
Seizures 91
Pathophysiology 91
Clinical presentation 91
Diagnostic data 92
Nursing care 92
Status epilepticus 92
Pathophysiology 92
Clinical presentation 93
V. Care Common to Neurological Problems 95
Increased intracranial pressure (ICP) 95
Pathophysiology: ICP 95
Monitoring ICP 96
Subarachnoid screw 96
Ventricular drain 96
Epidural catheter 96
Methods to decrease ICP 96
Postoperative care 96
Program Assessment: Science and Situation 99
Key Point Recognition Answers 111
PASS Answer Sheet 117
Survey Summary 119

Chapter Four—Pulmonary System 129

I. Pulmonary System: Overview 135
II. Anatomy 135
Respiratory tract 135
Lungs 138
Bony thorax 139
Muscles of respiration 139
Inspiration 139
Expiration 140
Pulmonary circulation 140
III. Physiology 141
Ventilation 141
Flow measurements 142
Alveolar ventilation (Va) 142
Regulation of ventilation 142

  Mechanics of breathing 144
  Compliance 144
  Airway resistance 145
  Diffusion 145
  Oxygen transport 146
  Carbon dioxide transport 147
  Arterial hypoxemia 148
  Acid-base 149
   Buffer systems 149
   Chemical buffers 149
   Respiratory component 150
   Renal component 152
   Acidosis 153
    Causes of primary respiratory acidosis 153
    Causes of metabolic acidosis 153
   Anion gap 154
   Alkalosis 154
    Causes for respiratory alkalosis 154
    Causes for metabolic alkalosis 155
    Relationship of potassium and alkalosis 155
   Compensation 155
   Mixed acid-base disturbances 156
  Treatment 157
   Respiratory acidosis 157
   Metabolic acidosis 157
   Respiratory alkalosis 157
   Metabolic alkalosis 157
  Signs and symptoms 157
IV. Assessment of the Pulmonary System 158
  Patient assessment 158
  Anatomical landmarks 159
  Lungs 161
  Inspection 162
  Palpation 162
  Percussion 162
  Auscultation 163
   Techniques of auscultation 163
  Laboratory and radiologic studies 163
V. Pathological States and Nursing Management 166
  Respiratory failure 166
   Pathophysiology 166
   Pathophysiology: specific 166
   Clinical presentation 167
   Diagnostic data 167
   Nursing care 168
  Adult respiratory distress syndrome (ARDS) 168
   Pathophysiology: general 168
   Clinical presentation 169

Diagnostic data   169
Nursing care   169
Chronic obstructive pulmonary disease (COPD)   170
  Pathophysiology: general   170
  Pathophysiology: specific   170
  Clinical presentation   171
  Diagnostic data   171
  Nursing care   172
Status Asthmaticus   172
  Pathophysiology   172
  Clinical presentation   173
  Diagnostic data   173
  Nursing care   173
Pulmonary embolism   174
  Pathophysiology   174
  Clinical presentation   174
  Diagnostic data   175
  Nursing care   175
Chest trauma   176
  Pathophysiology: general   176
  Pathophysiology-rib fractures   176
  Clinical presentation   176
  Diagnostic data   176
  Nursing care   176
  Pathophysiology-flail chest   177
  Clinical presentation   177
  Diagnostic data   177
  Nursing care   178
  Pathophysiology-hemothorax, pneumothorax and tension pneumothorax   178
  Clinical presentation   179
  Diagnostic data   179
  Nursing care   179
Cardiac tamponade   180
  Pathophysiology   180
  Clinical presentation   180
  Diagnostic data   180
  Nursing care   180
Injury to the diaphragm   180
  Pathophysiology   180
  Clinical presentation   181
  Diagnostic data   181
  Nursing care   181
Tracheal or bronchial rupture   181
  Pathophysiology   181
  Clinical presentation   181
  Diagnostic data   181
  Nursing care   181

         Esophageal rupture   182
            Pathophysiology   182
            Clinical presentation   182
            Diagnostic data   182
            Nursing care   182
   VI. Care Common to Respiratory Problems   182
         Airway obstruction   182
         Airway maintenance   183
            Complications associated with airway intubations   187
         Continuous ventilatory support   187
         Drug therapy   190
         Suctioning   190
         Weaning   191
         Intermittent mandatory ventilation (IMV)   191
         General nursing care   191
         Chest physiotherapy   192
         Intermittent positive pressure breathing (IPPB)   192
         Continuous positive airway pressure (CPAP)   192
         Humidification   192
         Oxygen therapy   192
            Complication associated with oxygen therapy   193
         Adjunctive oxygen equipment   193
         Complications   194
   Program Assessment: Science and Situation   197
   Key Point Recognition Answers   203
   PASS Answer Sheet   211
   Survey Summary   213

Chapter Five—Cardiovascular System   229

   I. Cardiovascular System: Overview   235
  II. Anatomy   235
         Functional and microscopic anatomy   235
         Coronary chambers, valves, conduction system   238
            Chambers   238
            Atria   239
            Ventricles   240
            Valves   241
            Conduction system   241
         Circulation   243
            Coronary circulation   243
            Conduction system blood supply   244
            Lymph supply   244
            Vascular anatomy   245
 III. Physiology   246
         Electrophysiology   246
         Nervous control of the heart   249
            Reflex responses   249
         Factors affecting blood flow and pressure   250
            Regulation of flow   250

       Principles of distribution 251
   Cardiac cycle 252
   Cardiac output 253
   Factors affecting cardiac function and output 256
       Preload 256
       Central venous pressure (CVP) 257
       Pulmonary capillary wedge pressure (PCWP) 257
       Afterload 258
       Contractility 258
       Heart rate 259
       Anemia, ion concentration, hypoxia 259

IV. Assessment of the Cardiovascular System 260
   Level of consciousness 261
   Inspection 261
   Palpation 262
   Percussion 262
   Auscultation 263
   Heart sounds 263
       Normal heart sounds 263
       Physiological splitting 264
       Fixed splitting 264
       Gallops 264
       Order of sounds heard 264
       Abnormal heart sounds 265
   Evaluation of vital signs 267
   Laboratory and special studies 267
       Laboratory studies 267
       Special studies 268
       Electrocardiography 269
       Axis-vectors 274
       Axis deviation 276
       Hemiblocks 278
       Electrolytes and EKG changes 282
       Arrhythmia methods 282
       Common methods for rate determination 294
       Invasive assessment methods 295

V. Pathological States and Nursing Management 297
   Arteriosclerosis 297
       Pathophysiology 297
       Clinical presentation 298
       Diagnostic data 298
       Nursing care 298
   Angina pectoris 298
       Pathophysiology 298
       Clinical presentation 298
       Diagnostic data 299
       Nursing care 299
   Myocardial infarction 299
       Pathophysiology 299

    Clinical presentation 299
    Diagnostic data 299
    Nursing care 300
   Congestive heart failure and pulmonary edema 301
    Pathophysiology 301
    Clinical presentation 302
    Diagnostic data 303
    Nursing care 303
   Pericarditis 303
    Pathophysiology 303
    Clinical presentation 303
    Diagnostic data 304
    Nursing care 304
   Hypertensive crisis 304
    Pathophysiology 304
    Clinical presentation 304
    Diagnostic data 305
    Nursing care 305
   Shock 305
    Pathophysiology 305
    Clinical presentation 306
    Diagnostic data 307
    Nursing care 308
   Pacemakers 308
    Pathophysiology 308
    Temporary pacemaker 308
    Clinical presentation 309
    Diagnostic data 309
    Nursing care 309
    Permanent pacemakers 310
    Clinical presentation 311
    Diagnostic data 311
    Nursing care 311
    Types of pacemakers 312
    Electrical complications 314
   Surgical intervention 315
    Nursing care 315
    Vascular surgery 316
VI. Care Common to Cardiovascular Problems 321
  Cardiac circulation 321
  Hemodynamics: monitoring and adjuncts 321
   Central venous pressure 321
   Pulmonary artery wedge pressure monitoring 321
   Intra-aortic balloon pump (IABP) 321
   Nursing care 322
 Program Assessment: Science and Situation 327
 Key Point Recognition Answers 335
 PASS Answer Sheet 311
 Survey Summary 345

Chapter Six—Renal System 359

- I. The Renal System: Overview 365
- II. Renal Anatomy 365
    - Location 365
    - Size 365
    - Renal fascia 365
    - Gross structures 366
        - Renal cortex 366
        - Renal medulla 366
        - Renal pelvis 366
    - Nephron 367
        - Glomerulus 367
        - Renal tubules 368
- III. Renal Physiology 369
    - Glomerular filtration 369
    - Constituents of glomerular filtrate 370
    - Tubular reabsorption and secretion 370
        - Proximal tubule 370
        - Henle's loops 371
        - Distal tubule 371
        - Collecting tubules 371
    - Regulation of water balance 372
    - Regulation of blood pressure 373
    - Regulation of electrolytes 375
        - Sodium 375
        - Potassium 375
        - Calcium and phosphate 375
        - Magnesium 376
        - Chloride 376
    - Excretion of waste products 377
    - The kidney and acid-base balance 377
        - Phosphates as renal buffers 378
        - Secretion of ammonia 379
        - Acidosis 379
        - Alkalosis 379
- IV. Assessment of the Renal System 380
    - Gross cerebral function 380
    - Specific cerebral function 380
    - Inspection 380
    - Palpation 380
    - Percussion 380
    - Auscultation 381
    - Renal assessment 381
        - Level of consciousness 381
        - Voiding pattern 381
        - Control of stream 381
        - Dysuria 381
        - Toilet habits 381

Evaluation of vital signs 382
Laboratory and radiologic studies 382
V. Pathological States and Nursing Management 384
Acute renal failure 384
Pathophysiology: general 384
Pathophysiology: specific 386
Clinical presentation 386
Diagnostic data 386
Nursing care 386
Chronic renal failure 387
Pathophysiology 387
Clinical presentation 388
Diagnostic data 388
Nursing care 388
Pyelonephritis 388
Pathophysiology 388
Clinical presentation 389
Diagnostic data 389
Nursing care 389
Glomerulonephritis 389
Pathophysiology 389
Clinical presentation 390
Diagnostic data 390
Nursing care 390
Nephrotic syndrome 391
Pathophysiology 391
Clinical presentation 391
Diagnostic data 391
Nursing care 391
Hypertension 392
Pathophysiology 392
Clinical presentation 392
Renal insufficiency 392
Pathophysiology 392
Clinical presentation 393
Diagnostic data 393
Nursing care 393
Dialysis 393
Peritoneal dialysis 394
Hemodialysis 395
Nursing care 396
VI. Care Common to Renal Problems 397
Maintenance of fluid balance 397
Monitoring fluid balance 398
Maintenance of electrolyte balance 398
Maintenance of nutrition 399
Maintenance of renal perfusion 399
Maintenance of acid-base balance 399
Prevention of complications 400

Program Assessment: Science and Situation   403
Key Point Recognition Answers   411
PASS Answer Sheet   417
Survey Summary   419

Chapter Seven—Endocrine System   427

I. The Endocrine System: Overview   431
II. Anatomy and Physiology   432
    Endocrine glands   432
        Pituitary (hypophysis)   432
        Thyroid   432
        Parathyroid   432
        Pancreas   432
        Adrenals   433
    Hormones   434
        Hormones associated with the hypophysis   434
        Hormones associated with the neurohypophysis   436
        Hormones associated with the thyroid gland   437
        Hormones associated with the parathyroid gland   437
        Hormones associated with the pancreas   438
        Hormones associated with the adrenal glands   438
III. Assessment of the Endocrine System   441
    Gross cerebral functions   441
    Specific cerebral function   441
    Level of consciousness   441
    Inspection   442
    Palpation   442
    Percussion   442
    Auscultation   442
IV. Pathological States and Nursing Management   444
    Diabetes insipidus   444
        Pathophysiology   444
        Clinical presentation   444
        Diagnostic data   444
        Nursing care   444
    Secreton of inappropriate ADH (SIADH)   445
        Pathophysiology   445
        Clinical presentation   445
        Diagnostic data   445
        Nursing care   446
    Thyrotoxic crisis   446
        Pathophysiology   446
        Clinical presentation   446
        Diagnostic data   446
        Nursing care   446
    Hypoparathyroidism   447
        Pathophysiology   447
        Clinical presentation   447
        Diagnostic data   447

Nursing care 447
Diabetic ketoacidosis 447
Pathophysiology 447
Clinical presentation 448
Diagnostic data 448
Nursing care 448
Hyperketotic hyperosmolar coma (HHNK) 449
Pathophysiology 449
Clinical presentation 449
Diagnostic data 449
Nursing care 449
Hypoglycemia 449
Pathophysiology 449
Clinical presentation 449
Diagnostic data 450
Nursing care 450
Adrenal crisis 450
Pathophysiology 450
Clinical presentation 450
Diagnostic data 450
Nursing care 450
V. Care Common to Endocrine Problems 453
Airway and ventilation 453
Fluid and electrolyte balance 453
Neurological status 453
Patient and family education 454
Program Assessment: Science and Situation 455
Key Point Recognition Answers 463
PASS Answer Sheet 469
Survey Summary 471

Chapter Eight—The Gastrointestinal System 481

I. The Gastrointestinal System: Overview 485
II. Anatomy and Physiology 486
Upper G.I. system 486
Oral cavity 486
Pharynx 487
Esophagus 487
Stomach 488
Lower G.I. system 493
Small intestine 493
Large intestine 497
Blood supply to the G.I. tract 501
Nervous innervation 501
Accessory organs of digestion 502
Gallbladder 502
Pancreas 504
Liver 505

III. Physical Assessment of the Gastrointestinal System 506
   History 506
   Inspection 507
   Auscultation 508
   Percussion 509
   Palpation 509
IV. Nursing Assessment of the G.I. System 510
   Evaluation of eating 510
   Evaluation of swallowing 510
   Evaluation of digestion 510
   Evaluation of elimination 510
   Evaluation of vital signs 510
   Laboratory and radiologic studies 511
V. Pathological States and Nursing Management 512
   Cirrhosis of the liver 512
      Pathophysiology 512
      Case study 513
      Diagnostic data 514
      Nursing care 514
   Hepatic failure 515
      Pathophysiology 515
      Clinical presentation 515
      Case study 516
      Diagnostic data 516
      Nursing care 517
   Bleeding esophageal varices 517
      Pathophysiology 517
      Clinical presentation 518
      Case study 518
      Diagnostic data 519
      Nursing care 519
   G.I. hemmorrhage from peptic ulcers 520
      Pathophysiology 520
      Clinical presentation 520
      Case study 521
      Diagnostic data 522
      Nursing care 522
   Acute pancreatitis 522
      Pathophysiology 522
      Clinical presentation 523
      Case study 524
      Diagnostic data 525
      Nursing care 525
VI. Care Common to Gastrointestinal Problems 527
   Fluid and electrolyte problems 527
      Pathophysiology 527
      Clinical presentation 527
      Nursing care 527

Nutritional maintenance   528
   Clinical presentation   528
   Diagnostic data   528
   Nursing care   529
Program Assessment: Science and Situation   533
Key Point Recognition Answers   543
PASS Answer Sheet   547
Survey Summary   549

Chapter Nine—Hematopoietic System   557

  I. Hematopoietic System: Overview   563
 II. Anatomy and Physiology   563
    Blood   563
      Components   563
      Odor, color, specific gravity, pH   563
      Function   563
      Volume and volume control   563
    Plasma   565
      Components   565
      Color   565
      Function   565
      Volume control   565
    Blood-forming organs   566
      Bone marrow   566
      Liver   566
      Spleen   566
      White pulp   567
      Marginal zone   567
      Red pulp   567
      Functions of the spleen   567
    Normal red blood cell production, function and destruction   568
      Erythrocytes   568
      Hemoglobin   569
      Producton stimulus   569
      Destruction   569
    Normal white blood cell production and function   570
    The inflammatory process   572
    Immunity   573
      Cellular immunity   573
      Humoral immunity   574
      Alterations in immunologic response   574
    Blood groups   576
    Hemostasis   577
III. Assessment of the Hematopoietic System   578
    History and general signs and symptoms   578
    Specific signs and symptoms   579
    Inspection   579
    Palpation   579

Percussion 579
Auscultation 579
Evaluation of vital signs 579
Laboratory and radiologic studies 580
IV. Pathological States and Nursing Management 582
   Anemia 582
      Pathophysiology 582
      Clinical presentation 582
      Diagnostic data 582
      Nursing care 583
   Leukemia 585
      Pathophysiology 585
      Clinical presentation 585
      Diagnostic data 586
      Nursing care 586
   Lymphomas 587
      Pathophysiology 587
      Hodgkin's disease 587
      Non-Hodgkin's lymphoma 589
   Polycythemia 589
      Pathophysiology 589
      Clinical presentation 589
      Diagnostic data 589
      Nursing care 589
   Anaphylaxis 590
      Pathophysiology 590
      Clinical presentation 590
      Diagnostic data 590
      Nursing care 590
   Disseminated intravascular coagulation (DIC) 591
      Pathophysiology 591
      Clinical presentation 591
      Diagnostic data 591
      Nursing care 591
   Hemophilia 592
      Pathophysiology 592
      Clinical presentation 592
      Diagnostic data 592
      Nursing care 592
   Sickle cell disease 592
      Pathophysiology 592
      Clinical presentation 593
      Diagnostic data 593
      Nursing care 593
   Multiple myeloma 594
      Pathophysiology 594
      Clinical presentation 594
      Diagnostic data 594
      Nursing care 594

      V. Care Common to Hematopoietic Problems 596
          Reduced erythrocytes 596
              Nursing care 596
          Reduced white blood cells 596
              Nursing care 596
          Decreased platelet functions 596
              Nursing care 596
          Administration of blood 597
              Types of blood 597
              Complications related to transfusion 597
              Nursing care 597
      Program Assessment: Science and Situation 599
      Key Point Recognition Answers 609
      PASS Answer Sheet 615
      Survey Summary 617

Chapter Ten—How to Prepare for and Take an Examination 625
      How to Prepare for and Take an Examination 627
          Why take the examination? 627
          The CCRN examination 627
          Physical changes related to the stress of test-taking 627
          Examination preparation 628

Chapter Eleven—Practice Examination 629
Bibliography 669
Index 679

CHAPTER ONE
INTRODUCTION

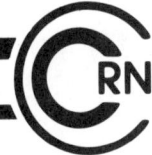

CRITICAL CARE NURSING: AN OVERVIEW

The professional nurse embarking on a career in critical care nursing has unprecedented challenges and opportunities. Nursing has been in a process of evolution for the past 20 years. One result of this evolutionary process is the concept of nursing specialists, or nurses with extended knowledge and skills. The critical care nurse is just such a specialist.

Critical care nursing demands specialized training in physiology and technology. But it also requires the personal attributes of intelligence, initiative, responsibility and integrity. Physiological assessment and parameters of care can be taught to professional nurses. But remember that skills and knowledge are only two components of the profession called nursing. Caring for the patient as an individual and sharing the hope of recovery or rehabilitation is the cornerstone of optimal nursing care.

Reviewing and reading this text will aid preparation for the critical care examination. It will also aid the nurse in caring more effectively for the critically ill patient. In these respects, rewards are immediate. But there are even more long-term rewards to be found in the critical care setting. The opportunity to work in many specialized settings—cardiac, trauma, surgical, renal, neuro and neonatal—is often a catapult into other career challenges.

All medical practice, including nursing care, is designed to observe the basic functions of life: inhalation, circulation, assimilation and elimination. Therefore, an understanding of these functions is a good starting point for the professional nurse. It is merely the varying parameters of these functions in relation to disease that distinguish the critical care nurse's orientation from that of the generalist. The basic nursing care is the same. The natural sciences are the same. Critical care nursing is merely the intensification of nursing practice—an evolutionary process!

CRITICAL CARE: YESTERDAY

The diversification of today's special care units offers the patient and practitioner a scope never before realized in the history of health care. It was the development in the mid-1950s of recovery rooms that initiated the concept of "special rooms" for "special care." This concept revolutionized health care and, within it, the nursing profession.

Recovery room nurses were given the extensive training and skills necessary to intervene in life-threatening situations due to complications of general anesthesia.

Recovery rooms proved effective, why not other areas for specialized needs? Surgical intensive care units were born. The patient who had major surgery was transferred from the recovery room to a specialized area where nurses, again on a reduced patient ratio, intervened in preventing and treating complications of major surgery.

Concurrently, bedside monitoring was being developed, as well as ventilatory assistance, in rehabilitative form for patients with post-devastating diseases, such as polio and tuberculosis. Thus, the surgical intensive care, coronary care and pulmonary rehabilitative units were the beginning of what are now widespread specialized units.

Most of these early innovations in critical care were developed at the university teaching hospital level. Teaching endeavors were directed primarily toward training the physician. Thus, the procedures and assessment skills were first within the domain of the physician, and then evolved into nursing skills. This two-tier system has persevered. The second tier has, at the community hospital level, evolved to the point that nurses accept much more of the responsibility for assessment and evaluation. They have become the ears and eyes of the non-hospital-based physician. The specialized care units of the hospital have directly influenced the nursing profession by accelerating the growth potential of the nursing staff. With the nurse alongside the physician as a teammate, nurse-physician relationships have been enhanced. Better communication between the nurse and physician has helped to facilitate the goal of health care innovations—patient care.

Struggling to establish an identity in the early years of critical care, nurses looked to other allied health disciplines for direction. It was not until 1969 that the critical care nurse was identifiable as a professional entity through the vehicle of a professional organization, the American Association of Critical Care Nurses (AACN). Appropriately at that time in the critical care evolution, AACN was the product of a group of coronary care nurses.

Early in its organization, the AACN began addressing the priorities of educational development and forming a national center for organization and reference. Specific methods to meet these goals were realized through the development of the core curriculum and certifying examination.

Through the realization of AACN's goals, critical care practitioners are being recognized, encouraged and assisted in professional growth. But with professional growth comes the responsibility of accountability.

A natural outgrowth of professional growth and accountability is an increased awareness of credentialing mechanisms. Certification is the strongest credentialing tool available for a voluntary professional organization. AACN has used the certification process to establish professional competency. This is the respected CCRN designation available to nurses who meet AACN's criteria for certification.

Other methodologies that can assure professional competency, and thereby meet the responsibility of accountability, include **in-depth interviews, skill assessments** and **case study interpretations.**

Return demonstration of psychomotor skills inherent in the care of the critically ill patient should be evaluated early in the employment of a critical care practitioner. With the legal climate of today's health care institutions, the increased expectancy of the consumer, the increase in the number of regulatory agencies, and the emphasis on accountability both by employer and practitioner, it can be expected that the credentialing process in nursing will evolve to the level of validation as the credentials-qualifications committees of present medical staffs review applicants.

ATTRIBUTES OF THE CRITICAL CARE NURSE

Experience shows that special care nurses come in all shapes, sexes, colors, sizes and ages. There are, however, some common identifiable characteristics. Critical care nurses usually are bright, caring individuals who have a sense of obligation to the patient, the family and the facility, as well as to their own professional growth. These nurses are usually well organized, can identify patient needs and can set priorities without the need for peer approval or direct intervention by others.

Critical care nurses must function well under pressure and demonstrate personal stability in all situations. The nurses in this setting must accept patients' values and attitudes without judgment. Professional nurses practicing in a specialty unit must take responsibility for their own convictions and decisions. The nurse must realize that many of the stressful situations in the unit are not to be taken personally.

A mature, caring nurse gains personal and professional satisfaction from the work in a critical care setting in spite of the ever present stress. Rewards are seen in a patient's smile, a family's appreciation or a physician's acknowledgment of a job professionally done.

Ultimately, the critical care nurse must be able to **care intensively,** allow the family to **intensively care** and not merely place the patient in **intensive care!**

PROFESSIONAL RELATIONSHIPS

The nurse in the critical care setting has an opportunity to work side by side with the physician as never before. Critical care nursing involves assessment and skills that once were totally within the realm of the physician. In the patient care process, the nurse is the **liason** between the hospital environment and the private physician.

The health care team may be captained by the physician, but it is navigated by the nurse. Good relationships with the multiple paramedical health care team members enhance patient care. Therefore, the navigator must understand the functions of the individual team members and assist in coordinating patient care in order for the team to maintain continuity, competency and coordination.

By the mere fact of proximity, the nurse often has the most impact on the patient and family. This constitutes a great deal of power and intervention in the lives of others. This power must be used wisely and consistently. Throughout the relationships with other team members, the nurse should **support care,** not replace it!

MULTIPLE SYSTEMS APPROACH

Assessment of the critically ill should be from the multiple system perspective, regardless of the specific unit to which the patient is admitted. The increased interest and use of systems charting provides additional validity to the multiple system concept. (See Fig. 1-1.)

SYSTEMS CHARTING ASSESSMENT FACTORS

1. Effects of the neurological system
   - pupil response
   - levels of consciousness
   - restlessness
   - confusion
   - syncope
   - pain

2. Effects of the circulatory system
   - blood pressure
   - peripheral pulses temperature
   - bruits when indicated
   - Homan's sign (calf tenderness)
   - capillary blood filling and nail bed color
   - petechiae, ecchymotic areas, pressure areas
   - skin color, moisture, temperature
   - edema
   - neck vein distention

3. Effects of the pulmonary system
   - respiratory rate and quality
   - chest expansion and configuration documented when abnormal
   - rales, rhonchi, breath sounds
   - shortness of breath, dyspnea nocturnal, dyspnea, exertional dyspnea
   - hemoptysis when present

4. Effects of the cardiac system
   - chest wall size and configuration documented when abnormal
   - apical/radial pulses; rate, quality, rhythm
   - heart sounds, murmurs
   - pericardial friction rub

5. Effects of the genitourinary system
   - urinary output
   - quantity
   - color
   - consistency
   - odor

6. Effects of the gastrointestinal system
   - inspection
   - auscultation
   - palpation
   - stool evaluation
   - N/V
   - appetite

7. Effects of laboratory results
   - ECG
   - x-ray studies
   - respiratory
   - laboratory studies

Fig. 1-1. Multiple Systems Charting

The multiple systems approach is well supported by the nursing process. The nursing process involves data collection, identification and prioritization of needs; formulation and implementation of an appropriate nursing approach; and evaluation.

Technology in critical care continues to increase at an astounding rate. The nurse has an obligation to stay abreast of these advances; but in this maze of instrumentation, it is imperative that the patient does not also become an object. The value of the individual as a person must be maintained. Human sensitivities must be perceived and valued. Technological advancements, which include many audio and visual parameters, are a constant threat to the sensory limitations of the patient. Therefore, the patient care plan should include compensation for this sensory and visual overload. Noise control, as well as repetitive orientation to person, place, time and anticipated procedures, should be components of the care plan developed via the nursing process.

Technological advancements that include monitoring and support devices for nearly every body system are prolific in the health care marketplace. The operating suite is the only care center that surpasses the critical care area in absorbing health care dollars spent on instrumentation. It is important that the practitioner be familiar with the normal values and pressures of technological assessments. However, the patient can be harmed as a result of inadequate correlation of technological data with data derived from physical evaluation. Therefore, multiple systems evaluation is a necessary component of technological evaluation.

Technological devices *must* be viewed within the clinical framework. The patient who is cardiographically and hemodynamically monitored, ventilated, Swan-Ganzed, dialyzed and balloon-pumped is an exquisite challenge to a technologically oriented critical care nurse. The nurse must remember that under the lines, tubes, dressings and monitors there is an individual with feelings, values and goals. Perhaps most important for the nurse to remember is that technology is meant to *enhance* patient care, not *replace* it.

COST CONTAINMENT IN THE CRITICAL CARE UNIT

Cost containment in critical care is an explosive issue. Consumers, health care providers and legislators agree that costs must be contained. But when it is a family member who needs critical care, then the request is for every available instrument and for only the best. Within the discussion of cost containment lurks the issue of quality of life versus dollars expended.

The critical care nurse has a responsibility in containing health care costs by controlling situations in which inefficiency, waste and redundancy occur. Coordinating physicians' orders to avoid duplicating diagnostic and therapeutic measures is an effective cost containment mechanism that can be controlled in the patient care setting. Evaluating capital expenditures to determine actual enhancement of patient care is easily performed by the nurse in the unit.

On the other hand, cost control measures should not be allowed to interfere with effective patient care, such as infection control practices. There must be a balance of health dollars and optimal care. The bedside nurse has a responsibility to help preserve health resources and dollars while providing quality patient care.

LEGAL RESPONSIBILITIES OF THE CRITICAL CARE NURSE

The legal responsibilities of the critical care nurse become more complex as the scope of practice broadens. Frequent causes of legal concern are the decisions, intervention and technological applications of assessments made daily by the critical care nurse. Legal implications are complex because they are matters of judgment, not emphatic rules of behavior.

From a legal standpoint, scope of practice issues are more easily resolved if the nurse adheres to policy, procedure and standing orders. The community standard is another parameter by which scope of practice is determined.

To legally assist the professional nurse, professional organizations and agencies have developed practice statements. However, a review of available literature indicates that the majority of legal claims against nurses are not scope of practice, but the result of carelessness and poor communication with colleagues, physicians and patients.

The best protection against legal claims is sound nursing judgment and adequate documentation. The patient's chart is the most visible document in court!

Nurses should protect their rights and be aware of their liabilities as well as the patients' rights. (See Fig. 1-2.)

> The health care consumer is more particularly referred to as the patient. The nursing profession today is constantly being challenged to join the consumer, or to become the patient's advocate. Once a patient or client has entered the health care system, it is considered a nursing function to coordinate the care he or she receives. In order for the nurse to perform this service, she must be familiar with what care, planning, and evaluation the patient is eligible to receive. The American Hospital Association, in November of 1972, adopted a statement of 12 principles which became known as the *Patient's Bill of Rights* [5]:
>
> (1) The patient has the right to considerate and respectful care.
>
> (2) The patient has the right to obtain from his physician complete current information concerning his diagnosis, treatment, and prognosis in terms the patient can be reasonably expected to understand.
>
> (3) The patient has the right to receive from his physician information necessary to give informed consent prior to the start of any procedure and/or treatment... Where medically significant alternatives for care or treatment exist, or when the patient requests information concerning medical alternatives, the patient has the right to such information (and) to know the name of the person responsible for the procedures and/or treatment.
>
> (4) The patient has the right to refuse treatment to the extent permitted by law, and to be informed of the medical consequences of his action.
>
> (5) The patient has the right to every consideration of his privacy concerning his own medical care program.
>
> (6) The patient has the right to expect that all communications and records pertaining to his care should be treated as confidential.
>
> (7) The patient has the right to expect that within its capacity a hospital must make reasonable response to the request of a patient for services.
>
> (8) The patient has the right to obtain information as to any relationship of his hospital to other health care and educational institutions insofar as his care is concerned...(and) any professional relationships among individuals, by name, who are treating him.
>
> (9) The patient has the right to be advised if the hospital proposes to engage in or perform human experimentation affecting his care or treatment...(and) has the right to refuse to participate.
>
> (10) The patient has the right to expect reasonable continuity of care.
>
> (11) The patient has the right to examine and receive an explanation of his bill regardless of source of payment.
>
> (12) The patient has the right to know what hospital rules and regulations apply to his conduct as a patient.

Fig. 1-2. Bill of Patients' Rights*

Critical care nursing has come to mean technology, skills, management, advanced knowledge and caring. As these evolve, critical care nursing evolves. With credentialing, the visibility of the specialty nurse is heightened. Tomorrow? The possibilities of growth are unlimited. Develop professional critical care nursing for your personal and professional growth, and for the ultimate reason, better patient care.

*Reprinted with the permission of the American Hospital Association.

THE NURSING PROCESS

OVERVIEW

The *nursing process* is the utilization of a scientific method to individualize the delivery of patient care. The increased complexity of patient problems has necessitated a systematic approach to patient care. The nursing process provides a vehicle for nursing professionals to *assess, plan, implement* and *evaluate* the quality of care their patients receive.

The critical care nurse is a health professional who has the opportunity to continually observe patients' needs and spend the majority of nursing time at the bedside. Therefore, the critical care nurse's primary goal should be fulfilling the patient's needs.

The four components of the nursing process are:

Assessment

Planning

Implementation

Evaluation

The nursing process provides the nurse with a systematic approach to caring for patients. A systematic approach is essential when working in a critical care unit, where patient care is complex and team members need to be well coordinated.

The process is *goal-directed* nursing care, which besides improving patient care, provides a higher level of satisfaction among health team members. For a critical care nurse to carry out an efficient plan of patient care, an adequate number of qualified staff members is essential. They are necessary to perform their assigned duties and to oversee the complexity of care in relation to predetermined criteria and goals.

The patient's records are concrete proof of the effectiveness of activities and are the critical source for evaluating the success of established goals. These records also provide a perpetual basis for new information in the continual revision of the patient's plan of care.

Assessment

The first step in the nursing process, assessment, should be viewed as an orderly, continual process of collecting and analyzing data to determine the patient's problem. Patient assessment is the responsibility of every professional nurse.

The nurse and the patient have open and dynamic communication. The basic principle from the beginning of the relationship is the acceptance of the patient as a person. The nurse can utilize knowledge and experience, personal sensitivity and personal values, beliefs and perceptions to assess the patient's needs.

The critical care nurse is constantly receiving new data on the patient. The data is received through formal and informal routes and is used primarily to help the nurse decide the patient's needs and appropriate nursing actions. Formal data is received through the nurse's skilled observation, patient history and diagnostic test results. Informal data is received through ongoing communication with the patient, family and other health team members. The nurse must analyze all the data and continually make decisions regarding its priority, reliability and usefulness. All data must be considered before making a decision, but the decision is based on the best information available at the time.

One constant problem to accurate assessments, especially in critical care units, is inadequate time to gather all the data. The nurse is pressed into implementing immediate patient care with a minimum data base. The nurse should try to obtain adequate data except in emergencies, where immediate intervention is essential.

Data should cover all aspects of the patient's body systems. Each system is related to the functioning of the whole person, just as separate steps make up the whole of the nursing process. The **nursing history** may be the foundation of information upon which other data can be developed. The history should include:

(1) Basic data: name, date, address

(2) History: chief complaint

(3) Previous illness: characteristics

(4) Previous history

(5) Review of systems

(6) Family history

(7) Personal-social history

(8) Expectations of hospitalization

The format used to obtain the history should be flexible enough to accommodate any situation, and allow sufficient time to focus on the patient as a person.

In an emergency situation, there may not be an opportunity to obtain a complete nursing history. Furthermore, hospital records and a complete previous history may not be available. The nurse's primary sources will become the patient's family, friends and physician. All data obtained must then be placed in perspective to other data.

The critical care patient is in a dependent position. The nurse must evaluate the immediate needs of the patient. Illness has different effects on each individual. One patient may experience dependency from separation anxiety, another may worry about the financial burden, while a third may fear impending death. The nurse should try to understand:

(1) How the patient and the family perceive the situation

(2) What they expect from the hospitalization

To minimize feelings of dependency, begin the patient's participation in the treatment program in the critical care unit. The patient must be involved in the planning and caring of health in order to lessen loss of control and identity.

A primary goal of the critical care nurse is the patient's progress from dependence to independence. This is best accomplished by providing the patient with all necessary information from which sound decisions can be made. The nurse must be skilled in recognizing the meaning of the patient's verbal and nonverbal communication. When formulating the plan of care, the patient's strengths and decisions regarding care should be utilized and supported. Using these principles limits unrealistic expectations that the patient is not capable of achieving.

Planning

The planning phase is essential to the nursing process. Planning is accomplished through a nursing diagnosis. This process begins when the critical care nurse first comes in contact with the patient, and it changes with the patient's condition. The objective of the planning phase is the expected patient outcome. **(The expected outcome may be a small task or overall patient progress.) Whatever the planned outcome, it must be specific and written in behavioral terms. It should determine the best course of action to attain the desired goal. Planning involves identification of potential problems and incorporates flexibility of nursing care.**

The more complex the patient's care, the more important planning becomes. Maslow's hierarchy of needs allows the nurse to prioritize the patient's problems and formulate a nursing diagnosis. A nursing diagnosis is an assessment of the circumstances and conditions surrounding the patient that are significant to restoring wellness.

In contrast, the medical diagnosis summarizes the patient's signs and symptoms and remains the same, regardless of the patient's progress. Just as a medical diagnosis is an independent function of the physician, a nursing diagnosis is recognized as an independent function of the professional nurse. It is important that the critical care nurse accept this responsibility, make nursing decisions and accept the outcome of those decisions. However, there must be a realization that the nurse cannot do everything for every patient. Consideration must be given to the staff's capabilities, available equipment and the motivation of the patient. Realistic goals that will resolve the patient's problem must be set. These goals should be based on a 24-hour period, ensuring continual evaluation, revision and continuity of care.

Implementation

The third step of the nursing process, implementation, is putting the plan into action. It is easier to plan care than it is to implement individualized patient care. The critical care nurse cannot physically provide all of the nursing care. The nurse's responsibilities also include delegating and coordinating other health team members. Successful implementation of an individualized plan of care is a dynamic process that involves communication among staff members, as well as staff development through formal and informal instruction.

The implementation of the care plan must be flexible enough to accommodate change, either in emergency situations or as the patient becomes more independent. As the patient becomes more independent, nursing intervention decreases. However, the critical care nurse should always be available to assist the patient. The implementation phase requires continual review to meet ever changing needs.

Evaluation

Evaluation is the final step in the nursing process. Evaluation is that part of the process used to determine the success of the plan. It allows for continuation of the specific care or addition of new data from which to base a revision. The evaluation is directly related to the nursing diagnosis and plan of care, with the end result being improvement of the patient's health and appropriateness of the nursing actions.

Evaluation is becoming more important as consumers of health care demand accountability from health care providers. Evaluation is accomplished predominantly through direct observation by the nurse, based on both objective and subjective data. However, other resources should be utilized, including laboratory results, team conferences, medical progress reports and nursing care plans.

The dynamic elements of the nursing process continue as evaluation cycles back to the beginning and becomes part of the new data that individualizes patient care.

CASE STUDY

The following case study demonstrates how the nursing process is used to formulate an individualized care plan.

Case History

A 63-year-old white male, Mr. R., was admitted through the emergency department for his fifth hospitalization. He was known to have a history of coronary artery disease, chronic obstructive pulmonary disease and a triple aortocoronary bypass graft, performed three years previously. His last admission, eight months ago, was for a sudden onset of pulmonary edema. At that time he was found to have severe systemic hypertension. He responded well to medical treatment and was discharged to his home on daily doses of digoxin 0.25 mg, Lasix (furosemide) 40 mg and nitropaste 1" every four hours. Mr. R. was seen routinely in the physician's office and considered to be doing reasonably well.

In the early morning, Mr. R. developed a sudden onset of respiratory distress and was taken to the emergency room by the paramedics and accompanied by his wife. On admission he was found to be unconscious, cyanotic, with severe dyspnea, and he deteriorated to a straight-line EKG. Cardiopulmonary resuscitation was initiated and rhythm was restored to atrial tachycardia with marked ST segment elevation. He received sodium bicarbonate to reverse the acidosis, furosemide and ethacrynic acid to initiate mobilization of fluid, with the resulting effect of returning him to a stable baseline. Mr. R's blood pressure rose throughout the procedure to 240/110, but returned to baseline after the above treatment was instituted.

A physical examination was performed post-resuscitation in the emergency room with the following results:

CNS: conscious, oriented, moving all four extremities

C/V: color—pale; skin—warm and dry
    atrial tachycardia at 110, no audible murmurs or pericardial friction rubs
    slight jugular vein distention
    B.P. 140/80

RESP: rales bilaterally in all lobes posteriorly
    slight expiratory wheezes
    no pleural rubs

ABD: no masses or tenderness palpated, bowel sounds present

Mr. R. was admitted to the coronary care unit with the tentative medical diagnosis of:

1. Rule out myocardial infarction
2. ASHD post ACB
3. Severe systemic hypertension
4. Pulmonary edema
5. Obesity

A Swan-Ganz catheter was inserted into his right subclavian vein to measure hemodynamics. The pulmonary capillary wedge pressure (PCWP) was 15 mm Hg (6 to 12 mm Hg is normal), with a pulmonary artery pressure of 36/17 mm Hg (20/10 mm Hg is normal).

Early lab results showed the following:

Radiograph: evidence of pulmonary congestion, early pulmonary edema with borderline heart size

ABG: pH 7.10
           pCO_2 64
           pO_2 73
           BE - 11
           HCO_3 18

SMA: K^+ 3.7 Na^+ 140
        BUN 26 K^+ 3.7
        NA 140 CO_2
        GLU 101 Cl^- 95

                         Bun 26
                         Glu 101

HEMOGLOBIN: Hgb 16.5
                  Hct 50.4
                  WBC 18, 100

The following orders were written for Mr. R., in addition to the routine CCU protocol:

IPPB with Bronkosol 4 gtts/3cc NaCl q4 hr. while awake

O_2 3 liters per nasal cannula

Nitropaste 1" q4 hr.

Lasix (Furosemide) 40 mg P.O. QD

Lanoxin (digoxin) 0.25 mg P.O. QD

morphine sulfate 4 to 6 mg I.V. Q3 to 4 hr. as necessary

I.V. 5% dextrose in water KVO rate
LDH, CPK, SGOT, ABG, SMA6, EKG in a.m. and daily for 3 days
2 gm Na, low-cholesterol diet
fluid restrictions of 1500 cc per 24 hr.

The coronary care nurse developed a care plan as soon as Mr. R. was stabilized, and he and his wife were interviewed. The nursing care plan was evaluated after the first 24 hours, and the necessary revisions were made.

INITIAL CARE PLAN

Nursing Diagnosis	Expected Goals	Nursing Activities	Evaluation
1. Alterations in breathing pattern	To ensure adequate lung ventilation as evidenced by clear lungs on auscultation	Turn, deep breathe and cough every hour; IPPB with Bronkosol every 4 hours while awake; continuous Swan-Ganz readings; auscultate lungs every hour; patient on bedrest in orthopneic position	Clear lungs
		O_2 at 3 liters per nasal cannula; intake and output every hour; fluid restriction, 1500 cc/24 hr.	
		Weight daily in a.m., medications as ordered (i.e. Lasix, Lanoxin, morphine sulfate); lab test as ordered (i.e. SMA, ABG); 2 gm sodium diet; rotating tourniquets on standby	
2. Alterations in cardiac output	To promote adequate cardiac output and myocardial oxygenation	Constant ECG monitoring; blood pressure and apical pulse every 4 hours; routine critical care unit orders (i.e. anti-arrhythmic, vasoconstricting, analgesic drugs and emergency procedures);	Free of chest pain; no arrhythmias
		daily test (i.e. 12 lead ECG, cardiac enzymes in a.m. and daily as ordered); low-cholesterol diet	
3. Alterations in tissue perfusion	Maintain blood pressure at baseline of 130/70 (±10 mm Hg)	Monitor blood pressure every 4 hours, lying and sitting; assess level of consciousness and peripheral circulation every 4 hours; medications as ordered (i.e. Nitropaste 1″ every hour)	Free of headache; maintain B.P. at 130/70
4. Anxiety due to being in an unfamiliar environment and fear of death	Reassure patient and encourage communication of fears and concerns	Provide verbal and non-verbal support; spend time allowing patient to express feelings; explain rationale for care to patient and family; sedate per critical care unit orders; encourage patient by communicating daily status changes	Free of anxiety, fear

SUMMARY

This brief overview of critical care nursing and summary of the nursing process illustrates how evolving medical technology and nursing care interface to provide individualized, quality patient care. The nursing process provides the means to develop a specific plan of care to insure attainment of the primary goal of the critical care nurse—fulfillment of the critical care patient's needs.

System	Technique	Assess
SKIN	Inspect	Color, vascularity, edema, lesions
	Palpate	Texture, moisture, turgor, temperature
HEAD	Inspect	Signs of trauma, scalp, skull, face
	Palpate	Texture of hair, face, cranial contour
EYES	Inspect	Position of eyebrows, eyelids, appearance of sclera, conjunctiva, cornea, irises, pupillary reaction, extraocular movement, visual acuity, visual fields
EARS	Inspect	Auricles, canals, drums, hearing
NOSE AND SINUSES	Inspect	Nares, mucosa, septum, turbinates, sinuses
MOUTH AND PHARYNX	Inspect	Lips, mucosa, gums, teeth, tongue, pharynx
NECK	Inspect	Symmetry
	Palpate	Tenderness, stiffness, cervical nodes, trachea, thyroid
BACK	Auscultate	Carotid arteries
	Inspect	Symmetry, alignment of spine, deformities, signs of trauma
	Palpate	Spine and muscles, pain
	Percuss	Costovertebral angle
CHEST	Inspect	Signs of trauma, symmetry, deformities, respiratory effort
	Auscultate	Breath sounds, heart sounds, adventitious sounds
	Palpate	Respiratory excursion, tenderness, symmetry, tactile fremitus, PMI
	Percuss	Flatness, dullness, resonance, tympany, chest periphery, cardiac silhouette
BREAST	Inspect	Symmetry, color, shape
	Palpate	Nodes, lesions, tumors, tenderness
ABDOMEN	Inspect	Distention, masses, signs of trauma, symmetry, peristalsis, pulsations
	Auscultate	Bowel sounds, bruit
	Percuss	Organ size, ascites
	Palpate	Tenderness, organ size, rebound, guarding, femoral pulses, aortic pulsations
GENITALIA	Inspect	Development
MUSCULOSKELETAL	Inspect	Clubbing, lesions, movement, symmetry, edema, deformities, vascularity
	Palpate	Vascularity, edema, pulses, neurological status, range of motion
NEUROLOGICAL	Inspect	Motor, position
	Percuss	Reflexes
	Palpate	Pain, tenderness, sensation, vibration, motor strength, muscle tone

Fig. 1-3. Overview of Body Systems

CHAPTER TWO
PSYCHOSOCIAL ASPECTS OF CRITICAL CARE

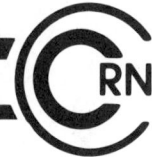

BEHAVIORAL OBJECTIVES

After reading *Psychosocial Aspects of Critical Care,* the nurse will be able to:
- Describe the psychosocial aspects of critical care nursing
- List Maslow's hierarchy of human needs
- List the three mental attitudes
- Identify coping mechanisms used by the patient and health care provider
- Identify situations that may be stress-producing to the nursing staff
- List the causes of sensory deprivation and sensory overload
- List the five stages of death and dying
- List intervention techniques used to assist the dying patient and family in dealing with death

TOPICAL OUTLINE
PSYCHOSOCIAL ASPECTS OF CRITICAL CARE

- I. Psychosocial Nursing   19
- II. Basic Human Needs   19
- III. Mental Attitudes   20
- IV. Stress   21
- V. Common Emotional States of the Critical Care Patient   22
  - Anxiety   22
  - Denial   23
  - Depression   24
- VI. Aggressive Sexual Behavior   24
- VII. Inappropriate Responses to Stress: Addiction/Suicide   25
- VIII. Crisis   26
- IX. The Stresses of Critical Care   27
  - The patient's viewpoint   27
    - Pain   28
  - The nurse's viewpoint   29
  - The family's viewpoint   29
- X. Death and Dying   30
  - Program Assessment: Science and Situation   33
  - Key Point Recognition Answers   39
  - PASS Answer Sheet   41
  - Survey Summary   43

PSYCHOSOCIAL NURSING

Nursing involves both physiological and psychological care of the individual. When ministering to a person's needs, the nurse's goal should be to think of the patient as a whole, complete person. However, to understand the interaction of the physiological, psychological and social selves, the nurse must separate the whole into individual parts. One important part is the psychosocial self. The psychosocial self is composed of complex processes developed through experiences and interactions with the environment. As varied as each life experience and social milieu may be, all individuals have the same basic needs. Furthermore, all persons utilize basic psychological and social methods. It is through analyzing these universal needs, psychosocial development and coping mechanisms that the nurse can most effectively assess and intervene when dealing with the psychosocial self.

KEY CONCEPT: Nursing care is concerned with both psychological and physiological needs.

KEY POINT RECOGNITION
Write true or false by each statement. Answers are at the end of this chapter.
_____1. Nursing care involves only the physiological needs of the patient.
_____2. The psychosocial being develops through life experiences only.
_____3. Individuals have different basic needs.
_____4. The nurse's goal is to think of the person as a whole.

BASIC HUMAN NEEDS

Basic physiological and psychological needs are common to all people. Everyone needs to eat, sleep and be loved. While basic needs are the same, they are fulfilled according to each person's abilities, environment and experiences.

Maslow's categorization of human needs makes it easier to understand need-fulfillment. Needs are satisfied by progressing from the lowest biological requirement of food to the highest cerebral fulfillment of self-actualization. Each level of need is achieved by meeting related goals. Attaining these levels can be analogized to the steps of a ladder (see Fig. 2-1). The needs or steps must be achieved in order, but people vacillate between the steps depending on their current life situation and status. Without a careful concentrated climb, movement can regress to lower levels, requiring the individual to start the climb again.

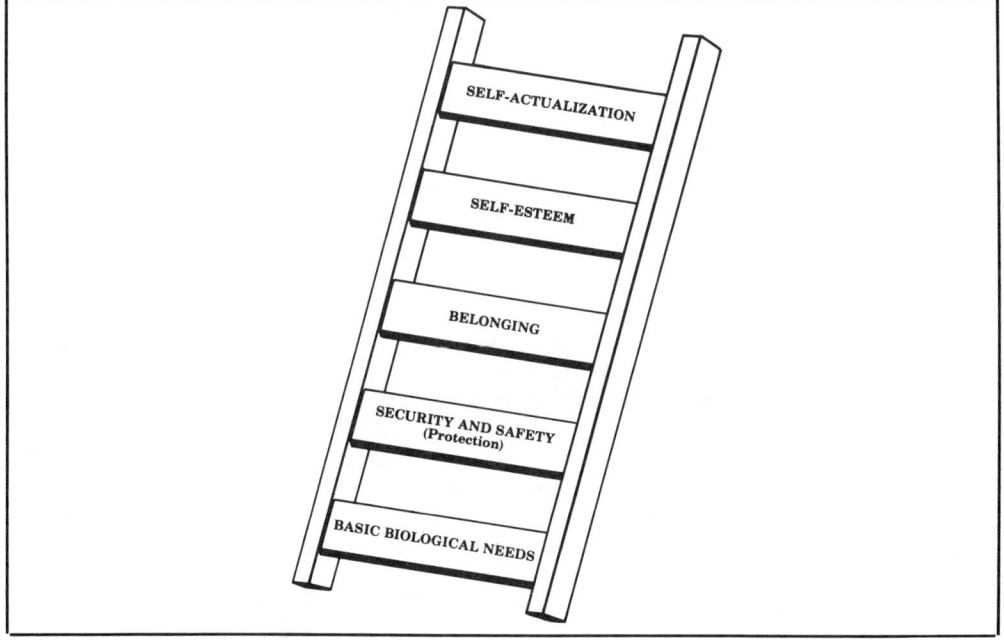

Fig. 2-1. Step ladder of human needs

Each step is important. The lowest rung on the ladder is the physiological step. This includes the basic biological need for food, shelter, recreation and rest. Some people achieve the basic biological needs by working and earning the money necessary to obtain the things required for fulfilling these needs. Once this step is reached, the individual progresses to the next step.

The next step of need is that of security and safety. Once security is achieved, individuals begin to fulfill the need to belong. For some individuals, participation in clubs and organizations may satisfy social interests. Others may satisfy the need by other social efforts.

As individuals develop self-confidence, the need for self-esteem surfaces. Individuals want to be independent and recognized for their own competence and knowledge. This is the level at which most adults remain. Lack of education, drive and finances prevent people from reaching the pinnacle of self-actualization or self-fulfillment.

When people are sick, they regress to basic physiological needs. These needs must be met before higher needs can be achieved. The nurse must be familiar with Maslow's hierarchy of needs in order to understand patient behavior and to assist the patient in achieving need-level goals.

KEY CONCEPT: Progressive achievement of Maslow's hierarchy of needs is necessary for psychosocial growth. Individuals may vacillate between the steps; however, lower levels of needs must be fulfilled before progressing.

KEY POINT RECOGNITION

Write true or false by each statement. Answers are at the end of this chapter.

_____ 1. Food, shelter, recreation and rest are basic biological needs.

_____ 2. Maslow's hierarchy of needs must be fulfilled in a progressive order.

_____ 3. Once goals for a level of need are achieved, the individual will never regress to a lower level.

_____ 4. Self-actualization is a level that all adults reach upon physiological maturity.

MENTAL ATTITUDES

An individual's mental attitude is directly related to one's overt behavior. Therefore, behavior can be anticipated, reacted to, or even better understood if an individual's mental attitude is defined.

Dr. Eric Berne, a well-known lecturer on social psychiatry and psychology of human relationships, has categorized mental attitudes: parent, child, adult.

By using these three categories, the nurse can understand a patient's behavior, react to the behavior and assist the patient in choosing appropriate behavior in stressful situations.

Each attitude has specific characteristics. The parent attitude is characterized by messages the individual has learned from people in authoritative positions. Examples of a parent attitude are statements such as: "I do," "I don't," or "I shouldn't." The parent attitude dictates the rules and values necessary for coexistence of an individual with society.

The child attitude is characterized by feeling. The child is cute, spontaneous and thinks only of personal needs. The development of the child attitude creates negative feelings because of contradictory messages. The child wants to explore and the parent refuses to allow it. For example, the child wants to urinate at will, and the parent confuses the child by toilet training. From these messages, children may sense that their feelings are wrong. The development of the child attitude creates negative feelings by the very nature of messages. Rules, whether helpful or harmful, are being developed. The rules and values learned at such an impressionable time will guide the individual throughout life. Thus, natural instincts are sacrificed for parental approval. The child attitude is often manifested in the angry adult.

Psychosocial Aspects of Critical Care—2

With the development of movement, the adult attitude emerges. As a baby begins to move and can experiment, the decision-making process begins to evolve. The synthesis of ideas or analytical process is characteristic of the adult attitude. An adult is capable of making rational decisions after collecting and analyzing data.

It is the balanced relationship of the three attitudes that embraces the total person. When people are sick, mental attitudes may change from adult to child or parent to child.

It is important to understand the mental attitudes of each individual. By recognizing the attitudes of patient, family, physician or colleague, the nurse is able to communicate more effectively. An angry individual will become more angry if responded to with a parent attitude. Communications should be with an adult approach to change the angry child attitude to an adult attitude.

In cardiac arrest situations, for example, the nurse or physician must exhibit the parent attitude. This life-threatening emergency requires the individual to direct, organize and control the scene. Family members may develop a child attitude as a result of the rules dictated by the nurse, physician or hospital. Sometimes the adult attitude may emerge, enabling the family member to make decisions.

By understanding the three mental attitudes, the nurse can anticipate, react to and guide the individual's behavior during stressful situations. The ultimate aim is to enable all three mental attitudes to cooperate in suitable fashion.

KEY CONCEPT: The patient's overt behavior is a reflection of mental attitudes.

KEY POINT RECOGNITION

Write true or false by each statement. Answers are at the end of this chapter. A score below 80% indicates the need for further study.

_____1. Mental attitudes cause negative or positive responses from others.

_____2. The nurse should identify the patient's mental attitude as a means to understanding behavior.

_____3. Only the adult attitude is necessary to balance a person's mental attitudes.

_____4. The parent attitude is one of rules and values.

_____5. The adult attitude is one of analyzing and reasoning.

STRESS

Stress is an emotionally, and sometimes physically, disruptive influence. Although stress is always disruptive, it does not always have a negative or counterproductive effect on the body. Stress can be described as either (1) **distress,** the condition present when an individual encounters threatening stimuli; or (2) **eustress,** the condition present when an individual encounters nonthreatening stimuli.

Whether a specific stimulus is perceived as threatening or nonthreatening relates to a person's self-concept. Each person has a self-image. Within this image are perceptions of stress-producing factors and abilities to cope with those factors. A situation that might create stress in one person may not create stress in another because the situation is perceived differently.

A person's self-image has significant influence on behavior. People who feel they can handle any situation will try to cope with it. They will not allow situations to cause debilitating stress. Learning to develop a positive self-image that is open to learning and self-improvement is important in handling stress.

Other people feel that each situation they face will cause much distress. They often become anxious, even before the situation presents itself, thus increasing stress to a point of loss of control or crisis.

Defense mechanisms are one method employed to deal with stressful and painful experiences. (See Fig. 2-2.) When defense mechanisms are used appropriately, stress is reduced. Inappropriate use of defense mechanisms can result in abnormal behavior.

Type	Definition
1. Denial	Unable to give validity to reality, can be constructive or destructive
2. Repression	Occurs automatically to effect a balance between emotional and environmental changes
3. Rationalization	Gives logical reason for what is done so it will seem appropriate
4. Projection	Inability to recognize faults, and transfers them onto others (empathy)
5. Reaction formation	Saying the opposite of what is believed
6. Intellectualization	Dealing with highly charged situations abstractly (objectivity)
7. Undoing	Tries to make good for impulsive act (confession)
8. Displacement	Reroute reason into different channel
9. Regression	Returning to a time when there were more pleasurable results, usually temporary

Fig. 2-2. Defense mechanisms

Abnormal behavior is behavior that is inappropriate to a situation or does not benefit the person. Understanding defense mechanisms can assist the critical care nurses in helping their patients accept and deal with stressful situations. By channeling stress appropriately, conflict can be avoided, and stress can be relieved.

KEY CONCEPT: Stress is perceived differently by each individual. Self-image influences behavior and one's perception of stress.

KEY POINT RECOGNITION

Write true or false by each statement. Answers are at the end of this chapter.

_____1. Stress can be emotionally or physically disruptive.
_____2. Stress always has a negative or counterproductive effect on the body.
_____3. The ability of the individual to perceive the stimuli as threatening or nonthreatening depends on one's self-concept.
_____4. Behavior is the end product of self-perception.

COMMON EMOTIONAL STATES OF THE CRITICAL CARE PATIENT

ANXIETY

Critical care patients often are extremely anxious, especially in the initial phase of their illness. Some of a patient's symptoms may be symptoms of anxiety rather than illness itself. Therefore, the nurse must be familiar with the symptoms of anxiety, such as excessive talking, inability to concentrate, crying, dry mouth, inability to move, perspiration, insomnia, nausea, increased heart and respiratory rate, and body tremors.

Fear often manifests itself in anxiety. Many patients fear death; some patients fear loss of independence; others fear the physical environment itself. It is important to recognize such fears and to alleviate anxiety.

At the adaptive level, anxiety and fear are effective responses to stress. By becoming anxious or fearful at the first sign of illness, the individual seeks medical attention. But in the critically ill, over-anxious states may develop. At this level, patients are unable to cope and become more debilitated.

The nurse should try to relieve anxiety by providing an environment conducive to enhancement of interpersonal communications. The patient's family should be involved whenever possible. The nurse should anticipate the patient's needs and provide comfort. This helps decrease fear and anxiety.

KEY CONCEPT: Anxiety is common among critically ill patients.

KEY POINT RECOGNITION
Write true or false by each statement. Answers are at the end of this chapter.

_____1. Excessive talking and insomnia are symptoms of anxiety.
_____2. A quiet, peaceful environment tends to relieve anxiety and heighten communication in a stressful situation.
_____3. Anxiety and fear are appropriate responses to stress.
_____4. By providing comfort and anticipating patient needs, fear and anxiety can be reduced.

DENIAL

Initially, many critically ill patients and their families deny the seriousness, or even the existence, of their illnesses. Denial as a coping mechanism is extremely important. The patient blocks out information that is too stressful. This provides the patient with the time needed to begin to accept reality.

The critical care nurse must be able to recognize denial as a coping mechanism and to intervene appropriately. (See Fig. 2-3). Many patients using denial as a defense are inappropriately labeled difficult or uncooperative.

Symptoms	Nursing Process
Shrugs off having symptoms of illness prior to hospitalization	Assess: Is denial interfering with patient care? Is it verbal or active?
Will not discuss illness or its prognosis	If denial is verbal, listen. Do not attempt to get patient to accept facts at this time. Never force more information than patient is ready to accept.
Minimizes the severity of both diagnosis and prognosis	Be empathetic.
Quotes others when talking about condition	Direct all staff members to offer positive information.
May verbalize illness, but ignores restrictions	If active denial: Do not allow actions to compromise nursing care. Allow patient more control of own care.
Overtly cheerful	Maintain an honest environment. Provide opportunities for expression of emotions.
Asks same questions of staff	Maintain correct and informative care plan so all staff members answer questions the same way. Privileges and restrictions should be the same on all shifts.

Fig. 2-3. Denial: symptoms and the nursing process

One cause of denial is loss of autonomy. Illness and hospitalization take over the patient's decision-making process. This process is important in maintaining a positive self-concept. Denial allows the patient time to accept the situation.

KEY CONCEPT: Denial is an important coping mechanism.

KEY POINT RECOGNITION
Write true or false by each statement. Answers are at the end of this chapter.

_____1. Denial blocks reality and can only harm the patient.
_____2. The patient who denies an illness appears extremely depressed.
_____3. Denial may allow the patient time to accept reality.
_____4. One cause of denial is loss of autonomy.

DEPRESSION

The critically ill patient often experiences depression and a sense of hopelessness as the reality of the illness becomes more evident. The patient feels totally dependent and unable to control the future. Signs and symptoms of depression include anorexia, crying, sadness and lethargy. The patient may exhibit negative feelings and speak in short sentences.

During a depressive state, the nurse must offer objective, easily understood information that identifies the patient's needs and helps visualize the future. The nurse's role is to identify depression by listening and observing the patient's behavior. The nurse can intervene by communicating and offering positive stimuli. The nurse should offer honest information and allow the patient to cry, but set limits when anger becomes abusive. (See Fig. 2-4.)

Symptoms	Nursing Process
Sad, not interested in anything, limp	Reflect what you see. Tell the patient he looks sad.
Feels despair, always negative	Communicate that this is a normal reaction.
Speaks in short sentences	Listen. Identify patient's feelings. Identify patient's perception of the illness.
Lethargic	Try to improve surroundings, such as providing a radio or reading materials, decrease visiting time.
Withdrawn	Offer positive stimuli.
No appetite	Make the food tray attractive; provide for visitors at meals. Assist with meals.
Cries a lot	Allow the patient to cry. Remain nonjudgmental.
Angry	Remain objective about the anger, do not personalize it. Set limits, if the patient is abusive.

Fig. 2-4. Depression: symptoms and the nursing process

KEY CONCEPT: Depression is a sense of hopelessness.

KEY POINT RECOGNITION
Write true or false by each statement. Answers are at the end of this chapter.

_____1. Patients feel totally helpless and unable to control their futures.

_____2. The nurse should offer honest information to the depressed critically ill patient.

_____3. The nurse should allow the depressed patient time to cry.

_____4. The nurse should set limits when the depressed patient becomes abusive.

AGGRESSIVE SEXUAL BEHAVIOR

Human sexuality is a very important part of the total individual. It is a part of a person's self-image. When the self-image is threatened, so is sexuality. The individual's reaction to this threat depends on many lifelong factors, such as development and environment.

One such reaction that can pose a threat to the nurse is aggressive sexual behavior. Fright, fear of impotence and loss of independence may result in aggressive behavior. The nurse must be able to identify such misplaced behavior and intervene appropriately. (See Fig. 2-5.) If the patient is critically ill, aggressive behavior may not manifest initially. But as the patient improves, this problem may emerge. Aggressive sexual behavior is seen as flirting, seductive comments, exposure of genitalia or open discussion of sexual encounters. Nursing intervention includes letting the patient know that the behavior is unacceptable. The nurse may offer alternative means of improving a damaged self-image by discussing sexual activities permitted during and after recovery.

Symptoms	Nursing Process
Many seductive comments	Attempt to identify what the patient is attempting to do.
Flirting, attempts to touch or kiss	If the behavior makes you uncomfortable, tell the patient.
Exposing self	Understand the actions are attempts to improve a tattered self-image.
Exaggerating about sexual encounters	Have the physician discuss sex with the patient and spouse prior to discharge. Set limits for behavior and discussion.

Fig. 2-5. Aggressive sexual behavior: symptoms and the nursing process

KEY CONCEPT: Patients who display aggressive sexual behavior need restoration of their self-image.

KEY POINT RECOGNITION
Write true or false by each statement. Answers are at the end of this chapter.

    ____1. A threat to one's self-image may also result in a threat to one's sexuality.

    ____2. The nurse should accept aggressive sexual behavior because it helps to improve the patient's self-image.

    ____3. Sexual activities during and after recovery should be discussed with the sexually aggressive patient.

    ____4. Human sexuality is a very important part of the total individual.

INAPPROPRIATE RESPONSES TO STRESS: ADDICTION/SUICIDE

Inappropriate responses to stress can result in an individual who stops growing and learning. Self-image is reduced and the person feels unimportant. The person feels that life is not worth living. Many of these individuals become addicted to drugs, alcohol or both. They may accidentally overdose or attempt suicide.

Interpersonal communication is important in the nurse-patient relationship if the patient is to be helped. The patient needs empathy and support. The nurse should remain nonjudgmental. Unrequested and unwanted moral standards should not be imposed on the patient. Both verbal and nonverbal behavior should be observed. Positive behavior should be reinforced with positive statements. The patient should be provided with a safe environment.

In the critical care unit, drug addiction and alcohol-related emergencies should be considered medical emergencies. Acute alcohol intoxication may result in death from an undiagnosed head injury, unavailable or unreliable history, or lack of a clear diagnostic picture. The chronically intoxicated individual is often in poor medical health. Chronic alcoholics have nutritional deficiencies, seizures, hepatitis, hallucinations, anemia, delirium tremens, tuberculosis and other medical problems.

Nursing intervention should be objective, empathetic and nonjudgmental. Observations should be made for verbal and nonverbal communications. During the critical phase, evaluation of the circumstances leading to the overall pattern may not be possible. As the patient's condition and memory improve, information can be obtained to provide the family and patient with support, ventilation, reality and referral.

Drug addiction and drug abuse patients feel vulnerable and are unable to deal with everyday activities. After the initial critical phase, nursing intervention includes helping the patient gain self-esteem, purpose, goals and a positive approach. The elderly need companionship, security and a feeling of need from family and community.

There is no difference between the patient who gestures suicide and the one who successfully completes the suicide. Suicidal thoughts are universal, from the child who wishes to punish a parent to the adult who overdoses on a lethal dose of drugs. Demographic and clinical characteristics common to suicide victims include:

Age. Younger persons attempt suicide more often. Older persons are more successful.

Lifestyle. Persons who live alone are a higher risk.

Occupation. Unemployed people, or those dissatisfied with their jobs, are a higher risk.

Crisis situation. People dealing with death, divorce, unemployment, loss of self-esteem or guilt are a higher risk.

Medical history. People with a family history of suicides, terminal disease or hormonal imbalances are a higher risk.

It often is difficult to deal with drug-addicted or suicidal patients. The nurse may feel anger and hostility toward the patient; but to help the patient, the nurse must come to terms with personal feelings about drug addiction and suicide.

KEY CONCEPT: Inappropriate responses to stress reduce self-image. As a result, many individuals become addicted to drugs, alcohol or both.

KEY POINT RECOGNITION

Write true or false by each statement. Answers are at the end of this chapter. A score below 80% indicates the need for further study.

_____1. Drug addiction or suicide is an appropriate response to stress.

_____2. The nurse should identify the patient's problem, pointing out that drug addiction is morally wrong.

_____3. Alcohol intoxication may mask other medical problems.

_____4. Family of the drug addict or suicidal patient may need support and referral.

_____5. *Attempted* suicide and suicide are two distinct entities.

CRISIS

Crisis is an acute state of stressful anxiety in which stimuli bombard the individual at such an intensity that the person feels an overwhelming inability to cope. Crisis is a self-limiting event. It usually lasts from four to six weeks. The individual begins to cope and the crisis passes. For many individuals, a catastrophic illness is a crisis situation. Any event can pose a threat to one's psychosocial balance. There are usually three events that will precipitate a crisis: an emergency, stress and an accumulation of minor incidents that cause a major problem. Not every patient experiences crisis. It depends on the patient's perceptions of an event. A person's response to a specific event is directly related to the current situation, past events, personality traits, socioeconomic status, religion and cultural influences. Crisis situations are of two types: *situational* or *maturational.* A situational crisis is caused by a situation or problem. The situation may cause a major crisis for the patient. For example, an elderly patient is to be admitted to the critical care unit. She is uncooperative and demands to be transferred. Nursing intervention discovers that her husband died in the same unit last year. She believes her admission will lead to her death. A maturational crisis involves difficulty in attaining a developmental task. For example, an adolescent may have problems accepting her physique, or an adult may still have difficulty achieving emotional independence.

When a person goes through a crisis, either real or perceived, many of the same patterns as those adapting to death or dying are seen. The patient disbelieves, denies, accepts and either changes or learns to live with the situation. Crisis intervention involves opening the lines of communication, preventing further disorganization of one's emotional equilibrium, preventing permanent psychosocial problems and providing support. The nurse should talk with the patient, listen and help the patient identify the perceived problem. The nurse should be empathetic but neither condoning nor patronizing. The patient may find support from family and close friends because they are usually a familiar and trusted source. The nurse should encourage their involvement and support. Remember, the patient and family must solve the problem, but the nurse can help the patient prioritize goals to solve specific problems.

Nursing intervention includes various techniques to maintain psychosocial equilibrium. The patient in the critical care unit is influenced by staff, other patients and the physical layout of the unit. Patients under stress become acutely aware of both verbal and nonverbal messages of staff and family members. Nonverbal communication by staff should include the appearance of confidence, warmth, good eye contact, friendly facial expressions, openness, calmness and control. Touching is a means of reassuring the patient. If physical touch is impossible, as in burns or quadriplegia, eye contact and facial expression may be the only nonverbal communication. The nurse should avoid facial expressions of distaste or askance, especially when faced with disfigurement or unpleasant smells. Physical touch can allay fear and anxiety and provide comfort.

Verbal communications in a calm, reassuring tone allay anxiety and reduce fear. In emergency situations, high tension levels are apparent from loud or rapid voices. Along with verbal communication, small courtesies help provide a pleasant environment. Both patient and family are less anxious when staff members introduce themselves and explain their roles. The patient recognizes faces and names. The strange environment becomes more familiar. Anxiety and stressful situations retard absorption of information. When explaining procedures, equipment, staff and policies, be brief and free of lengthy technical details.

KEY CONCEPT: Crisis is an acute state of stressful anxiety.

KEY POINT RECOGNITION

Write true or false by each statement. Answers are at the end of this chapter. A score below 80% indicates the need for further study.

_____1. A crisis can be a growth experience.

_____2. Crisis situations are usually self-limiting.

_____3. The nurse should identify the patient's problem and offer solutions to it.

_____4. Every patient experiences crisis.

_____5. Crisis intervention involves opening the lines of communication.

_____6. The nurse should not allow the patient to continue with the wrong perception.

_____7. The patient, not the nurse, must solve the problem.

_____8. Verbal and nonverbal communications are important techniques in communicating with the critically ill patient.

THE STRESSES OF CRITICAL CARE

THE PATIENT'S VIEWPOINT

Sensory Deprivation and Overload. Admission to a critical care unit can be frightening. Most patients are anxious. Their self-image is lowered as health care providers perform daily living tasks for them. Besides the initial fear and anxiety, patients have other emotional trauma if the length of their stay is prolonged. Nurses have jokingly labelled this syndrome "ICU-itis." Patients with ICU-itis syndrome can become dependent upon the staff for their psychological and physical needs. Being confined in a small area with no outside contact or sensory stimuli can cause an individual to lose all sense of time, and eventually, sense of place. Patients feel isolated and confined. Time becomes meaningless. The absence of normal stimuli will, if allowed to continue, cause changes in mentation, auditory and visual hallucinations, anxiety, depression and psychosocial disruption. Some individuals hallucinate in an unconscious effort to compensate for the lack of input from the outside world. This absence of stimuli is called sensory deprivation.

Nursing intervention for patients suffering from sensory deprivation should reacquaint the patient with the world. The patient should be offered information about significant events of the day. The nurse should explain the health care plan and procedures, and orient the patient to the time of day. For example, the nurse should say, "Here is your 10 a.m. medication." Even if patients are unconscious, the nurse should talk to them. Families should be encouraged to relay positive information from home, other family members and friends.

Another cause of ICU-itis is the noise level in the critical care unit. The monitors, respirators and lights, as well as tests and treatments, interfere with a patient's rest and sleep. This disturbance is called sensory overload. Sensory overload can leave a patient totally exhausted. The nurse must recognize the problem of overloading the senses and adjust nursing routines to compensate for the problem, allowing patients some uninterrupted time. The body needs three hours of uninterrupted sleep for adequate rest.

KEY CONCEPT: The critical care nurse should be cognizant of the deleterious effects of sensory deprivation and sensory overload in a critically ill patient.

KEY POINT RECOGNITION
Write true or false by each statement. Answers are at the end of this chapter.

_____1. Critical care units may cause patients to exhibit signs of anxiety and fear.

_____2. Providing the patient with a clock, newspaper or even bedside window may prevent symptoms of sensory deprivation.

_____3. Hallucinations may occur because of sensory deprivation.

_____4. Patients become used to the noise and light in a critical care unit. Turning the lights off at night may result in sensory deprivation.

Pain

The patient in a critical care unit often feels pain. Pain is a subjective symptom. The way a patient perceives pain is unique to each individual. Although all people have the capacity to experience pain, methods of dealing with it are individual. Reactions to pain are influenced by cultural and religious experiences, coping mechanisms and the nature of the pain. However, common to everyone are the feelings of vulnerability, loss of independence and fear of serious implications. Pain is a frightening, yet individual, experience.

The nurse can evaluate the pain by using open-ended questions. This enables the patient to describe location, quality, intensity and characteristics of the pain. Also, the nurse should observe facial expressions and behavior for clues of the degree and intensity of the pain. Patients may experience relief from pain by being provided with support and empathy, or basic nursing care, such as back rubs or change in position. The nurse should be aware of factors that influence pain, such as age, disease pathology and one's ability to cope. The elderly have diminished pain sensation because of the normal aging process. Nursing intervention may also include administering medication to relieve pain and reduce anxiety; changing the patient's position; helping the patient maintain proper body alignment; offering reassurance; and maintaining open communications.

KEY CONCEPT: The most important factor in reducing patients' anxieties are the people who care for them.

KEY POINT RECOGNITION
Write true or false by each statement. Answers are at the end of this chapter.

_____1. Experience influences the manner in which patients deal with pain.

_____2. Pain is subjective.

_____3. Pain should be described by patients in their own words.

_____4. A display of empathy by the nurse may cause the patient to feel relief from the pain.

THE NURSE'S VIEWPOINT

Critical care nursing is exciting, demanding and rewarding. It is a unique opportunity to combine medicine, surgery, psychiatry and nursing skills beyond the practice of a generalist. The critical care nurse must be skillful in physical assessment, hemodynamic monitoring and cardiopulmonary resuscitation. The critical care nurse must be sensitive to the needs of the patient, family, peers and others with whom there is daily contact. Critical care is a specialty that also produces anxiety and frustration. Nurses must be aware of the possible stressful situations that cause burnout and job dissatisfaction. The nurse should be aware of ways to alleviate or reduce the occurrence of stressful situations.

Listed below are some stress-producing situations encountered by critical care nurses:

(1) The nurse does not have the opportunity to follow the patient from illness to hospital discharge. There is sometimes a sense of lacking gratification of a job well-done.

(2) The nurse must always be alert, able to instantly recall information and maintain ever changing technical skills.

(3) Demands resulting from understaffing can result in tired personnel.

(4) The constant care of critically ill patients drains the nurse both physically and emotionally.

(5) Relationships with other hospital personnel are often strained. The critical care situation makes the patient more dependent than a patient on the nursing floor.

(6) Visitors often require as much psychosocial assessment and intervention as the patients.

Dealing effectively with these problems often means the difference between a frustrating, short-lived critical care nursing career and a satisfying one. Interpersonal communication among health care providers is the key to alleviating job stress. Inappropriate adaptive mechanisms often include frequent lateness, excessive absence from work, avoiding the patients and overemphasizing technological equipment in patient care.

KEY CONCEPT: Critical care nursing is intense. Stress factors must be alleviated before a crisis develops. Stressful situations cause the nurse to burn out and leave nursing.

KEY POINT RECOGNITION

Write true or false by each statement. Answers are at the end of this chapter.

_____1. If a nurse really enjoys critical care, then it will not become stress-producing.

_____2. Nurses should be able to identify their frustrations and reduce some stress-producing stimuli.

THE FAMILY'S VIEWPOINT

Admission to the critical care unit is very frightening to both the patient and family. The family and patient lose contact and support. The family is told to wait outside. Alone and separated from the patient, they begin to think the worst. They become angry and more frightened, and often even abusive. Most nurses agree that the family is important, but they must take a less important role than the patient.

There are ways to alleviate the breakdown in family structure and communication. Allow the family members into the unit during admission procedures. This orients them to the equipment, rules, staff and visiting hours. It also allows questions to be asked and establishes a rapport among the patient, nurse and family. The family can provide useful information, especially concerning the patient's medical history. The nurse has the opportunity to observe interaction between family members and the patient.

It is important for the nurse to be available during visiting hours. The family wants to communicate with the nurse. They need reassurance. This helps reduce fear and anxiety and makes them more willing to participate in giving support and a positive attitude to the patient.

KEY CONCEPT: The family is equally as frightened as the patient. The nursing goal is to provide support to the family and patient.

KEY POINT RECOGNITION

Write true or false by each statement. Answers are at the end of this chapter.

_____1. The family is as frightened as the critical care patient.

_____2. Family members become angry when separated from critically ill loved ones.

_____3. Allowing a family member in the critical care unit while admitting the patient may decrease anxiety and increase rapport.

_____4. It is important for the nurse to speak with the family during visiting hours.

DEATH AND DYING

Dying is a process. Elizabeth Kübler-Ross has identified five stages in the process of dying: denial, anger, bargaining, depression and acceptance. (See Fig. 2-6.)

Stages	Pertinent Facts
Denial	"No, it can't be me" is used by all patients; can also recur at later time in illness; gives patients time to collect their thoughts; is usually temporary.
Anger	"Why me?" exhibits rage and resentment; very difficult stage for patient, family, staff; angry at doctors, nurses, hospitalization; **do not personalize the anger.**
Bargaining	"If this...then I will" is an attempt to postpone the inevitable; offers a prize for good behavior; sets self-imposed deadlines.
Depression:	"What for?" replaces anger by sense of great loss.
Reactive depression	Associated with past losses, use cheerful nursing approach.
Preparatory depression	Takes in account impending losses; allow patient to express sorrow. Will find final acceptance easier; be grateful for those who can sit with patient without talking; silent depression, starts disassociating self.
Acceptance	Separated from things important to self; no feelings; sleeps a lot; talk is not important; sit and hold patient's hand. It is a time family needs more help than the patient.

Fig. 2-6. Stages of death and dying

The first stage of death and dying is **denial.** The patient and family members cannot believe it is happening to them. All terminally ill patients go through this stage. It allows the patient an opportunity to collect thoughts and develop coping mechanisms necessary to progress to the second stage. The nurse should not humor the patient or family, but should give honest and factual information. This is an excellent time to allow the patient to verbalize, "No, it can't be me." It is a temporary stage, although patients may come back to the denial stage.

The second stage is **anger.** The patient exhibits rage and resentment. This is an extremely difficult time for the patient, family, staff and friends. The patient's anger is projected to others. The nurse should not personalize this anger, but should show concern and empathy, even if the patient is unpleasant.

The third stage is called **bargaining.** It is an attempt to postpone the inevitable. The patient offers a prize for good behavior and even sets deadlines. For example, the patient states, "If I can make it to my grandson's wedding, I will not ask for anything else." During this stage, the nurse should listen and encourage the patient to have hope. The nurse should encourage the patient to set realistic goals, which include realizing that the patient is not in full control of the situation.

The fourth stage of death and dying is **depression.** It is exhibited by a sense of loss. This stage allows the patient and family to express impending loss and sorrow. It makes final acceptance easier. The nurse should use a cheerful approach and hold hands with the patient. Touching is very important. Words are not necessary.

The fifth and final stage is **acceptance.** The patient separates from things that are personally important. The dying patient expresses feeling. The patient sleeps and shows little, if any, communication. The nurse, or a family member, should sit and hold the patient's hand. In this stage, the family needs more help than the patient.

Nurses, family and the patient must work through the dying process. The process requires preparing for death (intraphysic stress), as well as preparing for death of a loved one (interpersonal stress). As the stages progress, a feeling or philosophy of death is also derived. Thus, while the nurse cannot intervene to stop the process, intervention can make the experience easier.

By understanding the five stages, the nurse should be able to recognize which stage the patient and family are in. The nurse can provide assistance as the family and patient move through the stages. Empathy, compassion and touching are important communication techniques available to the nurse. The nurse should be honest, yet focus on realistic hope. People must have hope.

Providing care for dying patients can be stress-producing. The nurse should develop a personal philosophy of death. Nurses should also be cognizant of their own coping mechanisms when called upon to deal with dying patients and families. Although intervention cannot result in changing the situation, it can mean comforting responses to patient needs within therapeutic parameters.

KEY CONCEPT: The five stages of death and dying as identified by Elizabeth Kübler-Ross are denial, anger, bargaining, depression and acceptance.

KEY POINT RECOGNITION
Write true or false by each statement. Answers are at the end of this chapter.

_____1. Dying is an instantaneous happening.

_____2. Denial is the first stage of the dying process.

_____3. Once the patient accepts the finality of death, hope is lost.

_____4. The nurse should disregard personal emotions when dealing with a dying patient.

PASS
Program Assessment: Science and Situation

1. According to Maslow's hierarchy of human needs theory, an individual must fulfill these needs by
   a. progressing through each stage, beginning with the lowest biological need and ending at the highest need of self-actualization.
   b. progressing randomly through each stage without regard to satisfaction.
   c. progressing from the lowest biological need directly to self-actualization in order to develop one's being at an early age.
   d. achieving safety and security needs as the first requirement before meeting other more esoteric goals or steps.

2. Social interests, such as participation in clubs, organizations, and meetings, can help fulfill which of the following needs in Maslow's hierarchy of needs:
   a. security
   b. belonging
   c. physiological
   d. self-esteem

3. In Maslow's hierarchy of human needs, independence and recognition are part of developing a sense of
   a. self-actualization.
   b. self-esteem.
   c. belonging.
   d. security.

4. Basic biological needs include which of the following:
   a. self-fulfillment
   b. trust
   c. socialization
   d. recreation

5. The highest attainable level of need, according to Maslow, is
   a. self-esteem.
   b. self-confidence.
   c. self-actualization.
   d. self-recognition.

6. Self-actualization may
   a. be reached very early in Maslow's hierarchy of human needs.
   b. never be reached by many individuals.
   c. be interchanged with self-esteem, allowing for independence.
   d. be equated with emotional maturity.

7. Factors such as stress and illness may cause individuals to
   a. progress rapidly to the next need level.
   b. reach the pinnacle of actualization sooner.
   c. regress to a previous level.
   d. none of the above.

8. Berne's child attitude is exemplified by
    a. emotions of anger and jealousy.
    b. rational reasoning.
    c. the synthesis of ideas.
    d. a and c.

9. Berne's parent attitude is characterized by
    a. natural and instinctive feelings.
    b. previously taught messages by individuals of authority.
    c. messages involving thought processes.
    d. negative feelings.

10. Berne's adult attitude is characterized by
    a. a synthesis of ideas.
    b. the development and transmission of negative feelings.
    c. the development of emotional responses.
    d. the employment of natural instincts.

11. The three mental attitudes known as adult, parent and child can be
    a. related to one's behavior.
    b. identified as one's ability to cope.
    c. effective if properly developed.
    d. significant in justifying one's feelings.

12. Of the following attitudes, which is the most desirous:
    a. child
    b. parent
    c. adult
    d. parent-adult

13. Stress can best be defined as
    a. a negative effect in the body.
    b. an emotional or physical disruption.
    c. always a threatening, but never nonthreatening, stimuli.
    d. an emotionally disruptive influence.

14. Stress can be dealt with by using
    a. Maslow's hierarchy of human needs.
    b. positive mental attitudes.
    c. Erik Erikson's developmental task.
    d. defense mechanisms.

15. A condition by which an individual encounters a stimuli as nonthreatening is called
    a. coping.
    b. distress.
    c. eustress.
    d. self-image.

16. Self-perception plays an important role in one's
    a. image.
    b. actualization.
    c. conception.
    d. behavior.

17. Defense mechanisms can be used in a painful situation to
    a. relieve stress.
    b. alter abnormal behavior.
    c. avoid conflict.
    d. all the above.

18. Anxiety is characterized by which of the following symptoms:
    a. bradycardia
    b. crying
    c. lethargy
    d. slowed speech

19. In the critical care setting, interpersonal communications can be more effective when
    a. the family is excluded from planning.
    b. comfort needs of the patient are met.
    c. the patient's anxiety level is high.
    d. the patient is permitted to deny the illness.

20. Denial is an important coping mechanism. It allows patients
    a. time to continue their lifestyles.
    b. time to concentrate on past events.
    c. the opportunity to cooperate with alterations in their lifestyles.
    d. time to negate reality.

21. One of the primary causes of denial is
    a. the inability of the patient to cope effectively.
    b. the timing of the illness.
    c. the severity of the illness.
    d. the ability of the patient to maintain a positive self-image.

22. As the reality of an illness becomes more concrete, critically ill patients
    a. become uncooperative.
    b. verbalize feelings regarding death.
    c. develop sudden independence.
    d. develop depression.

23. Depressive states are characterized by
    a. a sense of hopelessness and the emergence of abnormal use of defense mechanisms.
    b. the need for complex information regarding the illness from physicians and nurses.
    c. a sense of hopelessness and a dependency on physicians and nurses.
    d. the patients' ability to control their futures.

24. In the critical care unit, Mr. Jones, 47 years old, was admitted for rule out myocardial infarction (R/O MI). After two days, he started whispering sensual remarks to the female nursing staff. This is characteristic of
    a. depressive states.
    b. aggressive sexual behavior.
    c. hostility.
    d. denial.

25. Endangering one's self-image may also threaten one's
    a. ability to effectively use coping mechanisms.
    b. perception.
    c. sexuality.
    d. all the above.

26. In the critical care unit, a 32-year-old female constantly lowers the covers when the male RN and male physician enter the room. This behavior, based on the threat to her self-esteem, is most likely
    a. sexually aggressive.
    b. depressed.
    c. bizarre.
    d. passive aggressive.

27. Which of the following best defines crisis:
    a. self-perpetuating events
    b. stimuli deprivation
    c. acute state of stressful anxiety
    d. stressful events lasting from months to years

28. The primary focus in crisis intervention is
    a. helping the patient to identify the problem.
    b. opening the lines of communication.
    c. assisting the patient to solve the problem.
    d. all the above.

29. Patients in a critical care setting often feel isolated and confined. This may cause a condition known as
    a. sensory overload.
    b. sensory perception.
    c. sensory deprivation.
    d. sensory oppression.

30. Sensory deprivation is characterized by
    a. restless behavior.
    b. display of independence.
    c. sense of self-worth.
    d. sexually aggressive behavior.

31. In the critical care unit, if a patient exhibits signs of delusions, illusions or hallucinations, it may be due to
    a. sensory overload.
    b. sensory deprivation.
    c. sensory oppression.
    d. sensory stimulation.

32. Nursing intervention for patients suffering sensory deprivation includes which of the following nursing actions:
    a. orient to surroundings
    b. limit family visitation
    c. provide quiet, dark environment
    d. limit explanations to prevent confusion

33. Sensory overload can be caused by
    a. noise and lights in the critical care unit.
    b. sedatives used to induce sleep.
    c. the limitations placed on visitors.
    d. lack of stimulation.

34. Lack of sleep because of constant interruptions by nursing personnel may leave a patient exhausted. This exhaustion may cause a condition referred to as
    a. sensory deprivation.
    b. sensory overload.
    c. sensory perception.
    d. none of the above.

35. Stress and anxiety are often felt by critical care nurses. The nurse may display signs of stress by
    a. arriving late for work.
    b. allowing dependency by the patient.
    c. never being absent, even when ill.
    d. being autocratic in leadership, thereby discouraging flexibility.

36. Job-related stress can best be alleviated by
    a. providing nurses with the latest technological equipment.
    b. improving interpersonal communications.
    c. permitting absenteeism as needed.
    d. creating surroundings that are pleasant to the eye.

37. According to Kübler-Ross, the stages of death
    a. apply only to the dying person.
    b. apply to the dying person as well as the family.
    c. are a sequential process by both the patient and the family.
    d. are a process through which patient and family proceed at different degrees.

38. Patients experiencing a terminal illness should
    a. be given hope.
    b. never be given hope.
    c. be allowed to make funeral arrangements.
    d. a and c.

39. Families of critically-ill patients have needs that must be met. The most important need is
    a. to feel that the hospital personnel are concerned about their loved ones.
    b. to talk with the physician daily.
    c. to be referred to outside agencies for follow-up.
    d. to be allowed solitude.

40. Kübler-Ross has identified five stages of dying. They are
    a. denial, isolation, depression, acceptance, anger.
    b. denial, isolation, anger, acceptance, depression.
    c. denial, anger, bargaining, depression, acceptance.
    d. isolation, denial, bargaining, depression, acceptance.

41. Death and dying are everyday occurrences to the critical care nurse. However, the nurse should recognize that people deal with the death of a loved one
    a. by crying.
    b. by denying it.
    c. in different ways.
    d. by crying and denying it.

42. A patient's spouse is informed of his death. She begins to cry and begs the physician to continue resuscitative measures. This behavior is
    a. abnormal.
    b. normal.
    c. hysteria requiring treatment.
    d. guilt.

43. Physical complaints, such as anorexia, nausea and lethargy, are signs of
    a. depression.
    b. anger.
    c. denial.
    d. bargaining.

44. The first stage of death and dying is
    a. denial.
    b. anger.
    c. bargaining.
    d. depression.

45. By successfully progressing through Kübler-Ross's five stages of death and dying, death can be viewed as a
    a. negative experience.
    b. positive experience.
    c. frightening experience.
    d. repugnant experience.

46. Important communication skills utilized by the nurse in caring for dying patients include
    a. empathy.
    b. concern.
    c. compassion.
    d. all the above.

KEY POINT RECOGNITION ANSWERS

Psychosocial Nursing
1. False—Nursing involves caring for both physiological and psychosocial patient needs.
2. False—The psychosocial self-being develops through life experiences and environment.
3. False—All individuals have the same basic needs.
4. True

Basic Human Needs
1. True
2. True
3. False—Many factors, such as illness and stress, can cause the individual to return to a lower need level.
4. False—Self-actualization is a level to aspire for in continued psychosocial growth.

Mental Attitudes
1. True
2. True
3. False—All three (parent, adult and child) are necessary to balance a person's mental attitude.
4. True
5. True

Stress
1. True
2. False—It does not always have a negative or counterproductive effect on the body.
3. True
4. True

Anxiety
1. True
2. True
3. True
4. True

Denial
1. False—Denial is important in allowing the patient to come to grips with reality.
2. False—The patient may appear to be cheerful and without worry.
3. True
4. True

Depression
1. True
2. True
3. True
4. True

Aggressive Sexual Behavior
1. True
2. False—The nurse need not be uncomfortable. Therapeutic intervention will not be detrimental to the patient and will relieve the nurse's anxiety.

3. True
4. True

Inappropriate Responses to Stress: Addiction/Suicide
1. False—They are inappropriate and result in no growth.
2. False—A nonjudgmental attitude is necessary for therapeutic intervention.
3. True
4. True
5. False—There is no difference between the patient who gestures suicide and the one who successfully completes the suicide.

Crisis
1. True
2. True
3. False—The patient should identify the problem. The patient must solve the problem.
4. False—Not every patient experiences crisis.
5. True
6. True
7. True
8. True

Patient's Viewpoint
Sensation
1. True
2. True
3. True
4. False—Sensory overload robs the patient of rest.

Pain
1. True
2. True
3. True
4. True

Nurse's Viewpoint
1. False—Because of the critical environment alone, the job is stress-producing.
2. False—It is often impossible to identify one's own problems. Stress-producing stimuli may never be totally removed. Communication between staff is the key.

Family's Viewpoint
1. True
2. True
3. True
4. True

Death and Dying
1. False—Dying is a process.
2. True
3. False—Acceptance of death does not negate hope for survival.
4. False—Nurses must be aware of their feelings about death as well as their emotions at the moment.

PASS ANSWER SHEET

1. a	24. b
2. b	25. d
3. b	26. a
4. d	27. c
5. c	28. d
6. b	29. c
7. c	30. a
8. a	31. b
9. b	32. a
10. a	33. a
11. a	34. b
12. c	35. a
13. b	36. b
14. d	37. d
15. c	38. d
16. d	39. a
17. d	40. c
18. b	41. c
19. b	42. b
20. c	43. a
21. a	44. a
22. d	45. b
23. c	46. d

SURVEY SUMMARY
PSYCHOSOCIAL ASPECTS OF CRITICAL CARE

I. **Psychosocial Nursing**
   A. Nursing involves both physiological and psychological care of the individual.
   B. The nurse must explore the universal needs, psycho-social developments, and coping mechanisms in order to effectively assess and intervene when dealing with the psycho-social self.

II. **Basic Human Needs**
   A. Basic needs may be the same but the manner in which they are fulfilled is dependent upon personal abilities, environment, and life experience.
   B. Maslow's hierarchy of needs is progressive.
      1. need for food, shelter, rest, relaxation
      2. need for security and safety
      3. need to belong
      4. need for self-esteem
      5. need for self-actualization

III. **Mental Attitudes**
   A. An individual's state of mind is directly related to his behavior.
   B. Mental Attitudes can be described as the
      1. Parent attitude
      2. Child attitude
      3. Adult attitude

IV. **Stress**
   A. Stress is a disruptive influence of two types.
      1. Distress
      2. Eustress
   B. Self-concept is an important factor in the ability to deal with stress.
   C. Stress is dealt with by using defense mechanisms.

V. **Common Emotional States of the Critical Care Patient**
   A. Anxiety
      1. Critically ill people are often anxious.
      2. Anxiety can produce both psychological and physiological symptoms.
      3. Anxiety is relieved through developing self-esteem and interpersonal communications.
   B. Denial
      1. Denial is a mechanism which allows the patient to come to grips with reality a little at a time.
      2. Denial may be manifested by shrugging off symptoms; refusing to discuss the illness; appearing cheerful; and verbalizing the illness while ignoring restrictions.
   C. Depression
      1. Depression is characterized by a sense of hopelessness.
      2. The nurse should offer the depressed patient information necessary to identify his needs and to realistically visualize the future.

VI. Aggressive Sexual Behavior
A. A threat to one's self-image may also result in a threat to one's sexuality.
B. A threat to sexuality may result in aggressive sexual behavior.

VII. Inappropriate Response to Stress: Addiction/Suicide
A. Inappropriate responses to stress result in an individual who stops growing and learning.
B. The nurse must maintain a non-judgemental attitude while providing a physically safe environment and opening lines of communication.

VIII. Crisis
A. Crisis is an acute state of stress in which the person feels overwhelmed.
B. It is self-limiting and allows for growth.
C. Crisis may be either situational or maturational in focus.
D. Intervention is aimed at identifying the problem and developing a viable solution.

IX. The Stresses of Critical Care
A. Patient's viewpoint
  1. Admission to a critical care unit is frightening and anxiety producing.
  2. Sensory deprivation and sensory overload are stress factors within a critical care unit.
  3. Nursing intervention to relieve stress factors should include:
     a. maintaining a calm, restful environment.
     b. providing for as much independence of the patient as possible.
     c. providing contact with reality and the outside world.
  4. Pain is experienced and handled differently by all individuals. The nurse must intervene accordingly.
B. Nurse's Viewpoint
  1. Critical care nursing is often frustrating and stress producing.
  2. Recognition of stress producing stimuli and reduction through effective interpersonal communication among staff is necessary for continued job satisfaction and effective nursing care.
C. Family's Viewpoint
  1. Families are often frightened and angry.
  2. Nursing intervention to alleviate the frightened family should include:
     a. bring family into the unit
     b. brief explanation as to equipment and rules
     c. be available during visiting hours

X. Death and Dying
A. Kubler-Ross's 5 stages of dying include:
  1. denial
  2. anger
  3. bargaining
  8. depression
  5. acceptance
B. The nurse should develop a personal philosophy of death in order to deal effectively with dying patients and living families.
C. Compassion, empathy, and touch are important tools in caring for the dying.

CHAPTER THREE
NERVOUS SYSTEM

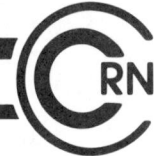

BEHAVIORAL OBJECTIVES

After reading the *Nervous System,* the nurse will be able to:

- Identify the anatomy of the nervous system
- Describe the functions of structures related to the nervous system
- Describe nerve impulse formation and transmission
- State the anatomical location and major functions of the following lobes: frontal, temporal, parietal and occipital
- Identify the names, functions and tests for the 12 cranial nerves
- Identify vessels related to the anterior and posterior segments of the Circle of Willis
- Identify characteristics related to cerebrospinal fluid
- Identify the types of seizures and the five parameters for observation of a seizure
- Identify two major complications resulting from cervical spinal cord damage
- Identify the differences between an epidural hematoma and a subdural hematoma
- Identify the level of function for spinal cord injuries and four major nursing considerations in spinal cord injury management
- Describe the pathophysiology of two types of spinal cord syndromes
- Describe six major nursing responsibilities in the management of acute head injuries
- Name the most common organism and the diagnostic findings related to the clinical picture of meningitis
- Identify tests and results indicative of myasthenic crisis and cholinergic crisis
- Identify clinical manifestations associated with:
  left middle cerebral artery infarct
  tetanus
  facial nerve paralysis
  subarachnoid hemorrhage
  Guillain-Barre
  upper motor neuron lesion
  Brown-Séquard Syndrome
  Parkinson's disease
- Identify the following drugs as to dose, indication and route of administration:
  amicar (aminocaproic acid)
  Decadron (dexamethasone)
  phenytoin sodium
  phenobarbital
  carbamazepine
  ethosuximide
  clonazepam
  Tensilon (edraphonium chloride)
  diazepam
- Describe the pathogenesis of tetanus
- Define the following terms:
  stereognosis
  aphasia
  decorticate
  decerebrate
  ataxia
  reflex action
  Broca's area
  Wernicke's area

dysmetria
Babinski reflex testing
dysphagia
opisthotonos
nuchal rigidity
hemiparesis
hemiplegia
quadriplegia

- Develop a nursing care plan for these conditions:
  cerebrovascular accident
  head injury
  spinal cord injury
  infectious meningitis process
  metabolic tetanus coma

  Be sure to include the following points:
  airway
  ventilation
  fluids and electrolytes
  bowel and bladder control
  skin care
  prevention of joint deformity
  patient/family teaching
  psychological support

TOPICAL OUTLINE
NERVOUS SYSTEM

I. The Nervous System: Overview 51
II. Anatomy and Physiology 51
    Skull 51
    Spinal column 53
    Nervous tissue: cells of the nervous system 55
    Transmission of nerve impulses 56
    Reflex action 59
    Cerebral metabolism 60
    Divisions of cerebral tissue 60
    Cerebral blood supply 63
    The ventricular system 66
    The spinal cord 67
    Autonomic nervous system 70
III. Assessment of the Neurological System 73
    Cranial nerve testing 73
    Cerebellar function testing 75
    Sensory system testing 76
    Motor system testing 76
    Reflex testing 76
    Level of consciousness 77
    Pupillary response 77
    Motor strength and equality 77
    Evaluation of vital signs 78
    Laboratory and radiologic studies 78
IV. Pathological States and Nursing Management 79
    Cerebral vascular accidents (CVA) 79
        Pathophysiology 79
        Clinical presentation 80
        Diagnostic data 80
        Nursing care 80
    Cerebral aneurysm 81
        Pathophysiology 81
        Clinical presentation 81
        Diagnostic data 81
        Nursing care 81
    Meningitis 82
        Pathophysiology 82
        Clinical presentation 82
        Diagnostic data 82
        Nursing care 83
    Guillain-Barre syndrome (acute polyneuritis) 83
        Pathophysiology 83
        Clinical presentation 83
        Diagnostic data 83
        Nursing care 84

Head injury 84
   Pathophysiology 84
   Clinical presentation 85
   Diagnostic data 85
   Nursing care 86
Spinal cord injury 86
   Pathophysiology 86
   Clinical presentation 87
   Diagnostic data 88
   Nursing care 88
Myasthenia gravis 89
   Pathophysiology 89
   Clinical presentation 89
   Diagnostic data 89
   Nursing care 90
Tetanus 90
   Pathophysiology 90
   Clinical presentation 90
   Diagnostic data 90
   Nursing care 90
Seizures 91
   Pathophysiology 91
   Clinical presentation 91
   Diagnostic data 92
   Nursing care 92
Status epilepticus 92
   Pathophysiology 92
   Clinical presentation 93

V. Care Common to Neurological Problems 95
  Increased intracranial pressure (ICP) 95
  Pathophysiology: ICP 95
  Monitoring ICP 96
    Subarachnoid screw 96
    Ventricular drain 96
    Epidural catheter 96
  Methods to decrease ICP 96
  Postoperative care 96

Program Assessment: Science and Situation 99
Key Point Recognition Answers 111
PASS Answer Sheet 117
Survey Summary 119

THE NERVOUS SYSTEM: OVERVIEW

Functionally, human beings are a product of their body systems. All of the systems are interdependent, even though each is specifically responsible for an independent function. In order for these systems to function together, a regulating system is necessary. The *nervous system* is the coordinating system of the multi-system organism.

The basic functions of the nervous system are those of intellectual abilities, coordination and orientation through the senses. There are three divisions of the nervous system:

Central nervous system (CNS)
(brain and spinal cord)
Peripheral nervous system (PNS)
(cranial nerves and spinal nerves)
Autonomic nervous system (ANS)
(sympathethic and parasympathetic systems)

Generally, the CNS is considered the *voluntary* system, while the ANS is referred to as *involuntary*.

The nervous system may also be conceptualized in terms of its *gross anatomy* (brain, spinal cord, spinal and cranial nerves, and parasympathetic and sympathetic nerves and ganglion chains) and its *functional anatomy* (motor and sensory neurons). Physiologically, transmission of nerve impulses and reflex action are the tasks of the nervous system. Anatomically, the structures necessary for support and protection are the skull, spinal column, ventricular system, cerebral blood supply and meninges.

KEY CONCEPT: The nervous system's functions are those of intellectual abilities, coordination and orientation.

ANATOMY AND PHYSIOLOGY

SKULL

Covering the *skull* are various layers of tissue: **skin, subcutaneous tissue, galea aponeurosa** (a thick band of fibrous tissue), **ligaments** and **periosteum.**

The skull is the bony, rigid box that houses the brain (Fig. 3-1). The four bones of the skull—the *frontal, parietal, temporal* and *occipital*—compose the external surface of the skull and the majority of the interior landmarks. An additional bone, the butterfly-shaped *sphenoid* bone helps divide the interior of the skull into three areas known as *fossae* (Fig. 3-2). The lesser wing of the sphenoid is the *posterior* landmark for the *anterior fossa*. The *anterior* landmark is the *frontal* bone. The anterior fossa contains *frontal lobes, sinuses* and *roof of the eye orbits*.

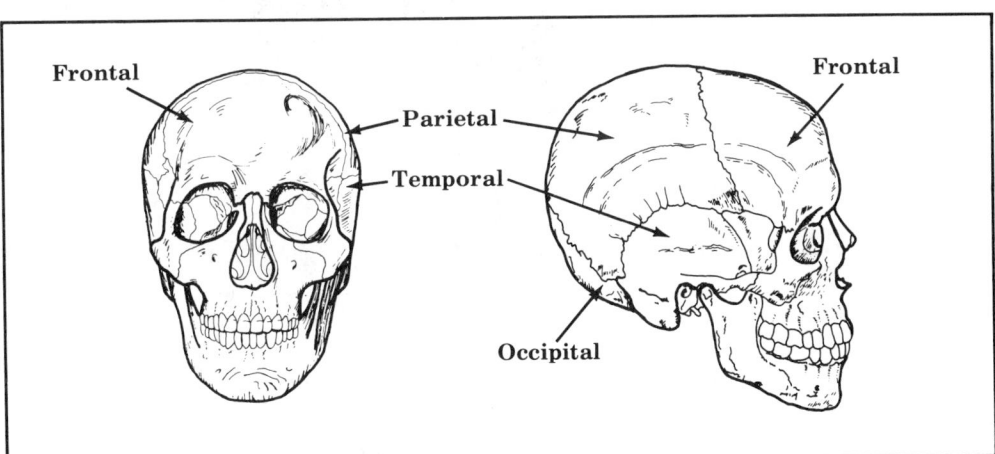

Fig. 3-1. Skull

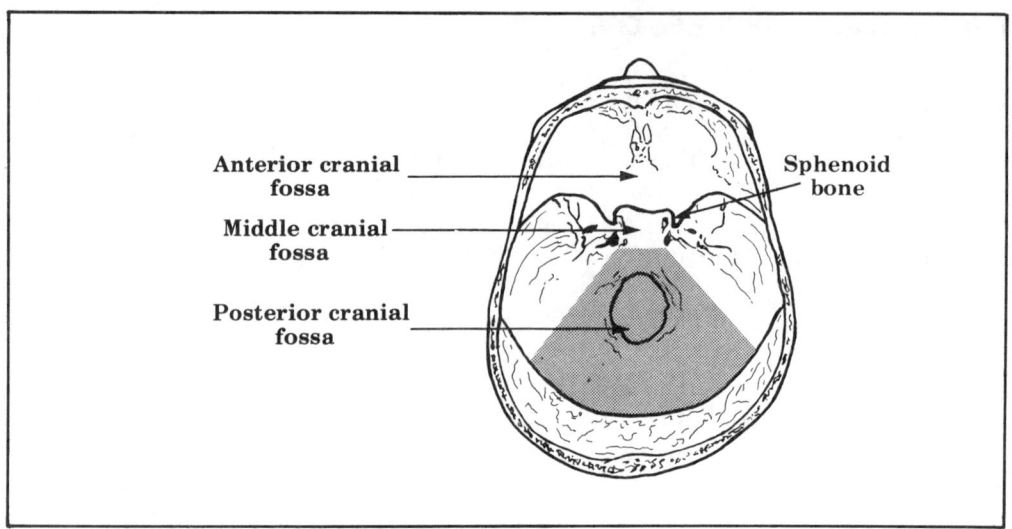

Fig. 3-2. Fossae

The **middle fossa,** found between the lesser and greater wings of the sphenoid, contains the temporal lobes. The ***posterior fossa,*** posterior to the greater wings, contains the ***brainstem, cerebellum,*** and ***foramen magnum.***

The posterior boundary of the posterior fossa is the occipital bone. Also found in the sphenoid bone in the central area is a concave depression, the ***sella turcica,*** which houses the pituitary gland. The greater wings of the sphenoid join with the petrous ridges at the posterior portion of the temporal bone to form a ridge, called the ***tentorium,*** covered by a layer of dura. The tentorium also separates the ***supratentorial*** contents (cerebrum) from the ***infratentorial*** contents (brainstem). The tentorium is the structure involved in tentorial (transtentorial) herniation. Under the skull lie the three layers of meningeal tissues known as the ***meninges*** (Fig. 3-3). They protect and cushion the brain, and assure the circulation of cerebrospinal fluid (CSF). The outermost layer is the ***dura,*** a tough fibrous membrane with two distinct layers: ***endosteal*** and ***meningeal.***

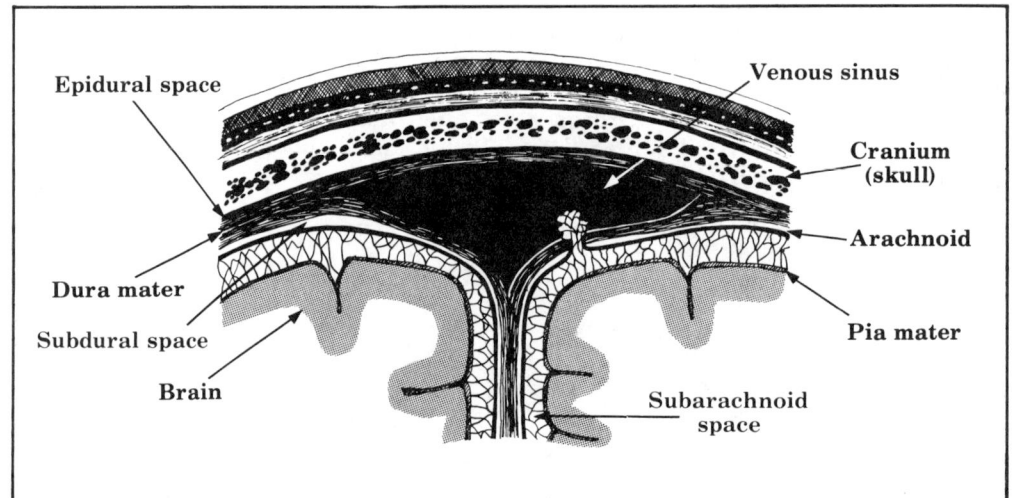

Fig. 3-3. Meninges

At various points the two layers separate, much like the layers of a facial tissue. The cavity formed between the two layers is the ***venous sinus.*** The space between the bone and the dura is the ***epidural space.*** In reality it is a potential space since under normal circumstances there is nothing in this space.

The layer of tissue below the dura is the *arachnoid membrane,* a spidery, delicate membrane networked by extracerebral blood vessels. The potential space between the dura and the arachnoid is the *subdural space.*

The most internal layer is the *pia,* a fine, delicate membrane directly adherent to the surface of the brain. Between the arachnoid and the pia is the *subarachnoid space,* a true space, since this is the space through which the spinal fluid circulates. The pia is directly attached to the brain and no space exists below it.

SPINAL COLUMN

The bones of the vertebral column provide a rigid support structure and housing for the spinal cord. The vertebral column is composed of 33 vertebrae. A typical *vertebra* (Fig. 3-4) consists of:

(1) The **body,** a solid bony area
(2) The **arch,** consists of a pair of pedicles and a pair of laminae and supports seven processes
(3) The **articular processes,** flattened areas that allow for articulation of vertebrae above and below, and contact with other areas (ribs)
(4) **Intervertebral foramina,** openings that accommodate the spinal nerves
(5) **Vertebral foramen,** a central opening through which the spinal cord runs
(6) **Intervertebral disk,** a two-layered structure that maintains space between vertebral bodies and acts as a shock absorber
    a. **Annulus fibrosus,** tough fibrocartilage outer layer
    b. **Nucleus pulposus,** gelatinous inner layer; herniates out through annulus when tear develops in annulus, resulting in herniated nucleus pulposus (HNP) or herniated disk syndrome

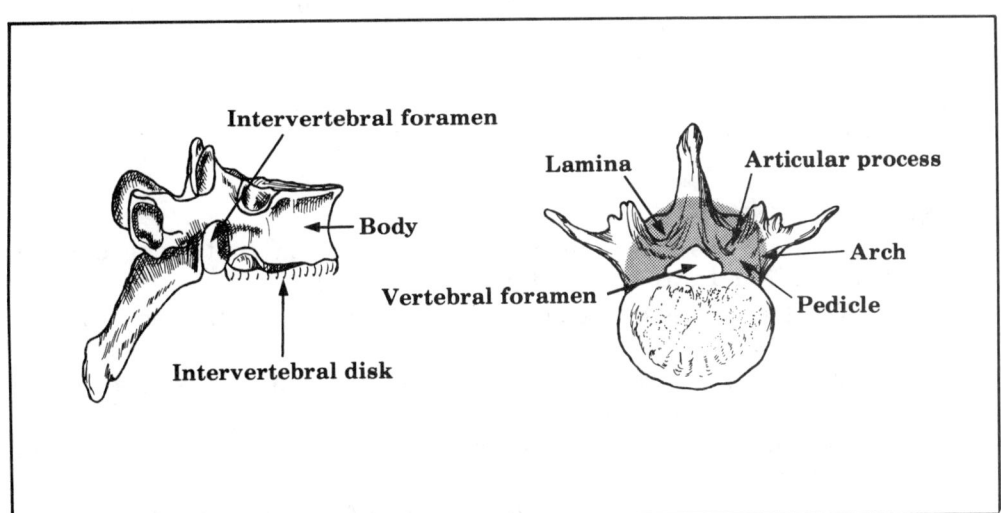

Fig. 3-4. Typical vertebra

The column (Fig. 3-5) is divided into the following five sections: cervical, thoracic, lumbar, sacral and coccygeal. There are seven *cervical vertebrae* that provide support for the head and neck. They are the smallest vertebral bodies. Two of the cervical vertebrae, the *atlas* (C1) and the *axis* (C2), differ significantly in structure from all other vertebrae.

The atlas is a small vertebra, with no body, that articulates directly with the occipital bone of the skull. The axis, also having a smaller body, articulates with the atlas and allows for head rotation. The axis has an upward projection, the odontoid process, that projects through the center opening of the atlas and permits flexion and extension (nodding) of the head and neck.

The 12 *thoracic vertebrae* provide for support of chest musculature and movement by articulation with the ribs. The five **lumbar vertebrae** are the largest vertebral bodies. They support the majority of the body weight. The *sacral vertebrae* are five small vertebrae fused to form a triangular structure called the sacrum. The **coccygeal vertebrae** are four rudimentary vertebral bodies composing the terminal portion of the vertebral column.

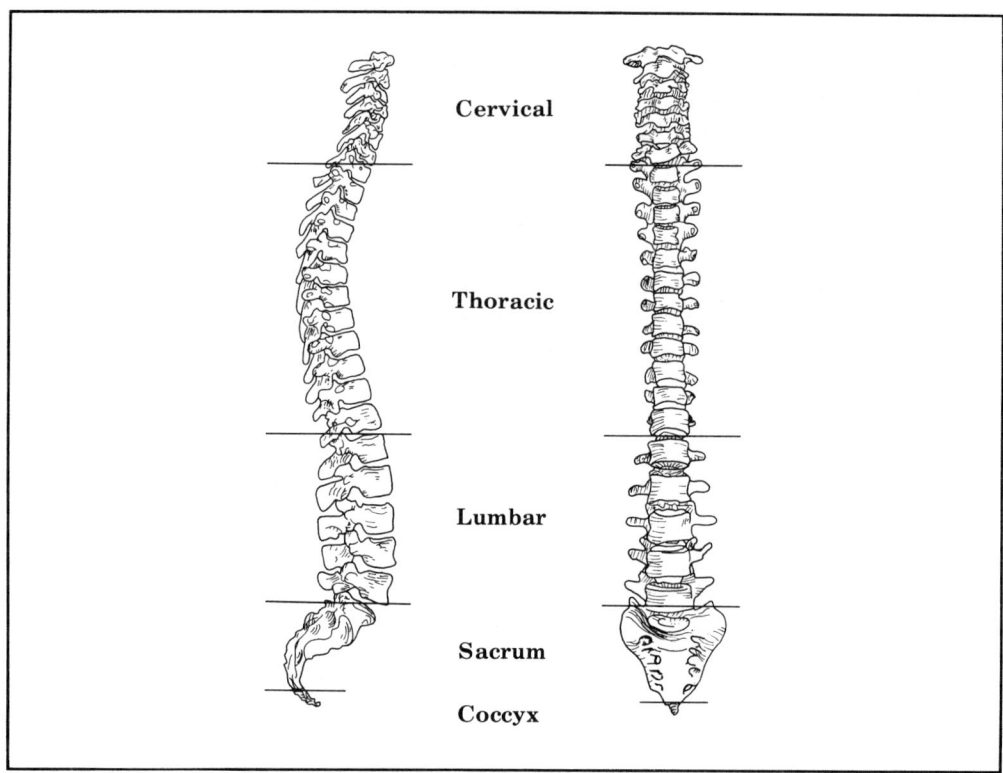

Fig. 3-5. Vertebral column

KEY POINT RECOGNITION

Write true or false by each statement. Answers are at the end of this chapter. A score below 80% indicates the need for further study.

_____ 1. The four bones of the skull are the frontal, parietal, temporal and occipital.

_____ 2. The zygomatic process divides the interior of the skull into three fossae.

_____ 3. The three fossae are called the anterior fossa, superior fossa and posterior fossa.

_____ 4. The tentorium separates the cerebrum from the brainstem.

_____ 5. The sella turcica houses the frontal lobes of the brain.

_____ 6. The outermost layer of meningeal tissue is the pia.

_____ 7. The epidural space is a potential space between the bone and dura.

_____ 8. The space between the dura and arachnoid is the subarachnoid space.

_____ 9. A potential space exists between the pia and the brain.

_____ 10. There are 33 vertebrae.

_____ 11. A typical vertebra consists of the body, arch, intervertebral foramina and intervertebral disk.

_____ 12. The vertebral column has six divisions.

NERVOUS TISSUE: CELLS OF THE NERVOUS SYSTEM

There are two types of cells that make up the cells of the nervous system. **Neurons** (Fig. 3-6) are the functional cells that transmit all information in the brain and spinal cord. There are more than 10 billion neurons in the average adult human brain. Their functions include transmission of nerve impulses, reception of impulses from other neurons and transference of information across the synaptic cleft to other neurons or selected muscle or organ cells. Each neuron is composed of:

1. **A cell body** that performs the metabolic functions of the cell
2. **Dendrites,** fibers extending from the cell body that receive and conduct impulses toward the cell body
3. An **axon,** a single sheath (one per cell body) that conducts impulses away from the cell body.

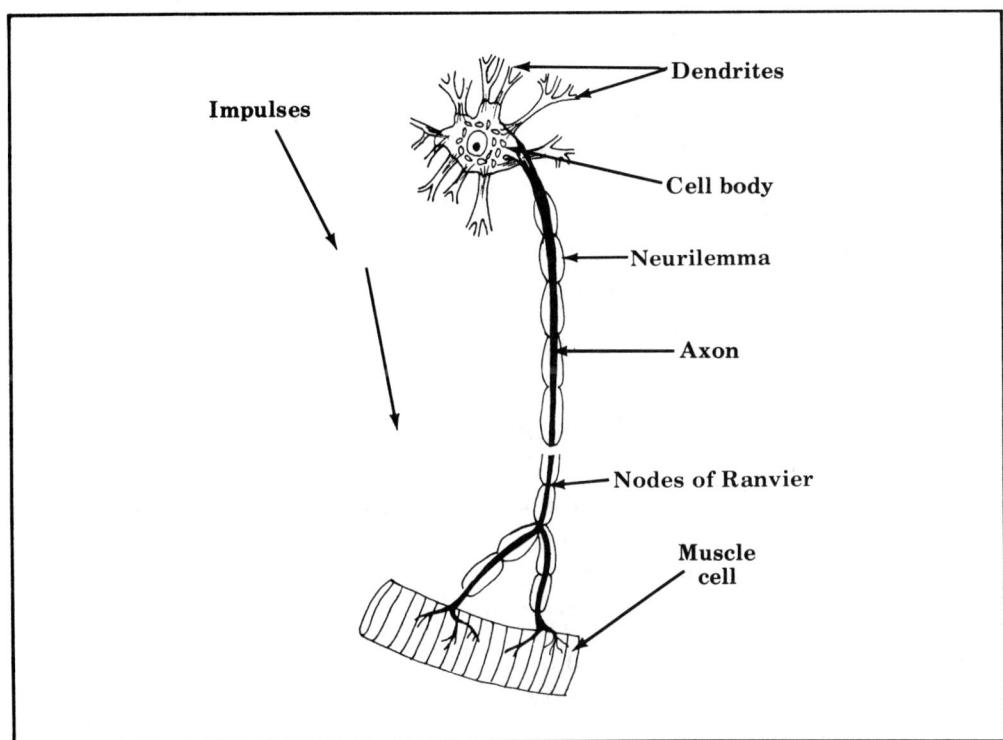

Fig. 3-6. Neuron

In addition, certain other characteristics may or may not be present. *Myelin,* a white phospholipid coating, is present on many axons in both the peripheral and the central nervous system. The purpose of myelin is to speed the conduction of impulses down the axon sheath. Not all myelination is completed at birth. It continues for many years after birth. Lack of myelin accounts for some of the jerky, uncoordinated movements seen in neonates. Demyelinating diseases, the classic example being multiple sclerosis, occur after puberty when the myelination process has been completed.

Myelination also occurs in the peripheral nervous system. The myelination of the peripheral nervous system is augmented by the formation of *neurilemma,* an additional phospholipid coating produced by Schwann cells. Neurilemma forms around the myelin sheath of the *axon.* There are periodic constrictions of the neurilemma called *nodes of Ranvier.* Impulses are conducted from node to node, by saltatory conduction, further speeding the rate of nerve impulse conduction. Saltatory conduction literally means skipping from node to node. This movement of the action potential along myelinated neurons is in a saltatory manner. Both myelin and neurilemma are capable of regeneration. However, it is the peripheral nervous system neurilemma that enables the entire peripheral nerve to regenerate if it has not been deprived of its blood supply for a prolonged period of time.

The second type of central nervous system cell is the **neuroglial cell.** There are four main types of **glial** cells, and each has a different supporting function: **oligodendrocytes, astrocytes, microglia** and **ependymal.**

Oligodendrocytes are support cells whose main function is the production of myelin in the central nervous system.

Astrocytes are support cells whose primary functions are provision of support for neurons and blood vessels, and the formation of the blood-brain barrier.

Microglia are phagocytic cells activated when there is inflammation within the nervous system.

Ependymal cells line the ventricles and the central canal of the spinal cord.

KEY CONCEPT: There are two types of nervous tissue: neuron and neuroglial cells.

KEY POINT RECOGNITION
Write true or false by each statement. Answers are at the end of this chapter. A scores below 80% indicates the need for further study.

_____ 1. The two main cell types found in the nervous system are the neuron and the microglial cell.
_____ 2. The neuron is composed of dendrites, an axon and myelin.
_____ 3. Dendrites conduct impulses away from the cell body.
_____ 4. The function of myelin is to speed conduction of impulses down the axon sheath.
_____ 5. Neurilemma is another name for myelin.
_____ 6. Myelin enables the peripheral nerve to regenerate.
_____ 7. There are four types of glial cells.
_____ 8. Oligodendrocytes are support cells with the main function of myelin production in the CNS.
_____ 9. Microglia line the ventricles.
_____10. Astrocytes line the central canal of the spinal cord.

TRANSMISSION OF NERVE IMPULSES

Nerves conduct impulses afferently from organs to the brain and efferently from the brain to the organs (Fig. 3-7). A **nerve impulse** is the term for the transient, excitatory process upon stimulation. The junction between neurons, where the axon of one and dendrite of another are relatively close, is called a **synapse.** At this point, the impulse is conducted from one neuron to the other. Impulse conduction can only proceed in one direction because of the polarization of the synapses.

The process by which impulses are conducted is physiochemical. Chemical transmitters, known as **neurotransmitters,** are released, changes occur in cell membrane permeability with resultant electrolyte movement, and electrical voltage becomes significant enough to initiate an action potential. **Action potential** is the temporary difference in voltage between the active and resting part of a nerve or muscle cell which takes place when depolarization has reached threshhold level. The action potential is self-propagating and spreads to the next cell, initiating the transmission of the electrical nerve impulse.

Repolarization occurs as in cardiac cells. Repolarization is the process by which a polarized state is re-established.

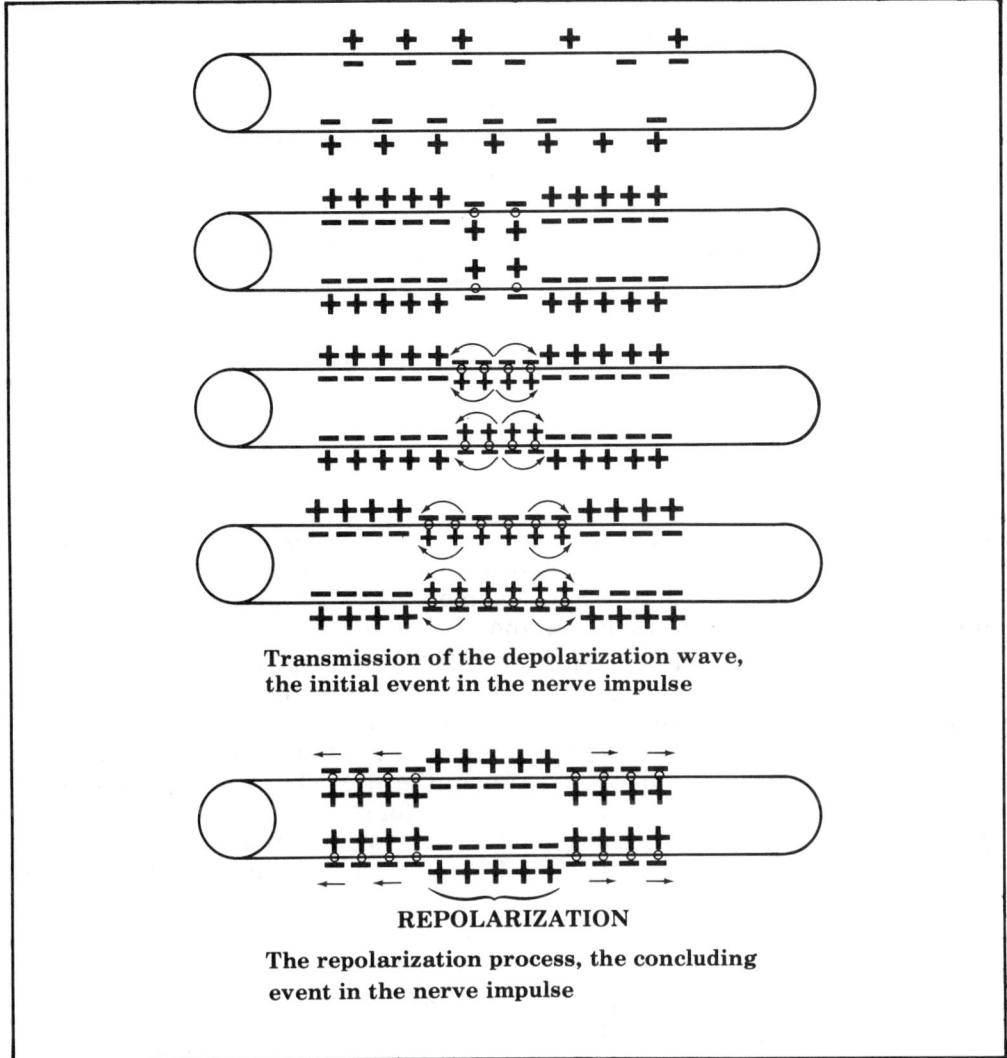

Fig. 3-7. Transmission of nerve impulses (Referenced from Guyton Functions of the Human Body p. 217 1966 W. B. Saunders)

The transmission of nerve impulses parallels the transmission of impulses in cardiac cells in several areas. Electrical activity at the cell membrane of muscle and nerve cells is critical to their ability to contract and transmit impulses. The electrical activity at the cell membrane is due to the presence of sodium and potassium in the intracellular and extracellular fluid, and the cell membrane's reaction to them. Active transport is also involved. Specifically, the electrical **resting potential** for nervous system cells is -70 to -90 mv. By the process of **depolarization,** the cell membrane becomes more permeable to sodium ions. When the cell has been sufficiently depolarized, the membrane is permeable to sodium (Na), and the sodium/potassium (Na/K) pump is activated. Sodium rushes into the cell, potassium diffuses out and the action potential is achieved.

The **neurotransmitters** (Fig. 3-8) are: **acetylcholine (ACh), norepinephrine (Ne), dopamine (DA), gamma amino butyric acid (GABA)** and **serotonin (5-HT).**

The major difference occurs at the synapse with the release of **neurotransmitters.** When the impulse reaches the synaptic knob, the current generates movement of the synaptic vesicles to the end-plate membrane. The **end-plate,** or neuromuscular junction, is where the motor axon flattens, plate-like in appearance, close to the muscle fiber's membrane. **Synaptic vesicles** are reservoirs for

Neurotransmitter	Site of Action	Actions
Acetylcholine (ACh)	Cholinergic fibers of ANS nerves to skeletal muscles	Motor movements
Norepinephrine (Ne)	Adrenergic fibers of ANS	Sleep, temperature regulation and eating behavior
Dopamine (DA)	Substania nigra	Eating, drinking, and sexual behavior; is an inhibitory transmitter
Gamma—aminobutyric acid (BABA)	Substania nigra and some synaptic junctions	Is an inhibitory transmitter
Serotonin (5-HT)	Brainstem, hypothalamus, midbrain and caudate nucleus	Sleep behavior

Fig. 3-8. Neurotransmitters

specific neurotransmitters. The impulse causes the *vesicles* to contact the membrane, and the vesicles open. The neurotransmitter is released from the vesicle and diffuses into the *cleft* through the open pores of the membrane. A *synaptic cleft* is the space between the nerve and muscle fiber membrane.

Once in the *cleft,* it diffuses across the cleft to the receptor site, initiating a change in membrane potential there. The action potential is then potentiated while the receptor cell releases antitransmitter enzyme, severing the neurotransmitter's attachment to the receptor and driving it back across the cleft into the vesicles. Some, but not all, of the transmitter is used up during this process (Fig. 3-9) and the remaining portion is available for reuse. This is the major site of dysfunction in diseases such as myasthenia gravis, which is believed to be production of an abnormal protein that blocks the binding of the neurotransmitter to the receptor site.

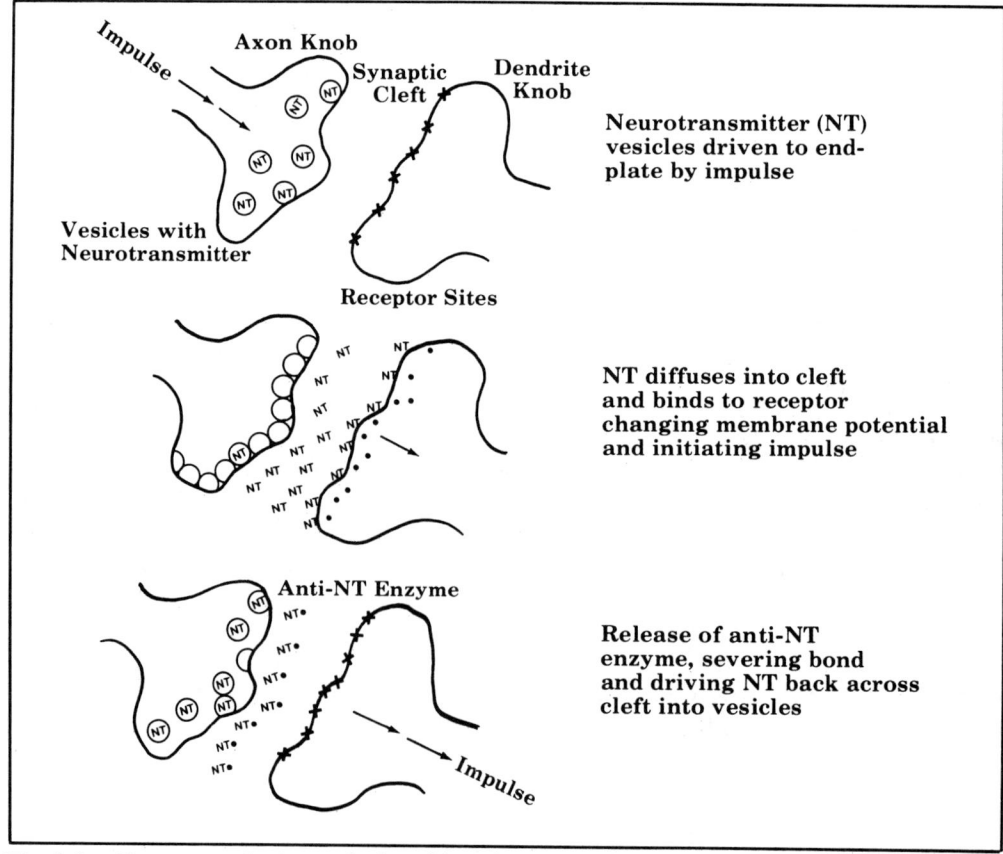

Fig. 3-9. Neuromuscular transmission of impulse

KEY CONCEPT: Transmission of nerve impulses is a physiochemical process. Chemical transmitters known as neurotransmitters are released and the cell membrane becomes more permeable. These changes result in electrolyte movement and increased electrical voltage that is significant enough to start an action potential.

KEY POINT RECOGNITION
Write true or false by each statement. Answers are at the end of this chapter. A scores below 80% indicates the need for further study.

_____ 1. Afferent nerve impulses move toward an organ.

_____ 2. A synapse is a junction between an axon of one neuron and a dendrite of another that are in close proximity.

_____ 3. A synapse allows nerve impulses to travel in either direction.

_____ 4. Neurotransmitters affect cell membrane permeability.

_____ 5. Action potential is a permanent change in electrical voltage occurring during depolarization.

_____ 6. The repolarization process re-establishes polarization.

_____ 7. During depolarization, the cell membrane becomes less permeable to sodium ions.

_____ 8. For the action potential to be realized, sodium rushes into the cell and potassium diffuses out of the cell.

_____ 9. Two of the neurotransmitters are acetylcholine and norepinephrine.

_____10. The space between the nerve and muscle fiber membrane is called the synaptic cleft.

REFLEX ACTION

When a sensory impulse is initiated it stimulates *afferent fibers* leading into the *posterior horn* of the *spinal cord*. (See Fig. 3-10.) When this impulse reaches the horn, it is transmitted, via an *internuncial* neuron, to the *anterior horn* cells which stimulate the motor fibers of the muscle from which the sensory impulses arose. This requires no voluntary or involuntary control from higher cortical areas and continues to occur even in states of coma. The best example of a reflex action is the knee jerk reflex. The hammer stimulates the sensory impulse and the final end motor result in involuntary jerking of the leg at the knee.

KEY CONCEPT: Reflexes are involuntary responses to stimuli. They depend on an intact neural pathway.

KEY POINT RECOGNITION
Write true or false by each statement. Answers are at the end of this chapter.

_____ 1. Sensory impulses first stimulate afferent fibers in the anterior horn of the spinal cord.

_____ 2. A knee jerk is an example of reflex action.

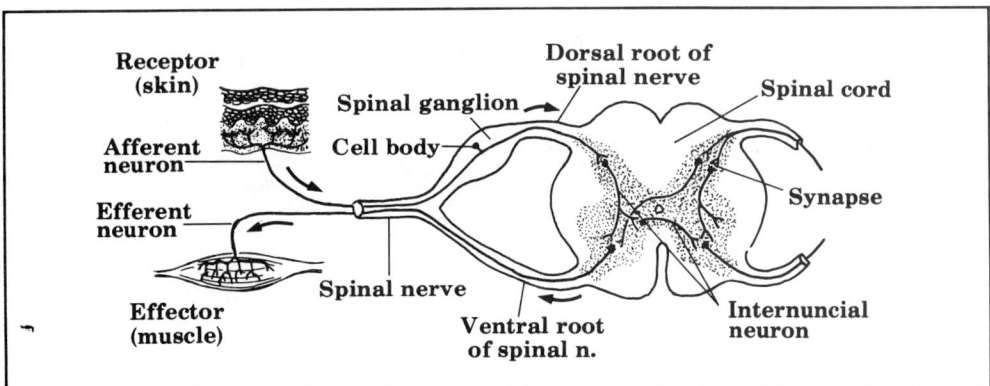

Fig. 3-10. Simple reflex arc

CEREBRAL METABOLISM

The **brain** consumes about 20 percent of the oxygen used by the total body at rest, and receives about 20 to 25 percent of each cardiac output volume. A constant supply of oxygen for the brain is essential since cytotoxic edema occurs within seconds if the brain is deprived of oxygen. Energy for the metabolic activities of the brain is derived from glucose and the oxidative metabolism of glucose. During hypoxia, oxidative metabolism and glycolysis decrease dramatically. Glucose is the major source of energy for ATP production and for the formation of amino and fatty acids, and carbon dioxide, which is used to regulate brain pH. Hypoglycemia severely depresses brain metabolism and leads rapidly to seizures, coma and death; but hyperglycemia has no known effect on brain cells.

The **cerebral blood flow (CBF)** is variable because of changes in **cerebral perfusion pressure (CPP)** (Fig. 3-11). CPP is the difference between the mean arterial pressure and the intracranial pressure (ICP). The brain is able to maintain perfusion pressure by autoregulating cerebral blood flow. This is accomplished by the brain's ability to change the diameter of blood vessels to accommodate changes in blood flow, and to maintain consistent resistance and blood flow. Arterial dilatation and subsequent increases in CBF occur when the pCO_2 rises about 45 mm Hg or the pO_2 falls below 50 mm Hg.

```
    MAP*         MAP = Mean arterial pressure
    -ICP         ICP = Intracranial pressure
    ─────        CPP = Cerebral perfusion pressure
    CPP

                 *MAP = (Systolic pressure + 2 × Diastolic pressure) / 3
```

Fig. 3-11. Cerebral perfusion pressure

KEY CONCEPT: The brain utilizes 20% of the oxygen demands of the body at rest. Oxygen for the brain is essential.

KEY POINT RECOGNITION

Write true or false by each statement. Answers are at the end of this chapter.

_____ 1. The brain consumes approximately 20 percent of the body's demand for oxygen.

_____ 2. Hyperglycemia severely depresses brain metabolism.

_____ 3. Cerebral perfusion pressure is the difference between the mean arterial pressure and intracranial pressure.

DIVISIONS OF CEREBRAL TISSUE

The brain is made up of **neurons** and **glial** cells. (See Fig. 3-12.) Gray matter is composed of nerve cell bodies.

For this discussion, the brain (Fig. 3-13) will be divided into the:

Cerebrum
(telencephalon)
(basal ganglia)

Cerebellum

Diencephalon
(thalamus/hypothalamus)

Brainstem
(midbrain)
(pons)
(medulla)
(reticular formation)

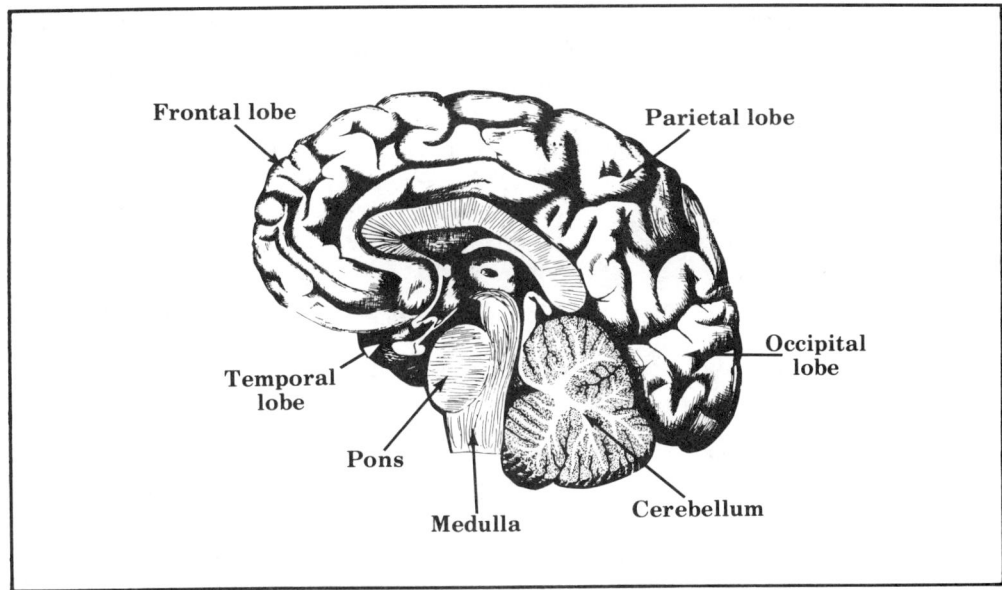

Fig. 3-12. Gross anatomy: division of the brain

Brain Part	Subdivisions	Size and Structure	Function
Cerebrum	Telencephalon basal ganglia	Largest part of brain; made up of 2 hemispheres, each divided into 4 lobes	Provides for sensations, emotions, voluntary actions, mental processes and consciousness; basal ganglia: extrapyramidal motor activity
Cerebellum		Second largest part of brain; composed of both gray and white matter	Coordination, equilibrium, synchronized muscle movement
Diencephalon	Thalamus	There is a right and left thalamus; made up of many cell bodies of neurons	Acts as relay station for sensory input; association of sensations and emotions
	Hypothalamus	Lies under the thalamus; one of smallest structures of the brain	Helps control many of the internal organs and vital functions; helps control endocrine performance; controls the waking state
Brainstem	Mesencephalon (midbrain)	Lies between pons and diencephalon, is connected to the cerebellum by the superior cerebellar peduncle	Some motor and sensory, as well as visual and auditory pathways
	Pons	Lies between the midbrain and medulla	Houses some motor and sensory pathways
	Medulla	Located at terminal portions of brainstem	Contains all the vital centers and is responsible for respiration, heartbeat and blood pressure; contains sensory and motor pathways
	Reticular formation (reticular activating system)	Diffuse network of fibers that project from brainstem to cortex	Ascending formation controls wakefulness and sleep; descending formation inhibits or enhances neurons controlling skeletal muscle activity

Fig. 3-13. Divisions of the brain

The *cerebrum* is composed of four lobes divided into right and left hemispheres by the longitudinal fissure. The two hemispheres receive information about each other via the ***corpus callosum.***

The *frontal lobe* is responsible for motor movement (voluntary motor strip) of the opposite (contralateral) side of the body and for mentation (intellect, insight, affect, judgment and personality).

The *parietal lobe* controls sensory function, also in a contralateral manner, and is concerned with sensory association and processing of general sensory information.

The *temporal lobe* is responsible for hearing, some aspects of behavior and emotion, and is associated with vestibular response, such as balance, and speech in the dominant hemisphere. (In all right-handed persons and the majority of left-handed persons, the left hemisphere is dominant.)

The *occipital lobe* is solely concerned with vision and the processing of visual information.

Further divisions of the cerebrum include ***Broca's*** and ***Wernicke's areas.*** ***Broca's area*** controls ***expressive speech.*** It is located in the ***dominant frontal-temporal area. Wernicke's area*** controls ***receptive speech.*** It is located in the ***dominant frontal-parietal area.***

The *basal ganglia* are composed of the putamen, globus pallidus, claustrum, caudate nucleus, subthalamic nucleus and substantia nigra. This is the major area concerned with involuntary (extrapyramidal) motor activity, regulating muscle tone, inhibiting muscle tone, and integrating motor responses and postural reflexes. Parkinsonism, a disease characterized by inadequate dopamine (basal ganglia neurotransmitter) in the substantia nigra, is the major disease process of the basal ganglia.

The *cerebellum* is found in the posterior fossa below the tentorium. It receives input from all other brain and spinal cord areas. The *cerebellum* controls equilibrium, balance, muscle tone, motion, posture and synchronized muscle movement. Cerebellar disorders include ataxia (staggering gait), dysmetria (overreach) and difficulty with rapid, alternating movements (disdiadochokinesia).

The *diencephalon* is composed of the thalamus, the hypothalamus and other structures with thalamus in their name (epi- and subthalamus).

The *thalamus* is a sensory relay station for all sensory input reaching the cerebral cortex. It also provides association areas for sensory input into motor function and consciousness.

The *hypothalamus* produces ***antidiuretic hormone (ADH),*** which is stored and released by the pituitary. It also produces releasing factors for the following hormones made by the pituitary: follicle stimulating hormone (FSH); luteinizing hormone (LH); growth hormone (GH), also called somatotropic hormone (STH); adrenocorticotropic hormone (ACTH); and thyroid stimulating hormone (TSH). It produces prolactin inhibiting factor to prevent release of prolactin from the pituitary. In addition, the hypothalamus plays a role in regulating body temperature, food and water intake and carbohydrate metabolism, and promoting parasympathetic responses. By interconnection with the limbic system, it is believed to affect aggressive and sexual behavior, and to play a part in maintaining the reticular activating system (RAS) and its control of consciousness.

The *brainstem* is made up of the ***midbrain, pons, medulla*** and ***reticular formation.*** The ***midbrain,*** located between the diencephalon and the pons, contains the third and fourth cranial nerve nuclei, some motor and sensory pathways, and the visual and auditory pathways. The ***pons*** lies between the midbrain and the medulla, and houses the sensory and motor pathways originating above and below the pons and coursing up to the cortex or down to the cord. It also contains the nuclei for the cranial nerves V, VI, VII and VIII. The ***medulla,*** located at the terminal portion of the brainstem just before the beginning of the spinal cord, houses the nuclei for cranial nerves IX, X, XI and XII and the cardiac and respiratory rate centers. Sensory and motor pathways also run through the medulla. The ***reticular formation*** (reticular activating system) is a diffuse network of fibers projecting from the brainstem to the cortex, spinal cord, cerebellum and thalamus. The ascending formation (ARAS) controls arousal, wakefulness and sleep. The descending formation (DRAS) may inhibit or enhance neurons controlling skeletal muscle activity.

KEY CONCEPT: Divisions of the brain include the cerebrum, cerebellum, diencephalon and brainstem.

KEY POINT RECOGNITION

Write true or false by each statement. Answers are at the end of this chapter. A score below 80% indicates the need for further study.

_____ 1. Gray matter consists of nerve cell processes.

_____ 2. The cerebellum is composed of four lobes.

_____ 3. The two hemispheres of the cerebrum receive information about each other via the corpus callosum.

_____ 4. The parietal lobe of the cerebrum is responsible for motor movement.

_____ 5. The temporal lobe of the cerebrum is responsible for hearing.

_____ 6. The cerebellum is a part of the midbrain and controls balance and equilibrium.

_____ 7. The diencephalon is composed of the thalamus and hypothalamus, as well as other structures.

_____ 8. The hypothalamus produces ADH.

_____ 9. The basal ganglia are concerned with extrapyramidal motor activity.

_____ 10. The brainstem is made up of the hypothalamus, pons and medulla.

_____ 11. The medulla houses the nuclei for cranial nerves V, VI and VII, and the cardiac and respiratory centers.

_____ 12. The reticular activating system is a diffuse network of fibers regulating sleep and waking cycles.

CEREBRAL BLOOD SUPPLY

The arterial blood supply to the brain is provided by the ***Circle of Willis***. The circle is supplied by a set of paired arteries, the ***internal carotids*** and the ***vertebral arteries*** (Fig. 3-14), which arise from the subclavian artery.

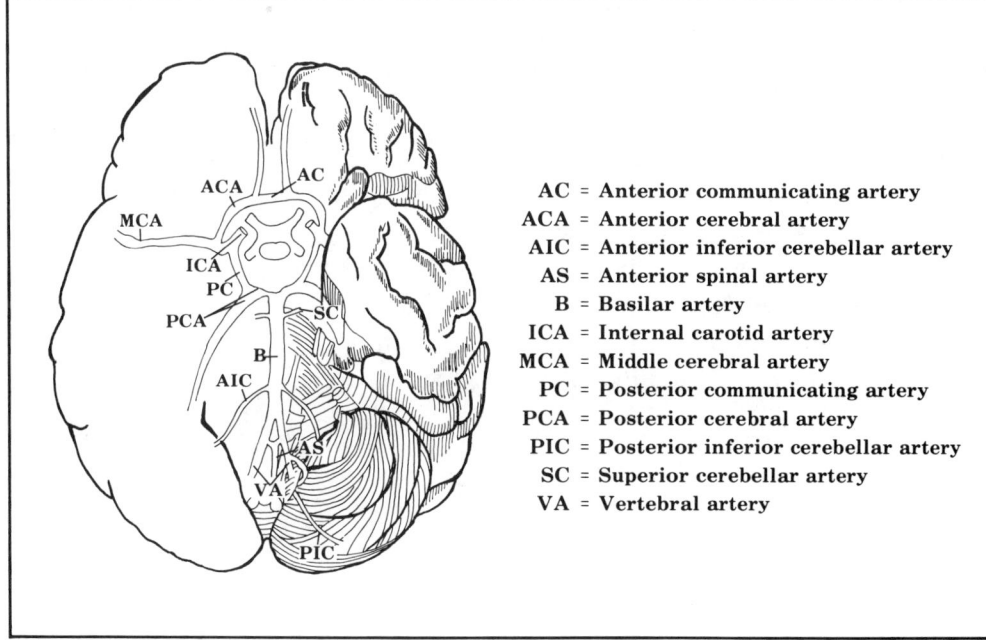

Fig. 3-14. Arterial cerebral blood flow

The *internal carotid* provides branches that compose the anterior Circle of Willis. They are the
  (1) *middle cerebral arteries,* which supply the lateral surfaces of the frontal, temporal and parietal lobes, as well as portions of the motor strip controlling movement of the face and upper extremities;
  (2) *anterior cerebral arteries,* which supply the corpus callosum, the medial portion of the frontal and parietal lobes, as well as the portion of the motor strip controlling lower extremities;
  (3) *anterior communicating artery,* which connects the right and left anterior cerebral arteries and provides for cross-flow from the opposite side should flow through the carotid on one side be slowly diminished; and
  (4) *posterior communicating arteries,* which connect the carotids with the posterior cerebral arteries and provide for cross-flow between anterior and posterior circulation.

The *vertebral arteries* (posterior system) join at the base of the pons to form the basilar artery. The branches of this system are the
  (1) *posterior inferior cerebellar arteries,* which perfuse the inferior and posterior aspects of the cerebellum;
  (2) *anterior spinal artery,* which perfuses the anterior segment of the spinal cord and the medial aspect of the brainstem;
  (3) *superior cerebellar arteries,* which supply the superior portion of the cerebellum;
  (4) *anterior inferior cerebellar arteries,* which supply the anterior and inferior aspects of the cerebellum; and
  (5) *posterior cerebral arteries,* which perfuse the posterior parietal lobes and the inferior aspects of the temporal and occipital lobes.

The *extracerebral blood supply* is provided by the **meningeal arteries,** which arise from the external carotid arteries. They supply the meninges and periosteum. The main branches are the
  (1) *anterior meningeal artery,* which supplies the anterior dura;
  (2) *middle meningeal artery,* which supplies the dura overlying the posterior frontal area, the temporal and parietal areas, and the anterior occipital area. (This is the artery that most frequently causes epidural hematomas.); and
  (3) *posterior meningeal artery,* which supplies the dura in the occipital area.

The *extracerebral blood supply* is drained by veins lying in the subdural space and the surface of the cerebral hemispheres. The internal circulation is drained via small capillaries within the cerebral hemispheres and cerebral tissue. Both internal and external systems empty into the venous sinuses formed by the separation of the layers of the dura.

The major venous sinuses and the areas they drain (Fig. 3-15) are the
  (1) *superior sagittal,* superior cerebral veins;
  (2) *inferior sagittal,* medial aspects of the hemispheres;
  (3) *straight sinus,* internal cerebral veins; and
  (4) *transverse sinus,* continuous with straight sinus.

The dural sinuses empty into the internal jugular veins.

Vessels	Branches	Area Supplied or Sinus Emptied Into
Internal carotid arteries	(Compose the anterior Circle of Willis)	(Arachnoid and pia)
	Middle cerebral arteries	Lateral surfaces of the frontal, temporal and parietal lobes; portions of the motor strip that controls movement of the face and upper extremities
	Anterior cerebral arteries	Corpus callosum; medial portion of the frontal and parietal lobes; portion of the motor strip controlling lower extremities
	Anterior communicating artery (connects the right and left anterior cerebral arteries)	Provides for cross flow of carotids
	Posterior communicating arteries (connects the carotids with the posterior cerebral arteries)	Provides for cross flow between anterior and posterior circulation
Vertebral arteries	(Posterior system)	(Arachnoid and pia)
	Posterior inferior cerebellar arteries	Interior and posterior aspects of the cerebellum
	Anterior spinal artery	Anterior segment of spinal cord; medial aspect of brainstem
	Superior cerebellar arteries	Superior portion of cerebellum
	Anterior inferior cerebellar arteries	Anterior and inferior aspect of cerebellum
	Posterior cerebral arteries	Posterior parietal lobes; inferior aspects of temporal and occipital lobes
Meningeal arteries	Anterior meningeal arteries	(Dura and periosteum) Anterior dura
	Middle meningeal artery	Dura over posterior frontal area; temporal and parietal areas; anterior occipital area
	Posterior meningeal artery	Dura in occipital area
Superior cerebral veins		Superior sagittal sinus
Small capillaries in medial aspects of cerebral hemisphere		Inferior sagittal sinus
Internal cerebral veins		Straight and transverse sinus

Fig. 3-15. Cerebral blood supply

KEY CONCEPT: Cerebral arterial blood supply is provided by the Circle of Willis. Extra-cerebral blood supply is provided by the meningeal arteries. Internal and external systems drain into venous sinuses.

KEY POINT RECOGNITION

Write true or false by each statement. Answers are at the end of this chapter.

_____ 1. The arterial blood supply to the brain is provided by the Circle of Willis.

_____ 2. The Circle of Willis is supplied by the internal carotids and the meningeal arteries.

_____ 3. The middle cerebral arteries provide for cross-flow between anterior and posterior circulation.

_____ 4. The meningeal arteries supply the frontal and temporal lobes.

_____ 5. The medial aspects of the hemispheres drain into the superior sagittal sinus.

THE VENTRICULAR SYSTEM

The *ventricular system* (Fig. 3-16) is composed of *four ventricles* and the *subarachnoid space* around the brain and spinal cord. This provides a continuous system for circulation of cerebrospinal fluid (CSF).

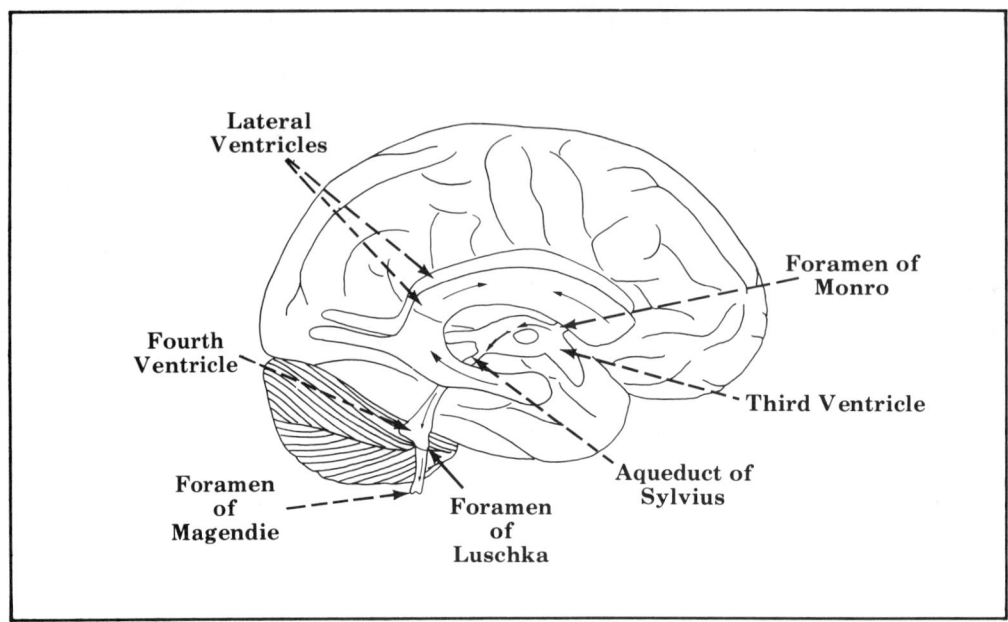

Fig. 3-16. Ventricular system

The *lateral ventricles* are the largest, extending into the frontal, temporal, parietal and occipital lobes in each hemisphere. One lateral ventricle lies in each hemisphere. The lateral ventricle is divided into the

(1) *anterior horn,* which is in the frontal lobe;

(2) *body,* which traverses the parietal lobe;

(3) *posterior horn,* which reaches to the occipital lobe; and

(4) *inferior horn,* which reaches across the temporal lobe.

Each ventricle is lined with specialized ependymal cells, called the *choroid plexus,* which filters the blood presented to it to form the cerebrospinal fluid (CSF). All ventricles participate in this filtration process but, because of size, the lateral and third ventricles provide the majority of the CSF. Each lateral ventricle drains into the third ventricle by way of the *foramen of Monro.*

The *third ventricle,* midline between the two lateral ventricles, is the second largest ventricle. It drains into the fourth ventricle via the *aqueduct of Sylvius.*

The *fourth ventricle,* the smallest, lies in the posterior fossa. The terminal portion forms the central canal, allowing spinal fluid to circulate downward around the spinal cord subarachnoid space. The other exits are the foramen of Luschka and the foramen of Magendie, permitting circulation around the subarachnoid space of the brain.

The functions of *cerebrospinal fluid* are to

(1) *cushion* and *protect* the brain and spinal cord;

(2) provide a fluid medium for flotation that *decreases* the *effective weight* of the brain and spinal cord; and

(3) help compensate for changes in *intracranial volume* and *pressure.*

After the CSF circulates around the brain and cord, it is reabsorbed by small projections of the arachnoid membrane *(arachnoid cranulations* or *villi)* bordering the dural sinuses. CSF is absorbed into the dural sinuses by way of the villi. It joins the venous circulation in the sinuses and is returned to the systemic circulation via the internal jugular veins. At any time there are about 150 cc of CSF in the system:

    25 cc in all four ventricles

    90 cc in the lumbar subarachnoid cistern

    35 cc in the remaining subarachnoid space

Normal CSF is clear, colorless and, with the patient lying on the side, has an opening pressure (OP) of about 80 to 180 mm H_2O. Lab normals include:

    Specific gravity—1.007

    pH—7.35

    Chloride—120 to 130 meq/L

    Sodium—142 to 150 meq/L

    Glucose—60 to 80 mg/l or 60% of serum glucose level

    Protein—lumbar 15 to 45 mg/dl
       cisternal 10 to 25 mg/dl
       ventricular 5 to 15 mg/dl

    White blood cells — polys = none   Lymphs = 0 to $10/cm^3$

KEY CONCEPT: The ventricular system, composed of four ventricles and the subarachnoid space around the brain and spinal cord, provides a continuous system for circulation of CSF. CSF is produced continuously by the choroid plexus in the ventricles and is returned to the systemic circulation via the arachnoid veins to the dural sinuses and finally emptied into the internal jugular veins.

KEY POINT RECOGNITION

Write true or false by each statement. Answers are at the end of this chapter. A score below 80% indicates the need for further study.

    _____ 1. The ventricular system provides continuous circulation of CSF.

    _____ 2. The lateral ventricles are the smallest.

    _____ 3. The lateral ventricle is divided into the anterior horn, posterior horn, inferior horn and body.

    _____ 4. The third ventricle drains into the fourth ventricle via the foramen of Monro.

    _____ 5. The lateral ventricles drain via the foramen of Luschka.

    _____ 6. There are about 175 cc of CSF in the ventricular system.

    _____ 7. Normally, opening pressure (in the side-lying position) is 80 to 210 mm H_2O.

THE SPINAL CORD

The *spinal cord* extends from the terminal border of the medulla to the L1-2 interspace. It is continuous with the medulla and covered by meninges that are continuous with the meninges covering the brain. The pia attaches to the cord and spinal nerve roots and ends at the filum terminale. The arachnoid extends to the level of S2, as does the dura.

The *conus medullaris* is the terminal end of the cord at L2. The *filum terminale* is the portion of meningeal covering after the conus and ending at the first coccygeal vertebra. The *filum* contains the *cauda equina,* the *nerves* of the *lumbar* and *sacral region* that exit after the conus medullaris, but no cord tissue since the cord ends at L2. Therefore, spinal punctures are performed at the L3-4 interspace to avoid the end portion of the cord and to avoid damaging central nervous tissue. Nerves of the *cauda equina* are classified as *peripheral nerves* and are capable of regeneration.

Gray matter, whether in the brain or cord, refers to tissue that is unmyelinated. White matter refers to tissue composed of axon sheaths that are coated with myelin. Spinal cord **gray matter** is the H-shaped interior arrangement of cell bodies making up the interior aspect of the cord tissue (Fig. 3-17). The **anterior (ventral) horns** of the cord contain the cell bodies of the **efferent** (motor from brain to body) fibers. The **posterior (dorsal) horns** contain the cell bodies of the **afferent** (sensory, from body to brain) fibers. Spinal cord **white matter** is the axon sheaths making up the various spinal cord tracts. **Ascending tracts** carry **sensory** information up from the periphery to the cortex. **Descending tracts** carry **motor** information down from the cortex to the end organs in the periphery. The direction of most tracts can be determined from their names, and hence their function deduced. (Example: spinothalamic—from spinal cord to thalamus, therefore, ascending and sensory; corticospinal—from the cortex to the spinal cord, therefore, descending and motor.) The **major spinal cord tracts** and their functions are listed below.

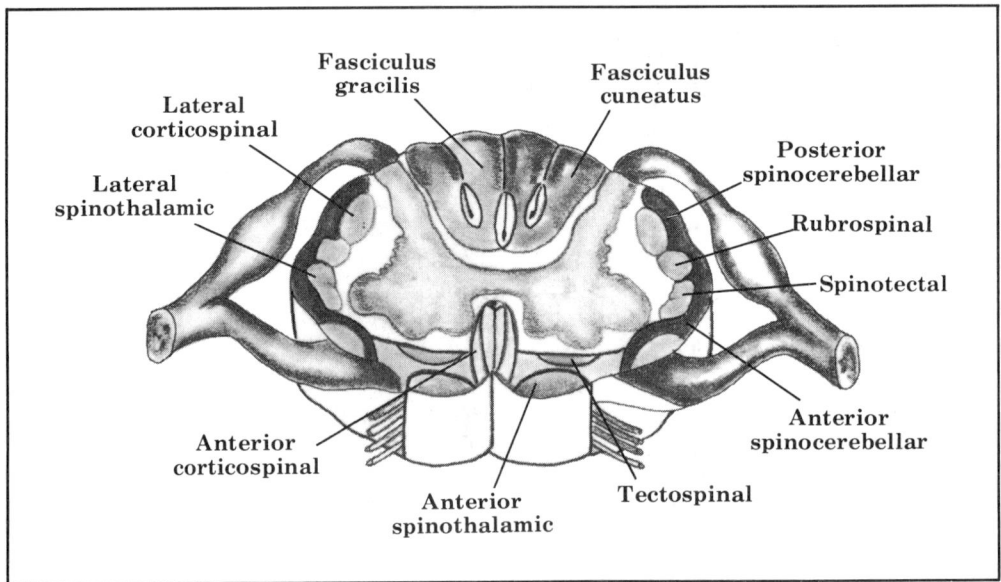

Fig. 3-17. Spinal cord

Ascending (sensory)—usually found in the posterior portion of the cord unless otherwise indicated in the name, such as lateral or anterior.
1. Fasciculus gracilis and fasciculus cuneatus—position and vibration, joint position and two-point discrimination
2. Lateral spinothalamic—pain and temperature sensation
3. Anterior spinothalamic—light touch, pressure and sensation
4. Dorsal and ventral spinocerebellar—proprioception affecting muscle tone
5. Spinotectal—carries sensory information to midbrain

Descending (motor)—frequently found in the anterior portion of the cord
1. Rubrospinal—impulses controlling muscle tone
2. Ventral and lateral corticospinal—impulses for voluntary movement (also known as pyramidal tracts, voluntary motor tracts that originate in the frontal motor strip)
3. Tectospinal—mediation of optic and auditory reflexes

The spinal and cranial nerves compose the **peripheral nervous system.** The **cranial nerves** arise from cerebral tissue (Fig. 3-18). The **spinal nerves** originate from the spinal cord. Thirty-one pairs exit the cord: **8 cervical, 12 thoracic, 5 lumbar, 5 sacral** and **1 coccygeal.**

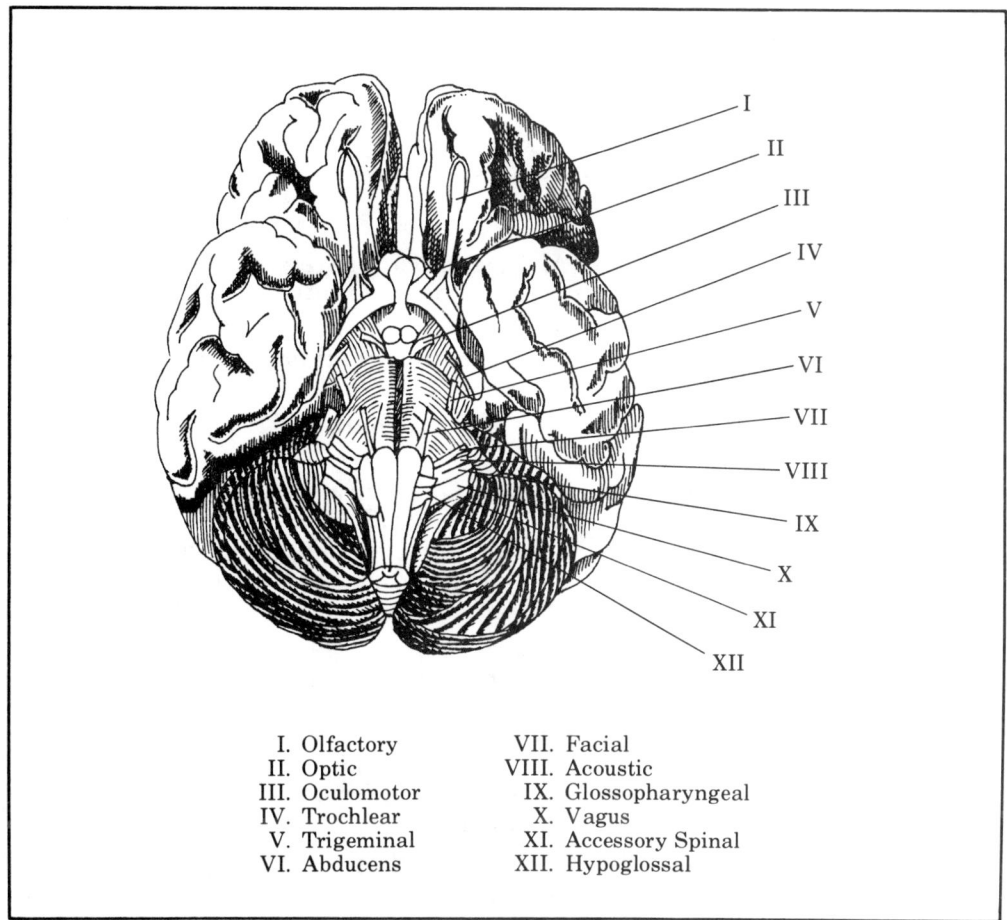

Fig. 3-18. Cranial nerves: origin

In the *cervical* region, they exit *above* the corresponding vertebra, hence the additional nerve that exits between C7 and T1. In the *thoracic, lumbar* and *coccygeal* regions, they exit *below* the corresponding vertebra. The *cauda equina* is composed of spinal nerves arising from the lumbarsacral portion of the cord. A *dermatome* is a single area of skin supplied by a single spinal nerve. Characteristic dermatome numbness or pain helps diagnose certain spinal cord syndromes, such as the HNP lumbar region. A *plexus* is a labyrinth of spinal nerves.

KEY CONCEPT: The peripheral nervous system comprises 31 pairs of spinal nerves and 12 cranial nerves. Nerves to the trunk and limbs originate from the spinal cord.

KEY POINT RECOGNITION
Write true or false by each statement. Answers are at the end of this chapter. A score below 80% indicates the need for further study.

_____ 1. The spinal cord extends from the terminal border of the medulla to the L1-2 interspace.

_____ 2. The cord ends at L2.

_____ 3. The cauda equina is composed of nerves of the lumbar and sacral area exiting after the conus medullaris.

_____ 4. The ventral horns of the cord contain efferent fibers.

_____ 5. Posterior horns contain sensory fibers.

_____ 6. Descending spinal cord tracts are frequently located in the anterior portion of the cord.

_____ 7. The ventral and lateral corticospinal tract is also known as a pyramidal tract.
_____ 8. There are 12 thoracic spinal nerves.
_____ 9. There are 12 pairs of spinal nerves.
_____ 10. A dermatome is a labyrinth of spinal nerves.

AUTONOMIC NERVOUS SYSTEM

The autonomic nervous system (ANS) is sometimes referred to as the involuntary nervous system because an individual has no control over the activities of the ANS.

The ANS comprises two divisions: **sympathetic** or thoracolumbar, and **parasympathetic** or craniosacral.

The two divisions may innervate the same organ but have an antagonistic effect on the organ (Fig. 3-19).

The ANS is composed of neuron chains. One neuron chain located within the lateral horns of the spinal cord's gray matter is called preganglionic cell bodies. The axons of these neurons exit from the spinal cord as part of the anterior root network. Upon exiting, the neurons divide and join the sympathetic trunk as white **rami communicans.** The white appearance comes from the myelinated covering on the neurons.

Sympathetic trunk ganglia lie on each side of the vertebral column from the first cervical vertebra to the coccyx. These chains of ganglia are connected by a fibrous network. Once the preganglionic fibers reach the sympathetic trunk, the neurons may synapse with collateral ganglia that are unmyelinated postganglionic neurons. These postganglionic fibers reach spinal nerves, cranial nerves, selective organs and blood vessels.

The second chain is the postganglionic axons that pass to the viscera by way of the sympathetic nerve network. Those which return to the spinal nerves make up the gray **rami communicans.** At this point gray rami join all spinal nerves. From the spinal nerve connection, the fibers continue to the walls of peripheral blood vessels, glands, hair follicles and certain muscles (Fig. 3-20).

The **sympathetic division** originates from the thoracolumbar segments of the spinal cord. The sympathetic division innervates the viscera, blood vessels, glands, smooth muscle tissue and the heart. It is referred to as the *fight or flight* response of the body. Stimulation of the sympathetic fibers produces a vasoconstriction to the affected body part. **Sympathetic stimulation** results in:

Increase in blood pressure
Dilation of bronchioles
Dilation of pupils
Salivation of thick secretions
Decrease in gastrointestinal motility
Increase in secretion of adrenal medulla
Increase in heart rate

These activities depend on the release of an agent from adrenergic neurons called **norepinephrine.**

The distribution of sympathetic fibers is as follows:

T1—sympathetic chain to head
T2—into neck
T3-6—thorax
T7-11—abdomen
T12-L1-2—legs

The **parasympathetic division** originates from the cervical and sacral region, hence craniosacral.

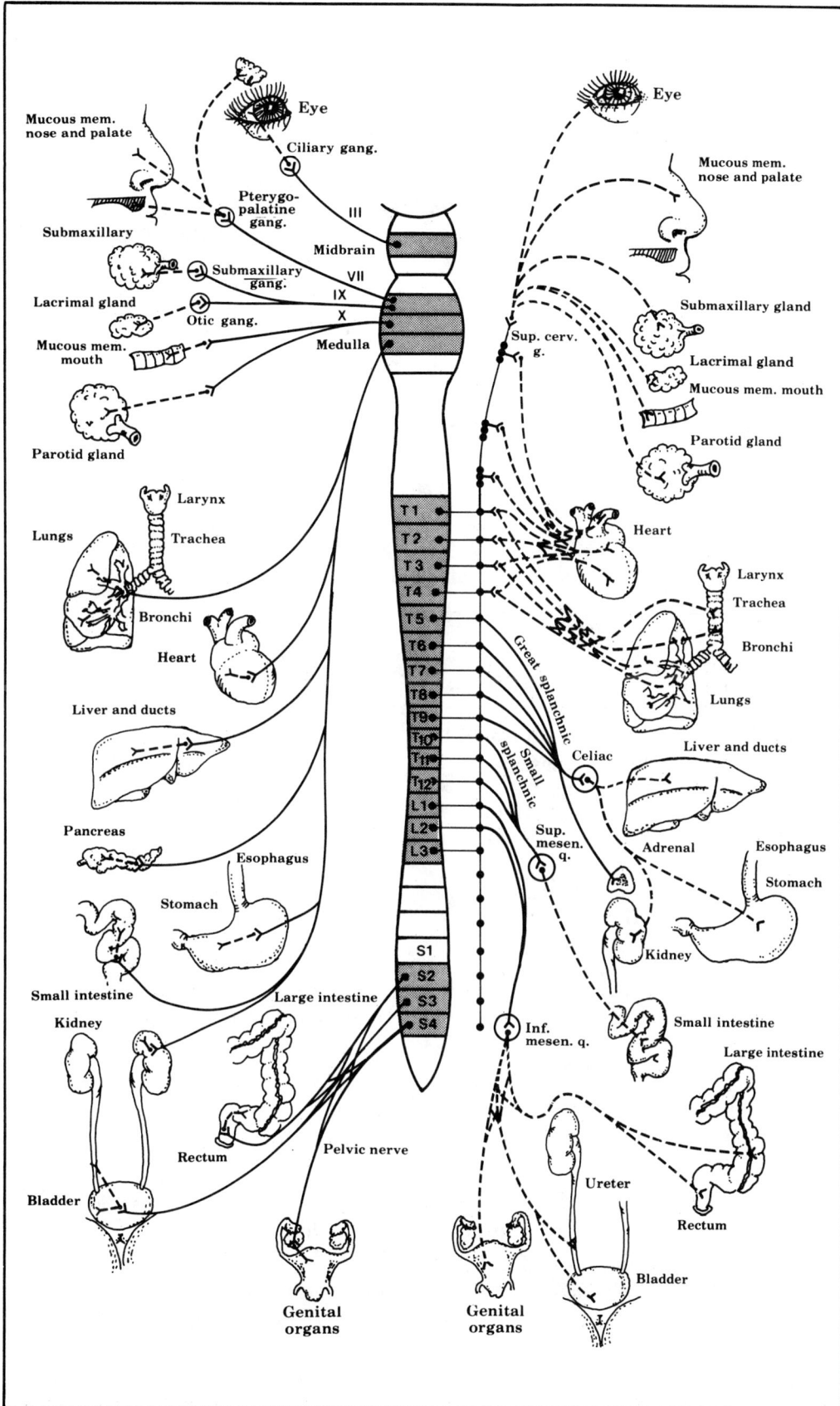

Fig. 3-19. ANS division

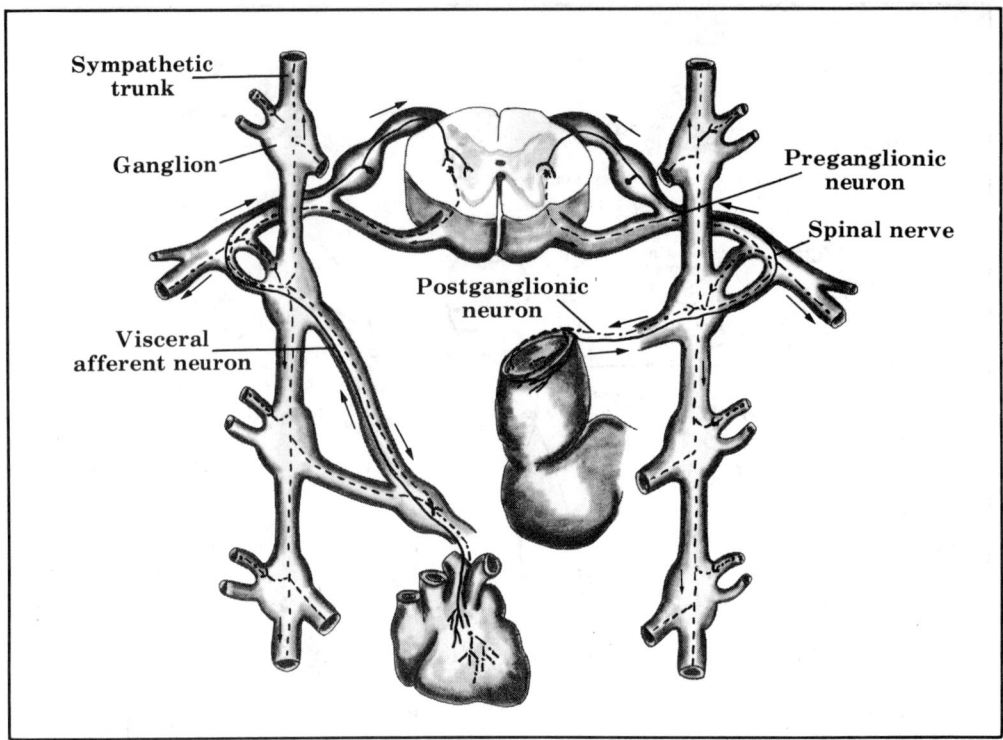

Fig. 3-20. Sympathetic division of ANS

The *parasympathetic division* is concerned with the management and functioning of the body's internal environment. Stimulation causes vasodilation. Parasympathetic stimulation results in:

Decrease in blood pressure
Constriction of pupils
Salivation of thin secretions
Increase in gastrointestinal motility
Decrease in heart rate

These activities depend on the release of an agent from *cholinergic neurons* called *acetylcholine*.

KEY CONCEPT: The autonomic nervous system is divided into sympathetic and parasympathetic systems. These divisions have antagonistic effects on organs and blood vessels. Each division releases a neurotransmitter: norepinephrine or acetylcholine.

KEY POINT RECOGNITION

Write true or false by each statement. Answers are at the end of this chapter. A score below 80% indicates the need for further study.

_____ 1. The involuntary nervous system is called the autonomic nervous system.
_____ 2. Preganglionic cell bodies arise from the spinal cord gray matter.
_____ 3. White rami communicans are unmyelinated.
_____ 4. Postganglionic fibers connect to spinal nerves and cranial nerves.
_____ 5. Gray rami communicans connect with spinal nerves from T1-L12.
_____ 6. The sympathetic division is called the thoracolumbar division.
_____ 7. The sympathetic division innervates viscera and blood vessels.
_____ 8. Sympathetic stimulation causes a decrease in heart rate and pupillary constriction.
_____ 9. Norepinephrine is a cholinergic neurotransmitter.
_____ 10. Two neurotransmitters of the ANS are acetylcholine and norepinephrine.

ASSESSMENT OF THE NEUROLOGICAL SYSTEM

Physical assessment of the patient experiencing neurologic dysfunction is not very different from the assessment of any other patient. Significant medical problems, current therapies, history and a review of systems are all included. Particular attention must be paid to the presenting complaint, its duration, character and the circumstances surrounding exacerbations and remissions. The following symptoms require further investigation: headache, fever, stiff neck, nuchal rigidity, neck pain, dizziness, visual changes, pupillary changes, loss of sensation, numbness, weakness, hemi- or monoparesis, changes in states of consciousness, personality changes, speech disturbances and acute memory changes.

Specific signs of altered functioning in specific brain areas may include:

Cerebellum—ataxia, dysmetria, uncoordinated motion

Frontal lobe—motor weakness, personality changes, speech distrubances, intellect changes

Parietal lobe—sensory loss, decreased ability to perceive touch

Temporal lobe—auditory loss, speech disturbances

Occipital lobe—visual disturbances

Cranial nerves—changes in pupil size/reactivity, loss of gag/swallow, loss of corneal reflex, facial droop

Brainstem—profound change of consciousness, cranial nerve dysfunctions, alterations in respiratory patterns

The physical examination should include assessment of the following:

(1) **Gross cerebral functions**
Overall behavior and appearance—consciousness, awareness, orientatation, memory, judgment, intellectual capacity
Emotional behavior—conversational ability, attention span, absence/presence of hallucinations, delusions

(2) **Specific cerebral functions**
Specific speech ability—evaluate for dysphasia, dysphonia (alteration in production of sound), dysarthria (alteration in articulation)
Sensory interpretation—ability to identify objects by touch
Motor interpretation—ability to carry out complex motor commands involving both sides of the body
Language usage and speech patterns

CRANIAL NERVE TESTING

Although they arise from the cerebral tissue, the cranial nerves are classified as peripheral nerves (Fig. 3-21).

I. **Olfactory**
Test each nostril with nonirritating odors, such as coffee, to check for anosmia.

II. **Optic**
Check visual acuity by testing with a standard eye chart.
Determine *visual fields.*
Examine *fundi* with an ophthalmoscope.

III. **Oculomotor**
Check pupils for *equality* of size and *reaction* to light.
Check *direct* (pupil constricts when light is shined in eye)
and *consensual* (pupil constricts when light is shined in opposite eye only) reaction to light.
Check ability to *elevate eyelid.*
Check ability to *move eye* in the four fields governed by the III nerve—*superior, inferior, medial* and *superior oblique*—by having the patient follow your finger with the eyes.

Nerve	Function	Innervation
I. Olfactory	Smell	Nasal mucous membranes
II. Optic	Vision	Retinal rods and cones

III. Oculomotor	Ocular movement	Ocular muscles:
		    levator palpebrae
		    rectus superior
		    rectus medius
		    rectus inferior
		    obliquus inferior

	Contraction of pupil and accommodation	Ciliary ganglion:
		    ciliaris pupillae
		    sphincter pupillae

IV. Trochlear	Ocular movement	Obliquus superior Muscle of eye
V. Trigeminal	Motor and main nerve of face for sensation	Skin of face, mucous membranes of face and head
	Mastication	Muscles of mastication
	Muscular	Sensory endings in muscles of mastication
VI. Abducens	Ocular movement	Lateral rectus muscle

VII. Facial	Facial expression	Muscles of expression:
		    stapedius
		    stylohyoideus
		    digastricus

VIII. Auditory	Hearing	Internal auditory meatus
	Cochlear hearing	Organ of corti cochlea

	Vestibular equilibrium; coordination of head and eye movement	Semicircular canals
		    Saccule
		    Utricle

IX. Glossopharyngeal	Taste	Pharynx and posterior third of tongue
	Reflex control of respiration, blood pressure and heart rate	Carotid bodies Carotid sinus Middle ear
X. Vagus	Involuntary muscle and gland control	Heart Lungs Esophagus G.I. tract
	Swallowing and phonation	Pharynx Larynx
	Visceral sensation: abdominal, thoracic	Carotid and aortic bodies Abdominal viscera
	Taste	Epiglottis Taste buds
	Cutaneous sensation	Auricular branch to external ear and meatus
XI. Accessory or spinal accessory	Swallowing and phonation	Muscles of pharynx and larynx
	Movement of shoulder	Sternomastoid and trapezius muscles
XII. Hypoglossal	Movement of tongue	Muscles of tongue

Fig. 3-21. Cranial nerves

IV. Trochlear
Check ability to move eye in *inferior oblique field* of gaze.

V. Trigeminal
Test sensation on forehead, cheeks and jaw bilaterally by using something soft for light touch, a pin for pinprick, and warm and cold objects for temperature.
Test corneal reflex bilaterally.
Check ability to chew and clench teeth.

VI. Abducens
Check for ability to *move eye* in *lateral* field.

VII. Facial
Test *strength* and *symmetry* of face by ability to raise the eyebrows, smile, frown, wrinkle the forehead and open eyes against resistance.
Check ability to *close* eyelid.
Test *taste* to *sweet* and *salt* on anterior two-thirds of tongue.

VIII. Acoustic
Check *auditory acuity* with *Rinne* (tuning fork on mastoid bone) and *Weber* (tuning fork on midline vertex of skull) test.
Check for absence of vertigo, nausea on movement, nystagmus, postural hypotension and vomiting.

IX. Glossopharyngeal
Check for *symmetry* of *arch* of *palate* on *phonation*.
Check for *gag* reflex.
Test for ability to *swallow* and *articulate*.

X. Vagus
Check *gag* reflex.
Test *carotid sinus reflex* by placing pressure over the carotid sinus. This should produce reflex bradycardia and decrease blood pressure.
Check for presence of hoarseness.

XI. Accessory spinal
Check *sternocleidomastoid* and *trapezius muscles* for *size* and *symmetry*.
Test ability to *hold head* to the *side against resistance*.
Test ability to *raise shoulder against resistance*.
Check *symmetry* and *position of scapulas*.

XII. Hypoglossal
Check *tongue* for *atrophy* and for *fasciculations*.
Test for *midline protrusion* of *tongue* (tongue will deviate toward side of lesion).

CEREBELLAR FUNCTION TESTING

To assess cerebellar function, the patient must have an intact motor system to the part being assessed.

Check for *dystaxia* by observing the patient for swaying when standing with feet together and eyes open; by observing for ability to walk heel-to-toe; by having the patient touch the nose and then the nurse's finger; or to bring the finger to the nose with eyes first opened and then closed; and by having the patient rub the heel down the shin.

Check for *nystagmus* by watching eye movements as the patient follows your finger through the fields of gaze.

Check for *hypotonia* by observing for rag doll gait and feeling for muscular resistance when passively moving a limb.

SENSORY SYSTEM TESTING

The **sensory system** is assessed for perception of tactile sensation, light pain, temperature, vibration, deep pressure, motion and joint position. It is important to determine if the sensory loss is along a nerve pathway. The nurse should be familiar with the larger dermatomal areas (Fig. 3-22). For cortical discriminatory sensation tests to be validly assessed, cortical area pathways and receptors must be functioning. Test the patient for **stereognosis, topognosia** and **graphognosia.**

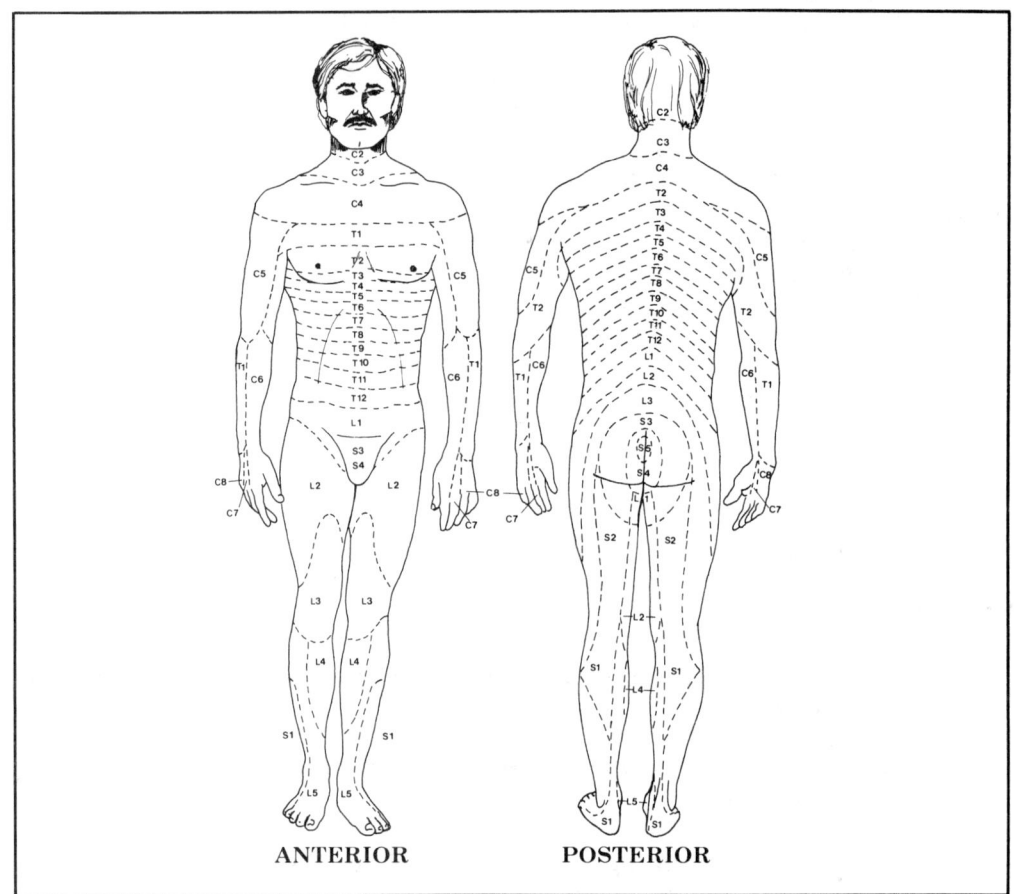

Fig. 3-22. Dermatonal areas

MOTOR SYSTEM TESTING

When assessing the **motor system,** the nurse must inspect the muscle as well as test for strength. Check the muscle for size, symmetry, tone and tenderness. Note any deviations from the norm, such as atrophy.

Strength is tested by having the patient grasp the examiner's hand or overcome the resistant force of the examiner's hand on a muscle or muscle group. Observe any patterns of weakness.

REFLEX TESTING

Deep tendon reflexes are assessed by using a reflex hammer. Responses on each side should be compared. Reflexes to check include the **jaw, biceps, brachioradialis, triceps, patellar** and **ankle**.

Cutaneous reflexes are assessed by using a sharp object on the skin. Reflexes to test include **abdominal** and **plantar.**

The Babinski sign is an abnormal plantar reflex. Upon stimulating the lateral aspect of the sole of the foot, the great toe extends. The normal response is flexion.

Grasping an object and not releasing it when instructed is indicative of cerebral dysfunction.

The corneal, gag, snout and glabellar reflexes should also be tested. Absent corneal and gag reflexes are abnormal findings. The presence of snout and glabellar reflexes are also indicative of cerebral dysfunction.

LEVEL OF CONSCIOUSNESS

Under any conditions, the **level of consciousness** is the single most important determinant of neurologic status and deterioration. Assessment of level of consciousness (LOC) evaluates a complex series of interactions between various brain components, including the cortex, brainstem, reticular activating system and hypothalamus. To assess LOC the following must be determined:

Arousability—to name, to shaking or to noxious stimuli. If unable to arouse, assess response to painful stimuli: purposeful withdrawal, nonpurposeful movement, decortication, decerebration or absence of any response (usually flaccid)

Orientation (if arousable)—to person, place, time and details of environment

Ability to follow commands—Test the ability to integrate and carry out verbal orders, not motor ability or strength.

PUPILLARY RESPONSE

After the LOC has been determined (it is much wiser to document what the patient can do rather than opt for subjective labels, such as comatose, stuporous, obtunded, lethargic), the *pupillary response* must be checked.

(1) Examine both pupils for *size* and *shape*. Are they *equal?* (Approximately 17 percent of the normal population will have a normal 0.5 to 1.0 mm inequality; however, both pupils will be equally reactive.) Are *both* pupils the *same shape?* Odd shapes frequently indicate eye surgery.

(2) With a bright light, shine the beam directly into the eye being tested. Watch for constriction; is it brisk, sluggish or nonreactive? Does the opposite eye constrict minimally when light reaches the eye being tested (consensual reaction indicating III cranial nerve is intact in the opposite eye)? Wait a few seconds, with both of the patient's eyes closed, for the pupils to readjust to the dark, then repeat the test in the other eye. The room should be as dark as possible when performing this test; no direct overhead lights should be in use.

(3) A blind eye has no direct reaction to light because of damage to cranial nerve II and failure to sense light by the retina; however, the consensual reaction is present since it is mediated by the third cranial nerve.

(4) Record pupil size in **millimeters** and reaction as **brisk, sluggish** or **absent** (fixed or nonreactive).

MOTOR STRENGTH AND EQUALITY

Next, the **motor strength** and **equality** are examined. Can the patient move all extremities? Are they equal in strength against both gravity and resistance? If unable to follow verbal commands, does the patient move all extremities equally in response to noxious stimuli? If unable to move the extremity, is the tone increased or is the extremity flaccid without reflexes? The classic upper motor neuron (UMN) lesion exhibits hyperreflexia, spasticity and lack of atrophy. The lower motor neuron (LMN) syndrome exhibits flaccidity, decreased or absent reflexes, atrophy and fasciculations. UMN lesions indicate damage in the cortex or prior to the first cord synapse; LMN lesions indicate damage in the cord or peripheral system.

Decortication is exhibited by flexor posturing with adduction of the upper extremities, and extension and plantar flexion of the lower extremities. *Decerebration* is seen when the upper extremities are extended, hyperpronated and adducted, with extension and plantar flexion of the lower extremities.

Grasp equality in the hands can be checked by asking the patient to forcefully squeeze one or two fingers of the examiner's hands. A more sensitive test for arm inequality is to have the patient extend arms, with palms facing up, at a 45 degree angle from the trunk. Ask the patient to maintain this position with the eyes closed. A minimal weakness causes the weak arm to turn in and down without the patient's awareness. This is referred to as a **pronator drift.**

EVALUATION OF VITAL SIGNS

The blood pressure may be normal or elevated. In neurologic dysfunction, **hypotension** is rarely seen; when it is present, it is usually a grave, preterminal sign. **Hypertension** may be seen as a compensatory mechanism to insure perfusion of a swollen, edematous brain. Intermittent hypertension may be seen with changes in cerebral edema or vascular spasm.

Bradycardia is common in mass lesions or edema, creating downward pressure on the brainstem. For unknown reasons, ST changes and T-wave inversion may be seen early in neurologic disease or injury; however, it appears to be benign and self-limiting.

Hyperthermia may be seen in injuries that cause compression of the hypothalamus. These elevated temperatures are usually accompanied by tachycardia and respond poorly to normal antihyperthermic measures. **Hypothermia** is rarely seen, except in profound injuries resulting in brain death. The use of hypothermia for controlling elevation of ICP is controversial and minimally effective, at best.

Respiratory changes are common with neurological disease. **Cheyne-Stokes** respirations are rhythmic hypo- and hyperventilations alternating with periods of apnea. The entire sequence is a crescendo-decrescendo response to alterations in pCO_2 levels. It frequently occurs with bilateral cortical lesions and damage in the midbrain. **Apneustic** (reversal of the inspiratory-expiratory ratio with inspiratory cramping) and **central neurogenic hyperventilation** (CNH) occur with lesions in the pons. **Ataxic** (irregular) and **cluster breathing** (irregular periods of respiration alternating with irregular periods of apnea) indicate lesions in the low pons or medulla.

LABORATORY AND RADIOLOGIC STUDIES

Laboratory studies in neurological disease are varied and tailored to the presumptive diagnosis at hand. A detailed discussion of all possible studies is beyond the scope of this review.

Radiologic studies are more distinct and are briefly discussed here:

Skull series—to determine bony abnormalities and fractures

Spinal films—to detect bony abnormalities and fractures of the vertebral column

Cerebral angiography—invasive injection of dye into the cerebral arteries to detect vessel patency, malformation, abnormality and rupture

Pneumoencephalography/ventriculography—injection of air into the subarachnoid space and/or ventricles to visualize CSF circulation and ventricle size and placement; replaced for the most part by CT scanning

Myelography—injection of dye into the spinal subarachnoid space to determine bony abnormalities and blocks

CT scan—a noninvasive radiologic procedure in which multiple films are interpreted by computer, based on density, to provide a three-dimensional view of the brain

Other tests, such as electroencephalography (EEG), brain scan and tomography are also useful diagnostic adjuncts.

KEY CONCEPT: Physical assessment of the neurological patient should include assessment of gross and specific cerebral functions and cranial nerves by performing cerebellar function testing, motor system testing, sensory system testing and reflex testing.

KEY POINT RECOGNITION
Write true or false by each statement. Answers are at the end of this chapter. A score below 80% indicates the need for further study.

_____ 1. Motor weakness and personality changes may be indicative of brainstem dysfunction.

_____ 2. Sensory loss and visual disturbances are indicative of temporal lobe dysfunction.

_____ 3. The II cranial nerve is evaluated by checking visual acuity and visual fields.

_____ 4. The VI cranial nerve is tested by checking ability to chew and checking for sensations on forehead, face and jaw.

_____ 5. The X cranial nerve is evaluated by checking the gag and carotid sinus reflexes.

_____ 6. The IX cranial nerve is the glossopharyngeal.

_____ 7. The XII cranial nerve is evaluated by checking the tongue for atrophy as well as midline protrusion.

_____ 8. The II cranial nerve is the oculomotor.

_____ 9. It is not necessary for cortical area pathways to be functioning in order to validly assess cortical discriminatory sensation.

_____ 10. Inspection of the muscle is not as important as assessing strength of the muscle.

_____ 11. Cutaneous reflexes are assessed by using a reflex hammer.

_____ 12. Absent corneal reflexes are abnormal findings.

_____ 13. The Babinski sign is a normal plantar reflex in the adult.

_____ 14. The pupillary response is the most important determinant of neurologic status.

_____ 15. Assessment of the LOC includes determination of arousability, orientation and ability to follow commands.

_____ 16. Pupils are checked for size, shape, equality and reactivity to light.

_____ 17. Decortication is seen when the upper extremities are extended, hyperpronated and adducted with extension and plantar flexion of the lower extremities.

_____ 18. Hypotension is a compensatory mechanism to insure perfusion of a swollen brain.

_____ 19. Hypothermia is seen in injuries that cause compression of the brainstem.

_____ 20. Central neurogenic hyperventilation occurs with lesions in the pons.

_____ 21. The presence of a pronator drift is established by having the patient extend arms at a 45 degree angle, with palms facing up from the trunk, and maintaining this position with the eyes closed.

PATHOLOGICAL STATES AND NURSING MANAGEMENT

CEREBRAL VASCULAR ACCIDENTS (CVA)

Pathophysiology

CVAs are generally caused by one of three etiologic factors:

Thrombus, embolus or **hemorrhage.** In the case of **thrombus** or **embolus,** the subsequent decreased blood flow causes decreased oxygen to the affected cerebral tissue, and the resulting anoxia leads to cell death and resultant functional loss. The area surrounding the anoxic area is also damaged, but it receives enough oxygen to maintain cell life. This leads to ischemic tissue surrounding the infarcted regions. The functional ability of the ischemic cells is not permanently lost and gradually returns, resulting in the improvement in neurological function seen in patients several days after the acute insult.

Hemorrhagic CVAs cause neurological deficit resulting from the pressure of the escaping blood (space-occupying lesion) on the surrounding tissue. This expanded volume adds pressure to the intracranial space, putting pressure directly on cerebral cells and vessels. The formation of a clot further increases the pressure, decreasing the blood supply and oxygen content available to cerebral tissue, and leading to cellular anoxia and cell death. Some ischemic cells in the perimeter may be spared and their function is not irreversibly damaged.

Precipitating factors leading to **thrombotic** or **embolic CVAs** are hypertension, vascular disease, thrombus/embolus formation history, valvular disease, obesity, sedentary lifestyle and elevated blood lipids. Precipitating factors for ***hemorrhagic CVAs*** may be vascular malformations, aneurysm, trauma, hypertension and clotting disorders.

Clinical Presentation

The clinical presentation is extremely variable and dependent on the area of brain involved. Changes in level of consciousness may occur, but are more common with extensive bilateral cortical lesions and brainstem lesions. Headache, hemiparesis, hemisensory loss, speech disturbances, visual changes, cranial nerve dysfunctions and any combination of the above may be seen. The most common preceding symptom of occlusive carotid artery disease is a transient ischemic attack (TIA) in which vision becomes blurred in the ipsilateral eye.

Diagnostic Data

CT scan is the best diagnostic aid, along with a complete history and physical, to determine the cause and extent of a CVA. There is little other definitive testing that can be done to document the etiology and extent of damage. EEG and angiography may be useful. Routine lab tests (CBC, electrolytes) are valuable to determine overall patient condition, but rarely add information of diagnostic value. Lumbar puncture (LP) may be done; but with the exception of hemorrhagic CVAs, it is usually clear, colorless and normal in other respects. (Opening pressure may be slightly elevated.)

Nursing Care

The major nursing responsibilities are listed below:

(1) **Airway:** Establish and maintain patent airway and ventilation. Apply suction as needed. Establish artificial airway and ventilation if needed. Prevent hypostatic pneumonia and aspiration if LOC is decreased or gag/swallow is impaired. Position the patient to prevent aspiration.

(2) **Circulation:** Monitor B.P., cardiac status and vital signs.

(3) **Neurologic status:** Monitor neruo signs. A flow sheet is useful to recognize trends. (Cushing's triad—increased systolic B.P., increased pulse pressure, bradycardia and respiratory changes are indicative of loss of compliance and imminent herniation; they are not the first sign of increased ICP.)

(4) **Fluid and electrolyte balance:** Maintain adequate hydration without overhydration leading to increased cerebral edema. Carefully assess gag and swallow before allowing P.O. intake.

(5) **Prevention of deformities:** To maximize rehabilitation potential, passive range of motion must be started immediately. Position to prevent contractures. Turn every two hours, or more frequently if needed. Begin planning for discharge, rehabilitation, follow-up and home care.

(6) **Monitor bowel and bladder functioning:** Retraining may be necessary. Avoid indwelling catheter whenever possible.

(7) **Skin care**

(8) **Maximize independence in ADL:** Involve the family in care.

(9) **Provide emotional support** to patient and family.

(10) **Devise communication methods** if speech and understanding are impaired. Devise adaptive devices to aid in self-performance of ADL.

(11) **Teach patient and family** about precipitating factors of CVA and modification of lifestyle.

KEY CONCEPT: Clinical presentation of CVA is varied. Nursing care is aimed at airway maintenance and prevention of complications.

CEREBRAL ANEURYSM

Pathophysiology

A cerebral aneurysm is a congenital defect in the medial layer of the arterial wall that leads to a weakening and an outward ballooning of the defect, with eventual rupture. It usually occurs at the bifurcation of the arteries in the anterior Circle of Willis.

Clinical Presentation

There are no prodromal symptoms prior to rupture. At rupture, there is severe, violent headache, nausea and vomiting. The patient may or may not lose consciousness. Focal neurological deficit may be present.

Diagnostic Data

The patient presents with a complaint of headache, possible change in LOC, and is usually hypertensive upon examination. Focal deficits may or may not be present. Physical examination may reveal a variety of the above mentioned signs. Lumbar puncture (LP) should be done unless signs of increased ICP are apparent. When done, CSF will be bloody, with elevated protein and cells. Opening pressure (OP) may also be elevated.

Radiologic studies include CT scan to detect area of bleeding, mass effect, cerebral edema, ventricular involvement and hydrocephalus, if present. A preoperative arteriogram is necessary to localize the aneurysm, and to determine the size, shape, orientation and position of the aneurysm neck, which is the site to be clipped.

Nursing Care

(1) **Rebleeding** is the most common cause of severe morbidity and death. The rebleed tends to occur between the 7th and 11th day post-initial bleed. This is when clot lysis peaks and the clot sealing off the weakened portion of the vessel begins to dissolve. Initial bleeds usually are into the subarachnoid space. However, rebleeds tend to be into the parenchyma of the brain because of the tendency of the clot to adhere to brain tissue. Grading the condition helps determine outcome and ideal time for surgical intervention. Surgery is usually deferred until 7 to 14 days post-bleed, before clot lysis, but after spasm subsides.

   Grade I—alert, without deficit, slight headache, nuchal rigidity

   Grade II—awake, minimal deficit, mild to severe headache, nuchal rigidity, no evidence of vasospasm

   Grade III—drowsiness, confusion, mild deficit, nuchal rigidity

   Grade IV—hemiplegic, unresponsive, nuchal rigidity, vasospasm may be present

   Grade V—comatose, moribund, decerebrate, vasospasm may be present

(2) **Specific nursing responsibilities:**
   a. Ensure complete bedrest and quiet environment. Eliminate all stress. Surgery is generally delayed until the patient reaches Grade I or II.
   b. Elevate head of bed 30 degrees.
   c. Limit fluids to decrease cerebral edema. Avoid dehydration.
   d. Sedation and antihypertensives may be necessary.
   e. Avoid Valsalva manuever.

f. Epsilon aminocaproic acid (Amicar) may be used as an antifibrinolytic to prevent clot lysis and minimize the chance of rebleeding. The medication prevents clot lysis; it does not promote clotting. A complication is the failure to dissolve existing clots, not thrombus formation. Be especially alert for signs of phlebitis.

g. Treatment of vasospasm, which occurs about 72 hours after initial bleed and increases cerebral ischemia, is controversial. Many experimental agents have been used. Hypervolemia with dextran is currently being studied. Reserpine and kanamycin (to deplete catecholamines that are believed to cause spasm), aminophylline and lidocaine, and Isuprel and lidocaine have also been used.

(3) **Monitor neurologic signs.**
(4) **Prepare patient and family for surgery.**
(5) **Offer emotional support.**
(6) **Prevent complications of immobility.**

KEY CONCEPT: Rebleeding is the most common cause of morbidity. Care should be aimed at preventing rebleeding.

MENINGITIS
Pathophysiology

Meningitis is an *inflammation* of the *meninges,* in contrast to encephalitis, which is an inflammation of the brain tissue itself. The most common agents causing meningitis are bacteria (meningococci in adults, hemophilus influenzae in children, also streptococci and pneumococci). Viral meningitis is less common. The organism gains entrance to the meningeal space via a depressed skull fracture, a penetrating head injury tearing through the dura (middle ear), or a sinus infection that erodes through the dura. Organisms may also gain entrance to the subarachnoid space through the bloodstream, as after sepsis. The organisms multiply and an exudate, composed of bacterial proteins and phagocytes, forms. This leads to edema, congestion of blood flow, tissue hypoxia and neuronal damage. In addition, the protein debris may block the arachnoid villi and result in hydrocephalus because of an inability to reabsorb CSF.

Clinical Presentation

The meningitis patient generally complains of a persistent headache, neck pain, nuchal rigidity and presents with an elevated temperature. Nausea, vomiting and dulled sensorium may be present. Photophobia (light sensitivity in the eyes), irritability, diplopia, tinnitus and seizures may also be present. If increased intracranial pressure is evident, the patient may have profoundly decreased LOC and present with papilledema on fundiscopic examination. Papilledema is generally a contraindication for LP.

Diagnostic Data

A patient history and physical examination may reveal a recent ear infection, sinus infection, bacteremia, pneumonia or penetrating head injury. However, this cannot always be elucidated by history. The patient will probably present with an elevated temperature and evidence of elevated WBC count. The definitive diagnosis is made by LP. The opening pressure is generally elevated. WBCs are elevated in bacterial meningitis, whereas lymphs are elevated in viral meningitis. CSF glucose is reduced in bacterial states because the bacteria utilize glucose as a substrate for growth. In viral meningitis, the glucose is normal or marginally decreased because viruses do not utilize glucose. Protein is elevated, reflecting foreign proteins from bacterial cell walls and phagocytes. The gram smear may show WBCs and organisms, enabling the clinician to begin presumptive treatment. Definitive treatment must be deferred until the results of cultures and sensitivities are obtained.

Nursing Care

The goal of nursing is to provide supportive care, as well as to prevent complications and further neurological deterioration.

(1) **Airway and breathing:** Maintain the patient's airway. Apply suction as needed. Establish an artificial airway and ventilation as required. Prevent aspiration and hypostatic pneumonia.

(2) **Administer appropriate antibiotic treatment.**

(3) **Fluid balance, hydration, electrolyte imbalance:** Monitor electrolytes, fluid intake and output. Assure gag and swallow before permitting P.O. intake. Avoid overhydration. Observe for signs of diabetes insipidus (DI) resulting from hypothalamic compression and dysfunction.

(4) **Control of temperature:** Every degree above normal of fever increases the brain's need for oxygen by about 7 percent because of increased metabolic rate. Control fever. Use of Thorazine (chlorpromazine hydrochloride) is advocated to control shivering when artificial hypothermia methods are utilized.

(5) **Monitor vital signs,** especially cardiac status since hyperpyrexia frequently causes tachycardia.

(6) **Monitor for seizure activity:** Prophylactic anticonvulsants may be given.

(7) **Give emotional support** to the patient and family.

(8) **Monitor** for the following complications:
>pneumonia
>hydrocephalus
>increasing cerebral edema
>brain abscess
>Waterhouse-Friderichsen syndrome (adrenal shutdown secondary to sepsis and stress, resulting in hemorrhage and shock)

(9) **Prevent complications** of immobility, develop skin care regimen and begin a physical therapy and deformity-prevention program.

KEY CONCEPT: Nursing must provide supportive care and prevent complications that would result in neurological deterioration.

GUILLAIN-BARRE SYNDROME (ACUTE POLYNEURITIS)

Pathophysiology

Much remains to be discovered about the pathology of *Guillain-Barre Syndrome (GBS)*. It is known, however, that almost all cases occur after exposure to viral infection or viral vaccine. The exposure commonly occurs two to three weeks before the onset of GBS. It is hypothesized that some sort of autoimmune process takes place and results in edema and inflammation of the spinal nerve roots. There is demyelination of the spinal nerve roots and the peripheral nerves. Capable of regeneration, these nerves can be expected to eventually repair themselves and regain function. However, the recuperative phase may last from several weeks to many months. Not all patients recover completely.

Clinical Presentation

Classically, the patient presents with symmetrical ascending muscle weakness. This weakness usually has a fairly rapid onset. It is not uncommon to also find weakness of the swallowing and breathing muscles, and a markedly decreased vital capacity. Other signs are paresthesias of distal extremities, muscle tenderness and aches, absent reflexes, slight sensory loss and cranial nerve dysfunction. When cranial nerves are involved, the impairment usually progresses through VII, VI, III, XII, V and IX, and resolves in the reverse order.

Diagnostic Data

A patient history and physical examination provide the objective data concerning presentation and may elicit the exposure to viral illness or vaccine. A useful diagnostic test is the LP. Characteristic findings are all normal except for elevation of protein. This is believed to be a result of the demyelination process.

Nursing Care

The goals of nursing care are supportive and restorative. Because of the prolonged period of dependence and loss of functional capacity, diversion and emotional support are essential. At the height of the acute phase, the patient often is totally immobile, mechanically ventilated and unable to provide for even the most elementary needs.

(1) **Airway and breathing:** Because of the high incidence of respiratory failure, most patients spend some time on mechanical ventilation. Prior to this event, frequent (every one to two hours, or more often) vital capacity measurements are necessary to detect impending failure. Pulmonary toilet, prevention of aspiration, suctioning and routine pulmonary care assume a high priority.

(2) **Prevention of deformity:** Develop a meticulous skin care regimen; provide for bowel and bladder functioning.

(3) **Monitor and assess vital signs.** Of special importance are arterial blood gas studies and checks of motor and sensory levels to detect improvement or deterioration.

(4) **Fluid and electrolyte balance** and **nutritional status** are a major area of importance since these patients are frequently unable to take P.O. nutrition because of tracheostomy or dysphagia. High calorie enteral feedings are recommended, with extreme caution. There is a high incidence of gastric dilatation and ileus in patients with GBS.

(5) **Prevention of all complications of immobility** is a must, especially pulmonary embolism. Patients frequently experience orthostatic hypotension as activity is increased; tilt tables and gradual position changes are recommended.

(6) **Provide emotional and psychological support** for the patient and family.

(7) **Symptomatic relief:** Warm, moist heat may be effective for relief of muscle pain and paresthesias. Whirlpool baths have also been reported to be effective. Some clinicians recommend the use of steroids to decrease edema and inflammation, but this is still controversial.

KEY CONCEPT: Nursing care is aimed at supporting vital functions and body parts through the illness, restoring functional capacity and rehabilitating the patient, both emotionally and physically.

HEAD INJURY

Pathophysiology

The particular pathology of head injury depends on the type of injury sustained. However, the most common problem concomitant with head injury is the increased intracranial pressure (ICP) that occurs as the brain swells in the tight, rigid skull. Normal ICP (0 to 15 mm Hg) increases as the volume of the intracranial contents increases. The intracranial volume is equal to the volumes of the brain, the blood and the CSF. When any of these components increases, the ICP rises unless a corresponding component is decreased. Increasing ICP causes compression on surrounding tissue and vessels, which leads to cellular anoxia and cell death.

Brain injury falls into several categories. The least severe is *concussion*, a stunning event similar to a precordial thump. A concussion is basically an electrical event, causing momentary depolarization, loss of consciousness and loss of immediate memory of the event. There are no gross brain tissue changes.

Next in severity is the *contusion*, actual petechial damage to the brain tissue. A common occurrence is the contrecoup contusion. In this condition, the brain, a gelatinous mass freely floating in the skull, strikes the interior surface of the skull at the point of impact. However, opposing forces are strong enough to drive the brain back against the opposite skull surface, resulting in a more severe injury directly opposite the point of impact.

Epidural hematomas are arterial bleeds, generally from the middle meningeal artery, occurring in the epidural space (between the bone and the dura). The usual cause is a fracture along the distribution of the middle meningeal artery (temporal area). Epidural hematomas may collect rapidly after a period of lucidity and lack of focal signs. Because the bleeding is arterial and under high pressure, extensive morbidity and mortality can occur within a short period of time. The extradural collection of blood becomes great enough to cause the uncus (tip) of the temporal lobe to begin to herniate down through the tentorium. Decreasing LOC, a fixed and dilated pupil (ipsilateral to the injury) and contralateral hemiparesis are signs of herniation. Epidural hematomas constitute a true neurosurgical emergency!

Subdural hematomas are collections of venous blood in the subdural space (between the dura and the arachnoid). They may be acute or chronic. They are less of an emergency than an epidural bleed, since the bleeding is venous in nature, but they still carry a high mortality rate. Symptoms may vary from changes in sensorium to herniation and death.

Intracerebral hematomas are the result of traumatic tearing of vessels. Unless they are confined to the surface of the brain, little can be done surgically, and the treatment is to wait for spontaneous reabsorption.

The common pathology of head injury is that the brain moves rapidly and abnormally within the skull. The tissue is bruised or lacerated, or hemorrhaging develops. The cells swell in response to the injury; the inflammation leads to increased ICP. Further compromise of cellular tissue ensues, herniation may occur and if the dura is torn, infection may develop because of invasion of organisms. Precipitating factors to head trauma are motor vehicle accidents, sports accidents, direct trauma, gunshot wounds, stab wounds and various fractures. Remember that the degree of fracture has no direct bearing on the degree of head injury. It is possible to receive a devastating head injury without any skull fracture. Conversely, it is possible to receive a large depressed skull fracture without any damage to the underlying brain.

Clinical Presentation

Any variety of symptoms may be present, depending on the severity and location of the trauma. Patients may present awake and alert, without focal signs, and rapidly slip into unconsciousness (common with an epidural hematoma). They may also present unconscious, but rapidly awaken with only a headache (common with a concussion and with some contusions).

Diagnostic Data

A history and physical examination, with particular attention to details of the accident, are important to the diagnosis. The history should be taken from an eyewitness. Be especially alert for any period of unconsciousness, no matter how short. This information is easiest to obtain from rescue squad personnel since patients frequently deny it or are unable to remember the event. Almost all concussions and contusions are preceded by short periods of loss of consciousness. Radiographs, CT scans and other radiologic tests must be tailored to the clinical history and presentation. It is wisest to assume, until otherwise ruled out, that all patients with head injuries have cervical spine injuries. Immobilize the head and neck in a neutral position and maintain the position until cervical spine radiographs have been taken and read. Spinal column injuries can occur, leaving the cord undamaged, until the patient moves in such a way as to extend the damage. Never assume that patients have no spinal injury just because they are able to move all extremities.

Nursing Care

Care is tailored to the particular type of injury. However, certain interventions are essential when dealing with head-injured patients.

(1) **Airway and breathing:** Monitor, suction and assist. If intubation becomes necessary prior to completion of the cervical spine radiographs, do not hyperextend the neck for oral intubation. Tracheotomy, or even intubation with an esophageal obturator, is preferable to extension of an occult spinal injury.

(2) **Monitoring and assessing** condition-serial examinations of vital signs and neurologic signs help to detect trends and deterioration.

(3) **Treatment of cerebral edema-increased ICP:** Elevate the head of the bed 30 degrees to promote venous drainage. Osmotic diuretics may be used (mannitol, urea). Use steroids to decrease edema (dexamethasone usually is preferred because of the lack of mineralocorticoid effect). Limit fluids. Monitor fluid/electrolyte balance.

(4) **Prophylaxis for seizures:** 18 to 20 percent of head-injured patients exhibit one or more seizures after the injury. Phenytoin is preferred because it does not alter the LOC and therefore invalidate the neurological exam. Phenobarbital may also be used, but it may affect the LOC and neurological exam.

(5) **Observe for drainage:** Anterior fossa fractures with puncture of the dura may result in CSF drainage from the nose. Ecchymotic rings around the affected eye may indicate anterior fossa fractures (raccoon's eye). Middle fossa fractures may result in leakage of CSF from the ear if the dura has been punctured. An ecchymotic area over the mastoid air cells is not uncommon with middle fossa fracture (Battle's sign). Never pack the nose or ear. Never insert anything into the nose or ear to clean it. Allow the orifice to drain naturally. Promote drainage by elevating the head 30 degrees. A sterile gauze placed lightly over the opening of the ear or nose may be used to collect drainage for testing. If the drainage is bloody and a clear halo forms around it within several minutes, this indicates CSF (halo test). CSF will also be Testape-positive because of its glucose content.

(6) **Prevent complications of immobility.**

(7) **Monitor for complications:** Diabetes insipidus is a common complication of bilateral cortical edema causing pressure on the hypothalamus. Monitor urine output and urine specific gravity. Stress ulcers may occur because of anxiety and use of steroids. Monitor stools for occult blood, check NG tube drainage for occult blood, monitor hemoglobin and hematocrit.

(8) **Family support:** Behavioral changes are common immediately after acute head injury. Prepare the family for obscene language, altered affect and loss of memory. Both patient and family require support while awaiting determination of prognosis, possible residual neurological deficits and alterations of future lifestyle.

KEY CONCEPT: In head injuries do not hyperextend the neck; maintain vital functions and monitor closely for increasing ICP.

SPINAL CORD INJURY

Pathophysiology

Spinal cord injuries can occur in the *cervical, thoracic* or *lumbar-sacral* regions. They can be fractures of the vertebral column without damage to the cord itself, stretching and disruption of the cord without damage to the vertebral bodies, interruption of blood supply to the cord or combinations of damage to both the cord and bony structures.

When the cord is damaged, pressure occurs either from compression of bone, disk, hematoma, tumor or actual cord tissue damage, and edema formation occurs at the site. In either case, there is damage to the structural cells of the cord.

The compression and edema cause decreased circulation which results in cellular anoxia and the production of norepinephrine by the cord itself. The norepinephrine actually causes autodestruction of the cord by internal autolysis. All functions of the damaged cells are lost. The loss may be motor, sensory or both, depending on the area of the cord involved. However, the loss is generally permanent. The permanency is due to irreversible cellular death in cells without the capacity to regenerate. Injuries rarely occur that result in anoxia for such short periods of time that the cells are not irreversibly damaged.

Spinal shock is a unique sequelae of spinal cord injury. Post injury, all motor, sensory and reflex responses below the level of the injury are lost. The cord seems to temporarily shut down below the level of the injury. There is also loss of autonomic control. Without autonomic control, there is systemic vasodilatation and pooling of blood in the distal extremities. This causes hypotension and the appearance of a shock-like state without the compensatory tachycardia that accompanies hypovolemic shock. Spinal shock may last from several days to months. The disappearance is heralded by the return of involuntary reflexes below the level of the lesion.

Spinal cord injuries commonly occur with trauma, such as fractures and dislocations; hyperflexion and hyperextension injuries during auto accidents, falls, diving accidents or sports; and stab and gunshot wounds to the neck. The most common patient is a 15- to 30-year-old physically active male.

Clinical Presentation

The presentation of the injured patient varies with the extent and location of the lesion. The occurrence of spinal shock may obscure the remaining functional capacity because these patients appear flaccid and flexible below the lesion. Determination of the functional capacity has to be delayed until spinal shock subsides.

Lesions in the high cervical region affect the ability to breathe spontaneously. Lesions of C1, C2 and C3 result in apnea because of loss of innervation to the muscles of respiration. Patients with lesions in this area require artificial ventilation for the remainder of their lives. Lesions of C4 and C5 also impair respiratory effort because of lack of intercostal innervation; therefore, abdominal breathing is rated. The ability to cough, breathe deeply or use the diaphragm is lost, but spontaneous respirations continue.

Any lesion in the cervical cord results in quadriplegia, as compared with thoracic lesions which result in paraplegia. The cervical nerves innervate the arm and hand muscles, and any cervical lesion results in some upper extremity impairment. The important landmarks (motor and sensory) are listed below:

Motor
  C1, C2, C3—muscles of respiration
  C4, C5—accessory muscles of respiration
  C5—deltoid innervation
  C6—biceps
  C7—triceps and medial hand
  C8—lateral hand

Sensory
  C5—shoulder tips and above clavicles
  T4—nipple line
  T10—umbilicus

Common spinal cord syndromes are as follows:

Central cord syndrome—There is damage to the central portion of the cord. The damage is generally vascular in nature. The motor loss is greater in the arms than the legs. Sensory loss is variable.

Anterior cord syndrome—The damage is to the anterior portion of the cord. There is complete motor loss below the level of the injury. This injury results in loss of pain and temperature sense below the level of the injury, with preservation of sense of proprioception (body position), vibration and touch.

Brown-Séquard syndrome—This syndrome results from hemisection of the cord, which is usually the result of a gunshot or stab wound. Motor function, position sense and vibration are lost below the level of the injury on the same side (ipsilateral). There is complete loss of pain and temperature sense below the level of the injury on the opposite side (contralateral). It must be remembered that the motor tracts cross at the medulla before entering the spinal cord; therefore, motor loss would be ipsilateral. However, tracts for pain and temperature enter the cord and then cross a level above their entrance; therefore, sensory impairment is contralateral.

Diagnostic Data

Again, the history and physical examination are of primary importance. Radiologic studies, such as skull and spine radiographs and tomograms, are usual adjuncts to establishing the diagnosis. Myelography may be used if the deficit is worsening and surgery is being considered.

Nursing Care

(1) **Maintenance of alignment/traction:** In most cases, reduction is achieved by the insertion of skeletal traction and the use of weights. The traction is frequently a Gardner-Wells or similar device, using pins in the scalp for stabilization. Daily pin and site care is necessary to prevent infection. Maintenance of proper neck alignment is paramount. Should the tongs accidentally slip free (a rare occurrence), maintain neutral alignment of the head and neck. Notify the neurosurgeon immediately!

(2) **Airway and breathing:** Provide supplemental oxygen and suctioning. Careful observation of respiratory effort (especially with midcervical injuries) is mandatory. The leading cause of death in the posttrauma period is respiratory related.

(3) **Urinary considerations:** A catheter is required until spinal shock has subsided, since even reflex voiding is impossible. Once spinal shock has passed, the catheter should be discontinued and a bladder regimen should begin. At this time, Crede's method, external catheterization (for males) or intermittent catheterization is preferable, since prolonged indwelling catheters cause atrophy of the bladder and detrimental changes in the lining of the bladder, as well as infection. Also, careful observation of bowel functions and bowel retraining programs should be instituted after spinal shock has subsided.

(4) **Fluid/electrolyte imbalance and nutrition:** Careful assessment of fluid intake and output is needed. High caloric intake should be given to meet bodily needs. It may become necessary to resort to frequent, small tube feedings with meticulous assessment of bowel sounds and abdominal status. Frequently, these patients are unaware of abdominal discomfort because of sensory loss. Postinjury ileus, due to autonomic disturbances, may make oral intake impractical. If enteral feedings are inadvisable because of gastric dilatation and ileus, then hyperalimentation must be used to meet caloric needs. Because of the high incidence of stress ulcer in cord-injured patients, frequent checks of gastric contents and stool for occult blood are necessary.

(5) **Skin breakdown and positioning:** The patient is totally dependent and unable to feel areas of redness or soreness. Circulatory changes due to loss of autonomic control also enhance the possibility of skin breakdown. Meticulous skin care, careful turning and repositioning are essential. Several devices (Kinetic Bed, Circ-O-Electric bed) aid in this care, but do not replace conscientious nursing care.

(6) **Emotional support:** Many patients require a year or more to come to terms with their disability. It is not uncommon for patients to ask when they will be allowed to walk in the halls or to seem oblivious to information regarding the permanency of their injury. Do not support patients in their refusal to accept disability, but provide for the time and place to discuss feelings, fears and perceptions.

(7) **Spasticity and contractures:** In spite of the best physical therapy and nursing care, spasticity and contractures may develop. Muscle relaxants and other medications may provide some relief. Warm, moist heat may also be beneficial.

(8) **Discharge and rehabilitation planning:** The needs of the spinal-cord-injured patient are lifelong. The sooner realistic plans are begun for home care, physical aids, equipment and rehabilitation, the better the prognosis is for a return to a satisfactory quality of life. The patient and family often benefit from professional psychiatric counseling to help overcome their fears, resentment and depression. Spinal-cord-injured patients are frequently young people with families to support. The families, as well as the paitent, feel anger and frustration since the entire framework of their lives has been irrevocably destroyed. Spouses resent having to be the sole financial support. The patient resents this enforced dependence, and children become insecure. The financial, emotional and psychological toll exacted by a spinal cord injury is tremendous.

KEY CONCEPT: Initial nursing care is aimed at maintaining vital functions without enhancing the injury. Discharge and rehabilitation planning must be initiated as soon as the life-threatening aspects of the injury have been stabilized. Realistic acceptance of the injury may take from months to years.

MYASTHENIA GRAVIS

Pathophysiology

The defect in myasthenia gravis (MG) is now believed to be an autoimmune process. An antibody is produced that inhabits the receptor site at the neuromuscular junction and prevents the attachment of acetylcholine during synaptic transmission. Drugs that prolong the amount of time acetylcholine remains in the synaptic cleft allow the acetylcholine to compete with the antibody for the receptor site. Given sufficient time, the acetylcholine will predominate and attach to the receptor, resulting in depolarization of the muscle end plate and propagation of the impulse. MG can occur in any voluntary muscle and the result, if untreated, is extreme weakness.

Clinical Presentation

Easy fatiguing of voluntary muscles, ptosis, voice changes (particularly hoarseness), respiratory difficulty, dysphagia, jaw weakness during chewing, diplopia and facial weakness are common presenting signs. Symptoms may be exacerbated by colds, flu, emotional stress, the menstrual cycle, pregnancy and many drugs (alcohol, -mycin antibiotics, quinidine, Pronestyl, quinine, phenothiazines, phenobarbital, narcotics and most anesthetics).

Diagnostic Data

A history and physical examination plus routine diagnostic workups are needed. The Tensilon (edrophonium chloride) test is useful in making the initial diagnosis in patients presenting with mystheniclike symptoms and in differentiating myasthenic crisis from cholinergic crisis. The symptoms are quite similar, but myasthenic crisis is due to inadequate medication, while cholinergic crisis is due to overmedication.

To give a Tensilon test, inject 2 to 5 mg of Tensilon I.V. and assess for improvement in muscle strength within one minute. If there is no improvement, repeat the 2 to 5 mg I.V. dose every two minutes until 10 mg have been given. Improvement in muscle strength indicates myasthenic crisis; lack of improvement or deterioration indicates cholinergic crisis. If the Tensilon test does not provide conclusive results, then neostigmine 0.5 to 1.0 mg I.V. may be used. Emergency respiratory equipment should be readily available when this testing is done, since respiratory arrest can occur with the use of these drugs in cholinergic crisis.

Nursing Care

(1) **Maximize neuromuscular transmission:** Administer anticholinesterase agents (neostigmine, Mestinon, Mytelase). Administration must be on schedule since the drugs have a very limited span of action. Note all responses to the medication, particularly improvement and side effects. Atropine may be used to counteract side effects of the medication but may mask symptoms of cholinergic crisis. ACTH or prednisone may be used in conjunction with other drugs to depress antibody formation. Watch for steroid side effects. Thymic tumors and thymic hyperplasia are associated with MG. Thymectomy or thymic irradiation may be used. Improvement is seen in many patients after these procedures. However, the most improvement is seen in young patients, and often, rather than curing the disorder, this treatment only succeeds in reducing the dose of medication required.

(2) **Maintain airway and breathing:** Assess the respiratory effort. Assist respirations if necessary. Frequent vital-capacity measurements will alert the clinician to the need for intubation. Meticulous pulmonary care is needed.

(3) **Anticipate problems:** Assess the patient's strength before meals. Plan independent activities to coincide with maximum effect of the drug. Observe for a weak cough, tiring of the jaw and dysphagia.

(4) Provide routine **skin care, positioning, nutrition, emotional support** and **patient education.**

KEY CONCEPT: Be alert to respiratory difficulty, Maintain breathing. Anticipate fatigue and provide support. Administer medications exactly on time and teach patients to be extremely punctual with medications.

TETANUS

Pathophysiology

Clostridium tetani, a gram-positive spore-forming anaerobe, is found in the soil and anywhere animal wastes are found. The organism produces a neurotoxin that attaches itself to CNS cells, specifically the motor nerve end plates and anterior horn cells in the cord and brainstem. The incubation period is from 5 days to 15 weeks. The result of neurotoxin attachment is exaggerated motor activity and death. Death is usually due to medullary involvement resulting in respiratory arrest. The organism gains access through burns, traumatic wounds (usually penetrating), cutaneous fistulas, abscesses, skin ulcers and injection sites during illegal use of narcotics. The organism requires anaerobic conditions and rarely flourishes in superficial surface wounds that are well-aerated.

Clinical Presentation

Signs and symptoms may vary from mild to generalized stiffness, dysphagia and head retraction with reduced vital capacity to severe opisthotonos, dysphagia, irritability, painful tonic convulsions, salivation, tachycardia, perspiration, hypertension, hyperpyrexia and cardiac arrhythmias.

Diagnostic Data

The history may elicit the event that allowed introduction of the organism. Physical examination reveals hyperactive, deep tendon reflexes; rigidity without pain in the abdominal muscles and painful muscle spasm on facial grimace or jaw closing.

Nursing Care

(1) **Airway and ventilation:** Intubation may be necessary, as well as suction, repositioning and monitoring of arterial blood gases.

(2) **Muscle spasm:** Muscle relaxants or anticonvulsants may be used. A quiet, dark environment with little auditory, visual or tactile stimuli is necessary.

(3) **Removal of toxin:** Administer tetanus antitoxin (TAT) I.M. to prevent further fixation of toxin to tissue. Removal of necrotic and contaminated tissue is required. Leave the wound open to air. Administer high doses of antibiotics.

(4) **Fluid/electrolyte balance and nutrition:** Maintain accurate I and O. While spasm persists, all fluids and nutrition must be given I.V.

(5) **Emotional and psychological support:** Offer both to the patient and family.

(6) **Prevention of skin breakdown, deformities and complications of immobility:** These tasks must be accomplished within the range of a quiet, nonstimulating atmosphere.

KEY CONCEPT: The pathology of tetanus involves a neurotoxin produced by the bacteria. Tetanus patients require a quiet environment. Maintain the airway and provide for respiratory assistance.

SEIZURES
Pathophysiology

Seizures are caused by paroxysmal high frequency/high voltage or synchronous low frequency/high voltage electrical discharges in neurons of the cortex and possibly the brainstem.

Epileptogenic neurons

- are capable of initiating autonomous electrical discharges;
- have increased electrical excitability;
- have a relative surface electrical negativity in comparison to surrounding neurons;
- are able to generate volleys of high frequency impulses by depolarization of the membrane resting potential;
- are capable of generating secondary epileptogenic foci in synaptically related cells.

Precipitating factors may include genetic factors, perinatal injury, trauma, cerebrovascular pathology, infections of the CNS, tumors, metabolic disorders, arteriovenous malformations and withdrawal of anticonvulsant medication.

Clinical Presentation
Generalized seizure disorders:

Grand mal—These are characterized by tonic-clonic symmetrical movements of the entire body, loss of consciousness, increased salivation, apnea, cyanosis and incontinence. They usually last less than five minutes. Postictal drowsiness and confusion are common. Less common is postictal hemiparesis (Todd's palsy).

Petit mal—These are characterized by a short loss of contact with the person's surroundings. The patient may experience repetitive minor motor movements such as lip smacking, twitching or eye rolling. Petit mal seizures generally last less than ten seconds. They end and begin abruptly. An initial occurrence is rare in patients over 12 years of age.

Akinetic—These are characterized by a sudden loss of muscle tone without loss of consciousness. They are also known as "drop attacks."

Myoclonic—These are characterized by sudden, repetitive muscle contractions. Usually only a single muscle group is involved. The arms are most often involved. Myoclonic seizures are of brief duration.

Partial seizure disorders:

Partial motor—These are motor seizures in a specific body area; however, they may progress and become generalized (Jacksonian).

Partial sensory—Partial sensory seizures are seizures without loss of consciousness. They are described as numbness or tingling in a specific body area. Vision, hearing and balance may be affected.

Partial seizures with complex symptomatology:

Psychomotor (temporal lobe seizures)—These are characterized by simple or elaborate alterations in behavior or sensation. Actions appear to be intentional, but the patient has amnesia for the entire seizure. Psychomotor seizures rarely last more than five minutes.

Diagnostic Data

The history is usually obtained by observing a seizure and the postictal period, or by obtaining the details of subjective events prior to and during onset of the seizure from the patient or by objective events from observers. Frequency and duration of seizures are an important part of the history.

A complete neurological and physical exam and lab data are necessary to rule out electrolyte imbalance, renal problems, hepatic disorders and metabolic causes of seizures.

Special studies include skull radiographs, CT scan and EEG.

Nursing Care

(1) **Observe, record and report seizure activity:**
   a. Special signs preceding attack (visual, auditory or olfactory are most common)
   b. Body parts involved; order of spread of involvement; type of movements
   c. Deviation of eyes and head; presence of nystagmus; pupillary size and reactivity
   d. Duration of seizure
   e. Duration of postictal phase; neurologic status with particular attention to speech and motor weakness

(2) **Prevent injury:**
   a. Protect the airway.
   b. Do not force objects into patient's mouth; use tongue blade only if you are able to insert it prior to seizure.
   c. Do not try to restrain the patient.
   d. Remove all objects that may cause injury.
   e. Protect the head.

(3) **Control seizure activity:**
   a. Drug therapy may be multi-agent to achieve adequate control; monitor blood levels.

(4)

Commonly used anti-convulsants	Therapeutic levels	Indications
Phenytoin	9 to 20 ug/ml	generalized/partial
Phenobarbital	20 to 40 ug/ml	generalized/partial
Carbamazepine	4 to 10 ug/ml	generalized/partial/partial-complex
Primidone	7 to 15 ug/ml	generalized/partial-complex
Ethosuximide	40 to 90 ug/ml	petit mal/partial-complex
Clonazepam	40 to 100 ug/ml	myoclonic/akinetic

(5) **Provide emotional support** to patient and family.

KEY CONCEPT: Observation of seizure activity is important for diagnosis and treatment. Prevention of injury is paramount during seizure activity.

STATUS EPILEPTICUS

Pathophysiology

This is a state in which continual seizure activity persists.

Grand mal status—There are recurrent grand mal seizures without full recovery between seizures. A prolonged status leads to hypoxia, hypoglycemia and hypothermia, which in turn precipitate additional seizure activity. Metabolic and physical exhaustion, as well as risk of aspiration, hypoxia and respiratory arrest, may lead to death.

Petit mal status—This is defined as 200 to 300 petit mal seizures within a 24-hour period.

Electrical status—This is characterized by a continual spike discharge (indicating electrical seizure activity) on an EEG with the absence or minimal clinical evidence of seizure activity.

Precipitating factors include withdrawal from anticonvulsants, withdrawal from alcohol, electroconvulsive therapy, brain tumors, trauma, cerebral edema, CNS infections, withdrawal from chronic use of depressants and sedatives, and metabolic conditions such as uremia, hyponatremia, hypoglycemia and hepatic dysfunction.

Clinical Presentation

(1) **Airway/ventilation:** Intubation and mechanical ventilation are necessary if seizures are not readily controlled.

(2) **Ablation of seizure activity:**
   a. Administer diazepam 5 to 10 mg I.V. over two minutes, and repeat as necessary. Monitor B.P. and respirations. Since this often results in respiratory arrest, intubation equipment should be at bedside.
   b. Administer phenytoin 13 mg/kg I.V. at the rate of 50 mg/min. Watch for cardiac arrhythmias, bradycardia or cardiac arrest. An adult generally requires about 1 gm to achieve an adequate blood level. Phenytoin does not act immediately and is incompatible with solutions containing dextrose. Phenytoin is given after status epilepticus has been arrested to prevent recurrence of further seizure activity.
   c. If diazepam does not control seizure activity, phenobarbital or paraldehyde may be used. Administer phenobarbital 5 to 8 mg/kg I.V. Observe for hypotension and respiratory arrest.

   Administer paraldehyde 0.1 to 0.5 ml/kg I.M., I.V. or rectally.

(3) **Prevention of complications:**
   a. Insert a nasogastric (NG) tube to prevent aspiration.
   b. Monitor cardiac status.
   c. Assess respiratory status.
   d. Assess neurologic status.
   e. Maintain fluid and electrolyte balance.

KEY POINT RECOGNITION

Write true or false by each statement. Answers are at the end of this chapter. A score below 80% indicates the need for further study.

_____ 1. CVAs are caused only by hemorrhage.

_____ 2. Precipitating factors leading to hemorrhagic CVA may be hypertension and obesity.

_____ 3. A change in the level of consciousness is the most common clinical presentation in a CVA of the cerebrum.

_____ 4. **Increased systolic B.P. and increased pulse pressure, bradycardia and respiratory changes are indicative of loss of compliance and imminent herniation.**

_____ 5. A severe, violent headache with loss of consciousness is indicative of a CVA.

_____ 6. Lumbar puncture should not be done if signs of increased ICP are present.

_____ 7. Rebleeding in a cerebral aneurysm tends to occur between the fifth and seventh day.

_____ 8. Epsilon aminocaproic acid (amicar) is used to stop thrombus formation in cerebral aneurysm.
_____ 9. In a cerebral aneurysm, vasospasm occurs about 72 hours after the initial bleed.
_____10. In a cerebral aneurysm, surgery is delayed until the patient reaches Grade III.
_____11. The most common causative agent in meningitis is a virus.
_____12. Presenting symptoms of meningitis include headache and nonreactive pupils.
_____13. Definitive diagnosis for meningitis is made by LP.
_____14. CSF glucose is greatly reduced and lymphs are elevated in viral meningitis.
_____15. The meningitis patient should be observed for signs of diabetes insipidus.
_____16. Thorazine is advocated to control shivering when hypothermia is instituted.
_____17. Waterhouse-Friderichsen syndrome is a complication of Guillain-Barre syndrome.
_____18. Symmetrical ascending muscle weakness is a presenting sign of cerebral aneurysm.
_____19. In Guillain-Barre syndrome, cranial nerve involvement usually progresses in the following order: VII, VI, XII, IX, III, V.
_____20. Prior to the need for mechanical ventilation, Guillain-Barre patients should have vital capacity measurements taken every shift.
_____21. Prevention of deformity is a major nursing responsibility in Guillain-Barre patients.
_____22. High caloric enteral feedings are important in Guillain-Barre syndrome both nutritionally and to help prevent gastric dilatation.
_____23. The most common complication of head injury is increased ICP.
_____24. A concussion is an electrical event resulting in momentary loss of consciousness.
_____25. A subdural hematoma is a true neurosurgical emergency.
_____26. Signs of herniation of the uncus of the temporal lobe down through the tentorium are a decreasing LOC, a fixed and dilated pupil ipsilateral to the injury, and contralateral hemiparesis.
_____27. Symptoms of brain injury are always severe and result in a decreased LOC.
_____28. Assume all patients with head injuries have cervical spine injuries until ruled out.
_____29. Intubation of head-injured patients should always be done orally.
_____30. Battle's sign is an ecchymotic area over the mastoid area and is common in middle fossa fractures.
_____31. The halo test is a test for identifying CSF in bloody drainage.
_____32. Diabetes insipidus may be a complication of head injuries that results in bilateral cortical edema sufficient to put pressure on the hypothalamus.
_____33. In spinal shock there is systemic vasoconstriction, hypotension and tachycardia.
_____34. The nurse must be alert to respiratory problems in high cervical spinal injuries.
_____35. A lesion in the thoracic cord results in quadriplegia.
_____36. Damage to the central portion of the cord results in greater motor loss in the legs than in the arms.

_____ 37. When there is hemisection of the cord, the patient usually has ipsilateral loss of motor function and position sense below the level of the injury.

_____ 38. In a spinal injury, if the traction tongs slip free, the nurse should maintain the head and neck in neutral alignment while awaiting the neurosurgeon.

_____ 39. Spinal injury patients may be unaware of abdominal discomfort.

_____ 40. Warm, moist heat should never be used to relieve muscle spasms.

_____ 41. Easy fatiguing of muscles, jaw weakness during chewing and ptosis are signs and symptoms of Guillain-Barre syndrome.

_____ 42. The Tensilon test is used to induce myasthenic crisis.

_____ 43. Thymic tumors are associated with myasthenia gravis.

_____ 44. Tetanus may result in respiratory arrest.

_____ 45. Mild muscle stiffness, dysphagia and a history of a recent traumatic injury should make the nurse suspicious of the presence of clostridium tetani.

_____ 46. In tetanus, severe muscle spasm can result in respiratory arrest.

_____ 47. The patient with tetanus should be nutritionally maintained by tube feedings while spasm is present.

_____ 48. Epileptogenic neurons are capable of initiating electrical discharges.

_____ 49. Grand mal seizures usually last less than two minutes.

_____ 50. Todd's palsy is a common occurrence after an akinetic seizure.

_____ 51. Myoclonic seizures are characterized by repetitive muscle contractions of a single muscle group.

_____ 52. Partial sensory seizures are often described as numbness or tingling.

_____ 53. Tongue blades should only be inserted prior to seizure activity.

_____ 54. Drug therapy for seizures should include only one agent to prevent severe CNS depression.

_____ 55. Prolonged seizure states lead to hypoxia, hyperglycemia and hyperthermia.

_____ 56. Intubation and mechanical ventilation are indicated in status epilepticus.

_____ 57. In status epilepticus, diazepam 5 to 10 mg I.V. over two minutes is given as necessary.

_____ 58. When giving phenytoin the nurse should observe for cardiac arrhythmias.

_____ 59. When administering phenobarbital, the nurse should observe for hypertension.

_____ 60. Epileptic seizures may be precipitated by brain tumors, trauma and metabolic conditions.

CARE COMMON TO NEUROLOGICAL PROBLEMS

INCREASED INTRACRANIAL PRESSURE (ICP)

Change in *level of consciousness* is the most sensitive sign of increased intracranial pressure. Focal motor signs may soon develop, as well as *fixed* and *dilated pupils.* Subjective signs include increased headache, diplopia, seizures, nausea and vomiting.

PATHOPHYSIOLOGY: ICP

The brain is enclosed in a rigid, bony vault without avenues for expansion beyond a limited amount. Pressure beyond the brain's ability to compensate causes the swollen brain to escape via the path of least resistance, which is herniation downward to an area of lower pressure—the brainstem.

MONITORING ICP
Monitoring of ICP may be done in three ways:

Subarachnoid screw
A bolt is placed into the subarachnoid space via a burr hole. This allows for accurate measurement of the ICP and is relatively noninvasive (nonpenetration of the brain). The disadvantage is that cerebrospinal fluid cannot be drained to alleviate ICP.

Ventricular drain
A drain is placed, via a burr hole, into the lateral ventricle. This allows for measurement of ICP and CSF drainage, but presents a slightly higher risk of infection because brain tissue is penetrated. Also, the drain cannot be placed if the ventricles are compressed or displaced.

Epidural catheter
The catheter is placed between the skull and dura without penetrating the dura. This placement is advantageous because the chances of serious infection are minimized. However, the accuracy is questionable because the pressure is transmitted through several layers of meninges and possibly dural sinuses. Disadvantages of this placement are that the catheter cannot be recalibrated when in place and CSF drainage is not possible.

METHODS TO DECREASE ICP
(1) Ventricular drainage
(2) Elevation of the head of the bed 30 degrees; maintaining the head in good alignment
(3) Hyperventilating to pCO_2 of 25 to 30 mm Hg; when suctioning the patient, hyperventilate and oxygenate both pre- and postsuctioning
(4) Osmotic diuretics to decrease brain edema
(5) Steroids to reduce cerebral swelling and cell damage
(6) Barbiturates to induce barbiturate coma in an effort to decrease metabolic rate of oxygen use
(7) Hypothermia to decrease metabolic requirements
(8) Surgery to remove part of the lobe

POSTOPERATIVE CARE
(1) **Continuous neurologic assessment and serial evaluation of changes**
(2) **Fluid/electrolyte balance:** Patients should be kept "dry." Allow only about 75 ml/hr. total fluids to limit cerebral edema. Avoid free water solutions. Monitor for diabetes insipidus, hypovolemia, hypotension and renal problems.
(3) **Pain control:** Avoid narcotics, as they mask neurological signs. Tylenol, aspirin or codeine, if necessary, are preferable.
(4) **Steroid use to treat ICP/cerebral edema by stabilization of the cell wall:** Concomitant use of antacids and/or cimetidine is recommended for prevention of stress ulcers related to steroid use. Test urine glucose as steroids promote hyperglycemia. Short-term steroids should be tapered for discontinuation of therapy, but may be stopped completely should G.I. hemorrhage occur.
(5) **Maintenance of adequate oxygenation and ventilation:** Proper maintenance prevents hypercarbia and increased ICP. Elevate head 30 degrees to promote venous drainage.
(6) **Checking head dressings for signs of leakage and bleeding**
(7) **Subgaleal and subdural drains:** Check amount and character of drainage. Drain may be in place for 24 to 48 hours.
(8) **Anticipating and recognizing complications from pre-existing medical problems**

KEY CONCEPT: Continous assessment for changes in LOC and maintenance of ICP are vital to managing neurosurgical problems.

KEY POINT RECOGNITION

Write true or false by each statement. Answers are at the end of this chapter. A score below 80% indicates the need for further study.

_____ 1. The most sensitive sign of increased ICP is increased headache.

_____ 2. The subarachnoid screw does not allow for drainage of CSF to alleviate ICP.

_____ 3. The epidural catheter cannot be recalibrated when in place.

_____ 4. ICP may be decreased by elevating the head of the bed 30 degrees, using osmotic diuretics, inducing a barbiturate coma and hyperthermia.

_____ 5. Postoperatively, the neurosurgical patient should be maintained on 75 ml/hr. of fluids.

_____ 6. Pain is controlled with Tylenol, codeine or aspirin.

_____ 7. Urine glucose should be checked for hyperglycemia if steroids are being given.

PASS
Program Assessment: Science and Situation

1. The three cranial nerves responsible for eye movement are
   a. trochlear, accessory and optic.
   b. oculomotor, trochlear and abducens.
   c. optic, oculomotor and trochlear.
   d. optic, trigeminal and facial.

2. Which of the following is the correct position to prevent further cervical cord damage?
   a. flexion of the neck with trochanter rolls
   b. rotation of the head to the side
   c. neutral position maintained with sandbags
   d. hyperextension of the neck to maintain a patent airway

3. Myasthenic crisis may be differentiated from cholinergic crisis by which of the following tests:
   a. measurement of vital capacity
   b. small doses of edrophonium chloride
   c. asking the patient to smile, raise eyebrows and show teeth
   d. arterial blood gases

4. Impairment of the right cranial nerve XII will result in
   a. the tongue deviating to the right.
   b. the tongue deviating to the left.
   c. inability to move the tongue from the midline.
   d. inability to move the neck to the right.

5. A lesion affecting the right optic tracts will result in
   a. left homonymous hemianopsia.
   b. bitemporal hemianopsia.
   c. right homonymous hemianopsia.
   d. right monocular blindness.

6. The spinal nerves exit in such a manner that there are
   a. 8 cervical, 13 thoracic and 6 lumbar nerves.
   b. 6 cervical, 11 thoracic and 4 lumbar nerves.
   c. 8 cervical, 12 thoracic and 5 lumbar nerves.
   d. 7 cervical, 12 thoracic and 5 lumbar nerves.

7. Which of following is true concerning production of CSF:
   a. 150 cc of CSF are produced per day and there are approximately 500 cc in the system at any time.
   b. CSF is produced by the arachnoid granules and reabsorbed by the choroid plexus.
   c. At any given time, there is approximately four times as much CSF in the ventricles as in the lumbar subarachnoid space.
   d. 500 cc of CSF are produced daily and there are approximately 150 cc in the system at any time.

8. Which best describes the CSF circulation?
    a. lateral ventricles to foramen of Monro to third ventricle to fourth ventricle to foramina of Luschka and Magendie
    b. lateral ventricles to foramen of Magendie to third ventricle to fourth ventricle to foramina of Luschka and Monro
    c. third ventricle to foramen of Magendie to lateral ventricles to fourth ventricle to foramina of Luschka and Monro
    d. lateral ventricles to foramen of Luschka to third ventricle to fourth ventricle to foramina of Magendie and Monro

9. The single most important indicator of neurologic status is
    a. pupillary reaction and size.
    b. motor ability.
    c. level of consciousness.
    d. respiratory pattern.

10. The Cushing triad is characterized by
    a. decreased B.P., increased heart rate and pupillary changes.
    b. increased pulse pressure, decreased heart rate and respiratory irregularities.
    c. decreased pulse pressure, decreased heart rate and respiratory irregularities.
    d. increased pulse pressure, increased heart rate and Cheyne-Stokes respirations.

11. A 54-year-old woman presents in the E.R. complaining of a headache. Photophobia and nuchal rigidity are noted upon physical examination and her temperature is 101°F orally. Her history is unremarkable, except for a severe otitis media several weeks ago, for which she stopped taking medication when she felt better. The most likely diagnosis is
    a. Guillain-Barre syndrome.
    b. subarachnoid hemorrhage.
    c. sinusitis.
    d. meningitis.

12. Death from tetanus is usually due to
    a. cardiac arrest caused by the action of neurotoxin on myocardial cells.
    b. dehydration due to inability to swallow.
    c. generalized sepsis.
    d. respiratory arrest due to medullary involvement.

13. The Circle of Willis is composed of which of the following?
    a. internal carotids, posterior cerebral and basilar arteries
    b. posterior and anterior communicating, posterior and anterior cerebral and middle cerebral arteries
    c. posterior and anterior communicating, posterior and anterior cerebral and middle meningeal arteries
    d. posterior and anterior cerebral, posterior and anterior meningeal and basilar arteries

14. The frontal lobe is associated with which of the following functions?
    a. speech and sensation
    b. vision and motor movement
    c. motor movement and mentation
    d. memory and mentation

15. A 62-year-old man presents in the E.R. with right hemiparesis (the arm is weaker than the leg, however) and a right facial droop. He is alert and appears oriented. He is able to follow commands involving his left side, but has expressive aphasia. The most likely cause of his problem is
    a. right internal carotid occlusion.
    b. left middle cerebral artery infarct.
    c. right anterior communicating artery infarct.
    d. ruptured cerebral aneurysm.

16. A 21-year-old man is admitted after a motorcycle accident. He is awake and alert and in no apparent respiratory distress. Pulse = 102, B.P. = 98/60, Resp. = 26 and regular. His extremities are flaccid and he has no sensation below the shoulders. Radiographs show a C7 dislocation fracture. The nurse should
    a. prepare for immediate intubation since cervical injuries result in impaired respirations.
    b. Prepare the patient for the O.R. since immediate reduction of the fracture will reverse the neurological deficit.
    c. anticipate that the patient will probably have Gardner-Wells tongs inserted to reduce the fracture with traction.
    d. realize that he will probably be permanently paralyzed.

17. After the appropriate action from #16 is taken, the patient is transferred to the intensive care unit. He has a stable night. The nurse arrives for work in the morning and begins to plan care for the patient. An appropriate action would be to
    a. request an order to remove the Foley catheter so the patient can void and feel more independent.
    b. institute a 1 to 2 hour turning schedule log-rolling the patient.
    c. request a clear liquid diet for the patient to hasten the return of bowel sounds.
    d. check the patient's lower extremities for volunatry movement every hour, checking for the disappearance of spinal shock.

18. After several days, the patient states that he cannot wait for the numbness in his arms and legs to go away so he can get up and move around. An appropriate response would be:
    a. "These things take a long time."
    b. "Have you discussed this with your doctor? Maybe we should mention it today."
    c. "Don't worry, you'll be your old self in no time at all."
    d. "What makes you think you'll ever walk again?"

19. This patient can eventually be expected to regain which level of functioning?
    a. quadriplegic with biceps and triceps, but no intrinsic hand muscles
    b. quadriplegic with deltoid innervation only
    c. paraplegic with arm movements intact
    d. quadriplegic with biceps only

20. A patient with a right facial droop involving the entire face above and below the eye has a lesion
    a. in the right facial nerve.
    b. in the left motor cortex.
    c. in the left trigeminal nerve.
    d. in the right trigeminal nerve.

21. The typical paralysis in Guillain-Barre is
    a. descending.
    b. ascending.
    c. more pronounced on one side of the body.
    d. more pronounced distally than proximally.

22. Sings of uncal herniation include
    a. deepening level of consciousness, dilated ipsilateral pupil and ipsilateral hemiparesis.
    b. deepening level of consciousness, constricted ipsilateral pupil and ipsilateral hemiparesis.
    c. deepening level of consciousness, dilated ipsilateral pupil and contralateral hemiparesis.
    d. lightening level of consciousness, dilated ipsilateral pupil and contralateral hemiparesis.

23. A nurse can check a patient's visual fields by
    a. asking the patient to read from a newspaper.
    b. testing the patient's ability to identify colors.
    c. touching the cornea with a cotton ball and watching to see if the patient reacts.
    d. observing to see which areas of the meal tray the patient appears to ignore.

24. When observing a seizure the nurse should take care to record which of the following?
    a. duration, aura, time of last meal, deviation of head or eyes and pupillary size and reaction
    b. duration, aura, focal onset and spread, the names and titles of others observing the seizure and the postictal state
    c. duration, aura, focal onset and spread, pupil size and reaction, deviation of head or eyes and postictal state
    d. duration, aura, focal onset and spread, temperature of room, pupil size and reaction, deviation of head or eyes and postictal state

25. Where would you expect the lesion to lie in the case of a unilateral sensory loss along a given dermatome?
    a. parietal lobe
    b. peripheral nerve or its entry point into the spinal cord
    c. ipsilateral thoracic cord below the level of T4
    d. right frontal lobe

26. A patient has no pupillary reaction at all to light in the left eye. There is reaction to light in both eyes when light is shined in the right eye. Where is the lesion?
    a. left cranial nerve II
    b. right cranial nerve II
    c. left cranial nerve III
    d. right cranial nerve III

27. The ability to recognize an object by touch is called
    a. stereognosis.
    b. apraxia.
    c. agnosia.
    d. agraphia.

28. A patient presents with a unilateral loss of all sensory modalities in a single extremity. Where is the lesion most likely located?
    a. ipsilateral sensory strip of the parietal lobe
    b. peripheral nerve or its entry point into the spinal cord
    c. cervical spinal cord
    d. contralateral sensory strip of the parietal lobe

29. A lesion of the left hemisphere in Broca's area results in a deficit of
    a. verbal comprehension.
    b. written comprehension.
    c. verbal expression.
    d. written expression.

30. Which set of symptoms would you expect to see with an upper motor neuron lesion?
    a. muscle atrophy, hyperreflexia, extensor plantar response
    b. spasticity, hyperreflexia, no fasciculations
    c. spasticity, fasciculations, extensor plantar response
    d. muscle atrophy, spasticity, hyperreflexia, fasciculations

31. The oculomotor nerve is responsible for all of the following, except
    a. elevating the eyelid.
    b. lateral eye movement.
    c. pupillary constriction to light.
    d. medial eye movement.

32. A 32-year-old man is admitted to the hospital following an automobile accident. He is awake and alert now, but was unconscious for several minutes after the accident. Physical examination is unremarkable except for a right linear temporal-parietal skull fracture. He should be assessed carefully each hour because
    a. he is at risk of developing an epidural hematoma.
    b. he will likely develop seizures within the next 24 hours.
    c. if he remains unchanged for four hours he may be sent home.
    d. he is likely to develop a CSF leak from his ear.

33. Which best describes the features of a facial nerve lower motor neuron paralysis?
    a. dysarthria, dysphagia and postural hypotension
    b. dysarthria, dysphagia and diplopia
    c. ipsilateral inability to close eye, control mouth or move lip
    d. ipsilateral inability to open eye, move tongue or move lip

34. The characteristic symptoms of Parkinson's disease are
    a. tremor, muscle rigidity and athetosis.
    b. tremor, muscle atrophy and akinesia.
    c. tremor, muscle wasting and athetosis.
    d. tremor, muscle rigidity and akinesia.

35. Characteristics of a cerebellar lesion are
    a. dystonia and tremor at rest.
    b. ataxia and dysmetria.
    c. ataxia and tremor at rest.
    d. dysmetria and dystonia.

36. Which statement is true concerning psychomotor seizures?
    a. The patient has complete recall of the event.
    b. The seizure begins in one extremity and gradually spreads.
    c. During the course of the seizure the patient retains motor function.
    d. The patient is incontinent and unconscious.

37. While talking, a patient's wife tells a nurse that she has been having episodes of blurred vision in the right eye several times a day. She describes it as "a veil covering my eye." An appropriate response would be to tell the wife that
    a. she has probably had a small stroke in her vision center and that she should see a doctor immediately.
    b. her problem sounds like TIAs and advise her to see a doctor immediately since it may be a warning sign of impending stroke.
    c. her problem sounds like TIAs and suggest that she mention it to her doctor at her next annual physical.
    d. since her problem only involves the eye, it is probably only eye fatigue and refer her to her opthalmologist.

38. With loss of pain and temperature sense on the left side of the body below the neck, and paralysis and loss of body position and vibration sense below the neck on the right, the lesion is
    a. Brown-Sequard syndrome, right cervical cord.
    b. anterior cord syndrome.
    c. Brown-Sequard syndrome, left cervical cord.
    d. central cord syndrome.

39. Nerve impulses in a single cell travel from
    a. axon to cell body to axon hillock to dendrite.
    b. axon to axon hillock to cell body to dendrite.
    c. dendrite to cell body to axon hillock to axon.
    d. cell body to axon hillock to axon to dendrite.

40. Neurons in the peripheral nervous system
    a. have myelin, but no neurilemma.
    b. are incapable of wallerian degeneration.
    c. have myelin and neurilemma, but lack nodes of Ranvier.
    d. are capable of regeneration.

41. The cerebrum is composed of
    a. 2 frontal lobes, 2 temporal lobes, 2 parietal lobes and 1 occipital lobe.
    b. 2 frontal lobes, 2 temporal lobes, 2 parietal lobes and 2 occipital lobes.
    c. 1 frontal lobe, 2 temporal lobes, 1 parietal lobe, 1 occipital lobe and the cerebellum.
    d. 2 frontal lobes, 2 temporal lobes, 1 parietal lobe and 1 occipital lobe.

42. The diencephalon is composed of
   a. the epithalamus, the subthalamus, the hypothalamus and the pons.
   b. the epithalamus, the thalamus, the hypothalamus and the reticular activating system.
   c. the epithalamus, the hypothalamus, the thalamus and the subthalamus.
   d. the epithalamus, the thalamus, the exothalamus and the hypothalamus.

43. Which of the following statements is incorrect:
   a. A subdural hematoma generally occurs after trauma, but an epidural hematoma may occur spontaneously in people with clotting disorders.
   b. A subdural hematoma may become symptomatic immediately after occurrence, or after several weeks or months.
   c. A subdural hematoma results from tearing of the bridging veins.
   d. There is a high correlation between linear fractures in the temporal area and epidural hematomas.

44. Mr. C., a 30-year-old man, presents to the emergency room complaining of a violent right frontal headache that began three days ago. He is afebrile, but has nuchal rigidity and photophobia. B.P. = 170/100, Heartrate = 86 NSR, Resp. rate = 22. He is to be admitted to the intensive care unit. The emergency room nurse should call the ICU to inform them that the patient
   a. probably has encephalitis and will need to be in isolation.
   b. probably has had a subarachnoid hemorrhage and will be going directly to the operating room for aneurysm repair.
   c. has an intracerebral bleed due to hypertension.
   d. appears to have had a subarachnoid hemorrhage due to either an aneurysm or an AVM, but is stable at this time.

45. Mr. C. arrives in the intensive care unit. He is awake and alert and without any focal neurologic deficit. His only complaint is the unrelieved headache. The doctor orders phenobarbital 30 mg three times a day, thorazine 10 mg q 6h, colace 100 mg twice a day and amicar 3 GM q 2h. Explain the rationale behind this therapy.
   a. Amicar lowers the B.P., while phenobarbital and thorazine sedate the patient, and colace prevents constipation.
   b. Amicar helps prevent clot lysis, phenobarbital lowers B.P. and acts as a sedative, thorazine potentiates phenobarbital and colace prevents constipation.
   c. Amicar and thorazine sedate the patient, phenobarbital lowers B.P. and colace prevents constipation.
   d. Amicar decreases cerebral spasm, phenobarbital lowers B.P., thorazine prevents the patient from becoming depressed and colace prevents constipation.

46. Mr. C. has been in the unit for four hours now. He is still complaining of a headache and requesting pain medication. The nurse examines him and finds that he now has a right ptosis and left arm weakness. The nurse should
   a. check him again in an hour since it is probably due to the effects of his sedation.
   b. ask him his religion and call a clergyman for him since he is probably having a rebleed of an aneurysm and the mortality rate for rebleeds is very high.
   c. call the physician immediately and report the change.
   d. call the physician immediately and report the neurologic change. Also tell the physician that the patient is in severe pain and that pain medication was not ordered.

47. The physician orders 10 mg Decadron® I.V. push stat and 4 mg I.V. q 6h because
    a. Decadron is anti-inflammatory and will relieve the pain.
    b. Decadron stabilizes the cell wall and reduces cerebral edema.
    c. Decadron stabilizes the cell wall and prevents further bleeding.
    d. Decadron reduces the possibility of the formation of a stress ulcer.

48. In myasthenia gravis
    a. thymic hyperplasia frequently develops after medical management has stabilized the symptoms.
    b. the presence of thymic tumor (thymonia) indicates advanced disease, which is usually refractory to treatment.
    c. thymectomy for thymonia or thymic hyperplasia may result in decreased medication requirements.
    d. thymectomy for thymonia or thymic hyperplasia usually results in complete remission in male patients.

49. Mr. C. is quite concerned about his family's ability to cope without him while he is hospitalized. His wife is chronically ill and both of his children have behavioral problems. The nurse might suggest to him that
    a. perhaps his family will be better off without him around for a while. They may learn to appreciate him more.
    b. it can be arranged for a social worker to meet with his wife and help her.
    c. he ask his doctor if he can go home and settle things and return the day before surgery.
    d. if he insists on discussing upsetting matters with his wife, she will be forced to stop all of his visitors.

50. Myelin is
    a. produced by oligodendrocytes and is completed before birth.
    b. produced by astrocytes and completed by the early 30s.
    c. produced by the oligodendrocytes in the CNS and the PNS, and is completed by puberty or late adolescence.
    d. produced by the astrocytes in the CNS and Schwann cells in the PNS, and continues to form until age 10, after which it disappears.

51. Neurilemma is
    a. the substance that forms the blood-brain barrier.
    b. the substance responsible for the mobilization of microglia.
    c. an autoimmune protein produced in multiple sclerosis.
    d. the outer covering of nerves in the PNS that aids in their regeneration.

52. At the synaptic cleft the neurotransmitter is
    a. totally destroyed after use.
    b. returned to the presynaptic vesicle with the majority still intact for reuse.
    c. converted to the neurotransmitter antagonist.
    d. incorporated into the receptor cell and passed along the axon with the electrical impulse.

53. The current theory of the cause of myasthenia gravis is
    a. an abnormal protein blocking the receptor sites.
    b. exposure to excessive radiation.
    c. related to tumors or hyperplasia of the adrenal glands.
    d. thought to be hormonal since it only occurs in women.

54. Which of the following are neurotransmitters:
    a. dopamine, norepinephrine, calcium, serotonin, GABA
    b. dopamine, GABA, norepinephrine, chloride, calcium
    c. dopamine, GABA, norepinephrine, serotonin, acetylcholine
    d. dopamine, GABA, norepinephrine, ceruloplasmin, acetylcholine

55. The brain
    a. receives 20 percent of the cardiac output.
    b. requires glycogen for direct synthesis to ATP.
    c. is able to withstand prolonged periods of hypoxia without significant damage.
    d. tolerates lactic acidosis and hypoglycemia well because of the protective effect of the blood-brain barrier.

56. The sella turcica is
    a. the area of the brain housing visual and auditory fibers.
    b. the area of the brain called the midbrain.
    c. the area of the skull through which the medulla passes to become the spinal cord.
    d. the area of the skull housing the pituitary gland.

57. Which statement is *not* true concerning the cervical spinal column?
    a. The atlas and the axis are the first two cervical vertebrae.
    b. The atlas and the axis are not part of the cervical vertebrae.
    c. The axis allows for rotation, flexion and extension of the head.
    d. The odontoid process is part of the axis.

58. The intervertebral disk
    a. is composed of the annulus fibrosus and the Edinger-Westphal nucleus.
    b. surrounds the vertebral bodies and holds them in position.
    c. is composed of the annulus fibrosus and the nucleus pulposus.
    d. is referred to as a ruptured disk when the annulus herniates through the nucleus pulposus.

59. The lumbar vertebrae
    a. are the smallest in the body.
    b. are fused into a triangular form.
    c. vary in number from five to seven.
    d. are the largest in the body.

60. The hypothalamus
    a. produces all the hormones released by the pituitary.
    b. is concerned with fat metabolism, temperature control and regulation of water intake.
    c. has connections with the occipital lobe and mediates visual information.
    d. is the sensory relay station.

61. The cranial nerves that exit in the pons are
    a. IV, V, VII, IX.
    b. III, V, VI, VII.
    c. II, III, IV, V.
    d. V, VI, VII, VIII.

62. The cranial nerves exiting in the medulla are
    a. V, VI, VIII, IX.
    b. IV, VII, VIII, IX.
    c. V, VI, X, XII.
    d. IX, X, XI, XII.

63. The anterior cerebral artery supplies
    a. the medial aspect of the frontal lobe.
    b. the occipital lobe.
    c. the lateral aspect of the frontal and temporal lobes.
    d. the superior aspect of the cerebellum.

64. Cranial nerves to be tested after posterior fossa surgey would be
    a. III, IV, VI, IX.
    b. VII, IX, XI, XII.
    c. II, V, VII, IX.
    d. V, VI, VII, VIII.

65. Decortication is
    a. posturing with arms flexed over chest and legs flexed at hips.
    b. posturing with arms flexed over chest and legs extended and feet plantar flexed.
    c. posturing with arms extended and legs flexed at hips.
    d. posturing with arms flaccid and legs extended.

66. Patients with CVAs may
    a. have variable motor signs, but are always alert.
    b. have variable motor signs, but are always comatose.
    c. have variable motor signs and levels of consciousness.
    d. have variable levels of consciousness, but are always hemiparetic.

67. The major nursing responsibilities for patients with CVAs are
    a. to ensure airway, ventilation and early physical therapy.
    b. to ensure airway, ventilation and postpone physical therapy until the patient has regained some motor control.
    c. to ensure adequate fluid balance, prevent the patient from performing any self-care to prevent overtiring and protect the airway.
    d. to involve the family in home care preparations, teach the patient about medications and encourage the family to be screened for diabetes.

68. Bacterial meningitis is
    a. highly contagious and requires strict isolation.
    b. an inflammation of the brain tissue itself.
    c. rarely caused by bacteria.
    d. characterized by increased white blood cells, elevated protein and decreased glucose in the CSF.

69. Guillain-Barre
    a. rarely occurs in men.
    b. is a CNS demyelinating process.
    c. is characterized by normal CSF except for elevated protein.
    d. is caused by a virus and is highly contagious.

70. Which is not true concerning patients with head injuries?
    a. Regardless of the severity, the patient is rarely able to return to pre-injury lifestyle.
    b. These patients should have the head of the bed elevated 30 degrees.
    c. Patients may exhibit radical, self-limiting personality changes after the injury.
    d. Patients will develop post-injury seizures in about 20 percent of cases.

71. Spinal shock
    a. develops only after extensive cervical injuries.
    b. occurs below the level of the injury.
    c. may recur many times during the post-injury phase.
    d. involves only loss of sensation below the level of the injury.

72. Tetanus
    a. is caused by a gram-negative virus.
    b. has an incubation period of 5 weeks to 15 months.
    c. is caused by an organism that produces a neurotoxin.
    d. causes muscle flaccidity and bradycardia.

73. Petit mal seizures
    a. frequently occur in adults.
    b. usually last less than ten seconds.
    c. are not amenable to drug therapy.
    d. precede the development of grand mal seizures.

74. Status epilepticus is best treated by
    a. intravenous diazepam.
    b. intubation and general anesthesia.
    c. Anectine® and curare.
    d. hyperventilation and phenytoin.

75. Diabetes insipidus is characterized by
    a. small quantities of dilute urine.
    b. small quantities of concentrated urine.
    c. large quantities of concentrated urine.
    d. large quantities of dilute urine.

KEY POINT RECOGNITION ANSWERS

Anatomy and Physiology: Skull and Spinal Column
1. True
2. False—It is the sphenoid bone.
3. False—Anterior, middle, and posterior fossa
4. True
5. False—The sella turcica houses the pituitary gland.
6. False—The dura is the outermost layer.
7. True
8. False—Between the dura and arachnoid is the subdural space.
9. False—The pia attaches directly to the brain.
10. True
11. False—It consists of six parts: body, arch, articular processes, intervertebral foramina, spinal foramina and intervertebral disk.
12. False—Five divisions: cervical, thoracic, lumbar, sacral and coccygeal

Nervous Tissue: Cells of the Nervous System
1. False—The two cell types are the neuron and neuroglial cells.
2. False—The neuron is composed of a cell body, axon and dendrites.
3. False—Dendrites receive and conduct impulses *toward* the cell body. The axon conducts impulses *away* from the cell body.
4. True
5. False—Neurilemma augments myelin.
6. False—Neurilemma
7. True
8. True
9. False—Ependyma lines the ventricles. Microglia respond to inflammation within the nervous system.
10. False—Ependymal line the central canal of the spinal cord. Astrocytes provide support for neurons and blood vessels and the formation of the blood-brain barrier.

Transmission of Nerve Impulses
1. False—The nerve impulses going toward the organ are called efferent. The nerve impulses going away from the organ are called afferent.
2. True
3. False—Impulse conduction can only proceed in one direction.
4. True
5. False—During depolarization, it is a temporary difference in the voltage between the active and resting part of a nerve or muscle cell.
6. True
7. False—The cell membrane becomes more permeable to sodium ions.
8. True
9. True
10. True

Reflex Action
1. False—Sensory impulses first stimulate afferent fibers in the posterior horn of the spinal cord.
2. True

Cerebral Metabolism
1. True
2. False—Hypoglycemia depresses brain metabolism.
3. True

Divisions of Cerebral Tissue
1. False—Gray matter consists of nerve cell bodies and white matter of nerve cell processes.
2. False—The cerebrum has four lobes.
3. True
4. False—The parietal lobe controls sensory function.
5. True
6. False—It does control balance and equilibrium, but is not a part of the midbrain.
7. True
8. True
9. True
10. False—Brainstem = midbrain, pons and medulla
11. False—It houses nuclei for cranial nerves IX, X, XI, and XII, as well as the cardiac and respiratory centers.
12. True

Cerebral Blood Supply
1. True
2. False—internal carotids and vertebral arteries
3. False—posterior communicating arteries
4. False—meninges and periosteum
5. False—inferior sagittal sinus

Ventricular System
1. True
2. False—Largest (The fourth ventricle is the smallest.)
3. True
4. False—The third ventricle drains via the aqueduct of Sylvius.
5. False—Each lateral ventricle drains into the third ventricle by way of the foramen of Monro.
6. False—150 cc
7. False—80 to 180 mm H$_2$O

Spinal Cord
1. True
2. True
3. True
4. True
5. True
6. True
7. True
8. True
9. False—31 pairs
10. False—A plexus is a labryinth of spinal nerves.

Autonomic Nervous System
1. True
2. True
3. False—White rami communicans have a white appearance from the myelinated covering.
4. True
5. False—Gray rami communicans join with all spinal nerves.
6. True
7. True
8. False—The sympathetic nervous system causes an increase in heart rate and pupillary dilation.
9. False—Norepinephrine: adrenergic
10. True

Assessment of the Neurological System
1. False—Frontal lobe; brainstem = changes in consciousness and respiratory patterns
2. False—Parietal lobe = sensory loss; occipital lobe = visual disturbance; temporal = auditory loss/speech disturbance
3. True
4. False—V = trigeminal; VI is abducens = check for ability to move eye in lateral field
5. True
6. True
7. True
8. False—II = optic; III = oculomotor
9. False—For cortical discriminatory sensation tests to be validly assessed, cortical area pathways and receptors must be functioning.
10. False—Motor system assessment includes both as vital for assessment.
11. False—Cutaneous reflexes = sharp object (pin); Deep tendon reflexes = hammer
12. True
13. False—Normal reflex is flexion of great toe.
14. False—Level of consciousness
15. True
16. True
17. False—Decerebration
18. False—Hypertension
19. False—Hyperthermia
20. True
21. True

Pathological States and Nursing Management
1. False—Thrombus, emboli, hemorrhage
2. False—Vascular malformations, aneurysm, trauma, hypertension and clotting disorders
3. False—More common in brainstem lesions
4. **True**
5. False—Cerebral aneurysm
6. True
7. False—Seventh to eleventh day

8. False—It is used to prevent clot lysis.
9. True
10. False—Grade I or II
11. False—Bacteria
12. False—Headache, stiff neck and elevated temperature
13. True
14. False—CSF glucose is normal, or slightly decreased, and lymphs are elevated.
15. True
16. True
17. False—Meningitis
18. False—Guillain-Barre syndrome
19. False—VII, VI, III, XII, V, IX
20. False—Every 1 to 2 hours, or more frequently
21. True
22. False—Enteral feedings must be used with caution since there is a high incidence of gastric dilatation and ileus in GBS
23. True
24. True
25. False—Epidural hematoma
26. True
27. False—A variety of symptoms may be present, from unconsciousness to a mild headache.
28. True
29. False—Nasal intubation, or tracheotomy, is preferable to extension of an occult spinal injury.
30. True
31. True
32. True
33. False—Systemic vasodilation, pooling of blood in the distal extremities and hypotension
34. True
35. False—Thoracic = paraplegia
36. False—Greater loss in the arms than in the legs
37. True
38. True
39. True
40. False—Muscle relaxants and warm, moist heat may be beneficial.
41. False—Myasthenia gravis
42. False—Myasthenic crisis from cholinergic crisis
43. True
44. True
45. True
46. True
47. False—Only by I.V. while spasm is present
48. True
49. False—Less than five minutes
50. False—Todd's palsy is postictal hemiparesis. It is seen, but not commonly, following grand mal seizures.

51. True
52. True
53. True
54. False—Multiple agents are often used to achieve control.
55. False—Hypoxia, hypoglycemia and hypothermia
56. True
57. True
58. True
59. False—Observe for hypotension and respiratory arrest.
60. True

Care Common to Neurosurgical Problems
1. False—Level of consciousness
2. True
3. True
4. False—All but hyperthermia; hypothermia is employed.
5. True
6. True
7. True

PASS ANSWER SHEET

1.	b	26.	a	51.	d
2.	c	27.	a	52.	b
3.	b	28.	d	53.	a
4.	a	29.	c	54.	c
5.	a	30.	b	55.	a
6.	c	31.	b	56.	d
7.	d	32.	a	57.	b
8.	a	33.	c	58.	c
9.	c	34.	d	59.	d
10.	b	35.	b	60.	b
11.	d	36.	c	61.	d
12.	d	37.	b	62.	d
13.	b	38.	a	63.	a
14.	c	39.	c	64.	b
15.	b	40.	d	65.	b
16.	c	41.	b	66.	c
17.	b	42.	c	67.	a
18.	b	43.	a	68.	d
19.	a	44.	d	69.	c
20.	a	45.	b	70.	a
21.	b	46.	c	71.	b
22.	c	47.	b	72.	c
23.	d	48.	c	73.	b
24.	c	49.	b	74.	a
25.	b	50.	c	75.	d

SURVEY SUMMARY
NERVOUS SYSTEM

I. **The Nervous System is divided into three parts.**
   A. The *central nervous system,* comprised of the *brain* and *spinal cord.*
   B. The *autonomic nervous system,* divided into the *sysmpathetic* and *parasympathetic* systems
   C. The *peripheral nervous system,* comprised of the *cranial* and *spinal* nerves.

II. **Anatomy and Physiology**
   A. The *skull* houses the brain.
      1. It is comprised of four bones
         a. frontal
         b. parietal
         c. temporal
         d. occipital
      2. The *sphenoid* bone helps to divide the interior of the skull into three fossae:
         a. anterior fossa
         b. middle fossa
         c. posterior fossa
      3. The *sella turcica* is a concave depression in the sphenoid bone and houses the pituitary gland.
      4. Three layers of meningeal tissue lie under the skull and are called the *meninges.*
         a. *dura* = outermost layer
         b. *arachnoid* = middle layer
         c. *pia* = inner layer
   B. The spinal column is composed of 33 vertebrae.
      1. A typical vertebrae consists of the
         a. body
         b. arch
         c. articular processes
         d. intervertebral foramina
         e. spinal foramina
         f. intervertebral disc
      2. The spinal column is divided into five sections.
         a. cervical vertebrae (7)
         b. thoracic vertebrae (12)
         c. lumbar vertebrae (5)
         d. sacral vertebrae (5)
         e. coccygeal vertebrae (4)
   C. Nervous Tissue: Cells of the Nervous System
      1. Two types of cells make up the nervous system
         a. *Neurons* are the functional cells which transmit all information in the brain and spinal cord.
            1. Each neuron is composed of a *cell body, dendrites* and an *axon.*

2. Some neurons are myelinated. Myelination speeds conduction of impulses down the axon sheath.
3. *Neurilemma* augment peripheral nervous system myelin and by saltatory conduction increase the rate of nerve impulse.
   b. *Neuroglial cells* provide the supporting structure within the nervous system.
      1. *Oligodendrocytes*—produce myelin
      2. *Astrocytes*—support for neurons and blood vessels and formation of blood-brain barrier
      3. *Microglia*—phagocytic cells
      4. *Ependymal*—line the ventricles and central canal of the spinal cord.
   2. The *neurons* transmit nerve impulses and the *neuroglial* cells form the nervous system's supporting structures.
D. Transmission of Nerve Impulses
   1. Conduction of nerve impulses travel afferently and efferently.
   2. Synaptic junctions permit travel of neurons in only one direction.
   3. Impulse conduction is a physio-chemical process.
      a. Changes begin with release of neurotransmitters such as *acetylcholine, norepinephrine, dopamine, gamma aminobutyric acid,* and *serotonin.*
      b. Cells become more permeable to sodium.
      c. Electrolyte movement and electrical voltage change initiating an action potential.
      d. Repolarization is followed by the re-establishment of polarization.
   4. *Eno-plate* or *neuromuscular* junction is to allow for axon flattening, and storage in the vesicle reservoir of specific neurotransmitters.
   5. Synaptic clefts are spaces located between the nerve and muscle fiber membrane.
E. Reflex Action
   1. Sensory impulses stimulate afferent fibers leading into the posterior horn of the spinal cord.
   2. The Posterior horn transmits the impulse to the Anterior horn.
F. Cerebral Metabolism
   1. The brain consumes approximately 20% of the oxygen demands of the body.
   2. The brain receives about 20-25% of the cardiac output.
   3. Cerebral blood flow changes according to cerebral perfusion pressure.
G. Divisions of Cerebral Tissue
   1. The brain is made up of neurons and glial cells.
   2. The brain consists of both white and gray matter.
   3. The brain may be divided into
      a. The *cerebrum* is composed of four lobes, which are divided into right and left hemispheres using the *corpus callosum* to receive information about each other.
         1. frontal
         2. parietal
         3. temporal
         4. occipital

b. The ***cerebellum*** controls equilibrium, balance, and synchronized muscle movement.

c. The ***diencephalon*** is primarily composed of the
1. ***Thalamus***—a sensory relay station
2. ***Hypothalamus***—regulates food and water intake and produces releasing factors for many hormones.

d. The ***basal ganglia*** is concerned with involuntary motor activity.

e. The ***brainstem*** is made up of the ***midbrain, pons,*** and ***medulla.***
1. The ***midbrain*** contains the third and fourth cranial nerve nuclei as well as motor and sensory pathways.
2. The ***pons*** lies between the midbrain and medulla. It contains the nuclei for cranial nerves V, VI, VII, and VIII.
3. The ***medulla*** contains the nuclei for cranial nerves IX, X, XI, XII. It also contains the cardiac and respiratory center.

f. The ***reticular formation*** is a diffuse network of fibers. It is also called the ***reticular activating system.***

H. Cerebral Blood Supply
1. Arterial blood supply to brain is provided by the **Circle of Willis.**
2. The Circle of Willis is supplied by the
   a. ***Internal carotids*** which branch into
      1. ***Middle cerebral arteries***
      2. ***Anterior cerebral arteries***
      3. ***Anterior communicating artery***
      4. ***Posterior communicating arteries***
   b. ***Vertebral arteries*** which branch into
      1. ***Posterior inferior cerebellar arteries***
      2. ***Anterior spinal artery***
      3. ***Superior cerebellar arteries***
      4. ***Anterior inferior cerebellar arteries***
      5. ***Posterior cerebral arteries***
3. Extra cerebral blood supply (periosteum and dura) is provided by the ***meningeal arteries*** which branch into
   a. ***Anterior meningeal arteries***
   b. ***Middle meningeal artery***
   c. ***Posterior meningeal artery***
4. The extra cerebral blood supply is drained by veins.
5. The internal circulation is drained by small capillaries within the tissue.
6. Internal and external systems drain into venous sinuses;
   a. superior cerebral veins into superior sagittal sinus
   b. medial aspects of hemispheres into inferior sagittal sinus
   c. internal cerebral veins into straight and transverse sinus.

I. Ventricular System
1. There are four major ***ventricles.***
   a. ***Lateral ventricles*** (2)
   b. ***Third ventricle***
   c. ***Fourth ventricle***

2. The choroid plexus forms CSF by filtering the blood presented to it.
3. The ventricles drain into:
   a. **Lateral ventricles**—drain into third ventricle via Foramen of Monro.
   b. **Third ventricle**—drains into the fourth ventricle via the aqueduct of Sylvius.
   c. **Fourth ventricle**—drains into the spinal cord subarachnoid space, the Foramen of Luschka, and the Foramen of Magendie.
   d. CSF cushions and protects the brain and spinal cord.
   e. CSF is absorbed into the dural sinuses by the arachnoid villi and returns to systemic circulation via the internal jugular veins.
   f. Normal CSF is colorless, clear, has an opening pressure (in a side-lying patient) of 80-180 mm H_2O, has a specific gravity of 1.007, a pH of 7.35, and a chloride of 120-130 m Eq/L, sodium of 142-150 m Eq/L, glucose of 60-80 mEq/L, and no WBC's.

J. Spinal Cord
   1. The cord extends from the terminal border of the Medulla to the L 1-2 interspace.
   2. The cord ends at L 2 but the Meningeal covering extends to the first coccygeal vertebra and contains the **cauda equina.**
   3. Spinal cord **gray matter** make up the interior cord.
      a. **Anterior horns** contain **afferent** fibers.
      b. **Posterior horns** contain **efferent** fibers.
   4. Spinal cord **white matter** make up the **tracts.**
      a. **Ascending** tracts carry **sensory** information.
      b. **Descending** tracts carry **motor** information.
   5. The **peripheral nervous system** is comprised of;
      a. 31 pairs of **spinal nerves**
         1. 8 cervical
         2. 12 thoracic
         3. 5 lumbar
         4. 5 sacral
         5. 1 coccygeal
      b. 12 **cranial nerves.**

K. The Autonomic Nervous System is the involuntary nervous system.
   1. It is comprised of neuron chains.
      a. preganglionic cell bodies
      b. pastganglianic axons
   2. **Divisions** of the **ans**
      a. The **parasympathic** innervates visera, blood vessels, glands, smooth muscle tissue and the heart.
         1. "fight or flight" response
         2. vasoconstrictive effect
         3. Cholinergic Neurons release a neurotransmitter called **acetylcholine**

III. **Assessment of the Neurological System should include:**
   A. Assessment of Gross Cerebral functioning
      1. overall behavior and appearance
      2. emotional behavior
   B. Specific Cerebral Functioning
      1. speech ability
      2. sensory interpretation
      3. motor interpretation
   C. Cranial Nerve testing
      1. Olfactory
      2. Optic
      3. Oculomotor
      4. Trochlear
      5. Trigeminal
      6. Abducens
      7. Facial
      8. Acoustic
      9. Glossopharyngeal
      10. Vagus
      11. Accessory spinal
      12. Hypoglossal
   D. Cerebellar function testing
   E. Sensory System testing
   F. Motor System testing
   G. Reflex testing
   H. Level of Consciousness
      1. arousability
      2. orientation
      3. ability to follow commands
   I. The Pupillary Response
      1. size, shape, equality
      2. consenual reaction, bilateral reaction to light
   J. Motor Strength and Equality
      1. ability to move extremities against resistance and gravity upon command
      2. ability to move extremities in response to noxious stimuli
      3. Decortication
      4. Decerebration
   K. Evaluation of Vital Signs
   L. Laboratory and Radiologic Studies

IV. **Pathological States and Nursing Management**
   A. CVA
      1. CVA's are caused by either a thrombus, embolus, or hemmorhage.
      2. The patient may present with
         a. headache
         b. hemi-paresis
         c. hemi-sensory loss
         d. speech and visual disturbances

3. CT scan is the best diagnostic aid.
4. Nursing Care includes
   a. Maintenance of airway and circulation
   b. Monitoring neurologic status
   c. Maintaining fluid and electrolyte balance
   d. providing emotional support and patient education
   e. prevention of deformities
   f. maintaining bowel and bladder functioning
   g. skin care

B. *Cerebral aneurysms*
   1. Cerebral aneurysms are caused by defects in the medial layer of the arterial wall.
   2. The patient presents with a violent headache, nausea, and vomiting.
   3. Diagnostic data includes LP and CT scan.
   4. Nursing Care includes:
      a. observation for and prevention of rebleeding.
      b. providing emotional support.
      c. monitoring neurologic signs.
      d. preventing complication.

C. *Meningitis* is an inflammation of the Meninges of the brain.
   1. The most common causative agent is bacteria.
   2. Presenting signs symptoms include headache, stiff neck, fever, diplopia, tinnitus and seizures.
   3. Definitive diagnosis is by LP
      a. **Bacterial** meningitis is manifested by elevated WBC's and reduced CSF glucose.
      b. **Viral** meningitis is manifested by elevated lymphs and normal CSF glucose.
   4. Nursing Care includes
      a. airway maintenance
      b. administration of appropriate medications such as antibiotics and anti-convulsants.
      c. maintenance of vital functions
      d. provision of emotional support
      e. prevention of complications

D. *Guillain-Barre Syndrome* is also known as acute polyneuritis.
   1. Presenting signs and symptoms include symmetrical ascending muscle weakness, parasthesis of distal extremities, muscle tenderness sensory loss and cranial nerve dysfunction.
   2. Nursing Care is mainly **supportive** and **restorative.**
      a. Maintain airway and respirations.
         1. Check vital capacity every 1-2 hours.
         2. Prevent deformities; maintain bowel and bladder function; provide good skin care.
         3. Maintain vital functions.
         4. Provide symptomatic relief.
         5. Provide emotional support.

E. The pathology of **head injury** and resulting nursing care is dependent upon the type of injury sustained.
   1. The most common problem in head injury is increased ICP.

2. Types of head injuries include:
   a. **Concussion** (least severe)
   b. **Contusion** (petechial damage to brain tissue)
   c. **Epidural hematoma** (arterial bleed and true emergency)
   d. **Subdural hematoma** (venous bleed)
   e. **Intracerebral hematoma** (tearing of vessels)
3. Nursing Care includes:
   a. Maintenance of **airway** and **vital functions**
      1. Do not hyperextend neck.
   b. Monitor and treat for cerebral edema.
   c. Administer medications for seizure control.
   d. Observe for CSF drainage.
   e. Observe for complications.

F. **Spinal cord injuries** can occur in the cervical, thoracic, or lumbar-sacral region.
   1. **Spinal shock** is a "shut down" of all motor, sensory, and reflex responses below the level of the injury.
      a. It may last several days to several months.
      b. Its disappearance is heralded by return of involuntary reflexes below the level of the lesion.
   2. The patient will present with varied symptoms due to the extent and location of the lesion.
      a. C1, 2, 3 = apnea
      b. C4, 5 = impaired respiratory effort.
      c. cervical lesions = quadriplegia
      d. thoracic lesions = paraplegia
      e. Common **cord syndromes**
         1. Central Cord Syndrome
         2. Anterior Cord Syndrome
         3. Brown-Sequard Syndrome
   3. Nursing Care is aimed at maintaining life and beginning a realistic plan for rehabilitation
      a. Maintenance of airway and vital functions
      b. Maintenance of alignment, positioning and skin care.
      c. Fluid and electrolyte control
      d. Maintenance of nutrition
      e. Bladder and bowel care
      f. Emotional support.

G. **Myasthenia Gravis** is believed to be an autoimmune process.
   1. Clinical presentation includes:
      a. fatigability of voluntary muscles
      b. ptosis
      c. voice changes
      d. jaw weakness during chewing
      e. diplopia
   2. Diagnosis is often determined by the **tensilon test.**
   3. Nursing Care includes:
      a. Maximizing neuromuscular transmission
         1. Neostigmine, Mestinon, Mytelose
         2. steroids

  b. Maintaining respirations
  c. Emotional support
  d. Anticipating weakness and planning ADL accordingly
  e. Maintaining nutrition
 H. ***Tetanus*** is caused by a gram positive bacteria called Clostridium tetani.
  1. Signs and symptoms of tetanus may vary from mile to generalized stiffness. Further signs and symptoms include:
   a. hyperactive deeptendon reflexes
   b. abdominal rigidity
   c. facial muscle spasm on grimace or closing of jaw
  2. ***Nursing care*** is aimed at preventing muscle spasm and maintaining an airway.
   a. Administer tetanus antitoxin
   b. Maintain fluid and electrolyte balance
   c. Provide nutrition
   d. Maintain a quiet, non-stimulating environment.
 I. ***Seizures*** are electrical discharges in the neurons of the cortex and possibly the brainstem.
  1. Seizures may be precipitated by
   a. genetic factors
   b. trauma
   c. tumors
   d. metabolic disorders
   e. infections
  2. Seizures may be classified as
   a. Generalized Seizure Disorders
    1. Grand Mal
    2. Petite Mal
    3. Akinetic
    4. Myoclonic
   b. Partial Seizure Disorders
    1. Partial Motor
    2. Partial Sensory
   c. Partial Seizures with Complex Symptomatology (Temporal lobe or Psychomotor)
  3. Nursing Care is aimed at:
   a. observing and reporting seizure activity
   b. preventing injury
   c. controlling seizure activity
 J. ***Status epilepticus*** is persistent seizure activity.
  1. It is life threatening and must be terminated.
  2. Nursing care includes:
   a. Airway maintenance and ventilation
   b. Termination of seizure activity with drug therapy
   c. Maintain vital functions.

V. Care Common to Neurological Problems
 A. Observe for signs of increased ICP
  1. changes in LOC

2. fixed and dilated pupil
3. increased headache
5. seizures
6. nausea and vomiting

B. ICP is monitored in three ways:
1. Subarachnoid screw
2. Ventricular drain
3. Epidural catheter

C. ICP may be decreased by
1. ventricular drainage
2. elevating the head of bed 30 degrees
3. using osmotic diuretics/steroids and barbiturates
4. hypothermia
5. hyperventilation to PCO_2 of 25 to 30 mm Hg

D. Post-op Care includes:
1. fluid/electrolyte maintenance at 75 Ml/hr total fluids
2. pain control without narcotics
3. steroids
4. checking dressings and drains
5. maintaining ventilation

CHAPTER FOUR
PULMONARY SYSTEM

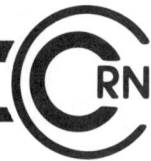

BEHAVIORAL OBJECTIVES

After reading the *Pulmonary System,* the nurse will be able to:
- Identify the anatomy of the pulmonary system
- Describe the function of structures related to the pulmonary system
- Describe inspiration and expiration
- Describe pulmonary circulation
- Describe pulmonary physiology
- State the components and physical assessment relating to the pulmonary system
- State laboratory and radiologic studies relating to pulmonary disorders
- Describe the pathophysiology of the following states:
  Respiratory failure
  Respiratory insufficiency
  Adult respiratory distress syndrome
  Chronic obstructive pulmonary disease
  Status asthmaticus
  Pulmonary embolism
  Chest trauma
- Identify clinical manifestations and diagnostic findings associated with:
  Respiratory failure
  Respiratory insufficiency
  Adult respiratory distress syndrome
  Chronic obstructive pulmonary disease
  Status asthmaticus
  Pulmonary embolism
  Chest trauma
- Develop a nursing care plan for these conditions:
  Respiratory failure
  Respiratory insufficiency
  Adult respiratory distress syndrome
  Chronic obstructive pulmonary disease
  Status asthmaticus
  Pulmonary embolism
  Chest trauma
- List the common problems associated with these pulmonary problems:
  Respiratory failure
  Respiratory insufficiency
  Adult respiratory distress syndrome
  Chronic obstructive pulmonary disease
  Status asthmaticus
  Pulmonary embolism
  Chest trauma

TOPICAL OUTLINE
PULMONARY SYSTEM

I. Pulmonary System: Overview   135
II. Anatomy   135
    Respiratory tract   135
    Lungs   138
    Bony thorax   139
    Muscles of respiration   139
      Inspiration   139
      Expiration   140
    Pulmonary circulation   140
III. Physiology   141
    Ventilation   141
    Flow measurements   142
    Alveolar ventilation (Va)   142
    Regulation of ventilation   142
    Mechanics of breathing   144
    Compliance   144
    Airway resistance   145
    Diffusion   145
    Oxygen transport   146
    Carbon dioxide transport   147
    Arterial hypoxemia   148
    Acid-base   149
      Buffer systems   149
      Chemical buffers   149
      Respiratory component   150
      Renal component   152
      Acidosis   153
      Causes of primary respiratory acidosis   153
      Causes of metabolic acidosis   153
      Anion gap   154
      Alkalosis   154
      Causes for respiratory alkalosis   154
      Causes for metabolic alkalosis   155
      Relationship of potassium and alkalosis   155
      Compensation   155
      Mixed acid-base disturbances   156
    Treatment   157
      Respiratory acidosis   157
      Metabolic acidosis   157
      Respiratory alkalosis   157
      Metabolic alkalosis   157
    Signs and symptoms   157
IV. Assessment of the Pulmonary System   158
    Patient assessment   158
    Anatomical landmarks   159
    Lungs   161

Inspection   162
Palpation   162
Percussion   162
Auscultation   163
    Techniques of auscultation   163
Laboratory and radiologic studies   163

V. Pathological States and Nursing Management   166
    Respiratory failure   166
        Pathophysiology   166
        Pathophysiology: specific   166
        Clinical presentation   167
        Diagnostic data   167
        Nursing care   168
    Adult respiratory distress syndrome (ARDS)   168
        Pathophysiology: general   168
        Clinical presentation   169
        Diagnostic data   169
        Nursing care   169
    Chronic obstructive pulmonary disease (COPD)   170
        Pathophysiology: general   170
        Pathophysiology: specific   170
        Clinical presentation   171
        Diagnostic data   171
        Nursing care   172
    Status Asthmaticus   172
        Pathophysiology   172
        Clinical presentation   173
        Diagnostic data   173
        Nursing care   173
    Pulmonary embolism   174
        Pathophysiology   174
        Clinical presentation   174
        Diagnostic data   175
        Nursing care   175
    Chest trauma   176
        Pathophysiology: general   176
        Pathophysiology-rib fractures   176
        Clinical presentation   176
        Diagnostic data   176
        Nursing care   176
        Pathophysiology-flail chest   177
        Clinical presentation   177
        Diagnostic data   177
        Nursing care   178
        Pathophysiology-hemothorax, pneumothorax and tension pneumothorax   178
        Clinical presentation   179
        Diagnostic data   179
        Nursing care   179

      Cardiac tamponade   180
        Pathophysiology   180
        Clinical presentation   180
        Diagnostic data   180
        Nursing care   180
      Injury to the diaphragm   180
        Pathophysiology   180
        Clinical presentation   181
        Diagnostic data   181
        Nursing care   181
      Tracheal or bronchial rupture   181
        Pathophysiology   181
        Clinical presentation   181
        Diagnostic data   181
        Nursing care   181
      Esophageal rupture   182
        Pathophysiology   182
        Clinical presentation   182
        Diagnostic data   182
        Nursing care   182
VI. Care Common to Respiratory Problems   182
    Airway obstruction   182
    Airway maintenance   183
      Complications associated with airway intubations   187
    Continuous ventilatory support   187
    Drug therapy   190
    Suctioning   190
    Weaning   191
    Intermittent mandatory ventilation (IMV)   191
    General nursing care   191
    Chest physiotherapy   192
    Intermittent positive pressure breathing (IPPB)   192
    Continuous positive airway pressure (CPAP)   192
    Humidification   192
    Oxygen therapy   192
      Complication associated with oxygen therapy   193
    Adjunctive oxygen equipment   193
    Complications   194
Program Assessment: Science and Situation   197
Key Point Recognition Answers   203
PASS Answer Sheet   211
Survey Summary   213

PULMONARY SYSTEM: OVERVIEW

The pulmonary system (Fig. 4-1) is responsible for all of the processes involved in delivering oxygen to the cells and removing carbon dioxide. It is not enough that the respiratory gases are moved through the system; the ultimate goal, at the cellular level, is the efficient *use* of the transported gases.

The work of the **pulmonary system** may be divided into three gas exchange phases. The first phase is the exchange between the atmosphere and alveoli; the second phase is the exchange between the alveoli and pulmonary capillaries; and the third is the exchange between the blood and the tissues.

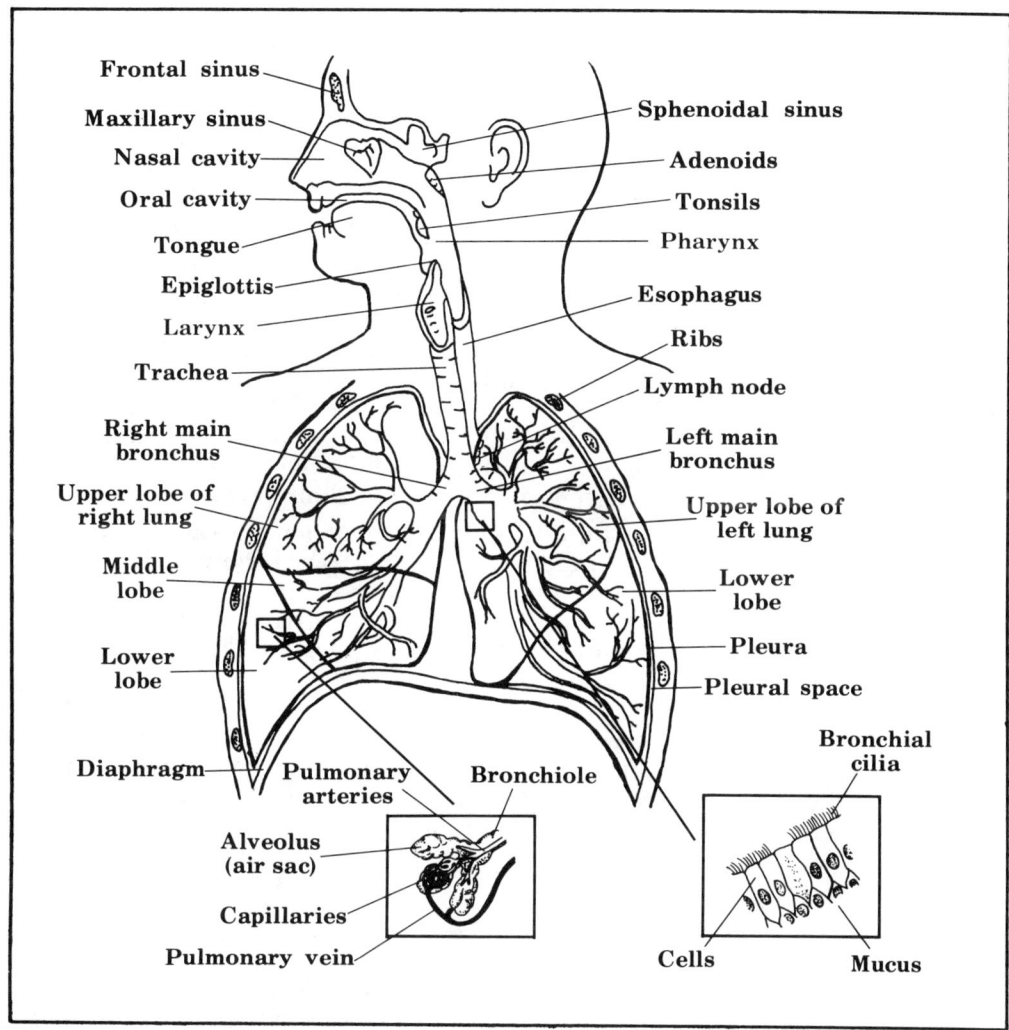

Fig. 4-1. Pulmonary system

ANATOMY

RESPIRATORY TRACT

The respiratory tract is divided into the **upper airway, lower airway** and **alveoli** (Fig. 4-1).

The **upper airway** consists of the **nasal cavity** and the **pharynx.**

The nasal cavity, which is lined with ciliated mucous membranes, allows air to enter the respiratory tract. Its functions include humidifying, warming and filtering the air. The nose also serves as the organ of smell and aids in phonation. The pharynx is about five inches long and extends from the base of the skull to the esophagus. It is composed of three parts: the **nasopharynx** (behind the nose); the **oropharynx** (behind the mouth); and the **laryngopharynx** (behind the larynx).

The pharyngeal tonsils are located in the nasopharynx. They are part of the lymphatic system that aids in controlling infection. The nasopharynx has two openings into the middle ear by way of the Eustachian tube, which equalizes pressure in the middle ear. Both food and air pass through the pharynx. These receptor areas cause the food to be propelled into the esophagus and, by closing the larynx, close off the trachea.

The *lower airway* consists of the *larynx, trachea, bronchi* and *terminal bronchioles.*

The *larynx* is cylindrical in shape and lies between the pharynx and the superior portion of the trachea. The outer framework of the larynx consists of a series of cartilaginous rings. The three most significant are the *thyroid cartilage, cricoid cartilage* and *epiglottis.* The *thyroid cartilage* consists of rectangular plates, or lamina, which give a characteristic protrusion referred to as the "Adam's Apple." Within the thyroid cartilage lie a pair of ligaments called the vocal cords. The *cricoid cartilage* is the only complete ring of cartilage in the respiratory tract. It is also the narrowest part of the airway in children, making cuffed tubes unnecessary. In adults, the narrowest part of the airway is the vocal cords.

The *epiglottis* is a small cartilage that is attached on one side to the thyroid cartilage and is free on the other sides. It acts as a hinge to form a lid over the larynx during swallowing. When the cough reflex is initiated, the vocal cords shut and the epiglottis closes. The cough reflex is initiated by foreign material in the throat. Contractions of the abdominal and intercostal muscles cause pressure to build up in the thorax. The epiglottis and vocal cords open and air is forced out under high pressure. The noncartilaginous bronchi and trachea collapse and air actually passes through a very narrowed airway, taking any foreign material with it. Disease processes or medications may interfere with the cough reflex, leaving the patient susceptible to aspiration.

The *trachea* is a 4½ inch long tube that extends from the distal end of the larynx to the bifurcation of the bronchi (carina). Both the larynx and carina are particularly sensitive to foreign matter and readily stimulate the cough reflex. The trachea is cylindrical in shape and is composed of cartilaginous rings. These rings are incomplete posteriorly and therefore are C-shaped. The trachea shares its posterior surface with the esophagus. The trachea is lined with ciliated epithelial cells that propel dust particles and mucus upward. The vagus nerve is responsible for nervous control of the trachea. Elective tracheostomy is performed by making an incision into the trachea between the second and third tracheal cartilages. Smooth muscle of the trachea is innervated by the parasympathetic branch of the autonomic nervous system.

The trachea divides at its lower end into two main branches, *right bronchus* and *left bronchus.*

The right main stem bronchus is shorter, wider and more vertical than the left. This accounts for aspirated materials frequently entering the lung via the right main stem. The walls of the large bronchi contain incomplete cartilaginous rings. These rings become complete as the bronchi enter the lung. Ciliated mucosa line the bronchi. Each main bronchus enters the lungs and divides into smaller branches, called secondary bronchi, and then further divide into small bronchioles.

The *terminal bronchioles* contain no cartilaginous rings and, therefore, collapse readily, increasing airway resistance. These bronchioles are also lined with ciliated mucosal cells. To this level, the respiratory tract acts as a conduit for air, but no exchange of gases take place. This area is known as *anatomical dead space.* The bronchioles are sensitive to calcium levels; with increased levels of calcium, the bronchioles dilate, and with decreased levels, they constrict.

Three to five terminal bronchioles compose the *lobule* of the lung (Fig. 4-2). The lobule consists of the terminal bronchioles, respiratory bronchioles, alveolar ducts, alveolar sacs, and vessels that supply this area. The respiratory bronchioles differ from the terminal bronchioles in their ability to participate in gas exchange. Respiratory bronchioles have some alveoli lining their surface. Respiratory bronchioles, alveolar ducts and sacs make up the acinus, or the respiratory unit of the lung. It is the unit where actual gas exchange takes place. This unit has a dual blood supply consisting of the bronchial and pulmonary arteries. The pulmonary artery carries unoxygenated blood from the right ventricle to be exchanged for oxygenated blood within the respiratory unit. The bronchial artery, a branch of the aorta, carries oxygenated blood to nourish the tracheobronchial structures and the lung tissue. The pulmonary veins, located at the periphery of the lobules, drain the areas supplied by the pulmonary and bronchial arteries. They carry the blood to the left atrium to be pumped into the systemic circulation.

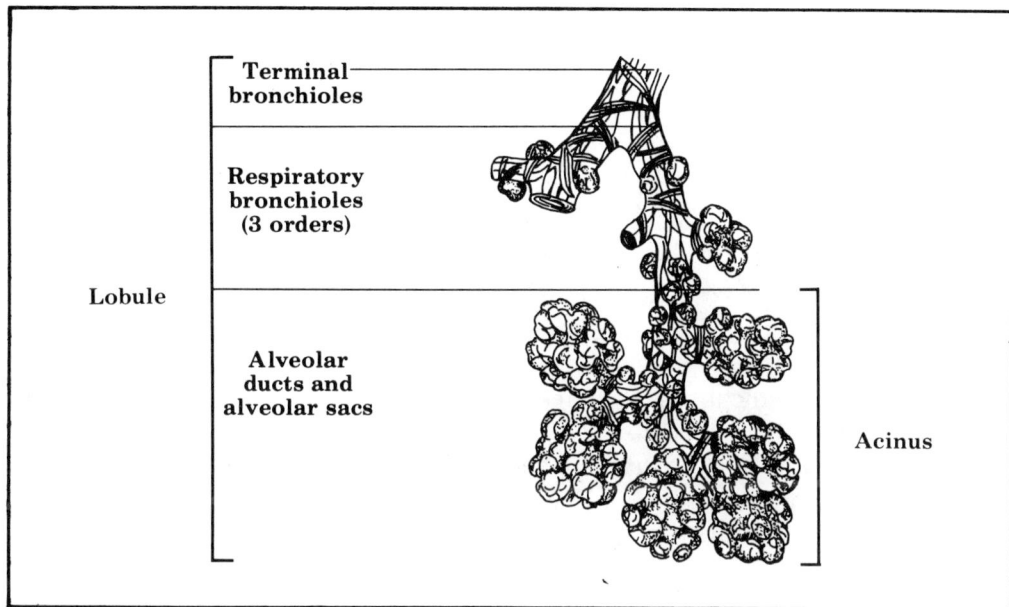

Fig. 4-2. Lobule of lung

The **alveoli** are lined with a continuous layer of epithelium. The average alveoli is approximately 0.2 mm in thickness. The alveolar walls contain capillaries, collagenous material, a basement membrane, and elastic connective tissue fibers. The entire lung parenchyma (respiratory bronchioles, alveolar ducts, air sacs) is covered with an epithelial fluid layer. This plasmalike fluid is constantly produced and mobilized. There are three types of cells that arise out of the membrane separating the alveolar air space and the capillary lumen. Type I cells have little, if any, metabolic activity. They provide the vast surface area for gas diffusion between the alveoli and the pulmonary capillaries. Type II cells are not as plentiful as Type I. They are also responsible for the constant production of epithelial fluid. This alveolar fluid is different than plasma in electrolyte composition. The nuclei of Type II cells have a great number of metabolic functions, few of which are clearly understood. Type II cells are thought to be the site of surfactant production.

Surfactant is a lipoprotein that has a detergentlike quality. It lowers the surface tension. Think of what occurs when a drop of water is placed on a flat surface. It remains in a compact mass because of tension that exists between the atmosphere and the surface of the water. If a detergent is added to the drop, the surface tension is lowered and it spreads out as a thin layer. Surfactant acts similarly on the alveoli. By acting as a detergent, it lowers the surface tension within the alveoli so they do not collapse during expiration. Any conditions causing diminished production or destruction of surfactant result in an increase in surface tension, making it more difficult for the alveoli to reinflate.

Type III cells, known as **macrophages,** originate in the bone marrow. Their nuclei are similar to those of white blood cells. They function as phagocytes, playing an important role in preventing respiratory infections. The thinness of the alveolar wall allows rapid diffusion of gases across its membrane. For an oxygen molecule to diffuse across this membrane from the alveolus to the capillary, it must pass through several layers: alveolar epithelium, alveolar basement membrane, interstitial space, capillary basement membrane, capillary endothelium, plasma, erythrocyte membrane and erythrocyte cytoplasm. At this point, the oxygen molecule attaches to the hemoglobin and is carried in the bloodstream.

KEY CONCEPT: The respiratory tract is divided into the upper airway, lower airway, and alveoli.

KEY POINT RECOGNITION

Write true or false by each statement. Answers are at the end of this chapter. A score below 80% indicates the need for further study.

_____ 1. The ultimate goal of the pulmonary system is the exchange of gas between the atmosphere and blood.

_____ 2. The pharynx has two divisions, the nasopharynx and oropharynx.

_____ 3. The cricoid cartilage is part of the larynx.

_____ 4. In adults, the cricoid cartilage is incomplete.

_____ 5. The trachea is innervated by the vagus nerve.

_____ 6. The right main stem bronchus is shorter, wider, and more vertical than the left.

_____ 7. Anatomical dead space in the respiratory tract acts only as a passage for air.

_____ 8. A lobule of the lung consists of three to five alveoli.

_____ 9. Terminal bronchioles participate in gas exchange.

_____ 10. Type II cells are probably the site of surfactant production.

LUNGS

The ***right lung*** (Fig. 4-3) is divided into three lobes and ten bronchopulmonary segments. The right upper lobe consists of three segments; the right middle lobe consists of two segments; and the right lower lobe consists of four segments. The ***left lung*** is divided into two lobes and eight bronchopulmonary segments. The left upper lobe consists of four segments and the left lower lobe has four segments. The bronchopulmonary segments are a group of lobules that are supplied by the same lobar bronchus. The lingula is a projection of the left upper lobe inferior to a notch caused by the impression of the heart.

Each lung is covered by a serous membrane, or ***pleura,*** and lies within the pleural space. There is a pleural space around each lung, except at the ***hilum***, which contains the main stem bronchi and pulmonary vessels. The mediastinum is the area between the two pleural spaces. Within the mediastinum lie the heart, great vessels, trachea, esophagus, and main stem bronchi. The pleurae are divided into the ***visceral*** pleura, which lines the lungs, and the ***parietal*** pleura, which lines the inner layer of the chest cavity. There is a potential space between the two layers, which are moist and glide easily against one another during respiration. The pleural lining extends about an inch above the clavicles. In the process of inserting subclavian lines, this area can be entered, causing a pneumothorax, especially in patients suffering from emphysema. Their lungs are hyperinflated and tend to extend farther above the clavicles. Although the pleural layers are moist, no measurable amount of fluid is present. In some disease processes, however, fluid accumulates in the pleural cavity. The fluid is of two types: ***transudates*** and ***exudates.*** The transudates have a specific gravity less than 1.015 and a protein content under 2 to 3 g per 100 ml. They are usually clear, but may contain RBCs. Transudates are seen in congestive heart failure, cirrhosis and nephritis. Exudates are usually thicker. They may be clear or cloudy, and they contain numerous cells and bacteria. Exudates are seen with pleural inflammations and infections. Pleural pain is usually associated with inflamed parietal

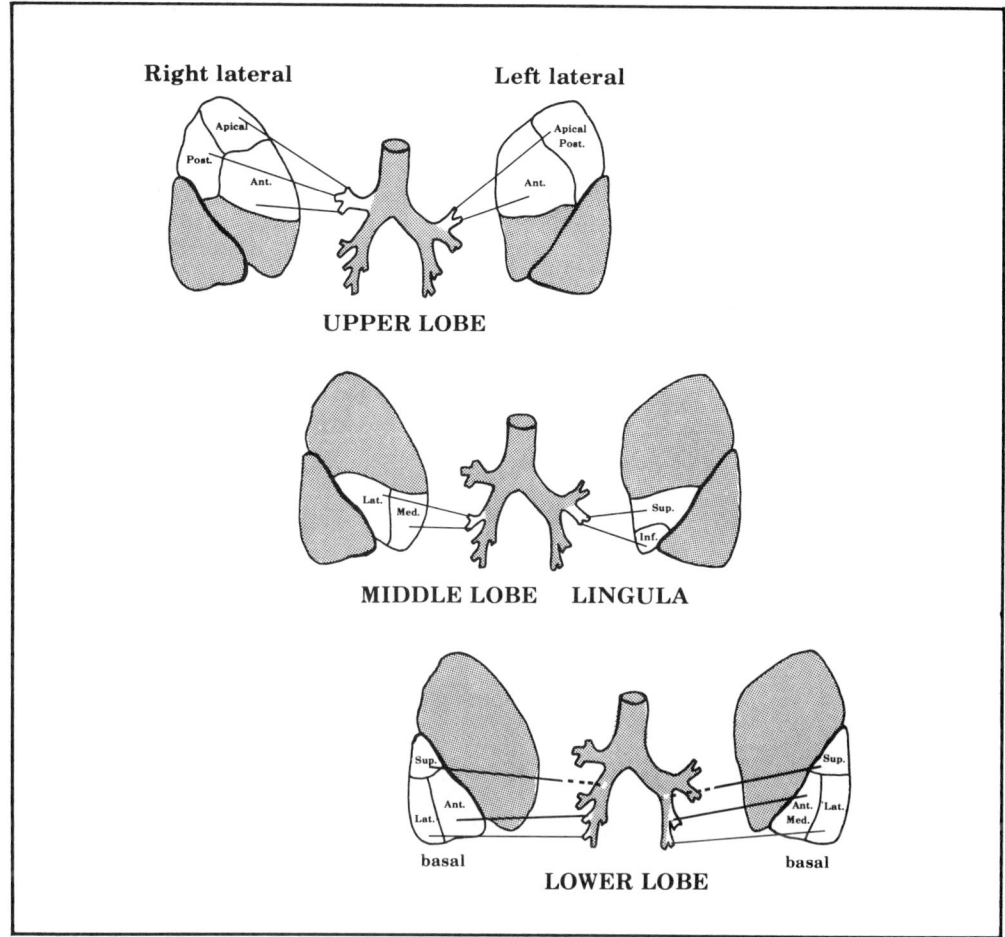

Fig. 4-3. Lobes of the lung

pleurae due to pneumonia, pneumothorax, tumors involving the pleurae, and fibrous pleurisy.

KEY CONCEPT: The lungs are covered by pleura. The right lung has three lobes; the left has two lobes.

BONY THORAX

The skeletal framework of the thorax consists of the 12 pairs of ribs and their cartilages, the sternum, and twelve vertebrae. The costal cartilages are hyaline cartilages. They articulate with the sternum, attaching the first seven ribs, or true ribs. The costal cartilages of the eighth to tenth ribs attach to the cartilage of the preceding rib, not to the sternum. They are called false ribs. The 11th and 12th ribs are free anteriorly, and are called floating or vertebral ribs. The attachment of the ribs to the vertebrae allows for expansion during inspiration. Anteriorly, the costal cartilage that attaches the first rib is fixed. The attachment of the costal cartilages and the other six true ribs are synovial joints that also allow for expansion during inspiration. Costochondritis is a common cause of chest pain and is sometimes initially confused with cardiac pain. The ribs are separated by the intercostal spaces that take their numbers from the rib above. The spaces become progressively wider.

MUSCLES OF RESPIRATION

Inspiration

The muscles of respiration are primarily innervated by the groups of neurons located in the pons and medulla. The inspiratory phase of respiration is the active phase, controlled by the diaphragm and intercostal and abdominal muscles. These muscles contract and the thorax expands. The diaphragm, which is dome-shaped at rest, contracts and flattens, thereby pulling the inferior boundary of the chest wall downward and elevating the lower ribs. The diaphragm is the principal muscle of inspiration. During normal respiration, the diaphragm provides for the movement of approximately two-thirds of the air entering the lungs. This results in the downward expansion of the lungs. The intercostal muscles pull the ribs forward anteriorly, increasing the anterior-posterior diameter. The sternocleidomastoid muscles elevate the sternum and, along with other muscles in the neck (accessory muscles), aid in inspiration and provide assistance in coping with disease processes or strenuous exercise.

Expiration

In contrast to inspiration, expiration is a passive act due to the natural recoil tendency of the lungs. The tendency for the lungs to recoil away from the chest wall and collapse is caused by two factors. First, many elastic fibers throughout the lungs attempt to shorten after being overstretched during inspiration. Second, the surface tension of the fluid lining the alveoli results in their tendency to collapse. Surfactant acts as a detergent in decreasing the surface tension and preventing total collapse of the alveoli. This is a critically important factor because the surface tension accounts for two-thirds of the lungs' recoil tendency. Any process or disease state interfering with the production of surfactant leads to widespread atelectasis and decreased lung compliance.

KEY CONCEPT: Inspiration is active; expiration is passive.

KEY POINT RECOGNITION
Write true or false by each statement. Answers are at the end of this chapter. A score below 80% indicates the need for further study.

    _____ 1. The right middle lobe of the lung consists of two bronchopulmonary segments.
    _____ 2. A bronchopulmonary segment is a group of lobules supplied by the same lobar bronchus.
    _____ 3. The lingula is a projection of the right lower lobe.
    _____ 4. There is a potential space between the layers of the pleura.
    _____ 5. The eighth to tenth ribs are not directly attached to the sternum.
    _____ 6. The muscles of respiration are innervated by neurons in the pons and medulla.
    _____ 7. Expiration is the active phase of respiration.
    _____ 8. During inspiration, the intercostal muscles pull the ribs anteriorly to increase the anterior-posterior diameter of the chest.
    _____ 9. The sternocleidomastoid muscles elevate the sternum.
    _____10. Ribs are separated by the intercostal spaces.

PULMONARY CIRCULATION

The pulmonary system has the ability to adapt in times of crisis and can increase its normal capacity up to 200 percent. Large volumes of blood can be expelled or shunted from the lungs into the systemic circulation in hemorrhagic states. In pathological states, such as left ventricular failure, pulmonary blood volumes increase, resulting in increased pulmonary pressures and decreased systemic pressure and volume. The opposite occurs in right-sided failure; pulmonary blood volumes decrease and systemic pressures increase. These shifts in volumes and pressures affect the pulmonary system more than the systemic circulation, since the blood volumes are normally much less in the lungs.

Because of variations in the hydrostatic pressures of the pulmonary vessels, blood flow distribution through the lungs tends to vary. In the upright position, blood flow into the apices is slight compared to the bases, where it is greater. In the supine position, blood flow tends to redistribute more evenly between the apices and bases.

A ventilatory maldistribution also exists within the lungs. The pleural pressure is more negative in relationship to the atmospheric pressure in the apices as compared to the bases. Normally, the alveoli are more expanded in the apices than in the bases.

During hypoxic states, the pulmonary vasculature constricts. The mechanism responsible for this action is not completely understood. However, as a result of this vasoconstriction, blood is shunted away from poorly ventilated alveoli. This maximizes blood flow to remaining alveoli and results in maximum gas exchange.

The pulmonary artery carries unoxygenated blood from the right ventricles to the lungs. It divides into right and left main branches and supplies both lungs. The walls of the pulmonary artery are thin, approximately one-third that of the aorta. All the pulmonary arteries, including the small arteries and arterioles, have large diameters. Both of these factors result in an increased compliance of these vessels and an ability to accept the right ventricular output. While this is true of the pulmonary arteries, the same does not hold true of the pulmonary veins, whose compliance matches that of the systemic circulation.

The systolic pulmonary artery pressures average 22 mm Hg, with the diastolic averaging 8 mm Hg. This results in an average pulse pressure (mean arterial pressure) of 14 mm Hg. This makes it a low pressure system. The left atrial pressure is 5 mm Hg. The pressure drop between the mean pulmonary artery pressure and mean left atrial pressure produces the blood flow through the lungs.

Both lungs contain about 12 percent of the total volume of the circulatory system. If the hypoxemia persists, right ventricular failure may result because of the chronic increase in pulmonary pressures.

KEY POINT RECOGNITION

Write true or false by each statement. Answers are at the end of this chapter.

_____ 1. The systolic pulmonary artery pressures average 8 mm Hg.

_____ 2. The drop between the mean pulmonary artery pressure and mean left atrial pressure causes blood to flow through the lungs.

_____ 3. In right-sided heart failure, pulmonary blood volumes decrease and systemic pressures increase.

_____ 4. In hypoxic states, blood is shunted away from poorly ventilated alveoli to maximize gas exchange in the remaining alveoli.

_____ 5. A chronic increase in pulmonary pressures may result in right ventricular failure.

PHYSIOLOGY

VENTILATION

The movement of gas volumes between the atmosphere and alveoli, which is necessary to maintain concentrations of CO_2 and O_2, is known as **ventilation.** Lung volume is important in ventilation. Lung volume has the following subdivisions:

Tidal volume (V_T): The volume of gas inspired and expired during a normal respiratory cycle. Tidal volume is further divided into two portions:

Dead space volume (Vd) fills the respiratory passages not participating in gas exchange;

Alveolar volume (Va) passages participate in gas exchange. The dead space volume averages 150 ml in an average adult. For every breath, approximately one-third is wasted and does not participate in gas exchange. Therefore, V_T = Vd + Va.

Inspiratory reserve volume (IRV): The volume that can be inspired above the tidal volume

Expiratory reserve volume (ERV): The maximal volume that can be expired below the tidal volume

Residual volume (RV): The volume of gas remaining in the lungs at the end of maximal expiration

There are four *lung capacities,* each of which includes two or more of the primary volumes:

Total lung capacity (TLC): The volume of gas contained in the lungs at the end of a maximal inspiratory effort; TLC = V_T + IRV + ERV + RV

Vital capacity: The volume of gas expelled from the lungs following a maximal inspiration and forced expiration; VC = V_T + IRV + ERV

Inspiratory Capacity (IC): The maximal volume of gas that can be inspired from the resting expiratory level; IC = V_T + IRV

Functional residual capacity (FRC): The volume of gas remaining in the lungs at the resting expiratory level; FRC = ERV + RV

FLOW MEASUREMENTS

Forced vital capacity (FVC) is the volume of gas forcibly exhaled.

Timed forced capacity (FEV_T) is the forced vital capacity over a set period of time.

Restrictive lung disease, such as pulmonary fibrosis and pleural thickening, causes a reduction in vital capacity and in all other lung volumes. There is, however, no restriction in the outflow of air. In obstructive diseases, such as emphysema and asthma, expiratory flow is decreased.

ALVEOLAR VENTILATION (Va)

Alveolar ventilation is the part of total ventilation taking part in gas exchange. *Minute ventilation* (Ve) is the total amount of air breathed in one minute. This includes dead space and alveolar ventilation. Therefore, Ve = Vd + Va; V = volume per minute.

There is no effective way to measure alveolar ventilation. It is indirectly measured by monitoring arterial pCO_2 levels. This is possible because the amount of CO_2 resulting from metabolizing cells is equal to the amount of CO_2 excreted in the lungs. Theoretically, if arterial pCO_2 levels are normal, alveolar ventilation is providing adequate oxygen levels. If alveolar ventilation is increased (hyperventilation) then pCO_2 levels are low because the lungs "blow off" CO_2. If alveolar ventilation is depressed (hypoventilation), then pCO_2 levels are increased.

KEY CONCEPT: Ventilation is the movement of effective concentrations of O_2 and CO_2 between the atmosphere and alveoli.

REGULATION OF VENTILATION

The *respiratory center* is divided into three major areas: the *medulla rhythmicity area,* the *apneustic area* and the *pneumotaxic area.*

The **medulla** is the center in which the basic rhythm of inspiration and expiration is established. It is postulated that two oscillating circuits exist, one for inspiration and one for expiration. These two cannot oscillate simultaneously because they mutually inhibit each other. Thus when one is activated, the other is inactive. This process, therefore, accounts for the rhythmic act of respiration.

The **apneustic** and **pneumotaxic** areas are located in the pons. Neither of these centers is necessary for the basic pattern of respiration. Normally, the inspiratory phase of respiration is ended by the pneumotaxic center and the Hering-Breuer reflex stimulating the expiratory neurons. Thus expiration begins when inspiration ends. The apneustic center stimulates the inspiratory neurons. If for some reason the pneumotaxic center is not functioning, the inspiratory phase is prolonged and increased in depth, while the expiratory phase is shortened. This is called **apneusis.**

Changes in respiration may occur as a result of stimuli arriving in the respiratory center from other parts of the nervous system. These include exercise, pain or any other stressful situation.

When the lungs become distended enough during inspiration, stretch receptors send inhibitory impulses via the vagus nerve to the respiratory center. These impulses cause the respiratory muscles to relax, and expiration follows. This is called the **Hering-Breuer expiratory reflex.** When the lungs sufficiently deflate to inhibit these receptors, inspiration begins again. This is the Hering-Breuer *inspiratory* reflex.

When the body temperature is increased, the respiratory center is stimulated to initiate a panting type respiration. This results in an increase of fresh air and humidity within the respiratory passages. This process cools the body by evaporation of water. Because the respirations are extremely shallow, most air entering the alveoli is dead space air. Therefore, an excessive amount of CO_2 is not lost, thus preventing respiratory alkalosis.

The major control of alveolar ventilation is the level of CO_2 in the body. Carbon dioxide causes an almost proportional increase in the hydrogen ion concentration in all body fluids. Hydrogen ion concentration is the major influence in stimulating the medullary center, but CO_2 also has a stimulating effect. This stimulation occurs in two ways: direct diffusion of CO_2 and H^+ ions from the blood to the respiratory center and, to a lesser extent, the hydrogen ion concentration of the cerebrospinal fluid (CSF) surrounding the brainstem. Carbon dioxide diffuses more rapidly across the blood-brain barrier than H^+ or HCO_3 ions. Therefore, the response of the respiratory center to metabolic acidosis (e.g. diabetic) or alkalosis (e.g. loss of HCl in vomiting) is slower than the effect of primary changes in alveolar ventilation. In metabolic acidosis, the CSF pH falls slowly, within hours. It stimulates the respiratory center to increase alveolar ventilation (Kussmaul respirations), which results in a drop in pCO_2 levels in an attempt to offset the decrease in arterial pH. In metabolic alkalosis, the CSF pH rises, causing alveolar ventilation to decrease, with a resulting rise in PCO_2 levels. This aids in offsetting the rise in arterial pH. Decreasing alveolar ventilation (increased pCO_2 levels) and increasing hydrogen ion concentration results primarily in rapid stimulation of the respiratory center. The result is an increase in alveolar ventilation and the return of the pCO_2 to normal. In contrast, when the pCO_2 levels drop, the effect on the respiratory center is diminished. The decreased levels of CO_2 and hydrogen ion concentrations cause reduced alveolar ventilation and a critical fall in the level of the pO_2. This in turn stimulates the peripheral chemoreceptors to stimulate alveolar ventilation and thus decrease the depressing effects of the low pCO_2 levels. This is frequently seen when overzealously ambulating a patient. The alveolar ventilation is increased, thereby decreasing the pCO_2 levels. The patient's respiratory drive is diminished and it takes a few seconds for spontaneous breathing to begin.

Under normal circumstances, oxygen plays a very small role in the control of respirations. Once reason is the ability of plasma pO_2 levels to stay relatively constant in the face of major ventilatory changes. Alveolar ventilation may decrease by half or increase ten times, and plasma oxygen concentration will stay fairly stable. Another reason is that even a slight increase in respiration resulting from hypoxia causes CO_2 to be "blown off," thereby inhibiting respirations. pCO_2 levels, on the other hand, change radically in response to changes in alveolar ventilation.

Peripheral chemoreceptors are located in the bifurcation of the carotid arteries and the arch of the aorta. They are responsive to changes in oxygen, carbon dioxide and hydrogen ion concentrations. When the arterial oxygen concentration ranges from 30 mm Hg to 60 mm Hg, receptors in the carotid bodies and the aortic arch stimulate the respiratory centers via the glossopharyngeal and vagus nerves, respectively. This results in increased alveolar ventilation. The CO_2 and hydrogen ion concentrations have the same stimulating effect on the respiratory center.

Factors that increase blood pressure also increase the respiratory rate. Baroreceptors located in the aortic arch and carotid bodies respond to elevations in arterial blood pressure and send signals to the central nervous system, resulting in decreased cardiac output and vasodilation. This has the effect of lowering the blood pressure. In turn, it lowers the respiratory rate.

Drugs that depress the respiratory center, such as morphine, depress not only the resting level of alveolar ventilation, but also decrease the ability of the respiratory center to respond to increases in alveolar pCO_2.

KEY CONCEPT: The respiratory center regulates ventilation.

KEY POINT RECOGNITION

Write true or false by each statement. Answers are at the end of this chapter. A score below 80% indicates the need for further study.

_____ 1. The volume of gas inspired and expired during a normal respiratory cycle is the residual volume.

_____ 2. Alveolar volume includes the passages that participate in gas exchange.

_____ 3. Expiratory reserve volume is the volume remaining in the lungs at the end of maximal respiration.

_____ 4. Vital capacity = V_T + IRV + ERV

_____ 5. Alveolar ventilation is measured indirectly by monitoring arterial pCO_2 levels.

_____ 6. The basic rhythm of respiration is established by the medulla.

_____ 7. The Hering-Breuer expiratory reflex causes the respiratory muscles to relax, resulting in expiration.

_____ 8. Oxygen level is the major control of alveolar ventilation.

_____ 9. Peripheral chemoreceptors stimulate alveolar ventilation in response to decreased CO_2 levels.

_____ 10. Chronic hypercapnea diminishes the effect of the CO_2 mechanism controlling respirations.

MECHANICS OF BREATHING

Because of the natural tendency of the lungs to recoil away from the chest wall and the tendency of the chest wall to recoil in the opposite direction, a negative pressure is created. Atmospheric pressure is approximately 760 mm Hg, and the intrathoracic pressure averages 765 mm Hg. This results in a negative pressure in the intrapleural space of -5 mm Hg. During inspiration, the thorax expands and the intrathoracic volume increases, dropping intrapleural pressures. Air flows into the lungs because of the gradient created between atmospheric and intrathoracic pressures. During expiration, pressures rise above atmospheric pressure because of the compression of the thorax and the decrease in volume. Air, therefore, flows out of the lungs. Maximal inspiratory efforts can decrease intrapulmonary pressures as low as -80 mm Hg.

KEY CONCEPT: The changes in pressure gradients are responsible for the mechanics of respiration.

COMPLIANCE

Both the lungs and thorax can expand. This expandability is called **compliance.** Any disease process or condition that increases compliance also increases the work of breathing. It is expressed as the volume increase in the lung for each unit increase in intra-alveolar pressure (cmH_2O). The relationship between pressure and volume is the amount of pressure required to exert a given pressure in lung volume. **Static compliance** is the change in lung volume per unit change in airway pressure when the lungs are motionless. The normal static compliance in an upright adult is 100 ml/cm H_2O. **Effective compliance** is particularly useful during mechanical ventilation. It is measured by dividing the tidal volume by the peak airway pressure. This is normally 50 ml/cm H_2O.

Compliance is decreased by any disease process that results in stiffer lungs, such as pulmonary fibrosis, atelectasis, pulmonary edema or pneumonia. Pneumothorax and pleural effusions diminish the space necessary for the lungs to occupy, thereby impeding lung expansion. Obesity, kyphoscoliosis and abdominal distention decrease the ability of the chest wall to expand. Compliance is increased in patients with COPD. Their lungs are easily expanded and stay expanded.

AIRWAY RESISTANCE

Airway resistance is the relationship between pressure and flow. A certain amount of pressure is needed to move the air along the respiratory passages. Normally, this energy is minimal, but when an obstruction is present (asthma, secretions, emphysema), a large amount of energy is needed by the muscles to move the air through the narrowed passages. Airway resistance depends on the viscosity of the gas, length of the airway, radius of the airway and velocity of the flow. Increased airway resistance can be detected by measuring expiratory flow rates. Disease processes causing increased airway resistance are called **obstructive ventilatory defects.**

DIFFUSION

Diffusion is the movement of gas from an area of higher concentration to a lesser concentration. In the lungs, the ability to exchange gases is called **diffusing capacity.** Several factors affect the ability of gases to diffuse across the respiratory membrane, including: the thickness of the membrane; the surface area of the membrane; the diffusion coefficient of the gas in H_2O; the pressure difference between the gases on the two sides of the membrane; and the amount of hemoglobin in the blood.

The diffusion coefficient is related to the solubility of a gas in liquid. Carbon dioxide is more soluble in a liquid (water) than oxygen and diffuses 20 times more rapidly than oxygen. The diffusion rate of a gas is dependent upon the difference of the partial pressures of that gas in the alveoli and capillary blood. This pressure gradient is the driving pressure, which causes gases to exchange across the alveolar-capillary membrane.

The force that causes a gas molecule to enter a liquid is the **pressure** of the gas. The force that causes gas molecules to escape from a liquid is called the **tension** of the gas in the liquid. In a steady state, the number of gas molecules leaving a liquid must be equal to the number entering the liquid. Therefore, during a steady state in a gas exposed to a liquid, pressure is equal to tension. In a mixture of gases, all gas molecules collide with the surface of the liquid with equal frequency. These collisions are responsible for the tendency of the gas molecules to dissolve in the liquid. In a mixture of gases, the pressure exerted by each type of gas molecule is called the **partial pressure** of that gas and is designated by the symbol "p".

Alveolar pCO_2 is normally 40 mm Hg. The pCO_2 in the pulmonary artery is approximately 45 mm Hg. Carbon dioxide moves into the alveoli because of this gradient and results in the pCO_2 in the pulmonary veins being 40 mm Hg (normal arterial pCO_2). Conversely, the alveolar pO_2 is normally 100 mm Hg, and the pO_2 in the pulmonary artery is 40 mm Hg. O_2 molecules move from alveoli to pulmonary veins, resulting in the arterial pO_2 of 100 mm Hg. The increased thickness of the alveolar membrane may be due to interstitial edema, fibrosis, consolidation or alveolar edema. The decrease in the surface area may be due to the removal of an entire lung or to emphysema due to the diminished alveolar surface area. The time it takes oxygen to combine with hemoglobin depends on the number of red blood cells and the amount of hemoglobin they contain. The distance the oxygen must travel to reach the hemoglobin is increased if the pulmonary capillaries are dilated, or if there is hemodilution with an increased percentage of plasma.

Because of interposing membranes and the distance between the alveoli and plasma, an A-a (A-aDO_2) gradient exists. This is simply the difference between the alveoli oxygen tension (PAO_2) and the plasma oxygen tension (PaO_2). This difference is normally 10 to 15 mm Hg with a patient breathing room air. This gives an indicator of how efficiently the oxygen is diffusing. The A-a gradient is increased by venous admixture, uneven ventilation in relation to perfusion, alveolar hypoventilation, and impaired diffusion. All of these, except venous admixture, may be corrected by breathing 100 percent O_2. By breathing 100 percent O_2, the alveolar pO_2 is increased, thereby increasing the driving pressure and increasing arterial pO_2. One method for determining adequate lung functioning is to calculate the A-a gradient or the alveolar-arterial oxygen difference. The following formula is used to calculate this difference. (Room air):

FIO_2 PB −47)− $PaCO_2$ ÷1.25)−PaO_2=A−a gradient

FIO_2 is the fraction of inspired oxygen.

PB is the barometric pressure of the atmosphere (760 mm Hg).

47 is water vapor temperature at body temperature (37°C).

$PaCO_2$ is arterial CO_2.

1.25 is the respiratory quotient, the estimated amount of CO_2 produced to O_2 consumed per unit time (40 x 1.25 = 50).

Therefore,

```
  760  PB                150
-  47  H2O             -  50
  ───                    ───
  713                    100  alveolar pO2
×  21% FIO2            -  90  PaO2
  ───                    ───
  713                     10  A-a gradient (A-a DO2)
 1426
  ─────
 149.7 = 150
```

KEY POINT RECOGNITION

Write true or false by each statement. Answers are at the end of this chapter. A score below 80% indicates the need for further study.

_____ 1. During inspiration the thorax expands, the intrathoracic volume increases and intrapleural pressures drop.

_____ 2. On expiration, air flows out of the lungs because of a rise in pressure above 760 mm Hg.

_____ 3. Compliance is expressed as the volume increase in the lung for each unit increase in intra-alveolar pressure.

_____ 4. Normal static compliance in an upright compliance is 200 ml/cm H_2O.

_____ 5. Compliance is decreased in atelectasis.

_____ 6. The relationship between pressure and volume is known as airway resistance.

_____ 7. The force that causes a gas molecule to enter a liquid is the tension of the gas in the liquid.

_____ 8. Alveolar pCO_2 is normally 40 mm Hg.

_____ 9. The difference between the alveolar oxygen tension and the plasma oxygen tension is normally 10 to 15 mm Hg on room air.

_____10. Alveolar hypoventilation decreases the A-a gradient.

OXYGEN TRANSPORT

Ninety-seven percent of the oxygen transported in the blood is bound to hemoglobin, and only 3 percent is dissolved in plasma. PO_2 is a reflection of dissolved oxygen only. The amount of oxygen combined with hemoglobin is dependent on the partial pressure of oxygen. The relationship between the amount of oxygen combined with hemoglobin and the partial pressure of oxygen in the blood is reflected in the oxyhemoglobin dissociation curve. The maximal amount of oxygen that can be carried by 1 g of hemoglobin is 1.34 ml. Oxygen capacity, therefore, is equal to the Hb x 1.34. This is expressed as ml of O_2 per 100 ml of blood (volume percent). The oxygen content is the actual amount of oxygen contained in blood.

O_2 content = O_2 capacity x O_2 saturation (volume percent)

The actual amount of oxygen in chemical combination with hemoglobin in relation to the maximal amount of oxygen the hemoglobin can carry is referred to as the

O_2 saturation (SaO_2) $\quad SaO_2 = \dfrac{O_2 \text{ content}}{O_2 \text{ capacity}} \times 100 \text{ percent}$

The oxygen saturation of arterial blood with a pO_2 of 100 mm Hg is approximately 98 percent.

Oxygen has a great affinity for hemoglobin. The upper flat portion of the oxyhemoglobin dissociation curve ensures that arterial oxygen content remains high and relatively constant despite reductions in the oxygen tension of the blood. The middle steep part of the curve allows the release of large quantities of oxygen from hemoglobin at lower oxygen tensions in the capillary blood. When the pO_2 is high, as in pulmonary capillaries, oxygen-hemoglobin binding is strong. When the pO_2 is low, as in tissues, hemoglobin gives up oxygen quite easily. The curve shifts to the right (more O_2 given up for a given pO_2) when pH decreases, pCO_2 increases (acidosis) and temperature increases. The curve shifts to the left (O_2 not dissociated from Hb readily) when the pH rises, pCO_2 decreases (alkalosis) and temperature decreases.

A state of alkalosis can prove to be more dangerous to the patient than a state of acidosis. Acidosis is often more easily reversed. Once a patient is alkalotic, it takes a longer period of time to correct the abnormality. In the face of an adequate pO_2 and high pH, even though there is adequate oxygen circulating, little might be diffusing into the tissues because of the strong bond with hemoglobin. Caution must be used in calculating the amount of $NaHCO_3$ given to correct acidosis to prevent producing a severe alkalosis. Overventilation on a respirator through a large tidal volume or increased rate can also cause severe alkalosis. Frequent blood gases and correction of the alkalosis should be undertaken as soon as possible.

The normal levels of 2, 3-dephosphoglycerate (DPG) keep the hemoglobin dissociation curve constantly shifted slightly to the right. In hypoxic conditions, the concentration of DPG increases, thus shifting the curve further to the right. This shift allows more O_2 to be released from the hemoglobin. Although this seems to be an excellent compensatory mechanism for hypoxia, it has also been shown that increased DPG makes it more difficult for the blood to absorb oxygen in the lungs. This often creates as much harm as benefit.

KEY CONCEPT: Ninety-seven percent of O_2 transported is bound to hemoglobin. Three percent is dissolved in plasma. The amount of oxygen combined with Hgb is dependent on the partial pressure of oxygen and is reflected in the oxyhemoglobin dissociation curve.

CARBON DIOXIDE TRANSPORT

Carbon dioxide is carried in the blood in a number of ways: physically dissolved (arterial pCO_2), chemically combined with hemoglobin, and in the form of bicarbonate (HCO_3). Only 7 percent of the body's total CO_2 content is transported in a dissolved state.

The dissolved CO_2 reacts with H_2O to form carbonic acid (H_2CO_3). Carbonic anhydrase (red blood cell enzyme) catalyzes the reaction between CO_2 and H_2O. This allows tremendous amounts of CO_2 to react with the red cell water even before the blood leaves the tissue capillaries. The carbonic acid (H_2CO_3) rapidly dissociates into hydrogen and bicarbonate ions. Only a small fraction of carbonic acid remains in the undissociated form. Most of the hydrogen ions formed inside the red blood cell are buffered by hemoglobin. The hydrogen ions leave the red blood cell and large quantities of bicarbonate ions remain. Many of these ions then diffuse into the plasma in exchange for chloride. This phenomenon is called the ***chloride shift.*** It results in the chloride level of venous blood being higher than arterial blood.

$$CO_2 + H_2O \xrightarrow{Ca} H_2CO_3 \longrightarrow H^+ \text{(Hb buffer)} + HCO_3^-$$

Carbon dioxide transported in this manner accounts for 60 to 70 percent of the CO_2 in the body.

CO_2 also reacts directly with hemoglobin to form a loose bond. In this form, it is called carbaminohemoglobin. CO_2 can combine more readily with reduced hemoglobin than with oxyhemoglobin. In the tissues, the Haldane effect causes increased pickup of CO_2 because of oxygen removal from the hemoglobin; in the lungs, it causes increased release of CO_2 because of O_2 pickup by the hemoglobin.

KEY CONCEPT: CO_2 is carried in the blood physically dissolved, chemically combined with Hgb and in the form of bicarbonate.

ARTERIAL HYPOXEMIA

Low inspired oxygen tension is usually due to high altitudes and, even with normal ventilation, results in hypoxemia. This leads to hyperventilation and a lower-than-normal pCO_2 level. If the lungs are normal, the A-a gradient will be normal.

Primary alveolar hypoventilation is hypoxemia due to hypoventilation and is always accompanied by hypercapnea (increased CO_2). It is most often associated with airway obstruction, such as emphysema or chronic bronchitis, or with pulmonary edema. Other causes include depression of the respiratory centers, abnormalities of the chest wall and respiratory muscle weakness or paralysis.

In ventilation (V) perfusion (Q) abnormalities, the most common cause for hypoxemia is the mismatching of ventilation and perfusion. Under normal conditions, the lung has an average alveolar ventilation of approximately 4 L/minute and a perfusion of approximately 5 L/minute, so the average V/Q for the entire lung is 0.8. Ideally, this would be 1.0 if each alveoli were ventilated and accompanied by the maximal amount of perfusion. For example, blood pools in the bases, but alveolar ventilation is lower, resulting in an excess of perfusion to ventilation.

If any areas of the lung are underventilated, as in atelectasis, there is too little ventilation (relative shunt) for the amount of perfusion. An absolute shunt occurs when no alveolar ventilation occurs. Usually the V/Q ratio is decreased (less than 0.8), similar to a right-to-left shunt, because the blood in these areas does not have the opportunity to pick up its supply of O_2 and returns to the left atrium. Hypoxemia results because the areas of functioning alveoli cannot be supersaturated with oxygen to compensate for underventilated areas. When the V/Q is increased (greater than 0.8), there is normal ventilation with diminished blood flow, as in pulmonary emboli. This is called ***wasted ventilation*** and is usually associated with excessive respiratory work. The physiologic dead space includes not only what is in the airways, but also gas contained in alveoli that are ventilated with no perfusion. Neither takes part in gas exchange. Both absolute and relative shunts result in venous admixture.

Right to left shunting occurs when blood goes from the right side of the heart to the left side without being oxygenated. Shunting occurs in many disease processes, such as end arteriovenous malformations, ARDS, pneumonia, pulmonary edema, intracardiac right-to-left shunts and vascular lung tumors. Normal physiologic shunting is approximately 2 to 5 percent of the cardiac output. Arterial pO_2 cannot be elevated by breathing 100 percent O_2 because the blood does not come into contact with ventilated alveoli. The pCO_2 levels are not normally elevated because of increased alveolar ventilation due to stimulation of the respiratory center. Shunting may be measured by comparing mixed venous blood O_2 (pulmonary artery) and arterial O_2. The shunt is estimated by allowing the patient to breathe 100 percent O_2 for 15 minutes. Breathing 100 percent O_2 usually raises the pO_2 to over 550 mm Hg. Lesser values may indicate a right to left shunt. The patient's cardiac output must also be considered.

Diffusion problems result from a thickened alveolar capillary membrane, usually due to disease processes such as interstitial pulmonary fibrosis and sarcoidosis. Pulmonary edema may cause diffusion problems because of the accumulation of fluid in the interstitial space and often in the alveoli. Normally, these defects are not associated with an increase in arterial pCO_2. However, secretions may accumulate in pulmonary edema to the extent that air flow is obstructed. This results in an elevated pCO_2. Aside from pulmonary edema, giving the patient 100 percent O_2 can correct diffusion defects.

KEY POINT RECOGNITION
Write true or false by each statement. Answers are at the end of this chapter. A score below 80% indicates the need for further study.

_____ 1. Ninety-seven percent of oxygen transported in the blood is dissolved in the plasma.

_____ 2. The amount of oxygen combined with Hgb is dependent on the partial pressure of oxygen.

_____ 3. The maximal amount of O_2 that can be carried by 1 g of Hgb is 1.34 ml.

_____ 4. Oxygen saturation is the actual amount of O_2 in the blood.

_____ 5. Sixty to 70 percent of CO_2 in the body is known as carbaminohemoglobin.

_____ 6. Low inspired oxygen tissue due to high altitudes may result in hypoxemia.

_____ 7. Hypoxemia due to hyperventilation is accompanied by hypercapnea.

_____ 8. Shunting may occur in pulmonary edema.

_____ 9. Normal physiologic shunting is about 2 to 5 percent of the cardiac output.

_____ 10. Diffusion problems result from a thickened alveolar capillary membrane.

ACID-BASE

Some definitions are necessary to the understanding of acid-base balance:

Acid—a proton (H+) donor; ex. H_2CO_3 (carbonic acid)

Base—a proton (H+) acceptor; ex. HCO_3 (bicarbonate)

pH—a term used to describe hydrogen ion concentration; the more hydrogen ions present in solution, the lower the pH for that solution. If the hydrogen ion concentration is low, the pH is higher. The pH is equal to the negative log of the hydrogen ion concentration. A neutral solution has a pH of 7.00. Normal range is 7.35 to 7.45, although 7.40 is considered normal.

pO_2—partial pressure of oxygen dissolved in plasma

pCO_2—partial pressure of carbon dioxide dissolved in plasma; normal pCO_2 is 40 mm Hg.

Acidemia—an acid condition of the blood—pH < 7.35

Alkalemia—an alkaline condition of the blood—pH > 7.45

Acidosis—the process causing the acidemia; that is, high hydrogen ion concentration

Alkalosis—the process causing the alkalemia; that is, low hydrogen ion concentration

Buffer Systems

A buffer is a substance that reacts to diminish the change in pH decrease that occurs when hydrogen ions are added to a solution. There are basically three types of buffering systems:

Chemical buffers

pCO_2 (respiratory component)

HCO_3 (renal component)

Chemical buffers include the bicarbonate, phosphate and protein buffer systems.

Chemical Buffers

The ***bicarbonate buffer system*** usually consists of carbonic acid (H_2CO_3) and sodium bicarbonate ($NaHCO_3$). Carbonic acid is a very weak acid. It rapidly dissociates into CO_2 and H_2O, leaving a high concentration of dissolved CO_2 and a weak concentration of acid. It does not readily dissociate into $H+$ and HCO_3^-.

The following reaction takes place when a strong acid, such as hydrochloric acid (HCl), is added to a solution with bicarbonate salt:

$$HCl + NaHCO_3 \rightarrow H_2CO_3 + NaCl$$

As a result of this reaction, a strong acid (HCl) is transformed into a weak acid (H_2CO_3).

When a strong base, such as sodium hydroxyl (NaDH), is added to a solution containing carbonic acid (H_2CO_3), the following reaction takes place:

$$NaOH + H_2CO_3 \rightarrow NaHCO_3 + H_2O$$

This reaction changes a strong base (NaOH) into a weak base ($NaHCO_3$). The pH will rise slightly.

The **phosphate buffer system** consists of two elements, hydrogen monophosphate (HPO_4) and phosphate (H_2PO_4). This system functions in much the same way as the bicarbonate buffer system. In the following reaction, a strong acid (HCl) is added to a solution containing $HPO_4 + H_2PO_4$:

$$HCl + Na_2HPO_4 \rightarrow NaH_2PO_4 + NaCl$$

Hydrochloric acid has been replaced by the weak acid, sodium phosphate (NaH_2PO_4). The pH will drop only slightly in response to this weaker acid.

If a strong base, sodium hydroxide (NaOH), is added to a similar solution, the following response takes place:

$$NaOH + NaH_2PO_4 \rightarrow Na_2HPO_4 + H_2O$$

Sodium hydroxide is changed to form water and sodium monophosphate (Na_2HPO_4), a weak base. Thus the pH will rise only slightly in response to the weaker base.

The **protein buffer system** consists of the proteins of the cells and plasma, which constitute the most plentiful buffers in the body. Carbon dioxide can diffuse through the cell membrane, as well as bicarbonate ions, although not to the same extent. As a result, the pH within the cells changes in proportion to the extracellular fluid. These buffer systems within the cells aid in buffering the extracellular fluid.

Respiratory Component

Cell metabolism produces and consumes acid. Complete combustion of the by-products of metabolism yields $CO_2 + H_2O$. Carbon dioxide is considered a potential acid because when it is combined with water, carbonic acid is produced:

$$CO_2 + H_2O \rightleftharpoons H_2CO_3 \rightleftharpoons H+ + HCO_3$$

This equation is reversible and is closely associated with the bicarbonate buffer system. The carbon dioxide produced by metabolism is excreted by the lungs. Fixed volatile acids are also produced during metabolism and are not combusted to $CO_2 + H_2O$. These acids must be excreted by the kidneys.

The partial pressure of carbon dioxide (pCO_2) is the partial pressure of CO_2 in a gas phase. The normal pCO_2 level is 40 mm Hg. Dissolved carbon dioxide is the concentrate of physically dissolved carbon dioxide and includes carbonic acid. Normal dissolved carbon dioxide concentration is 1.2 mm/L. This number is derived by multiplying $pCO_2 \times S$. S is equal to the solubility factor of CO_2. Therefore: $40 \times .03 = 1.2$ mm/L.

The **Henderson-Hasselbalch equation** relates the pH level of acid and the concentration of base.

$$pH = pK + \log HCO_3 \text{ (base) } 24$$
$$H_2CO_3 + \text{dissolved } CO_2 \text{ (acid) } 1.2$$

The pK relates to the pH at the level that dissociated substances are equal to the concentration of associated substances. The release of a hydrogen ion in solution is an example of dissociation. ($H^+ \rightarrow H^+ + Cl^-$)

The removal of a hydrogen ion from a solution is an example of association. ($NH+3 + H^+ \rightarrow NH_4$.) Both dissociation and association occur simultaneously in solution. In an equation, this is indicated by arrows in both directions. The arrows may be drawn so that their relative sizes show the tendencies for dissociation and association. The larger arrows point to the substance in greater quantity at equilibrium.

$$H_3PO_4 \rightleftharpoons H^+ + H_2PO_4^-$$
$$H_xCO_3 \rightleftharpoons H^+ + HCO_3^-$$

The pH at which carbonic acid is in equalibrium is 6.1. Therefore, the pK of H_2CO_3 is 6.1.

There is a direct or linear relationship between the log (logarithm) of bicarbonate to dissolved CO_2 and carbonic acid.

Abbreviated Logarithm Table
   log of 10 = 1.00 because 10^1 = 10
   log of 20 = 1.30 because $10^{1.3}$ = 20
   log of 30 = 1.56 because $10^{1.56}$ = 30

Example:

$$pH = pK + \log \frac{HCO_3^-}{\text{dissolved } CO_2 + H_2CO_3} \quad pCO_2 = 40 \text{ mm Hg}$$

$$pH = 6.1 + \log \frac{HCO_3^-}{pCO_2 \times 0.03} \quad HCO_3 = 24 \text{ meq/L}$$

$$pH = 6.1 + \log \frac{24}{40 \times 0.03}$$

$$pH = 6.1 + \log \frac{24}{1.2}$$

pH = 6.1 + log 20 (ratio of 24 to 1.2 = 20:1)
pH = 6.1 + 1.3
pH = 7.40 (neutral pH)

The body attempts to keep this 20:1 ratio at all times and under any circumstances, but the numbers are not the key factors. It is the ratio that must remain constant.

Example:

$$pH = pK + \log \frac{HCO_3}{\text{dissolved } CO_2 + H_2CO_3} \quad pCO_2 = 40 \text{ mm Hg}$$
$$HCO_3 = 12 \text{ meq/L}$$

$$pH = pK + \log \frac{12}{pCO_2 \times 0.03}$$

$$pH = 6.1 + \log \frac{12}{40 \text{ mm Hg} \times 0.03}$$

$$pH = 6.1 + \log \frac{12}{1.2}$$

pH = 6.1 + log 10 (ratio of 12:.2 = 10:1)
pH = 6.1 + 1.00
pH = 7.10 (acidotic pH)

Example:

$$pH = Pk + \log \frac{HCO_3}{\text{dissolved } CO_2 + H_2CO_3} \quad \begin{array}{l} pCO_2 = 40 \text{ mm Hg} \\ HCO_3^- = 36 \text{ meq/L} \end{array}$$

$$pH = pK + \log \frac{HCO_3}{pCO_2 \times 0.03}$$

$$pH = 6.1 + \log \frac{36}{40 \times 0.03}$$

$$pH = 6.1 + \log \frac{36}{1.2}$$

$pH = 6.1 + \log 30$ (ratio of 36:1.2 = 30:1)

$pH = 6.1 + 1.56$

$pH = 7.66$ (alkalotic pH)

The lungs have the ability to blow off CO_2. The relationship between the rate of alveolar ventilation and the level of alveolar pCO_2 must be examined in order to understand the significance of the arterial pCO_2 level. When the rate of alveolar ventilation increases, the level of pCO_2 decreases. The opposite occurs with a decreased rate of alveolar ventilation. There is an increase in the pCO_2 level. These changes only affect the denominator (dissolved CO_2 + H_2CO_3) of the Henderson-Hasselbalch equation, thereby changing the ratio. The lungs may also respond to changes in plasma HCO_3 levels to maintain this ratio. If the HCO_3 level rises, alveolar hypoventilation results to increase pCO_2. If the HCO_3 level decreases, alveolar hyperventilation results.

Renal Component

The respiratory system aids in controlling acid-base balance by increasing or decreasing CO_2 excretion. Feedback mechanisms limit this system's ability to adjust acid-base balance. The kidneys play the most important role in acid-base balance, in spite of the fact that excretion of acid and alkali occurs slowly over hours to days. The kidneys are responsible for excreting hydrogen ions, reabsorbing bicarbonate and the synthesis of new bicarbonate in response to changes in plasma levels (HCO_3). This mechanism for the excretion of acid and reabsorption of HCO_3 is illustrated in the following reaction. Acids may be excreted by either the phosphate buffer system or in the form of **ammonium.**

Hyperkalemia is the relationship of potassium and acidosis. The cellular response to an acidotic state, such as ketoacidosis, is for potassium to shift out of the cell and hydrogen to shift into the cell. Clinically, high serum potassium levels represent this shift. Physiologically, there is a potassium deficiency due to diuresis and loss of ECF volume. The shift that does occur may do so in response to a gradient change that is due to loss of extracellular potassium or as a compensatory mechanism in response to the acidosis (Fig. 4-4). Hydroxide is formed in the reaction. More base is created to neutralize acids in the plasma. The opposite response occurs with correction of the acidosis. Potassium shifts back into the cell. Clinically, there is hypokalemia, and potassium replacement is required. In both, HCO_3 reabsorption takes place.

NaH_2DO_4 is an acid salt and renders the urine acidic. The majority of HCO_3 is reabsorbed into the plasma. Primary changes in bicarbonate levels change the numerator of the Henderson-Hasselbalch equation.

Hydrogen ions, excreted by the kidney, are buffered by either HPO_4 or ammonia in the form of ammonium chloride. Very little acid is excreted into the urine as free hydrogen ions. Most is excreted as ammonium and the rest as titratable acid (H_2PO_4).

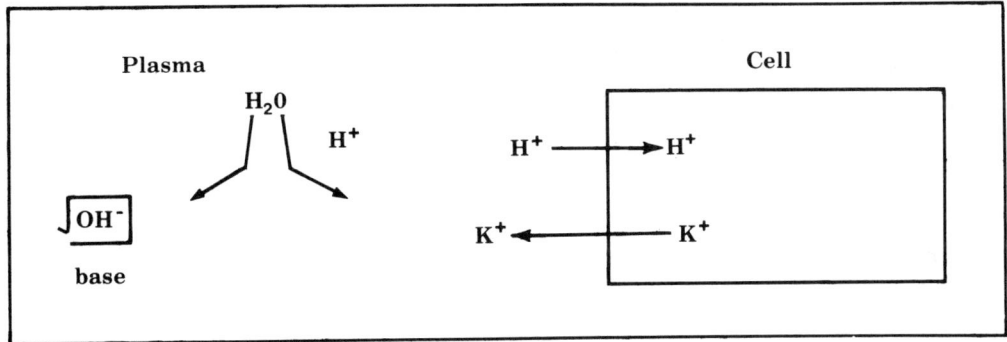
Fig. 4-4. Formation of hydroxyl

Acidosis

Acidosis may be a result of a primary respiratory disturbance with hypoventilation resulting in an increase in the pCO_2 level. It may also be the result of a primary metabolic disturbance causing a lowering of the HCO_3^- level. The results of both of these abnormal conditions are to lower the ratio of the Henderson-Hasselbalch equation and to lower pH.

Causes of Primary Respiratory Acidosis
Generalized lung disease
  COPD
Airway obstruction
  tongue
  secretions
  foreign body
Thoracic cage malfunction
  respiratory muscle paralysis
    Guillain-Barre syndrome
    myasthenia gravis
  chest trauma and splinting
    fractured ribs
    flailed chest
Respiratory center depression
  overdose of narcotizing drugs
Inappropriate mechanical ventilation

Causes of Metabolic Acidosis
Direct loss of HCO_3
  G.I. fluids distal to the pylorus
    fistula
    diarrhea
  Renal tubular acidosis due to HCO_3 wasting
Increased acid loading
  Ketoacidosis
    diabetic ketoacidosis
    starvation ketosis
  Lactic acidosis
    shock
    severe hypoxia
  Renal failure
    chronic and acute
  Drugs
    salicylate
    ethylene glycol
    methyl alcohol
    paraldehyde

Anion Gap

Metabolic acidosis is due to either acid loading (nonvolatile acid by ingestion, increased production or decreased excretion) or to loss of HCO_3^-. Determining the anion gap is useful in distinguishing between these two etiologic factors. There are unmeasurable anions in the extracellular fluids, including sulfates, phosphates and organic acid ions. Increased unmeasurable ions may be due to intoxication with salicylates, paraldehyde, methanol and ethylene glycol, or to ketoacidosis or lactic acidosis, renal failure or diabetes.

Determining the anion gap

$Na - (Cl + CO_2)$

$140 - (103 + 27)$

$140 - 130$

$10\ meq/L$

The normal anion gap is 8 to 10 meq/L. The normal range is 5 to 15 meq/L. Anion gap increases with an accumulation of one or more of the above acids (Fig. 4-5). When metabolic acidosis is due to direct loss of HCO_3 for chloride, it is frequently referred to as hyperchloremic acidosis. This category includes diarrhea, loss of intestinal fluid and renal tubular acidosis.

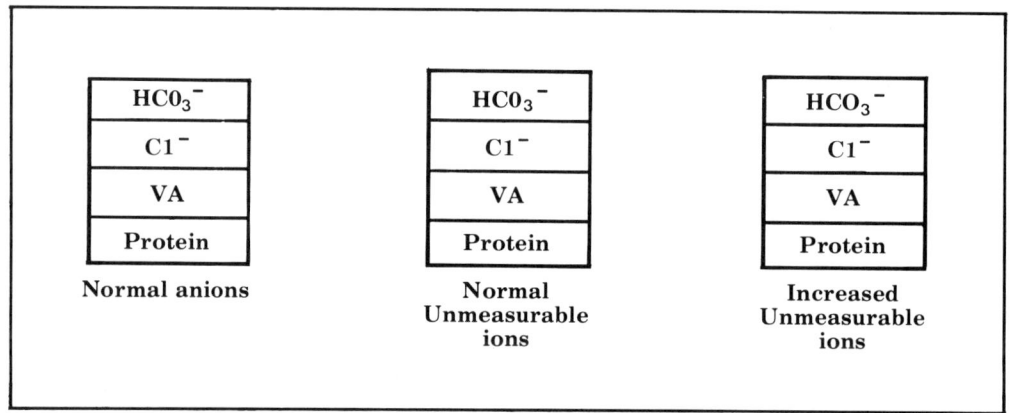

Fig. 4-5. Anion gap

Alkalosis

Alkalosis may be the result of primary respiratory disturbance with hyperventilation resulting in a decrease in the pCO_2 level. It may also be the result of a primary increase in the bicarbonate level. Either of these disturbances results in an increase in the ratio of the Henderson-Hasselbalch equation and an increase in the pH.

Causes for Respiratory Alkalosis

Acute hyperventilation
  anxiety
  fever or sepsis
  exercise
  acute hypoxia (pneumonia, acute pulmonary edema, asthma)
  salicylate intoxication
  mechanical hyperventilation

Chronic hyperventilation
  CNS disease (tumor, encephalitis)
  chronic hepatic insufficiency
  chronic hypoxia (lung disease, high altitudes)

Causes for Metabolic Alkalosis

Associated with chloride depletion
vomiting or suction of gastric secretions
alkalosis caused by loss of chloride
loss of gastric secretions without loss of lower intestinal secretions

With excessive vomiting or suctioning of gastric secretions, large amounts of HCl acid are lost. This results in a loss of chloride and the formation of a base in the plasma (Fig. 4-6).

Diuretic therapy produces loss of water and K^+. Chloride is lost with K^+ resulting in retention of HCO_3

Severe potassium depression

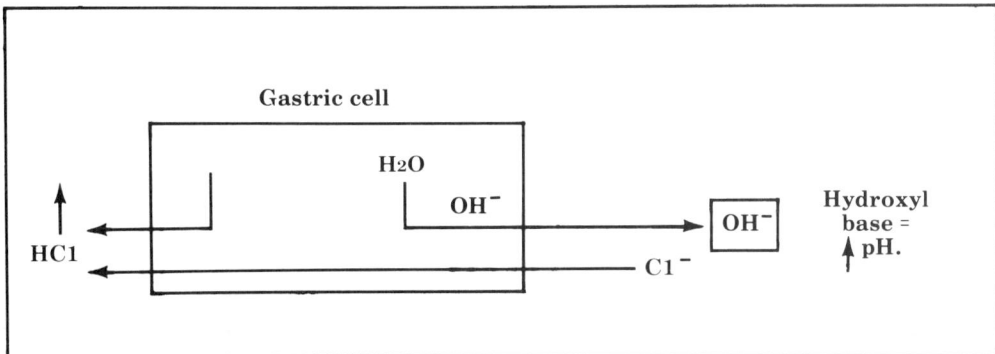

Fig. 4-6. Alkalosis caused by loss of chloride

Excessive Alkali Intake

antacids

excessive administration of $NaHCO_3$

Relationship of Potassium and Alkalosis

When a state of alkalosis exists, potassium shifts into the cell in exchange for hydrogen. Hydrogen shifts out of the cell because of a gradient that exists with the loss of free hydrogen ions in the plasma (Fig. 4-7).

The decrease in the serum potassium levels does not necessarily represent a total body depletion of potassium, but just the shift that occurs. With correction of the alkalosis, this process will reverse itself.

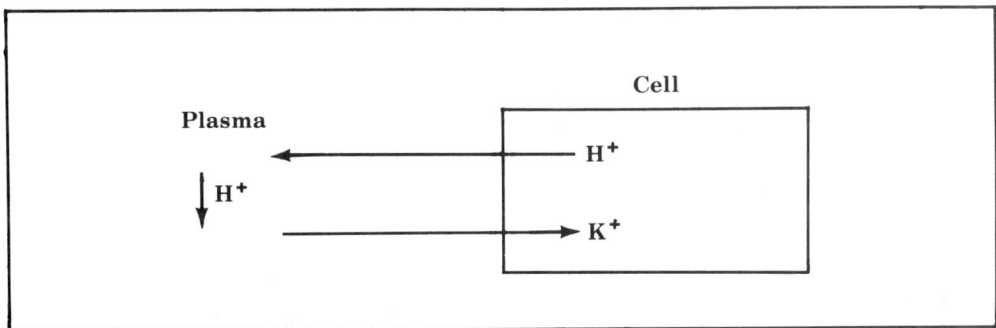

Fig. 4-7. Relationship of potassium and alkalosis

Compensation

With a primary change in either the numerator or denominator of the Henderson-Hasselbalch equation, the body attempts to compensate and maintain a 20:1 ratio between base and acid. Therefore, with a reduction in pCO_2 levels (loss of acid), the kidney excretes HCO_3 to maintain the ratio. With an increase in

pCO_2 levels (gain of acid), the kidney reabsorbs and synthesizes new bicarbonate from the renal tubular cells. The kidney restores the pH to within a normal range over a period of hours or days.

When the plasma HCO_3 level falls, the lungs release CO_2 (hyperventilate) and retain acid, restoring the ratio. With the addition of HCO_3, the lungs retain pCO_2 (hypoventilate). Although the lungs can respond rapidly to changes in HCO_3 levels, they cannot always completely compensate because the neuro response does not allow pCO_2 levels to increase or decrease beyond a certain point.

Examples:

Respiratory acidosis	Compensated
pH 7.10	pH 7.36
pCO_2 80	pCO_2 80
HCO_3 24	HCO_3 44

If the pH is toward the alkalotic side, an alkalotic process is occurring.

Respiratory alkalosis	Compensated
pH 7.70	pH 7.45
pCO_2 18	pCO_2 18
HCO_3 24	HCO_3 12
Metabolic acidosis	Compensated
pH 7.10	pH 7.35
pCO_2 38	pCO_2 20
HCO_3 12	HCO_3 12
Metabolic alkalosis	Compensated
pH 7.54	pH 7.42
pCO_2 40	pCO_2 50
HCO_3 31	HCO_3 31

A clue to interpreting ABGs with compensatory mechanisms taking place is to check the pH. Usually, if it is toward the acidic side, an acidotic process is taking place.

Mixed Acid Base Disturbances

Frequently, both respiratory and renal abnormalities occur simultaneously in the same patient. Classically, a combined disturbance is present in arrest situations.

Example:

pH 7.10
pCO_2 50   Combined respiratory and metabolic acidosis
HCO_3 15

Patients who are being hyperventilated with bag-valve-mask devices during codes, following administration of $NaHCO_3$, may have the following blood gas values:

pH 7.60
pCO_2 30   Combined respiratory and metabolic alkalosis
HCO_3 32

Other mixed disturbances include:

Respiratory acidosis and metabolic alkalosis

This disturbance may be present in a patient who has been on diuretics at home and presents in pulmonary edema:

pH 7.36
pCO_2 80
HCO_3 44

The kidneys would not have had time to respond to this acute increase in pCO_2 level; therefore, a primary metabolic disturbance is occurring simultaneously.

Respiratory alkalosis and metabolic acidosis

There are several clinical situations that might reflect this combination. Acute renal failure with a concomitant primary respiratory disturbance, such as Legionnaire's disease, resulting in a severe hypoxic state and hyperventilation is one such condition.

pO_2 7.30
pCO_2 19
HCO_3 12

These blood gas values reflect a very low pCO_2 because of the acute metabolic acidosis and the primary response to the hypoxia.

Calcium

$$Ca^{++} + \text{proteinate} \underset{\text{acid pH}}{\overset{\text{alkaline pH}}{\rightleftarrows}} \text{Protein-bound calcium}$$

Total calcium = ionized calcium (Ca^{++}) + protein-bound calcium

Increasing blood pH (alkaline) *decreases* the amount of ionized calcium and increases the amount of bound calcium. *Decreasing blood pH* (acidotic) increases the amount of ionized calcium and decreases the amount of bound calcium. It is the *decrease in ionized calcium* that *increases muscular irritability* in alkalotic states. Neuromuscular irritability is decreased in acidotic states.

TREATMENT
Respiratory Acidosis

The approach to the treatment of respiratory acidosis is the correction of the underlying problem. Support respirations by mechanical ventilation as needed.

Metabolic Acidosis

Protocol includes the administration of HCO_3 and treatment of the underlying cause. When the acute acidosis is due to endogenous metabolic acids, such as ketones and lactic acid, treating the causes will result in their conversion to bicarbonates. In addition, exogenous HCO_3 is given to the patient. Care must be taken in the dosage of HCO_3 administered to avoid a severe alkalosis.

Respiratory Alkalosis

Elimination of the underlying disorder is the only successful treatment.

Metabolic Alkalosis

Potassium chloride administration is helpful in treating alkalosis caused by diuretics. In patients with severe gastric losses, acidifying agents such a ammonium chloride or arginine hydrochlorides may be given.

SIGNS AND SYMPTOMS
Acidosis
confusion, stupor, coma
vascular collapse
hypercalcemia
hyperkalemia
ventricular fibrillation

Alkalosis
restlessness, irritability
tetany
convulsions
arrhythmias
hypocalcemia
hypokalemia

KEY CONCEPT: Acid-base balance is the relationship of hydrogen ion concentration within the body. When an imbalance occurs, the buffer systems react to diminish the change in pH. The renal system reacts by excreting hydrogen ions, reabsorbing bicarbonate and synthesizing new bicarbonate.

KEY POINT RECOGNITION

Write true or false by each statement. Answers are at the end of this chapter. A score below 80% indicates the need for further study.

_____ 1. An acid is a proton donor.

_____ 2. pH describes hydrogen ion concentration.

_____ 3. A buffer is a substance that reacts to diminish the change in pH that occurs when hydrogen ions are added to a solution.

_____ 4. The bicarbonate buffer system usually consists of carbonic acid and sodium bicarbonate.

_____ 5. The phosphate buffer system consists of hydrogen monophosphate and phosphates.

_____ 6. The protein buffer system aids in buffering intracellular fluid.

_____ 7. Cell metabolism produces acid without consuming acid.

_____ 8. The by-products of complete metabolic combustion are CO_2 and H_2O.

_____ 9. The Henderson-Hasselbalch equation relates the pH level to the concentration of acids and the concentration of base.

_____10. The respiratory system aids in controlling acid-base balance by decreasing CO_2 excretion only.

_____11. The kidneys play a minor role in acid-base balance.

_____12. The cellular response to an acidotic state is for potassium to remain in the cell.

_____13. Diuresis and loss of extracellular fluid volume result in potassium deficiency, as in ketoacidosis.

_____14. Acidosis may be a result of a primary respiratory disturbance with hypoventilation and an increase in the pCO_2 level.

_____15. Primary causes of respiratory acidosis are airway obstruction, lung disease, thoracic cage malfunction and respiratory center depression.

_____16. Causes of metabolic acidosis include direct loss of HCO_3, keto-acidosis and renal failure.

_____17. Normal anion gap is 20 to 30 meq/L.

_____18. When metabolic acidosis is due to direct loss of HCO_3, the level of chloride increase is due to the exchange of HCO_3 for chloride.

_____19. The body attempts to compensate by maintaining a 20:1 ratio between base and acid.

_____20. Increasing blood pH decreases the amount of ionized calcium and increases the amount of bound calcium.

_____21. Confusion, hypercalcemia and ventricular fibrillation may be signs and symptoms of alkalosis.

_____22. Tetany is a sign of alkalosis.

ASSESSMENT OF THE PULMONARY SYSTEM

PATIENT ASSESSMENT

Physical assessment of the patient experiencing respiratory dysfunction is similar to the assessment of any other patient. Significant medical problems, current therapies, family history and review of systems are all included. Particular attention must be given to the presenting complaint, its duration, and the character and circumstances surrounding exacerbations and remissions. The following symptoms require further investigation: dyspnea, fatigue, weight changes, fever, sleep patterns, energy levels, nervousness, temperature intolerance, general appearance, skin color, appetite and nutritional state.

Specific signs of altered functioning may include:

Cough: symptoms, duration, productivity

Sputum: character, amount, alleviating and aggravating factors

Dyspnea: onset, severity, exercise tolerance, wheeze, rales, rhonchi, cyanosis

Nose: discharges, bleeding

Sinuses: pain, tenderness

Throat: tenderness, infections

Chest pain: onset, duration, aggravating and alleviating factors, relationship to respirations

The general examination should include assessment of the following:

Gross cerebral functions: consciousness, awareness, orientation, memory, judgment

Level of consciousness: Under any condition, the level of consciousness is the single most important determinant of neurological status. To assess level of consciousness, the following must be determined:

Arousability

Orientation

Ability to follow commands

ANATOMICAL LANDMARKS

To locate abnormalities, it is necessary to know the exact location of underlying structures.

Anterior thorax: Lines of reference and landmarks commonly used are the midsternal and midclavicular lines (Fig. 4-8).

Midsternal line: runs downward through the middle of the sternum

Midclavicular line: runs vertically through the midpoint of the right and left clavicles, respectively

Suprasternal notch: located between the two sternocleidomastoid muscles; marks the upper border of the sternum

Manubrium: the superior portion of the sternum; triangular shape

Angle of Louis: formed by the junction between the manubrium and the body of the sternum; is a visible angulation about 5 cm below the suprasternal notch

Xiphoid process: located at the lower end of the sternal body in the triangular depression

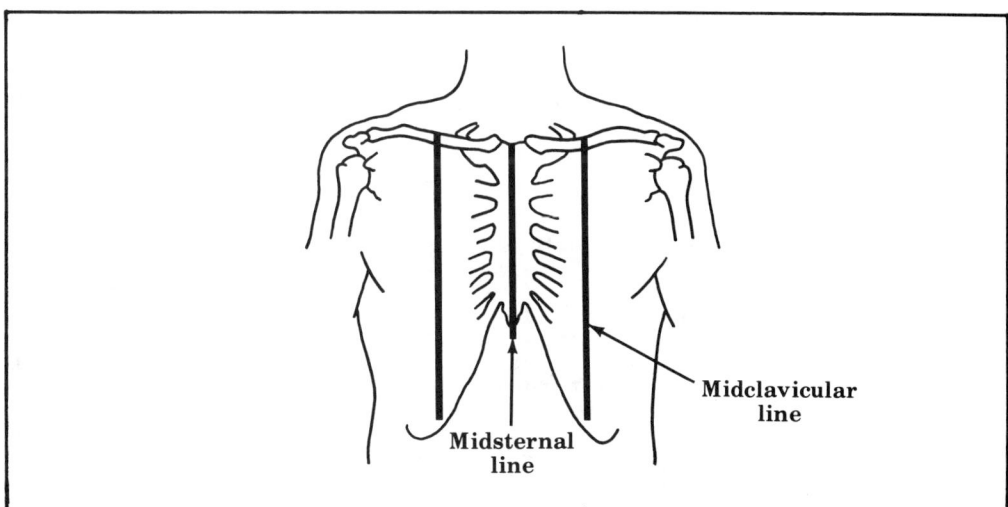

Fig. 4-8. Lines of reference: anterior thorax

Lateral chest

Anterior axillary line: runs downward from the origin of the anterior fold along the anterolateral aspect of the chest wall

Posterior axillary line: runs downward from the origin of the posterior axillary fold along the posterolateral chest wall

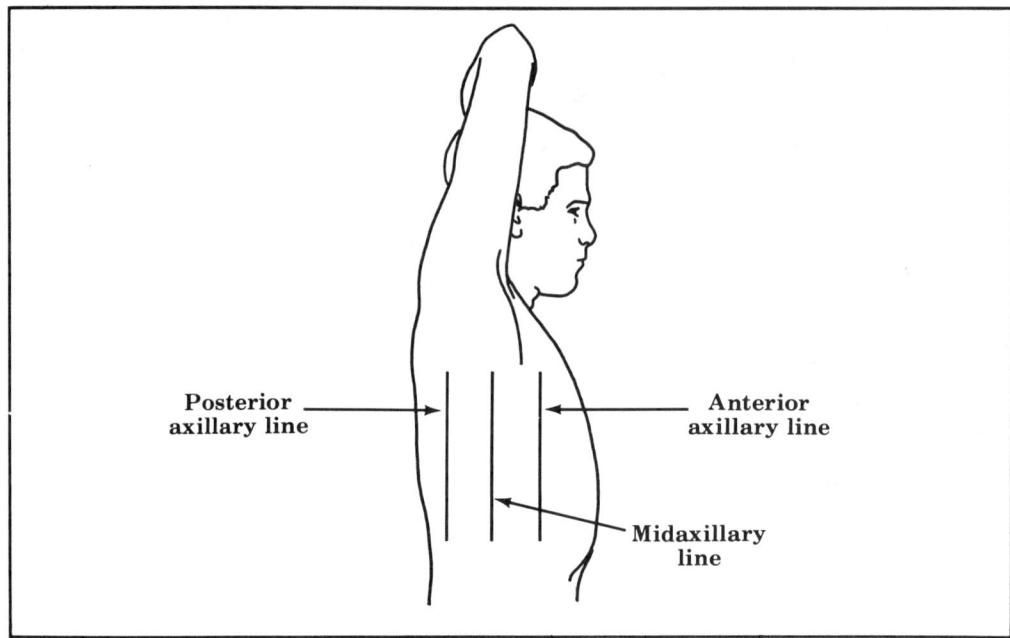

Fig. 4-9. Lines of reference: lateral thorax

Posterior thorax

Midspinal line or vertebral line: runs vertically along the spinous process of the vertebrae

Midscapular line: runs vertically from the midpoint of the scapula

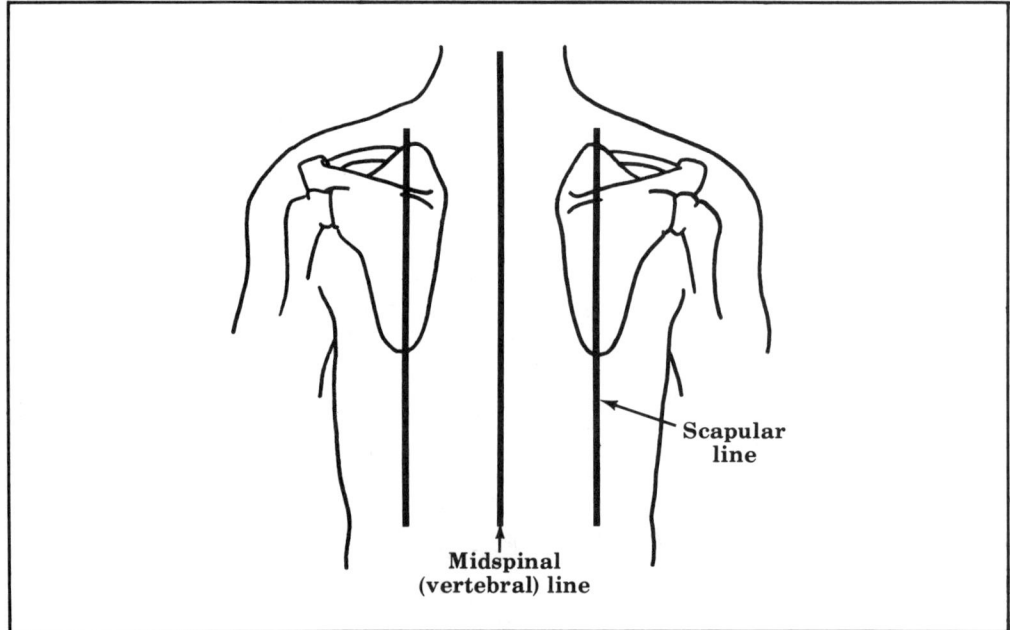

Fig. 4-10. Lines of reference: posterior thorax

LUNGS

The *apices* of the lungs (Fig. 4-11) extend approximately one inch above the medial one-third of the clavicles, on the right. The *oblique* or *diagonal fissure* divides the upper and lower lobe, extending from the fourth vertebra downward and laterally, and crossing the fifth rib at the midaxillary line. The fissure continues anteriorly to the sixth rib near the midclavicular line. On the anterior thorax, the fissure separates the middle and lower lobes. The middle lobe is located only on the anterior thorax.

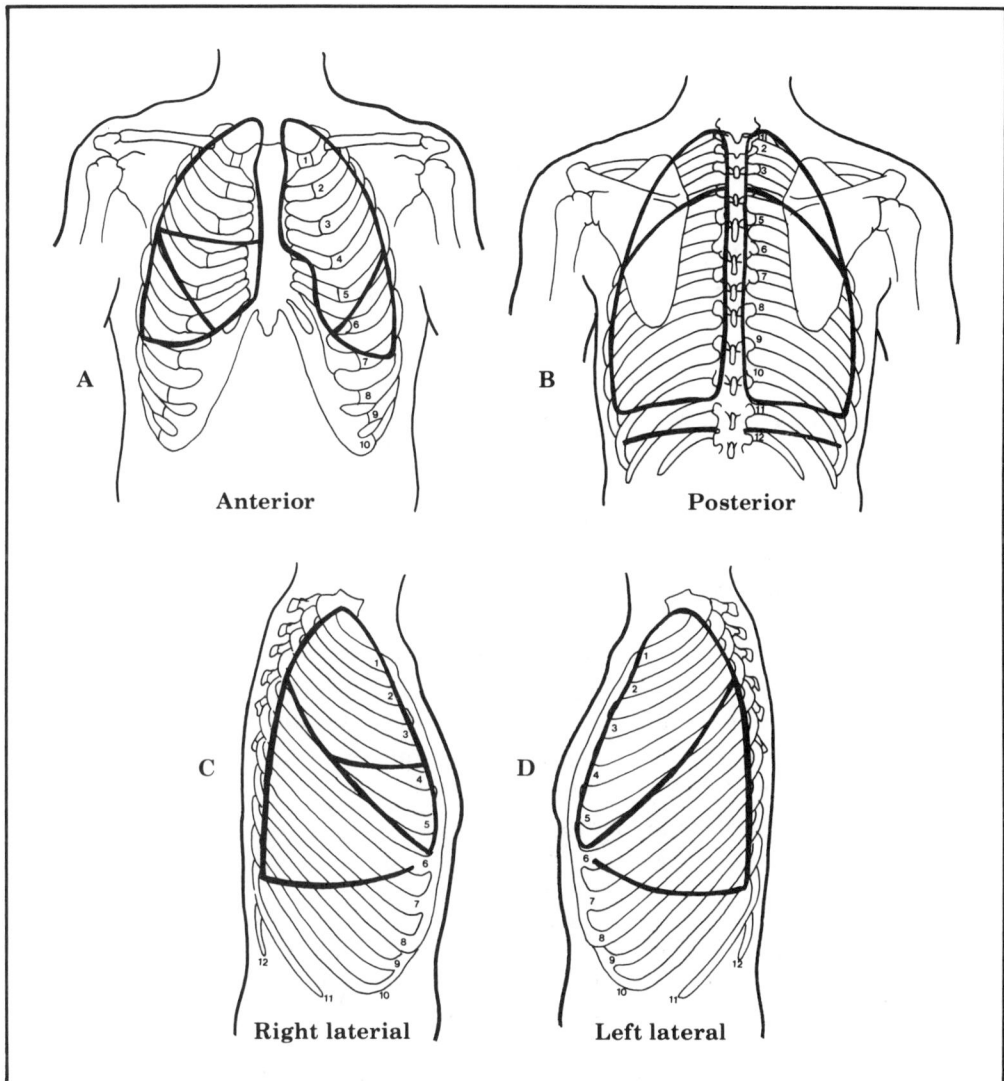

Fig. 4-11. Lungs: topographic anatomy

The *horizontal fissure* separates the upper and middle lobe. It begins at the oblique fissure and runs horizontally to the third interspace at the right sternal border. Since the left lung has only two lobes, it does not have a horizontal fissure.

The *left oblique fissure* is similar in location to the fissure of the right lung.

The lungs extend inferiorly from the apices to the diaphragm, with the lungs lying on both diaphragms. The *right diaphragm* rests at the level of the fifth rib, midclavicular line. The dome of the *left diaphragm* is one inch lower, at the level of the sixth rib in the midclavicular line.

The diaphragm separates the base of the left lung and the fundus of the stomach and the spleen.

INSPECTION

Observe for apparent health, general nutrition and musculoskeletal development.

Observe for thorax configuration: kyphosis, scoliosis, barrel chest, pectus carinatum (pigeon chest), pectus excavatum (funnel chest).

Observe for respiratory rate: pattern, type and rate of breathing—tachypnea, hyperventilation, bradypnea, eupnea, orthopnea, labored, or flared nares.

Observe movement of chest during ventilation—abdominal, diaphragmatic, costal, upper thoracic, symmetry, or intercostal retractions.

Check for cyanosis, capillary density and cherry-red coloring of carbon monoxide poisoning.

Observe for retraction or bulging of interspaces.

Observe for shortness of breath and respiratory effort.

Check for symmetry of chest during inspiration and expiration.

Check for clubbing of fingers.

Observe for restlessness, pain and mental alteration.

PALPATION

Palpate side to side and compare.

Palpate for symmetry of the chest.

Palpate for tenderness: rib fractures, costochondritis, masses, subcutaneous emphysema.

Palpate for fremitus: vibrations transmitted from the vocal cords through the trachea, bronchi and alveoli to the examiner's hand.

Palpate for vocal fremitus: transmission of sound, such as 99, to the examiner's hand.

Alterations in vocal fremitus may be described as:

Increased: palpated disorders causing consolidation of lung tissue, such as lobar pneumonia, lung tumors, pulmonary infarction, and pulmonary fibrosis

Decreased: palpated in airway obstruction, pleural thickening, pleural effusion, pneumothorax and emphysema

Absent: same disorders as in *decreased* above

Palpate point of maximal impulse (PMI): This is the impulse at the apex of the heart caused by the forward rotation of the heart at the beginning of ventricular systole. The PMI is located at the fifth intercostal space medial to the midclavicular line. Deviations of the PMI to the left are usually due to cardiac dilatation or hypertrophy and mediastinal shift. PMI deviation to the right may be due to massive atelectasis of the right side due to loss of lung volume.

Palpate for subcutaneous crepitus: This is due to an air leak in the trachea, mediastinum or abdomen or to a pneumothorax.

Palpate for tracheal deviation: The trachea will deviate toward the ***affected*** side in atelectasis, pulmonary fibrosis, pneumonectomy, paralysis of one side of the diaphragm, and during inspiration in a flail chest. Tracheal deviation to the opposite or ***unaffected*** side may be observed in neck tumors, thyroid enlargements, tension pneumothorax, mediastinal tumors, pleural effusion and in a flail chest during expiration.

PERCUSSION

Percuss for tenderness, pain and masses.

Percuss for breath sounds: resonant, tympany, dull, flat.

Percuss for diaphragmatic excursion at the diaphragmatic level at inspiration and expiration. Decreased excursion is observed in emphysema, pleurisy, pain, abdominal disorders and oversedation.

AUSCULTATION

Auscultation is performed with the stethoscope. High-pitched sounds are amplified best with the **diaphragm** of the stethoscope. The **bell** is the most effective when auscultating for low-pitched sounds.

Normal breath sounds are classified as: ***vesicular, bronchial*** and ***bronchovesicular.***

Abnormal or adventitious breath sounds may be classified as: ***absent, diminished, bronchial*** and ***bronchovesicular*** heard over lung fields, and ***voice sounds*** heard on ***auscultation.***

Techniques of Auscultation

Listen for **normal** breath sounds. ***Vesicular*** breath sounds are normally heard over the lung periphery. Inspiration is heard longer than expiration.

Bronchial breath sounds are heard over the trachea and large bronchi. Expiration is louder than inspiration. ***Bronchovesicular*** breath sounds are heard normally over or near major airways and are a combination of vesicular and bronchial sounds.

Listen for ***abnormal*** breath sounds. Absent or diminished breath sounds may be heard with: decreased air flow, pleural thickening, obesity, complete airway obstruction, pleural fluid, muscular weakness, chronic obstructive pulmonary disease and pneumothorax.

Pneumonia, tumors, pulmonary infarction and atelectasis may produce bronchial and bronchovesicular breath sounds over lung fields.

Adventitious sounds are abnormal, superimposed breath sounds. Examples include: rales, wheezes and friction rubs. Rales are indicative of fluid in the alveoli and airways. They have a crackling sound. Coarse rales produce a bubbling sound indicating large airway involvement. Wheezes or rhonchi are heard when there is obstruction of air flow. This may be intermittent or fixed and usually is associated with increased airway resistance. Rhonchi are usually heard during expiration, but may be heard during inspiration. Pleural friction rub is due to pleural inflammation. This is a leathery sound due to lack of lubricating fluid. Voices heard during auscultation are normally soft and barely audible. Bronchophony is heard over lungs that have less air than normal. The spoken word "99" becomes clear and audible. Egophony is the changing of the spoken word "E" to "A." This may be heard near pleural effusion. Whispered pectoriloquy is the whispered "99" that becomes more distinct and audible through the stethoscope.

Check vital signs. The blood pressure may be normal or elevated.

Hypertension may be observed in acute respiratory failure. ***Hypotension*** may be observed in adult respiratory distress syndrome or chest trauma.

Tachycardia and ***pyrexia*** may be present if there are pulmonary emboli or adult respiratory distress syndrome. Respiratory distress and cyanosis are common. Dyspnea may be seen in adult respiratory distress syndrome, chronic obstructive pulmonary disease, pneumothorax or pulmonary embolism. Hyperpnea may be seen in status asthmaticus. Narrowed pulse pressure and pulsus paradoxus may be seen in chest trauma, particularly cardiac tamponade. Any illness that reduces oxygen concentration and perfusion may alter vital signs. The reduction in oxygen concentration producing abnormal blood gases is a causative factor leading to hypoxia. Hypoxia may be secondary to hypovolemia, cardiac failure, respiratory distress and chest trauma.

LABORATORY AND RADIOLOGIC STUDIES

Laboratory studies in respiratory disorders are varied and tailored to the presumptive diagnosis at hand.

Sputum specimens are collected after deep cough has produced thick purulent sputum. Saliva is unacceptable.

Culture and sensitivity is the identification of the bacteria and determination of the sensitivity to specific drugs after initial gram stain analysis. The analysis may reveal bacterial or fungal infections.

Sputum cytology is used for detecting malignant diseases of the lung.

Occasionally, fiberoptic bronchoscopy is done to remove secretions and mucus plugs. The pliable tube can be directed toward the left bronchus, which is difficult to reach with other conventional methods. This is an effective procedure for atelectasis and protracted hypoxia. Even the mechanically ventilated patient can undergo fiberoptic bronchoscopy.

Serum protein reflects the amount of albumin, serum globulins, fibrinogen, prothrombin and plasminogen. Serum globulins are alpha, beta and gamma fractions. The alpha fraction is concerned with steroid, lipid and bilirubin transport. Serum albumin aids in the regulation of intravascular plasma volume.

Blood gas analysis reflects the respiratory oxygen transport function. Abnormal findings support the presence of pathology, the acid-base status and respiratory failure. The components include PAO_2, $PACO_2$, pH, base excess, bicarbonate, oxyhemoglobin saturation, O_2 content Hb_1 FIO_2, and body temperature.

PAO_2 is a measurement of the tension or the pressure of oxygen in the blood. Normal PAO_2 is arterial 80 to 100 mm Hg on room air.

$PACO_2$ measures the tension or the pressure of CO_2 in the blood. Normal is arterial 35 to 45 mm Hg. **pH** measures the acidity or alkalinity of the blood. Normal is 7.35 to 7.45. **Base excess** and **bicarbonate** (HCO_3) are influenced by metabolic changes. Base excess refers to bicarbonate and other bases in the blood. Normal is base excess -2 to +2. Normal is HCO_3 22 to 26 meq/L. **Oxygen saturation** measures oxygen carried by hemoglobin in percentage. This measurement is compared to the amount of O_2 that the hemoglobin could carry. Normal is 95 percent.

Radiologic studies are distinct and briefly discussed in the following:

Routine chest: The posteroanterior and lateral chest are radiographed to determine size, shape and position of the heart and lung.

Decubitus radiograph: This is performed to determine effusions.

Apical lordotic radiograph: This is performed to determine apices and diagnosis tuberculosis.

Right and left anterior oblique radiograph: This is performed to determine lesion location of the lungs visualizing the mediastinum and areas of the lung often obscured by thoracic structures.

Laminography, tomography, planography: These are noninvasive x-rays used to show cavities, neoplasms and densities of the lung.

Fluoroscopy: This is an invasive x-ray to detect diaphragmatic motion, size and contour of the heart.

Bronchography: This is an invasive procedure, injecting radiopaque material to detect obstruction and malformation of the tracheobronchial tree.

Pulmonary angiography: This is an invasive injection of dye to detect pulmonary tissue patency, embolism malformation, congenital and acquired abnormalities and rupture of the pulmonary vessels.

Lung scan: This is a procedure used to determine lung ventilation and perfusion and to aid in the diagnosis of **parenchymal lung** diseases and vascular disorders.

Bone survey: This is a procedure used to detect tumors and abnormalities of the bones.

Other studies include:

Skin test for PPD (Purified Protein Derivative): This is a highly purified product containing protein from tubercle bacilli, injected intradermally. A reaction is considered positive when it is 10 mm or more.

Endoscopy: This is an invasive procedure to detect masses, obstructions and malformations in the hepatic system, gallbladder, duodenum and biliary tract, esophagus and gastric mucosa.

Laryngoscopy: This is an invasive procedure used to visualize the larynx.

Bronchoscopy: This is an invasive procedure used to visualize the trachea, major bronchi and their branchings.

Mediastinoscopy: This is an invasive procedure used for the localization or diagnosis of masses in the hilar and mediastinal area.

Thoracentesis: This is an invasive procedure used to aspirate fluid from the pleural space or obtain biopsies of the pleura. Diagnostic studies are done on the fluid for specific gravity, white blood cells, red blood cells, protein, differential cell count, glucose, amylase, malignant cells and culture.

Biopsy: This is an invasive procedure used to diagnose histologic changes. The examination may be done on the tracheobronchial tree and lymph nodes of the chest.

Pulmonary function test: This is a noninvasive procedure used to assess lung function and to diagnose nonorganic causes of dyspnea, and to differentiate diseases of the lungs.

KEY CONCEPT: Physical assessment of the patient with a respiratory problem should include assessment of gross and specific cerebral functions in addition to inspection, palpation, percussion and auscultation of the respiratory system.

KEY POINT RECOGNITION
Write true or false by each statement. Answers are at the end of this chapter. A score below 80% indicates the need for further study.

_____ 1. Anterior thorax lines are midsternal and midclavicular.

_____ 2. The midsternal line runs downward through the middle of the sternum.

_____ 3. The suprasternal notch is located between the two sternocleidomastoid muscles marking the upper border of the sternum.

_____ 4. The Angle of Louis is 5 cm above the suprasternal notch.

_____ 5. The xiphoid process is the upper end of the sternal body.

_____ 6. The lung apices extend approximately one inch above the medial one-third of the clavicle.

_____ 7. The right oblique fissure divides the upper and lower lobe.

_____ 8. The horizontal fissure separates the upper and middle lobe of the right lobe.

_____ 9. Pectus carinatum is "pigeon chest."

_____10. Pectus excavatum is "funnel chest."

_____11. Decreased vocal fremitus may be palpated in lobar pneumonia.

_____12. The point of maximal impulse is located in the third intercostal space medial to the midclavicular line.

_____13. Deviation of the PMI to the left may be indicative of cardiac hypertrophy.

_____14. Tracheal deviation to the affected side can be seen in neck tumors and tension pneumothorax.

_____15. Decreased diaphragmatic excursion may be seen in emphysema.

_____16. Bronchial breath sounds are heard over the trachea and large bronchi.

_____17. Rales are indicative of fluid in the alveoli only.

_____18. Pleural friction rub is caused by pleural inflammation.

_____19. Whispered pectoriloquy is the whispered word "99" that becomes inaudible.

_____20. In egophony the word "A" is heard as "E."

_____21. Sputum analysis for culture and sensitivity may reveal bacterial or fungal infections.
_____22. A fiberoptic bronchoscopy may be done to remove secretions and mucous plugs.
_____23. Hypertension may be present in acute respiratory failure.
_____24. Pulmonary emboli or adult respiratory distress syndrome may cause tachycardia and pyrexia.
_____25. Narrowed pulse pressure and pulsus paradoxus may be seen in chest trauma.
_____26. Hypoxia may develop secondary to respiratory distress, chest trauma or hypovolemia.
_____27. Serum protein level only reflects the amount of albumin in the blood.
_____28. Blood gas analysis reflects the respiratory oxygen transport mechanism of the body.
_____29. PAO_2 is a reflection of the pressure of oxygen in the blood.
_____30. Normal arterial $PACO_2$ range is 85 to 95 mm Hg.
_____31. Base excess refers to oxygen saturation in the blood.
_____32. Flouroscopy is used to detect diaphragmatic motion, size and contour of the heart.
_____33. Endoscopy is used to detect masses, obstructions and malformations in the hepatic, biliary and gastrointestinal system.
_____34. Laryngoscopy is an invasive procedure used to visualize the larynx.
_____35. Pulmonary function tests assess lung function.

PATHOLOGICAL STATES AND NURSING MANAGEMENT
RESPIRATORY FAILURE
Pathophysiology

Respiratory failure is defined as failure of the respiratory system to provide for an exchange of oxygen and carbon dioxide between the environment and tissues of the body in quantities sufficient to sustain life. Adequate respiration requires not only lungs and upper airways, but also an integrated feedback control system involving the central and peripheral nervous system, thoracic cage and respiratory muscles. Respiratory failure can occur without the presence of disease. Respiratory failure requires a series of events: hypoxemia, hypoxia and excessive carbon dioxide.

Hypoxemia leads to hypoxia. Hypoxia causes an increase in sympathetic nervous system stimulation, which responds by producing vasoconstriction, an increase in peripheral resistance and tachycardia. Hypoventilation or circulatory impairment may result in hypoxia and hypercapnia. Uncorrected hypercapnia leads to cerebral depression, hypotension and circulatory failure. When an excessive amount of carbon dioxide accumulates, the sympathetic nervous system responds by increasing cardiac output or by the development of an acidotic state.

Respiratory failure may be chronic or acute. In chronic respiratory failure, the renal system responds to the hypercapnia. The arterial pH remains relatively normal because of an increase in serum bicarbonate levels. Acute respiratory failure is detectable by the fall in pH.

Pathophysiology: Specific

Alveolar ventilation is a reflection of how well the body's ventilation is being met. Therefore, **respiratory failure** is a condition of inadequate alveolar ventilation in relationship to the metabolic rate. An arterial pCO_2 of above 50 ml/Hg reflects the clinical state. This may be chronic or acute.

Acute respiratory failure is a sudden rise in arterial pCO_2 level with a fall in pH, and the occurrence of respiratory acidosis.

Chronic respiratory failure occurs over a time period sufficient to permit renal compensation. The pH remains near the normal range.

Respiratory insufficiency is a condition in which alveolar ventilation is inadequate, resulting in unmet metabolic demands. The respiratory center is stimulated and hyperventilation occurs. The hypoxemia is diagnosed by a pO_2 of less than 50 mm Hg.

Acute respiratory insufficency is the occurrence of alveolar hyperventilation with an increased pH and respiratory alkalosis.

Chronic respiratory insufficiency is the occurrence of alveolar hyperventilation that has taken place over a period of time. There is renal compensation and a normal pH.

Patients will continue to hyperventilate as long as they possess muscle power. However, once fatigued, hypoventilation develops, followed by respiratory failure. Frequently, signs and symptoms of carbon dioxide retention and hypoxemia develop, which makes it difficult to distinguish between acute and chronic conditions. At times, patients in acute respiratory failure are misdiagnosed as congestive heart failure or primary neurologic disease. The only reliable diagnostic test is arterial blood gases (Fig. 4-12).

Acute ventilatory failure:	pH 7.20 pCO_2 78 pO_2 50
Acute respiratory insufficiency:	pH 7.60 pCO_2 25 pO_2 65
Chronic respiratory insufficiency:	pH 7.44 pCO_2 24 pO_2 58
Chronic ventilatory failure:	pH 7.38 pCO_2 76 pO_2 50

Fig. 4-12. Arterial blood gases

Impaired ventilation decreases circulating oxygen through the lungs and decreases perfusion to the tissue. Precipitating factors leading to respiratory failure are impaired ventilation, including chronic airway obstruction and restrictive defects, neuromuscular defects and respiratory center damage. Also, impaired gas exchange and diffusion, and ventilation-perfusion abnormalities are factors to be considered.

Clinical Presentation

The clinical presentation is extremely variable and dependent upon manifestation of the primary disease and the extent of hypoxia. Changes in mentation such as confusion, lethargy and stupor may occur. Dizziness, muscle twitching, asterixis, papilledema, engorged fundal veins, diaphoresis, tachycardia and bradycardia, cardiac arrhythmias, cyanosis, and hypertension or hypotension may be observed. The most common preceding symptom of respiratory failure is a change in arterial blood gases. Complications associated with respiratory failure include cardiac arrhythmia, infections, psychosis, renal failure, hypotension, abdominal distention, paralytic ileus, gastrointestinal bleeding, thromboembolism and alkalosis.

Diagnostic Data

Patient history is an important diagnostic aid when determining the etiology of respiratory failure. Routine laboratory tests, CBC and urinalysis are done. The most valuable test for assessing respiratory status is arterial blood gases. Radiologic studies may be ordered.

Nursing Care

The major nursing responsibilities are:

(1) Maintain ventilation, open airways; maintain bronchial hygiene; intubate as needed; mechanical ventilation; and PEEP as needed.

(2) Provide oxygenation; correct shunting; maintain adequate hemoglobin.

(3) Prevent infection; use strict aseptic technique.

(4) Monitor arterial blood gases; PAO_2 above 50 mm Hg; pH range 7.36 to 7.44.

(5) Maintain nutritional status.

(6) Provide meticulous skin care.

(7) Monitor hypertensive states.

(8) Prevent complications.

KEY CONCEPT: Respiratory failure may present different clinical pictures according to specific etiology; but the overall nursing goals are to maintain the patient during the acute stage and to prevent further complications.

KEY POINT RECOGNITION

Write true or false by each statement. Answers are at the end of this chapter. A score below 80% indicates the need for further study.

_____ 1. Respiratory failure is defined as a failure of the respiratory system to provide an exchange of oxygen and carbon dioxide between the environment and tissues in quantities sufficient to sustain life.

_____ 2. Adequate respirations require lungs, upper airways, central and peripheral nervous system, thoracic cage and respiratory muscles.

_____ 3. Respiratory failure only occurs with lung disease.

_____ 4. Hypoxemia leads to hypoxia.

_____ 5. Hypoxia causes a decrease in sympathetic nervous system stimulation.

_____ 6. In chronic respiratory failure, the renal system responds to hypercapnia.

_____ 7. In chronic respiratory failure, the arterial pH falls.

_____ 8. In acute respiratory failure, the arterial pCO_2 rises and the pH falls.

_____ 9. Respiratory insufficiency is diagnosed by a pO_2 less than 35 mm Hg.

_____10. In chronic respiratory insufficiency, the pH is abnormal.

_____11. The most reliable diagnostic test used for assessing respiratory status is arterial blood gases.

_____12. Complications associated with respiratory failure include cardiac arrhythmia, psychosis, thromboembolism and renal failure.

ADULT RESPIRATORY DISTRESS SYNDROME (ARDS)
Pathophysiology: General

Adult respiratory distress syndrome (ARDS) is the term applied to acute and chronic conditions that cause injury to the alveolar-capillary unit. Other terms frequently encountered are shock lung, traumatic wet lung, white lung syndrome, acute alveolar failure, congestive atelectasis, pump lung and acute hyaline membrane disease.

Injury to the alveolar-capillary membrane increases the permeability of the capillary endothelium. This increase in permeability results in leakage of fluid into the interstitial space and eventually into the alveoli. The accumulation of fluid produces edema and a decrease in functional residual capacity (FRC). Atelectasis results from the presence of alveolar fluid, a decrease in surfactant activity and a reduction in surfactant production. Therefore, the atelectasis causes a decrease in overall lung compliance, leading to closure of airways, pulmonary congestion and a reduction in compliance.

Hypoxemia is caused by two basic mechanisms: shunting of blood through collapsed or congested lung tissue and the ventilation-perfusion imbalance. The major cause of arterial hypoxemia is right-to-left shunting. This leads to elevated A-a DO_2, even with 100 percent oxygen. The continuous use of 100 percent oxygen turns relative shunt to absolute shunt, therefore eliminating the nitrogen content of inspired air. The hypoxia results in pulmonary capillary constriction.

In the early stages of ARDS, hypercapnia is not a problem. Carbon dioxide diffusion remains unhampered. As ARDS progresses, gas exchange becomes abnormal and fibrotic changes develop in pulmonary tissue.

The precipitating factors are viral or bacterial pulmonary infections, aspiration, inhalation of toxic substances, drug abuse, trauma, fatty embolism, amniotic fluid embolism, gram negative septicemia and post cardiopulmonary bypass.

Clinical Presentation

The clinical presentation begins with dyspnea and tachycardia. As the disease progresses, the patient becomes increasingly cyanotic, hypotensive and hypoxic. Auscultatory findings are minimal with scattered rales. In later stages, rales become more evident.

Diagnostic Data

Patient history is an important aid in diagnosing ARDS. The patient develops a sudden marked respiratory distress. Radiological studies reveal bilateral interstitial and alveolar infiltrates. Arterial blood gases reveal a decreased pCO_2. Pulmonary studies reveal a reduction in compliance, volume and residual capacity. Shunt studies demonstrate right to left shunting. Also, an increase in A-a gradient is seen.

Nursing Care

The major nursing responsibilities are:

(1) Correct arterial hypoxemia; maintain ventilation; correct cause.

(2) Monitor ventilators; deliver a set tidal volume that reduces arterial pCO_2 levels; add dead space, if necessary, to raise pCO_2.

(3) Maintain PEEP; increase FRC; reduce shunting; improve gas exchange.

(4) Restrict fluids; monitor intravenous fluids; keep wedge-pressure below 12 mm Hg.; diuretics.

(5) Monitor respiratory status and arterial blood gases.

(6) Administer corticosteroids (controversial issue), which may reduce lung injury and edema.

(7) Prevent infection; use strict aseptic technique; antibiotics.

(8) Maintain nutritional status.

(9) Provide meticulous skin care.

(10) Prevent complications.

KEY CONCEPT: Nursing care is aimed at maintaining alveolar ventilation and oxygen transport in an effort to prevent further damage.

KEY POINT RECOGNITION

Write true or false by each statement. Answers are at the end of this chapter. A score below 80% indicates the need for further study.

_____ 1. ARDS is a term applied to acute, not chronic, respiratory conditions.

_____ 2. ARDS causes injury to the alveolar-capillary unit.

_____ 3. Injury to the alveolar-capillary unit increases the permeability of the capillary endothelium.

_____ 4. Leakage of fluid into the interstitial space produces edema.

_____ 5. Atelectasis causes a decrease in overall lung compliance leading to pulmonary congestion.

_____ 6. Shunting of blood may cause hypoxemia.
_____ 7. Ventilation-perfusion imbalance may cause hypoxemia.
_____ 8. As ARDS progresses, fibrotic change in pulmonary tissue occurs.
_____ 9. Widespread rales are heard early in ARDS.
_____ 10. In ARDS, the patient slowly develops respiratory distress.
_____ 11. In ARDS, arterial pCO_2 is decreased.

CHRONIC OBSTRUCTIVE PULMONARY DISEASE (COPD)
Pathophysiology: General

Chronic obstructive pulmonary disease is a condition defined as chronic obstruction of air flow caused by asthma, chronic bronchitis or emphysema. Emphysema and chronic bronchitis result in airway narrowing. This narrowing decreases maximal expiratory flow rates and increases airway resistance. Since elastic recoil provides support to airways during breathing and determines maximal expiratory flow rate, if diminished, the result is an increase in compliance, FRC and respiratory effort.

An increase in residual volume and functional residual capacity (FRC) are usually present. When the expiratory phase is prolonged, as seen in obstructive disease, inspiration begins before the respiratory system reaches its static balance point, resulting in a higher FRC. Total lung capacity is often elevated because of the loss of elastic recoil and airtrapping. Therefore, there is mismatching of ventilation and blood flow, resulting in arterial blood gas changes.

Patients with normal to low pCO_2 levels have an increased ventilatory drive. Patients with high pCO_2 levels and lower pO_2 levels have a decreased ventilatory drive. Other factors affecting the difference may be sensitivity to chemoreceptors.

Mild to severe pulmonary hypertension is often present. Reduction in the total pulmonary vascular bed is attributed to anatomic changes and constriction of smooth muscle in arteries and arterioles. Also contributing to this reduction is the obstruction of alveolar septa and loss of capillaries. Alveolar hypoxia leads to constriction of pulmonary vessels. Increased afterload on the right ventricle leads to right ventricular failure and, ultimately, cor pulmonale.

Pathophysiology: Specific

Chronic bronchitis is characterized by excessive tracheobronchial mucus production. Chronic bronchitis is associated with hyperplasia and hypertrophy of the mucus-producing glands of the submucosa of large cartilaginous airways. Changes in small noncartilaginous airways include goblet cell hyperpasia, edema, inflamed mucosa and submucosa, peribronchial fibrosis, loss of cilia, mucus plugs and an increase in smooth muscle. The major site of airway obstructive disease is the small airways. Most patients with COPD have chronic bronchitis and emphysema.

The most common obstructive disease is *emphysema.* Emphysema is defined as distention of the alveoli distal to the terminal bronchioles with destruction of the alveoli septa. There are two categories of emphysema: *centriacinar emphysema* and *panacinar emphysema.* In centriacinar emphysema, the destructive changes are limited to the respiratory bronchioles and alveolar ducts with less destruction in the peripheral acinus. Mild forms are found in patients over fifty years of age. Many lung units must be involved in order to be symptomatic.

Panacinar emphysema involves the central and peripheral portions of the acinus, which results in loss of surface area gas exchange capacity. The lung's elastic recoil properties are diminished.

In patients presenting with severe symptoms of emphysema, it becomes impossible to delineate between the two forms. Most emphysemic patients have elements of both types.

In *asthma,* the tracheobronchial tree is more sensitive to various stimuli. Asthma causes narrowing of the air passages, which may be relieved spontaneously or by therapy. Marked dyspnea, coughing and wheezing are indicative of asthma. Asthma may be divided into two categories, allergic and idiosyncratic. Allergic asthma is associated with a family or personal history of allergies. However, idiosyncratic asthma presents with a negative allergy history. The asthmatic attacks may be triggered by infections, drugs, environmental conditions and pollutants, exercise, smoking or stress.

Asthma reduces airway diameter because of smooth muscle contraction, edema and thick tenacious secretions, which result in an increase in airway resistance, respiratory effort and hyperinflation of lungs and thorax, and a decrease in expiratory forced volume, flow rate and elastic recoil. Alterations in ventilation and perfusion ratios are also seen.

Precipitating factors include air pollution, occupational irritants, infections, smoking, heredity, age and allergy.

Clinical Presentation

The clinical presentation is extremely variable and dependent upon cause. The patient presents with dyspnea and a cough. Wheezing may be present with or without pursed-lip breathing. The use of accessory muscles is observed if there is underlying respiratory infection and severe airway obstruction.

In emphysema, the clinical presentation includes scant mucoid sputum, weight loss, use of accessory muscles with prolonged expiration, pursed-lip breathing and grunting with each expiration. Neck vein distention and hyperresonance are also seen. Breath sounds are diminished or absent. High-pitched rhonchi are heard. Hypoxia, if present, is mild. Hypercapnia is unusual with pCO_2 levels normal to low. Vital capacity is low. Total lung capacity and residual volumes are increased. Maximal expiratory flow rates are diminished, with a severe loss of elastic recoil. The findings correlate with hyperinflation associated with emphysema.

Emphysemic patients tend to be less susceptible to complicating respiratory infections associated with sputum production. Therefore, they present less frequently in acute respiratory failure. Clinically, a marked increase in dyspnea is seen.

Bronchitis produces a history of cough associated with copious sputum production, which is often purulent. Initially, the symptoms are intermittent, but progress in frequency and severity. Dyspnea on exertion and severe airway obstruction are seen. However, dyspnea may not be evident at rest. Often, the patient is overweight and cyanotic. Percussion reveals a resonant note with coarse rhonchi. Auscultation may reveal wheezing. Cor pulmonale may be seen with chronic bronchitis. Right ventricular failure aggravates the existing cyanosis and produces peripheral edema.

Chronically, a rise in arterial carbon dioxide levels (50 to 60 mm Hg) and a falling pO_2 level (45 to 60) develop. Chronic hypoxia leads to erythropoiesis and hemoglobin desaturation with pulmonary vascular constriction. Total lung capacity is normal, but residual volume is slightly elevated. Expiratory flow rates are low.

Diagnostic Data

Radiologic studies reveal an increase in A-P diameter, flattening of the diaphragm, and narrowing and lengthening of the cardiac silhouette. The lungs become hyperradiolucent with retrosternal translucency on lateral chest radiographs. Also, the sternodiaphragmatic angle on lateral radiographs is over 90 degrees.

Laboratory studies may show polycythemia and eosinophilia. Gram stain sputum studies for gram positive or gram negative organisms are done. The common organisms found are ***streptococcus pneumonia*** and ***hemophilus influenza.***

Spirometry studies identify airway obstruction not revealed by physical examination. This includes vital capacity, flow rate, FEV_1 and total lung capacity.

Arterial blood gases show the degree of hypoxemia, hypercapnea, acidosis and renal compensation.

Nursing Care
The major nursing responsibilities are:
(1) Teach the patient to live with the condition, physiologically and psychologically.
(2) Restrict or remove irritants.
(3) Teach postural drainage, breathing exercises, chest physiotherapy.
(4) Correct arterial hypoxemia.
(5) Monitor respiratory quality, oxygenation.
(6) Administer drugs, antibiotics, mucolytic agents, expectorants, bronchodilators.
(7) Maintain adequate hydration.
(8) Prevent infections.
(9) Prevent complications.

KEY CONCEPT: Chronic obstructive pulmonary disease includes chronic bronchitis, asthma and emphysema. The clinical picture may vary depending on the specific cause.

KEY POINT RECOGNITION
Write true or false by each statement. Answers are at the end of this chapter. A score below 80% indicates the need for further study.

_____ 1. COPD is defined as chronic obstruction of air flow.
_____ 2. Emphysema results in enlarged airways.
_____ 3. Obstructive disease usually produces a prolonged expiratory phase.
_____ 4. A high FRC may be indicative of obstructive disease.
_____ 5. Loss of elastic recoil of lung tissue elevates total lung capacity.
_____ 6. Airtrapping reduces total lung capacity.
_____ 7. COPD may produce mild to severe hypertension.
_____ 8. Chronic overload in the right ventricle may lead to ventricular failure and cor pulmonale.
_____ 9. Chronic bronchitis is characterized by excessive tracheobronchial mucus production.
_____10. Chronic bronchitis is associated with hyperplasia.
_____11. Emphysema is defined as distention of the alveoli.
_____12. In asthma, the air passages are enlarged.
_____13. The only cause of asthma is allergies.
_____14. Infection may trigger an asthma attack.
_____15. In asthma, airway resistance is decreased.
_____16. Asthma does not produce changes in ventilation and perfusion ratios.
_____17. Dyspnea and cough are characteristic of COPD.
_____18. Bronchitis may produce wheezing sounds.
_____19. COPD may lead to cor pulmonale.
_____20. In COPD, radiologic studies reveal a hyperradiolucent lung with the sternodiaphragmatic or lateral radiograph angle under 90 degrees.

STATUS ASTHMATICUS
Pathophysiology
Status asthmaticus is defined as a severe asthmatic attack. The bronchi and bronchioles develop mucosal edema with thickening of the basement membrane. Also, tenacious secretions, mucus plugs and smooth muscle hyperplasia are seen. These changes lead to an increase in airway resistance and respiratory effort. Atelectasis develops from the mucus plugs, resulting in decreased alveolar ventilation. Bronchi constrict in response to the antigen-histamine production.

With advanced airway obstruction and atelectasis, severe ventilation-perfusion deficits occur. Changes in arterial oxygen levels and carbon dioxide tensions are seen. Severe hypoxemia occurs without a significant rise in carbon dioxide levels. When severe and rapid decompensation occurs, severe respiratory acidosis and hypoxemia are seen.

An increase in A-P diameter develops. Both inspiration and expiration become difficult. Expiration is usually prolonged. Hyperresonance, wheezing and rhonchi are heard. The chest may become silent, which indicates little or no air exchange. Coughing becomes ineffective, exhaustion increases and gasping respirations develop. Rising pCO_2 levels, hypoxemia, exhaustion and apnea establish the need for mechanical ventilation support.

Precipitating factors are respiratory infection, allergic stimuli, toxic and irritative stimuli, improper use of asthmatic medications, stress or environmental changes.

Clinical Presentation

A sudden onset of severe respiratory distress, hypercapnia and physical exhaustion is indicative of status asthmaticus. When status asthmaticus is complicated by dehydration, the viscosity of secretions increases. Cyanosis or pallor may or may not be present. Labored breathing, wheezing, rhonchi and tachycardia may be observed.

Diagnostic Data

Patient history is an important diagnostic aid when determining precipitating factors. Arterial blood gases are the single most important determinant of respiratory function. Radiologic chest studies may be ordered to determine hyperlucency.

Nursing Care

The major nursing responsibilities are:

(1) Maintain airway; clear airway obstruction; reduce bronchospasm.
(2) Provide oxygenation.
(3) Support ventilation.
(4) Reduce stress.
(5) Reduce secretions by chest physiotherapy and suctioning.
(6) Maintain fluid and electrolyte balance.
(7) Prevent infection; use strict aseptic technique.
(8) Administer antibiotics, bronchodilators, corticosteroids and sedatives.
(9) Prevent complications, cardiac arrhythmias, respiratory failure, pneumothorax.

KEY CONCEPT: Status asthmaticus is a severe asthmatic attack that decreases alveolar ventilation.

KEY POINT RECOGNITION

Write true or false by each statement. Answers are at the end of this chapter. A score below 80% indicates the need for further study.

_____ 1. Status asthmaticus causes the bronchi and bronchioles to become edematous.

_____ 2. Status asthmaticus leads to an increase in airway resistance.

_____ 3. In status asthmaticus, severe hypoxemia occurs with a marked decrease in carbon dioxide.

_____ 4. In status asthmaticus, expiration is shorter than inspiration.

_____ 5. Hyperresonance, wheezing and rhonchi may be indicative of status asthmaticus.

_____ 6. In status asthmaticus, mechanical ventilation support may be necessary.

_____ 7. Precipitating factors leading to status asthmaticus include toxic irritants, stress and respiratory infections.

_____ 8. When status asthmaticus is complicated by dehydration, secretions become more viscous.

_____ 9. Respiratory distress, hypercapnia and physical exhaustion may be indicative of status asthmaticus.

_____ 10. The most important determinant of respiratory function is arterial blood gas analysis.

PULMONARY EMBOLISM

Pathophysiology

Pulmonary embolism is a sudden occlusion of the pulmonary artery or one of its branches. It is the leading cause of pulmonary complications in the hospitalized patient. It is not uncommon for a pulmonary embolism to be undiagnosed because of vague symptoms. It is a combination of predisposing factors, clinical presentation and diagnostic findings that diagnose pulmonary embolism.

Thrombogenesis is defined as the formation of a blood clot. The causes of thrombogenesis are stasis of blood, abnormalities in the walls of blood vessels and alterations in blood coagulation. Oral contraceptives, the postoperative phase, abrupt cessation of anticoagulants and certain malignancies (sickle cell anemia) cause the blood to hypercoagulate. Trauma to the integrity of the blood vessel wall by the use of invasive procedures or from vascular disorders may cause thrombus formation or dislodgment of the clot. In general, clots form in the deep veins of the legs and pelvis. Superficial thrombophlebitis rarely leads to emboli; however, it may be indicative of deep vein thrombosis.

Emboli may cause increased pulmonary circulatory resistance and right ventricular failure. Thromboembolism is the most common cause of pulmonary embolism. Other causes of thromboembolism are sepsis, fatty formation, foreign bodies and air. Precipitating factors are age, recent surgery, pregnancy, oral contraceptives, immobility, heart disease, vasculitis and trauma to vessel walls.

Older people are more susceptible to thromboembolism, especially in the presence of congestive heart failure or heart disease. Postoperative periods following hip, pelvic or abdominal surgery increase the likelihood of thromboembolism because of immobility, and fatty particle and bone marrow dislodgment. Red blood cell disorders, such as polycythemia and sickle cell anemia, produce abnormal cells which lead to thrombosis. During pregnancy and the postpartum period, women are more susceptible because of hypercoagulation of the blood.

Clinical Presentation

Any variety of symptoms may be present, depending on the severity and location of the pulmonary embolism. A sudden onset of shock, cyanosis, respiratory distress, tachypnea, tachycardia, right ventricular gallop and changes in mentation are indicative of massive pulmonary embolism. Diffuse multiple pulmonary emboli present in a similar manner.

Signs and symptoms of pulmonary embolism are often vague and nonspecific. It is usually diagnosed after the patient presents with symptoms of tachycardia, substernal pressure or chest discomfort, tachypnea, hemoptysis, restlessness, syncope and dyspnea.

The clinical presentation for pulmonary infarction includes hemoptysis, pleural friction rub, sudden onset of pleuretic pain and pleural effusion.

Other physical findings are atelectasis, wheezing, and systolic murmurs. A wide, fixed splitting of S2 may be indicative of pulmonary hypertension and right ventricular failure. Fever is rarely seen without infection or infarction.

Pulmonary embolism may lead to cerebrovascular occlusion, acute myocardial infarction, cardiac arrhythmias, hepatic damage, pulmonary abscess, shock, bronchopneumonia and ARDS.

Diagnostic Data

A history and physical with particular attention to detail of predisposing factors are important to the diagnosis. Laboratory studies are usually not helpful in confirming the diagnosis. Leukocytosis and elevated sedimentation rate are present with pulmonary infarction. EKG changes are rarely seen except for tachycardia. Signs of pulmonary hypertension, right axis deviation, tall peaked P-waves and ST-T-wave changes are indicative of right ventricular failure and ischemia.

Radiologic studies, such as chest x-rays, are used to establish evidence of pleural effusion and parenchymal infiltrates.

Arterial blood gases are one of the important determinants in establishing a diagnosis. Hypoxemia, hypocapnia and respiratory alkalosis are frequently present.

The most important determinant in diagnosing pulmonary embolism is pulmonary angiography or lung scan. Pulmonary angiography provides information concerning anatomy of the pulmonary vasculature. A complete obstruction by the embolus is rare. Usually, a filling defect is noted as blood attempts to flow around the embolus.

A lung scan records radioactive uptake. This provides a visual image of blood flow in the lungs and distribution of ventilation. Valuable information is obtained about the ventilative-perfusion pattern.

Nursing Care

The major nursing responsibilities include:

(1) Prevent thrombosis; ambulation, passive and active exercises, elastic stockings, deep breathing exercises.
(2) Monitor fluid and electrolyte balance; correct and maintain adequate hydration; correct electrolyte imbalance.
(3) Maintain acid-base balance; correct acid-base imbalance.
(4) Maintain oxygenation and adequate ventilation.
(5) Administer anticoagulants.
(6) Administer thrombolytic therapy; streptokinase, urokinase.
(7) Provide postoperative care; pulmonary embolectomy; inferior vena cava, ligation, clipping, or percation; intracaval umbrella.
(8) Reduce stress and anxiety.
(9) Prevent complications.
(10) Provide patient and family education.

KEY CONCEPT: Pulmonary embolism may present different clinical pictures according to the degree and severity; but overall the nursing goals are to maintain the patient during the acute stage and to prevent further complications.

KEY POINT RECOGNITION

Write true or false by each statement. Answers are at the end of this chapter. A score below 80% indicates the need for further study.

_____ 1. Thrombogenesis is defined as clot formation.
_____ 2. Pulmonary embolism is a sudden occlusion of the pulmonary artery or one of its branches.
_____ 3. A pulmonary embolism is easy to diagnose by history.
_____ 4. Stasis of blood may cause thrombogenesis.
_____ 5. Injury to blood vessel walls may cause thrombogenesis.
_____ 6. Sickle cell anemia may cause hypercoagulation of blood.
_____ 7. Superficial thrombophlebitis always leads to deep vein thrombosis.
_____ 8. Sepsis is the most common cause of pulmonary embolism.
_____ 9. Taking oral contraceptives may prevent thromboembolism.

_____10. Profound shock may be indicative of a massive pulmonary embolism.

_____11. Diffuse multiple pulmonary embolism clinically presents with vague and nonspecific symptoms.

_____12. Hemoptysis, dyspnea and tachycardia may be indicative of pulmonary embolism.

_____13. Pulmonary embolism may lead to cerebrovascular occlusion.

_____14. A lung scan aids in the diagnosis of pulmonary embolism.

_____15. Arterial blood gases are of little value in establishing a diagnosis of pulmonary embolism.

_____16. The major nursing responsibilities are to maintain the patient during the acute stage and to prevent further complications.

CHEST TRAUMA
Pathophysiology: General

Chest injuries can occur as a result of penetrating, blunt or deceleration injuries. Chest trauma is usually present in multisystem injury.

Penetrating or open injuries are the most obvious. The injury causes penetration of the chest wall integrally, as seen with stabbings, gunshot wounds and industrial injuries. The injury may cause hemothorax, pneumothorax, contusions, cardiac tamponade, vessel trauma and esophageal injury. Since the pleura has been entered, a continuous exchange of air between the atmosphere and pleural cavity is created.

Blunt trauma or closed injury is nonpenetrating. There is no communication between the atmosphere and the pleural cavity. A direct injury results in fractured ribs, pulmonary contusions, pneumothorax and hemothorax. Crushing injuries produce multiple rib fractures, pulmonary contusions, sternal fractures and rupture of the diaphragm or blood vessels. Blunt trauma is often associated with abdominal and head injuries.

Deceleration injuries are the result of sudden forces hitting the body. The forces cause internal organs to continue to move, inflicting vessel and organ tearing and rupture. This type of injury is common following high speed auto accidents.

Pathophysiology - Rib Fractures

Rib fractures often follow crushing or penetrating injuries to the chest wall. Crushing injuries may cause multiple eggshell fractures. Penetrating injuries may cause comminuted fractures with bone fragments driven into the lung parenchyma. In steering wheel injuries, the sternum is separated from the ribs by multiple fractures. Bone fragments may override or push a sharp fragment inward, causing tearing of the pleura, lung tissue, heart or great vessels.

Complications of rib fractures are pulmonary contusions, pneumothorax, hemothorax, aortic rupture, vessel tears, splenic injuries, hepatic injuries and brachial plexus injury.

Clinical Presentation

The presentation of the chest-injured patient varies with the extent and location of the rib fracture. Clinical evidence includes dyspnea, tenderness and/or pain, ecchymosis and self-splinting to prevent chest movement.

Diagnostic Data

The single best determinant of rib fracture is through chest x-ray.

Nursing Care

The major nursing responsibilities include:

(1) Minimizing pain through intercostal nerve block or analgesics.

(2) Preventing excessive movement.
(3) Restoring adequate cardiopulmonary function.
(4) Preventing complications.
(5) Monitoring fluid and electrolyte balance.
(6) Maintaining acid-base balance and/or correcting acid-base imbalance.
(7) Reducing anxiety.

KEY CONCEPT: Rib fractures are diagnosed by history, pain and radiologic studies. The overall nursing goal is to restore adequate cardiopulmonary function.

Pathophysiology - Flail Chest

Flail chest (Fig. 4-13) is defined as the fracture of two or more ribs in two or more places that creates a detached or floating segment of the anterior chest wall. Paradoxical respirations occur as the floating section moves in with inspiration and out with expiration. Paradoxical respirations diminish the effectiveness of the chest wall, create severe pain and leave the patient unable to mobilize secretions.

If the crushing injury occurs head-on, the sternum may be fractured, leading to bilateral costochondral fractures that result in separation of the ribs and sternum.

If the flailed segment is large, ventilation is impaired.

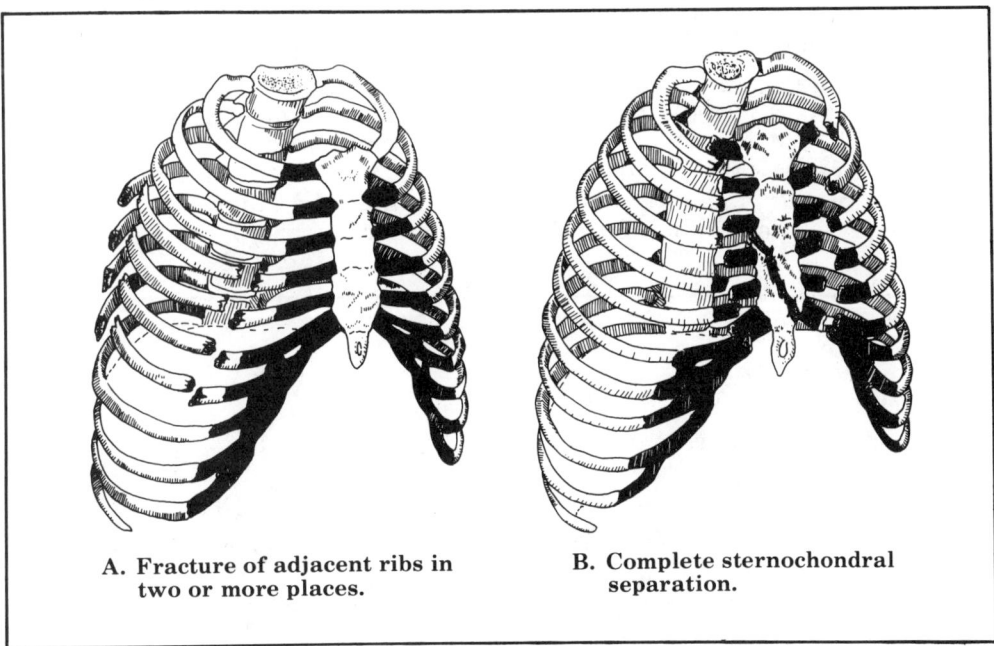

Fig. 4-13. Flail chest

Clinical Presentation

The clinical presentation varies, depending on the extent of damage.

Respirations are rapid and shallow. Skin color is cyanotic. The patient becomes hypoxic and hypercapneic. Coughing is ineffective. Palpation and inspection reveal a detached segment. The patient is in shock and complains of severe chest pain.

Diagnostic Data

A chest x-ray is the most important diagnostic aid.

Nursing Care

The major nursing responsibilities are:

(1) Promote adequate cardiopulmonary function.

(2) Stabilize chest wall; apply adhesive, sandbags.

(3) Provide airway maintenance; intubation, mechanical ventilation.

(4) Monitor cardiac status; EKG-V.S.

(5) Maintain acid-base balance; correct acid-base imbalance.

(6) Maintain fluid and electrolyte balance; correct fluid deficits; correct electrolyte imbalance.

KEY CONCEPT: The overall nursing goal in flail chest is to restore adequate cardiopulmonary function.

Pathophysiology - Hemothorax - Pneumothorax and Tension Pneumothorax

A hemothorax is a condition caused by bleeding into the pleural cavity. The blood accumulates, reducing ventilatory ability. Because of respiratory action, anticoagulant enzyme action and the smooth surface of the pleural cavity, blood does not clot. Therefore, shock ensues. Chest tubes are inserted to evacuate blood that has accumulated. If bleeding is due to vessel tearing, surgical intervention may be necessary.

A *pneumothorax* is a condition caused by an open or closed injury. An open pneumothorax is caused by a penetrating injury that exposes the affected lung to atmospheric pressure. This communication between intrapleural pressure and atmospheric pressure causes the lung to collapse (Fig. 4-14). Air passes during inspiration, but has difficulty leaving during expiration. Therefore, pressure rises within the affected side, causing the mediastinum to shift toward the unaffected side. Mediastinal shifting leads to compression of the functioning lung or unaffected side. To prevent movement of air into the pleural cavity, an occlusive dressing is placed over the open wound. Chest tubes are inserted to evacuate air and reestablish intrathoracic pressure.

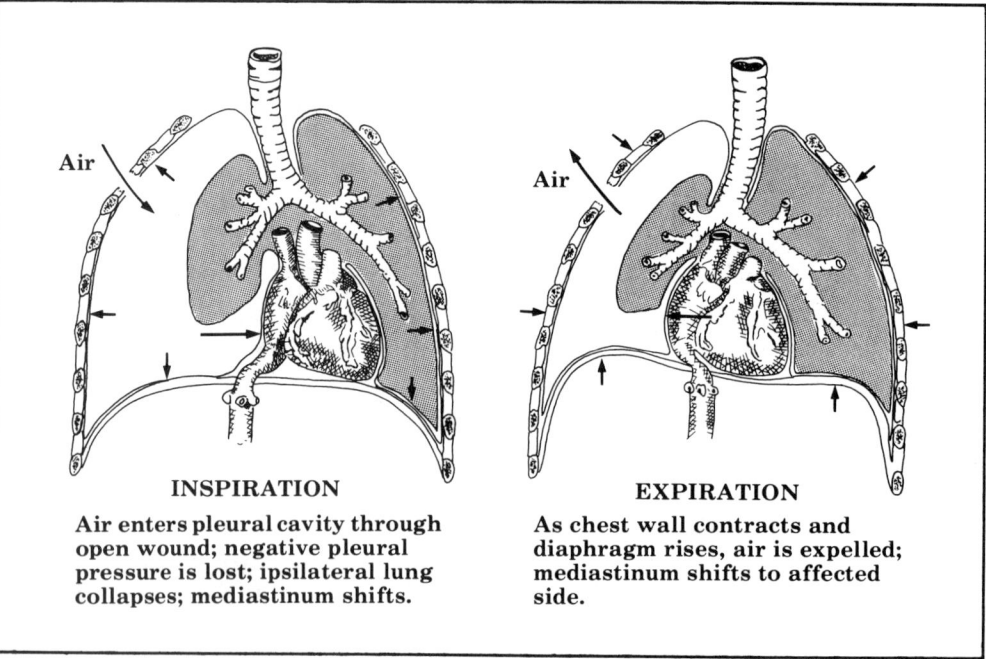

Fig. 4-14. Open pneumothorax

Tension pneumothorax is the result of rib fractures, volume ventilators, thoracentesis or emphysematous blebs. In tension pneumothorax, air leaks into the pleural space. During each inspiration, pressure rises and is unable to escape. The mediastinum shifts away from the affected side, compressing great vessels and reducing cardiac output. As a result, shock develops. To correct tension pneumothorax, a large bore needle is inserted between the second and third intracostal space at the midclavicular line. Then a chest tube is inserted.

Clinical Presentation

The clinical presentation is extremely variable and dependent upon the cause. All three may be characterized by respiratory distress, shock, cyanosis, chest pain, and absent or diminished breath sounds on the affected side. Dullness to percussion on the affected side may be seen in hemothorax. Increased resonance to percussion of the affected side may be seen with pneumothorax. Progressive cyanosis, mediastinal tracheal displacement and shift of the PMI away from the affected side may be seen in tension pneumothorax. Also, hyperresonance to percussion and widening of the intercostal spaces on the affected side may be present with tension pneumothorax.

Diagnostic Data

Laboratory studies revealing arterial blood gas imbalances are diagnostic aids. The best diagnostic aid is radiologic studies coupled with physical findings.

Nursing Care

The major nursing responsibilities are:

(1) Maintain cardiopulmonary functions.
(2) Maintain chest tube drainage.
(3) Maintain fluid and electrolyte balance; administer blood; correct fluid deficits; correct electrolyte imbalance.
(4) Monitor cardiac status.
(5) Maintain acid-base balance; correct acid-base imbalance.
(6) Maintain airway maintenance; suction; intubation, mechanical ventilation.

KEY CONCEPT: Hemothorax, pneumothorax and tension pneumothorax have similar, but varying, clinical presentations. Nursing care is aimed at restoring and maintaining cardiopulmonary function.

KEY POINT RECOGNITION

Write true or false by each statement. Answers are at the end of this chapter. A score below 80% indicates the need for further study.

_____ 1. Rib fractures never cause pleural damage.
_____ 2. Brachial nerve plexus injury may be a complication associated with rib fractures.
_____ 3. Deceleration injuries often are seen following auto accidents.
_____ 4. Chest injury is usually present with multisystem trauma.
_____ 5. Closed injuries are caused by blunt trauma.
_____ 6. A flail chest creates paradoxical respirations.
_____ 7. Respirations resulting from a flail chest are shallow and slow.
_____ 8. Nursing care is centered around restoring adequate cardiopulmonary function.
_____ 9. Tension pneumothorax is caused by bleeding into the pleural space.
_____10. A pneumothorax may be caused by an open or closed injury.
_____11. In pneumothorax, the inspiratory phase of respiration is the most difficult.
_____12. In pneumothorax, the mediastinum shifts toward the affected side.

_____13. Blood clots readily in the pleural space.

_____14. In tension pneumothorax, the mediastinum shifts away from the affected side.

_____15. In percussing for a hemothorax, dullness is heard on the affected side.

_____16. In percussing for a pneumothorax, increased resonance is heard on the affected side.

_____17. In percussing for a tension pneumothorax, hyperresonance is heard on the affected side.

CARDIAC TAMPONADE
Pathophysiology
Cardiac tamponade is the accumulation of fluid in the pericardium. Rapid collection of 250 ml of blood or less results in serious impediment of blood flow into the ventricles. Cardiac tamponade may be associated with rib fractures, stab wounds, gunshot wounds or hemopneumothorax. Pericardiocentesis or surgical intervention is necessary to repair the damage.

Clinical Presentation
The clinical picture is a result of venous congestion and decreased cardiac output. Changes in mentation, such as confusion, restlessness and unconsciousness, may occur. Distended neck veins, elevated central venous pressure, muffled or distant heart sounds, narrowed pulse pressure, pulsus paradoxus and shock may be present.

Diagnostic Data
History and physical provide the objective data. Radiologic studies may be useful. Aspiration of pericardial fluid confirms the diagnosis.

Nursing Care
The major nursing responsibilities are:
(1) Observe carefully for cardiopulmonary changes.
(2) Assist with pericardiocentesis.
(3) Prepare for surgery; thoracotomy, pericardiotomy.
(4) Provide postoperative care.

KEY CONCEPT: Cardiac tamponade is a life-threatening situation. The prognosis is dependent upon immediate recognition and intervention.

KEY POINT RECOGNITION
Write true or false by each statement. Answers are at the end of this chapter. A score below 80% indicates the need for further study.

_____ 1. Cardiac tamponade is due to excessive air in the pericardial sac.

_____ 2. Cardiac tamponade reduces blood flow into the ventricles.

_____ 3. Cardiac tamponade increases cardiac output.

_____ 4. Distended neck veins, elevated central venous pressure and muffled or distant heart sounds may be indicative of cardiac tamponade.

_____ 5. Pulsus paradoxus and shock are seen with cardiac tamponade.

INJURY TO THE DIAPHRAGM
Pathophysiology
Diaphragmatic injuries are caused by auto accidents, penetrating wounds or blunt trauma. Tearing or herniation of the diaphragm allows abdominal contents to enter the thorax. Pressure within the abdominal cavity is higher than pressure within the thoracic cavity. This pressure difference is responsible for the upward movement. Surgical intervention is necessary to correct the damage and replace abdominal contents.

Clinical Presentation

The patient with a diaphragmatic injury presents with severe respiratory distress, chest pain or shoulder pain on the affected side, and cyanosis. Signs of shock are present. Also, it becomes impossible to pass a nasogastric tube.

Diagnostic Data

Radiologic studies reveal an elevated hemidiaphragm and air-filled viscus in the thorax.

Nursing Care

The major nursing responsibilities are:

(1) Provide ventilatory support.

(2) Prepare for surgery.

(3) Provide postoperative plan of care.

KEY CONCEPT: Diaphragmatic injuries may result in rupture or herniation of the diaphragm.

KEY POINT RECOGNITION

Write true or false by each statement. Answers are at the end of this chapter. A score below 80% indicates the need for further study.

_____ 1. Abdominal contents may herniate into the thoracic cavity as a result of diaphragmatic rupture, because abdominal pressure is higher than thoracic pressure.

_____ 2. Diaphragmatic injuries may present with shock and respiratory distress.

_____ 3. To repair a rupture of the diaphragm, surgery is required.

_____ 4. In diaphragmatic injuries, a nasogastric tube is easily inserted.

_____ 5. In diaphragmatic injuries, shoulder pain is present on the same side as the tear.

TRACHEAL OR BRONCHIAL RUPTURE

Pathophysiology

Rupture of the trachea or major bronchi is usually associated with blunt trauma or deceleration injury. These injuries carry a high mortality rate. Most ruptures are within the carina. Major bronchial ruptures are on the right side.

Clinical Presentation

The clinical presentation is dependent upon two factors: communication between the rupture of the tracheobronchial tree and the pleural cavity, and the size of the pneumothorax. Other signs are hemoptysis, dyspnea, subcutaneous-mediastinal emphysema and shock. If there is no communication between the torn bronchus and the pleural cavity, the pneumothorax is usually small and expansion rapidly occurs following chest tube insertion.

Diagnostic Data

The most reliable diagnostic aid is bronchoscopy. Radiologic studies do not reveal bronchial rupture. If bronchoscopy reveals a bronchial tear of less than one-third of the lumen, and re-expansion is accomplished by a chest tube with underwater seal, treatment may be conservative. Often, surgical repair is indicated. Intubation and ventilatory support are then required.

Nursing Care

The major nursing responsibilities are:

(1) Maintain cardiopulmonary function.

(2) Maintain ventilatory support.

(3) Prepare for surgery.

(4) Provide postoperative care.

KEY CONCEPT: Rupture of the trachea or bronchi carries a high mortality rate. Early recognition and intervention are essential.

KEY POINT RECOGNITION
Write true or false by each statement. Answers are at the end of this chapter.

_____ 1. A large pneumothorax occurs following rupture of the tracheobronchial tree which communicates with the pleural cavity.

_____ 2. If there is no communication between rupture of the tracheobronchial tree and the pleural cavity, the pneumothorax is usually small.

_____ 3. Chest x-ray confirms the diagnosis of bronchial rupture.

_____ 4. Bronchoscopy confirms the diagnosis of tracheal or bronchial rupture.

ESOPHAGEAL RUPTURE
Pathophysiology

Rupture or tear of the esophagus may result from blunt or penetrating trauma or instrumentation of the esophagus. Esophageal rupture usually accompanies fracturing of the first or second rib. It is often fatal. Surgical intervention is necessary to repair the damage.

Clinical Presentation

The presenting complaint is onset of severe substernal midline chest pain, back pain or upper abdominal pain, dyspnea and a change in voice tone. Other symptoms include hematemesis, mediastinitis, cyanosis, pain on swallowing, pleural effusion, thirst, subcutaneous emphysema and gastric contents or bile in the chest tube.

Diagnostic Data

Diagnosis is by observation of sudden onset of severe chest pain or severe upper abdominal pain and history.

Nursing Care

The major nursing responsibilities are:

(1) Establish intravenous lines.
(2) Maintain fluid balance.
(3) Provide oxygenation.
(4) Prepare for surgery.
(5) Plan postoperative care.

 KEY CONCEPT: The major focus is airway maintenance and circulation.

KEY POINT RECOGNITION
Write true or false by each statement. Answers are at the end of this chapter.

_____ 1. Esophageal rupture may result from blunt or penetrating trauma.

_____ 2. Esophageal rupture is seen with fractures of the third and fourth ribs.

_____ 3. Hematemesis and subcutaneous emphysema may be indicative of esophageal rupture.

_____ 4. Severe onset of midline substernal chest pain, upper abdominal pain, dyspnea and change in voice may be indicative of esophageal rupture.

CARE COMMON TO RESPIRATORY PROBLEMS
AIRWAY OBSTRUCTION

Airway maintenance is the responsibility of the critical care nurse. It is a potential problem in any patient, regardless of diagnosis or physical status. The most common cause of upper airway obstruction is occlusion of the hypopharynx by the relaxation of the tongue. The debilitated, lethargic, comatose or heavily sedated patient is particularly susceptible to upper airway obstruction. Mucus, blood, dentures, and laryngeal spasms are also causes of upper airway obstruction. Lower airway obstruction involves movement of air from the larynx to the alveoli. Foreign bodies, secretions, hemorrhage, pneumonia, lesions, tumors, COPD and bronchospasm may cause lower airway obstruction.

Partial obstructions are characterized by snoring, retractions, stridor, wheezing and coughing. Limited air exchange takes place. This restrictive air flow results in hypoxia and hypercapnea. When the obstruction is complete, no air is exchanged. The patient becomes restless and has severe retractions and tracheal tugging. Obstruction involving the upper airways occurs during the inspiratory phase. Lower airway obstruction occurs during the expiratory phase.

AIRWAY MAINTENANCE

The easiest way to correct most obstructions is to hyperextend the neck and pull the mandible forward. Placing the head on a pillow may cause the head to fall forward, therefore producing airway obstruction.

An oropharyngeal airway is a rubber, plastic or metal device that curves over the tongue. The purpose of an oropharyngeal airway is to hold the tongue away from the posterior wall of the pharynx, thus facilitating suctioning of oral and tracheal secretions. Insertion of the airway can be accomplished by one of two methods:

(1) Place the airway so that it enters the mouth with the distal tip up. As the distal tip approaches the posterior pharyngeal wall, gently rotate and seat it into position.

(2) Press a tongue blade against the anterior surface of the tongue. The oropharyngeal airway is placed over the tongue. Slide it into position. Caution should be taken to prevent pushing the tongue backward against the pharyngeal wall. Also, proper size is essential to ensure good air flow. Aspiraton of vomitus may result from stimulation of the gag reflex. Airways are secured into position by tape to prevent accidental displacement.

Nursing care includes frequent mouth care. Humidification should be provided to prevent drying of mucous membranes.

Nasopharyngeal airways are soft, pliable, rubber or latex tubes. They are approximately six inches in length and are available in various sizes. They are useful in facial and jaw injuries, and in semiconscious patients. A lubricated nasopharyngeal airway is carefully inserted through the nose. Care must be taken to avoid mucosal damage and epistaxis.

Nursing care is aimed at maintaining a patent tube. Since the tube is soft and pliable, the nurse must watch for kinking. Also, humidification prevents occlusion of the lumen caused by secretions. The airway should be changed to the other side frequently to avoid mucosal erosion.

Mouth-to-mouth ventilation may be necessary as the first step in CPR until adjunctive equipment is available. Mouth-to-mouth ventilation is performed with the head hyperextended. A tight seal is made with the ventilator's mouth over the patient's mouth. The chest is observed for movement. If no air is moved, suspect airway obstruction. Reposition the head and try again. Whenever possible, leave dentures in place. This makes ambu masks more effective in achieving a tight seal. Effective mouth-to-mouth ventilation can deliver 17 to 18 percent oxygen.

Occasionally, mouth-to-nose ventilation is more effective than mouth-to-mouth ventilation, especially in injuries to the mouth and jaw. The head is tilted back and the mouth is closed. The ventilator forms a seal around the patient's nose. Observe for chest movement.

Direct mouth-to-stoma ventilation is used for patients with laryngectomies and tracheostomies. If the tracheostomy tube is temporary, seal the nose and mouth to prevent air leakage.

Bag-valve-mask equipment delivers an oxygen concentration of 90 percent or better with the use of an adaptor and oxygen reservoir. A bag-valve-mask provides immediate ventilation with a high concentration of oxygen. A tight seal is made with the mask following the insertion of an oropharyngeal airway. It also allows the ventilator to feel lung compliance in order to adjust the volume of air to be delivered. An overzealous ventilator may not allow for passive expiration, therefore producing a hyperventilation state. Complications, such as gastric distention, vomiting and aspiration, may occur. Also, the inability to form a tight seal with the mask may result in hypoventilation.

Demand-triggered pressure devices deliver oxygen under a pressure of 40 mm Hg and will continue to deliver as long as the control button is depressed. The chest is observed for expansion and adequate ventilation. This device is most effective during CPR and may be easily interspaced with chest compressions. Demand positive pressure devices may be used with spontaneously breathing patients. The negative pressure created during inspiration triggers the apparatus. The flow stops when the negative pressure ceases. Air escapes through the nonbreathing valve. Complications include an inadequate seal and gastric distention.

The esophageal obturator airway is a pliable, latex tube approximately 15 inches long. It is inserted into the esophagus and is inflated with 30 to 35 cc of air. The cuff inflates just below the level of the carina. Several openings are located above the cuff. Air flows through the tube and is deflected from the cuff into the trachea. The upper end is inserted into a special mask that allows for attachment of the ambu bag. The mask is fitted tightly on the face to prevent air escape. Occasionally, the cuff is inflated above the level of the carina, causing air obstruction. Also, the tube may pass directly into the trachea. Since the distal end of the esophageal obturator is blunt, no air will move. After insertion, observe the chest for bilateral symmetrical chest movement. This device is more often used in prehospital emergency situations by trained EMTs and paramedics. Other complications include esophageal rupture or tear, vomiting, aspiration and incorrect placement. This device is used on a short-term basis for unconscious patients. Endotracheal intubation may be performed with the esophageal obturator in place. Since vomiting occurs following removal of the esophageal obturator, it is recommended that the patient be intubated prior to removal. Suction should be available following removal.

Endotracheal tubes are soft rubber or latex and are available in various lengths and diameters. Most endotracheal intubation tubes have low pressure cuffs. Uncuffed tubes are used only for infants and children. This is a skilled procedure requiring dexterity and timing. Prior to endotracheal intubation, the patient is well oxygenated with 100 percent oxygen. This avoids severe hypoxia during the procedure. Following insertion of the endotracheal tube, the patient is again oxygenated and suctioned, if necessary. If the patient is spontaneously breathing, check for air movement by observing chest expansion. Breath sounds are checked bilaterally and in the lung periphery. A chest x-ray confirms tube position. The distal tip should be approximately 3 cm above the carina.

Nasotracheal intubation is used for patients with fractured jaws, oral trauma or alert individuals unable to tolerate an orotracheal tube.

Complications of endotracheal intubation include esophageal placement, laceration of the lips or mucosa, aspiraton of secretions, traumatic loss of teeth or damage to teeth. In nasotracheal intubation, specific complications include bleeding due to nasal mucosa trauma, lung infection due to nasal bacteria and dislodgment of a polyp, causing obstruction. Complications associated with endotracheal tubes are obstruction due to secretions and mucous plugs. High humidification can minimize the accumulation of secretions. Kinking occurs as a result of poor positioning of the patient's head. This is especially associated with orotracheal tubes. Occasionally, shortening the tube eliminates kinking. Pressure areas may form at the side of the mouth or nose, causing mucosa erosion. Moving the orotracheal tube from side to side every 24 hours prevents oral erosion. Frequent mouth care is important for comfort and prevention of infection. Carefully secure endotracheal tubes to prevent irritation and pressure.

Cuff herniation is less likely with the use of low pressure cuffs that are bonded to the tube. Temporary or permanent laryngeal damage may occur. Infections are due to poor aseptic technique or contaminated equipment. Patients often gag and wretch because of discomfort. This may require sedation. Slippage of the tube into the right main stem bronchus is a problem. Check for slippage after mouth care and suctioning. Following initial x-ray confirmation, mark the side of the tube at the level of the mouth. This mark can be used as a quick reference or guideline following manipulation of the tube. Routine auscultation of breath sounds will assist the nurse in discovering any position change. Clinical indications of tube slippage into the right main stem bronchus include diminished breath sounds on the left side, excessive coughing and decreased excursion on the left. Frequently, the tube slips to the level of the carina. Clinical signs include bilateral diminished breath sounds, excessive coughing and difficulty in introducing the suction catheter.

Adult-sized endotracheal tubes contain either a high or low pressure cuff. Both inflation and maintenance of the endotracheal tube are critical to avoid complications and to ensure delivery of an appropriate tidal volume. The initial amount of air instilled into the cuff should be recorded, followed by routine checks for leakage. A minimal leak avoids overinflating, while still providing protection from aspiration. This may be accomplished by placing the stethoscope on the neck area while instilling only enough air to allow for a minimal leak during peak inspiration. Broken cuffs may be easily detected if the patient is alert and able to speak. Diminished expiratory volumes on the ventilator's spirometer will occur. If the patient is ventilator-dependent, hypoxia will develop rapidly. Pressure changes associated with diminished expiratory volumes and hypoxia are indicative of a ruptured cuff. By monitoring the cuff for potential minor leaks, the nurse can quickly recognize and correct the situation. The competency of the cuff should be checked prior to intubation. This aids in preventing insertion of defective endotracheal tubes.

Low pressure cuffs prevent tracheal damage by conforming to the tracheal wall. This allows for even distribution of cuff pressure in the tracheal wall. If increasing amounts of air must be instilled into the cuff to maintain an adequate seal, a leak or tracheal dilatation should be suspected. Corrective slips should be instituted. With a low pressure cuff, periodic deflation is not necessary. Intermittent deflation of hard cuffs has not proven to be effective in preventing tracheal complications. Each time the cuff is deflated, the likelihood of aspiration increases. When indicated, extubation is performed when vital signs are stable and the patient is alert and capable of maintaining an open airway. Arterial blood gases are taken after the patient has been on a nebulizer T-tube at 40 percent oxygen for 30 minutes. If ABGs are acceptable, the tube is removed. Arterial blood gases are repeated 20 minutes post-extubation and periodically, as indicated by the clinical state.

A cricothyroidectomy is performed by skilled personnel. A transverse stab incision is made through the cricothyroid membrane, which is located just below the cricoid cartilage. A blunt object or tube may be used to maintain patency. Complications include permanent laryngeal damage, bleeding into the tracheobronchial tree and life-threatening subcutaneous emphysema. Although rarely used, it may be successful when no other means are available.

A tracheostomy is usually performed in an operating room using strict aseptic technique. Frequently the patient has an endotracheal tube in place and is well ventilated. When done under emergency conditions at the bedside, the incidence of complications increases. With the head extended, a transverse incision is made at the level of the second tracheal ring. If the incision is made lower, the tube may rest on the carina. Selection of proper size is essential. The largest cannula that will fit comfortably is used. Inserting a larger size decreases airway resistance. After insertion, the tracheostomy tube is securely tied with fabric tape looped through the flange and double knotted on the side of the neck. Tube position is confirmed by x-ray.

Indications for a tracheostomy in patients associated with acute respiratory failure include upper airway obstruction that prevents endotracheal intubation. Upper airway obstruction may be caused by allergic edema, croup and laryngeal or pharyngeal obstruction. A tracheostomy is more comfortable when a patient needs prolonged ventilation. Because the patient is more comfortable, less sedation is necessary. When secretions are copious or tenacious, tracheostomy facilitates adequate bronchotracheal toilet. Occasionally, a tracheostomy is performed for psychological reasons, especially if the patient does not tolerate an orotracheal tube. It may be necessary to bypass the normal amount of anatomical dead space, specifically in patients who are difficult to oxygenate.

Complications associated with tracheostomies can be minimized if the procedure is elective. Complications include hemorrhage, mediastinal pneumothorax, perforation of the esophagus and cardiac arrest. Also, cardiac and respiratory collapse may occur if the patient is ventilated too vigorously after cannula insertion. Severe hypercapnea causes sympathetic nervous system stimulation. If reversed too rapidly, sympathetic stimulation is suddenly removed, leading to cardiac arrest. Severe hypercapnea should be reversed gradually.

The cannula may be occluded by secretions or mucous plugs. By using humidification, this may be minimized. If the secretions are tenacious, frequent instillation of sterile saline can facilitate removal. Also, obstruction may be caused by cuff slippage over the distal end of the tracheostomy tube. If the tube is not positioned or secured properly, kinking inside the trachea may occur. Displacement of the ***tracheal tube*** is recognized by mediastinal or subcutaneous emphysema. However, the most common complication is infection due to poor suctioning technique and nosocomial transfer of organisms. Late complications include erosion of the cannula tip through the anterior wall of the trachea into the innominate artery, resulting in massive hemorrhaging. When the cannula erodes through the posterior wall of the trachea, a tracheoesophageal fistula develops, causing aspiration pneumonia. Tracheal erosion and stenosis may lead to airway obstruction. Selection of proper tube size, properly securing the tube and low pressure cuffs help minimize complications.

Various types of cuffed tracheostomy tubes are available. A common cuffed tube is the Portex, with or without an inner cannula. Double-cannula tracheostomy tubes can be made of metal or plastic. The inner cannula is removed for cleaning. It is securely locked to the outer cannula. This manipulation can cause irritation and severe coughing. Metal tracheostomy tubes are seldom used because of the rigidity involved. A cuff is employed for mechanical ventilation. Since it is not bonded to the tube, the likelihood of herniation increases.

Uncuffed fenestrated tracheostomy tubes are often used during the weaning process, especially after prolonged tracheal intubation. It is a double cannula with openings in both the inner and outer cannula. This has advantages during the weaning process. When the opening is plugged, it allows the patient to breathe through the larynx and cough effectively. It also allows the patient to speak. Plugging and unplugging the tube is a simple procedure enabling the patient to be weaned with minimal mechanical difficulty. It can easily be replugged if the patient has difficulty mobilizing secretions.

Successful weaning takes patience and sensitivity to the needs and dependencies of the patient. Following prolonged mechanical ventilation or tracheal intubation, the patient is psychologically dependent and may fear removal.

Probably the most important aspect of weaning is the attitude and approach of the nurse. Empathy will put the patient at ease, enhancing the nurse-patient relationship.

For the patient on a ventilator, the first step is placement on a T-tube setup with close monitoring of arterial blood gases and clinical changes. Either a fenestrated tube or a tracheostomy button may be inserted. Once the psychological bond has been reduced and arterial blood gases are stable, the tracheostomy tube may be removed. The tracheostomy incision closes in approximately 72 hours. After the closure is complete, the patient can produce an adequate cough.

Complications Associated with Airway Intubations

Endotracheal or tracheostomy intubation creates an artificial airway. The physiologic alterations may produce complications that are damaging to pulmonary and mucous membranes. The plastic or metal tubes act as a foreign body, producing additional mucous secretions. This accumulation of secretions provides a medium for bacterial invasion. Also, since the larynx is bypassed, aphonia develops. An ineffective cough is due to the elimination of pressure below the epiglottis.

Complications associated with the placement of an endotracheal tube include tooth damage and tearing or laceration to mucous membranes. Nasotracheal intubation may cause epistaxis, submucosal resection, rupture of polyp, infection or obstruction caused by dislodgement of the polyp. A tracheostomy procedure causes fewer problems if performed as an elective procedure. Complications associated with tracheostomy are cardiac arrest, hemorrhage, pneumothorax, damage to structures of the neck and mediastinal emphysema.

Obstructions can occur at any time and are usually caused by plugging of dried secretions. Rarely does herniation of the cuff or kinking of the tube occur.

Occasionally, the tube will dislodge or slip out of the trachea. This may cause a mediastinal or subcutaneous emphysema or pneumothorax. Clinical signs of displacement include poor arterial blood gases, poor chest excursion, inability to properly introduce the suction catheter and poor air movement. If the tube slips into one bronchus, usually the right main stem, the clinical picture includes asymmetrical chest movement, diminished breath sounds to the opposite side, coughing and expiratory wheezing. If the tube sits at the level of the carina, clinical signs include coughing, expiratory wheezing, difficulty in introducing the suction catheter and bilateral diminished breath sounds.

Other complications associated with tracheostomy tubes are wound infection, massive hemorrhaging from erosion of the innominate vessels, disconnection from the ventilator, leaks due to faulty cuffs and tracheal ischemia, necrosis or dilation.

Early complications following removal of artificial airways are laryngeal edema, hoarseness and aspiration of gastric contents. Later complications include tracheal stenosis, tracheoesophageal fistula and laryngeal stenosis.

CONTINUOUS VENTILATORY SUPPORT

Cuirass, or the iron lung, is a negative external pressure ventilator that encases the patient, covering the anterior thorax and abdomen. A negative pressure is created, pulling the chest wall outward and allowing air to flow in. This type of a ventilator is not effective for respiratory diseases, but is used primarily for neuromuscular disease.

Positive pressure ventilators apply positive pressure during the inspiratory cycle. A variable volume is delivered for each breath, depending on changes in lung compliance, lung resistance, chest wall compliance, position and changes in level of consciousness. Pressure-limited ventilators are for short-term situations because of the monitoring necessary to maintain constant parameters.

Volume-cycled ventilators provide constant ventilation, despite changes in resistance and compliance. These ventilators adapt to changes by increasing or decreasing peak airway pressures, therefore delivering a preset tidal volume. Accurate oxygen concentrations are delivered by the rise of air-oxygen blenders. The major disadvantage to a volume-cycled ventilator is its ability to deliver excessive pressures.

Assisted ventilation is synchronized to the patient's inspiratory effort. The amount of negative pressure required to trigger the machine is preset by adjusting the sensitivity. The assist mode may be used with either pressure-limited or volume-limited ventilators. The control mode on the ventilator allows delivery of a set volume and rate, regardless of the patient's respiratory effort. A combination of assist and control pressure will deliver a tidal volume when the appropriate negative pressure is reached. It will also deliver a backup rate if the patient's respiratory effort is decreased or ceases.

Before regulating ventilator settings, baseline arterial blood gases are drawn and tidal volume and rate are estimated. The normal tidal volume is 8 to 10 ml/Kg of body weight. The minute volume is 6 to 10 L per minute. Tidal volume for patients on ventilators is frequently 10 to 15 ml/Kg of body weight. Respiratory rate is varied. Normally, the expiratory phase exceeds the inspiratory phase by a ratio of 1:2. The rate is controlled by the time of the inspiratory and expiratory cycle and by the desired minute and tidal volume.

Tidal volume x rate = Minute volume

The baseline pO_2 and underlying etiology determine the oxygen concentration. Excessively high oxygen concentration leads to oxygen intoxication.

With the use of volume ventilators, patchy atelectasis may develop. It is usually not visible on a chest radiograph. Alveolar units collapse in a random fashion. In a normal individual, patchy atelectasis is prevented by the varying volumes in spontaneous respirations. The sigh mechanism of the ventilator attempts to vary the volume, thereby producing a more normal ventilatory pattern. The frequency and volume of sighs are preset. The average rate is six per minute, with a volume twice the normal preset tidal volume.

By adjusting the inspiratory-expiratory time ratio, time is allowed for the tidal volume to be delivered. Pressure limit settings are dependent upon the normal pressure required to deliver the tidal volume. Usually, the setting is 20 to 30 cm above the required pressure.

Alarm systems are designed to trigger as a result of a loss in pressure. Relying on the alarm systems may lead to a potentially dangerous situation.

Pulmonary pressure dynamics are altered during mechanical ventilation. Normally, intrapleural pressure is negative (~-5cm H_2O). With chest expansion it becomes more negative (-10 cm H_2O), thus allowing air to flow into the lungs. Air flows in as a result of the pressure gradient between the atmosphere and the lungs. A decrease in the size of the thorax during expiration causes the intrapulmonary pressure to reverse, allowing air to flow out of the lungs. During mechanical ventilation, air is forced into the lungs under positive pressure. Intrapulmonary pressure changes from -5 cm H_2O at rest to a positive pressure of +15 cm H_2O. Expiration remains a passive process during mechanical ventilation (Fig. 4-15).

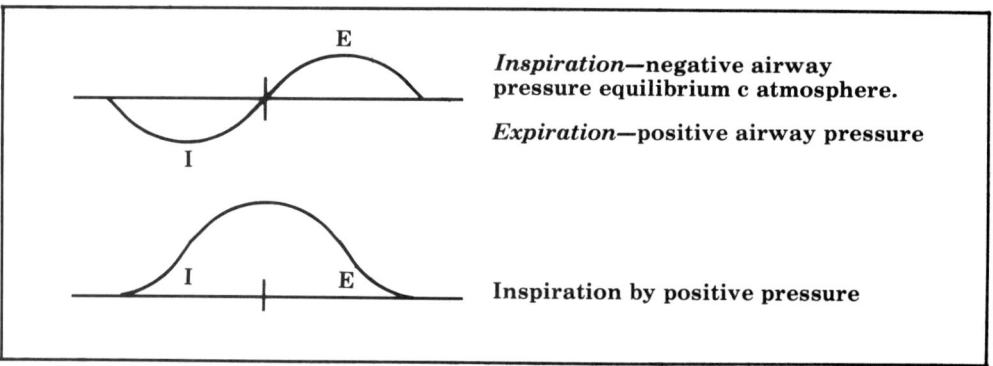

Fig. 4-15. Pressure equilibrium curve

Complications related to positive-pressure ventilators include compromised cardiovascular changes. An increase in positive pressure within the pulmonary system decreases venous return. This change is transitory until the body adjusts physiologically. Adjustment is dependent upon cardiac function fluid volume and ventilator volume setting. Clinical indications of decreased cardiac output include tachycardia, decreased blood pressure, decreased urinary output, cardiac arrhythmias, hypoxemia and acid-base imbalances. A pneumothorax may develop. Tension pneumothorax or mediastinal shifts may also develop. Atelectasis is usually the result of underlying disease or low tidal volumes. Atelectasis can be avoided by higher settings, adequate suctioning, pulmonary toilet, repositioning, chest physiotherapy and adequate humidification.

Subcutaneous emphysema occurs from an air leak into the interstitial space and mediastinum. Causes are tears in the pleura and air leaks around a tracheotomy tube. Humidification by cascade may cause fluid overload or pulmonary edema. This may be in response to stimulation of ADH caused by a low cardiac output. Clinical signs and symptoms include weight gain, hemodilution, increased A-a DO_2, reduced compliance and increased dead-space tidal volume ratios.

Mechanically induced alkalemia or acidosis may develop as a result of overzealous or inadequate ventilation. Often the alkalosis is caused by attempting to reverse acidosis. Inappropriate ventilator settings may precipitate a severe alkalosis. The ratio is slowed and tidal volume is reduced. Occasionally, mechanical dead space is added to increase pCO_2 levels. Hypoventilation may be caused by inappropriate settings or worsening of the disease process. Certain disease processes, such as COPD and cystic fibrosis, tend to make patients more dependent upon ventilators. With prolonged ventilation, muscles weaken and nutritional deficiencies develop. Dependency may be physiological or psychological.

Increased pressure is exerted on the abdomen and thorax, leading to decreased gastric motility, such as ileus and gastric distention. Stress ulcers and bleeding may be related to stress, starvation, hypersecretion of gastric acids and steroid therapy. Antacid therapy reduces gastric ulcer formation by controlling the pH.

Positive-end expiratory pressure, or PEEP, increases the functional residual capacity (FRC). The FRC represents the volume of gas left in the alveoli at the end of expiration. End-expiratory alveolar volume must remain above the critical level to keep alveoli from collapsing. As the FRC decreases, alveoli collapse increases the risk of hypoxemia and decreased compliance. An intrapulmonary shunt results from the continuous flow of blood around the collapsed alveoli. Hypoxemia develops and is unresponsive to oxygen therapy.

Collapsed alveoli decrease lung compliance, requiring a greater opening pressure. This increases respiratory effort.

PEEP is used primarily in disease processes caused by a decreased FRC, including ARDS, acute respiratory failure and pulmonary edema. The goal of PEEP is to restore FRC, which will in turn maintain arterial oxygenation with an FIO_2 below 50 percent. The lower FIO_2 will prevent O_2 intoxication.

The amount of PEEP is dependent upon the disease process and clinical condition. The hazards of PEEP include barotrauma due to high pressures causing lung damage, decreased venous return and reduced cardiac output. To achieve optimum oxygenation, a careful balance between the level of PEEP and the cardiac output is required.

Monitoring PEEP involves clinical observations to detect changes in cardiac output. This includes blood gases with oxygen levels, pulmonary artery pressure and arterial pressure. If cardiac output is reduced, then the continued need for PEEP, volume replacement, vasopressors and volume expanders may be necessary.

Controlling the ventilator is aimed at keeping the patient in phase with the machine. The term "out-of-phase" means the patient is allowing the machine to control the ventilatory pattern. This restricts the inspiratory cycle by actively pushing out while the machine is pushing in. The results of this fight are an increase in intrathoracic pressure and a decrease in alveolar ventilation, with an increase in oxygen demands. Sedation may eliminate the problem. Checks should be made to determine if there is a physiological basis for restlessness or agitation. This is especially important if the behavior has a sudden onset as opposed to the stage of an underlying disease process. The nurse should plan care to eliminate hypoxemia, CO_2 retention, hypotension, cerebral edema due to hypoxia and lack of sleep.

The aim of therapy is to keep the patient in phase while correcting respiratory abnormalities. Sedation, narcotics and paralyzing agents are frequently employed.

DRUG THERAPY

The principal effect of **morphine sulfate** is depression of the respiratory center. Morphine causes vasodilation and hypotension especially in those who are borderline hypovolemic. Morphine is titrated intravenously until the desired effect is reached. Doses may be repeated as often as every hour. Morphine is an excellent narcotic analgesic with the potential to cause dependency.

Paraldehyde has a rapid hypnotic effect. It acts as a central nervous system depressant with minimal analgesic effects. The route of choice is through the G.I. tract via a nasogastric tube. If given through the G.I. tract, it must be mixed with milk or syrup to prevent gastric irritation. Rectal administration is achieved by suspending the drug in an oil or isotonic solution to avoid local irritation and expulsion. Paraldehyde is not given intramuscularly because of the occurrence of sterile abscess formation. Sloughing and neuritis may occur. Intravenous administration is unpredictable and may cause cardiovascular collapse. Paraldehyde is detoxified in the liver and should not be administered in patients with liver impairment. The majority of the drug is exhaled, unchanged by the lung. Side effects include dependency, renal impairment and central nervous system depression.

Diazepam: Valium is a nonbarbiturate sedative-hypnotic drug with anticonvulsant and muscle-relaxant qualities. Valium affects the central nervous system. Side effects include hypotension, localized irritation, phlebitis, thrombus formation and addiction. Other side effects include physical and psychological dependency, increased cough reflex, laryngospasm, muscle weakness and urinary retention. Metabolites of valium are excreted via the kidney, so care should be used in patients with compromised kidney function. Volume is titrated intravenously at 1 mgm per minute until the desired effect is achieved.

Pavulon is a neuromuscular blocking agent that induces skeletal muscle relaxation. The dose is compiled by kg/body weight with the average 1 to 4 mgm intravenous every hour until the desired effect is reached. Subsequent doses prolong the duration of the block. Pavulon is excreted via the kidneys, therefore close observation is warranted in patients with kidney impairment. Side effects include tachycardia and prolongation of the blocked effect. Since Pavulon has no effect on consciousness or pain, it is given in combination with sedatives and narcotics.

SUCTIONING

If the patient is unable to mobilize secretions or develops an ineffective cough mechanism, suctioning is an important procedure for airway maintenance. When a ventilator patient needs to be suctioned, the pressure alarm should sound. The alarm sounds if pressure within the airway increases or if the ventilator volume decreases.

Side effects of suctioning include hypoxemia, which may lead to mucosal damage, cardiac dysrhythmias, bradycardia or cardiovascular collapse.

Suctioning requires strict aseptic techniques and preoxygenation. Adequate preoxygenation is accomplished by ambu ventilation with 100 percent oxygen for several seconds. The catheter is introduced without suction until an obstruction is felt. Suction is applied and the catheter is removed using a swirling motion or 360 degree rotation. The catheter should be of sufficient length to permit deep bronchi suctioning. The diameter should not be more than one-third of the tube's diameter. Withdrawal of the suction catheter should take no more than ten seconds. After the suction catheter is removed, the patient should be ambu ventilated at 100 percent oxygen for several seconds. While suctioning, monitor for dysrhythmias. If dysrhythmias develop, discontinue and begin 100 percent oxygen ventilation. If secretions are tenacious, small amounts of sterile saline may be introduced to facilitate aspiration.

Suctioning causes severe apprehension. Remember to explain the procedure and reassure the patient prior to and during the suctioning.

WEANING

Discontinuation of ventilatory support and extubation requires patient preparation. Preparation guidelines include both psychological and physiological readiness.

Ventilatory measurements include A-aDO$_2$, vital capacity, inspiratory force and Vd/V$_T$. Also, arterial blood gas measurements are analyzed frequently to monitor progress.

Decreased V$_T$, increased respiratory rate, increased PACO$_2$, diaphoresis and cardiac dysrhythmias may develop following ventilatory removal. If complications develop, immediately place the patient on the ventilator. When the patient can tolerate being off the ventilator for 20 to 30 minutes, blood gases are drawn. Gradually, the length of time off the ventilator is extended. Each patient is individually weaned according to personal response.

Extubation requires monitoring for spontaneous respirations. Adjunct airway equipment should remain at the bedside for emergency use. Post extubation complications are minimized by providing oxygenation. Humidification is administered to reduce laryngeal edema. If obstructive stridor or respiratory distress occurs, intubation is required. Hoarseness usually develops because of prolonged intubation but resolves spontaneously. Aspiration may occur as a result of the loss of the laryngeal reflex response.

INTERMITTENT MANDATORY VENTILATION (IMV)

IMV allows the patient spontaneous breaths augmented by mandatory ventilation. The intermittent mandatory inspiration is independent of the patient's inherent respiration. The ventilator's increased volume is not given on patient demand, but from a predetermined mandatory setting. The advantage to IMV is that it is universally adaptable and technically simple. IMV avoids the necessity for controlling the ventilatory cycle in situations in which the patient is capable of assuming some respiratory work. Other advantages include maintenance of spontaneous respiratory muscles, preventing uncoordinated movements between the chest wall and diaphragm. This is an advantage in COPD since weaning is a problem following total ventilator control for prolonged periods. Spontaneous respiratory activity aids in diminishing side effects associated with positive pressure ventilation and requires less sedation and muscle relaxants. The weaning process is enhanced and less traumatic since the number of controlled respirations may be diminished slowly. It also provides a safety mechanism, if the patient does not tolerate weaning.

The disadvantages to IMV include easy disconnection if the ventilator does not have a built-in IMV mode; inadequate delivery of humidification; the need for more water; and CO$_2$ buildup.

Nursing responsibilities include monitoring patient response; checking oxygen concentration levels; checking water levels; and monitoring V$_T$, the inspiratory rate, and minute ventilation.

GENERAL NURSING CARE

Nursing responsibilities for patients with respiratory impairment include general care, daily observations and ventilatory management.

General care includes careful observation, careful administration of prescribed medication and proper setting of the ventilating alarms. Early observations include pressure and cardiac monitoring, pulmonary function studies, laboratory studies, cardiac output, fluid and electrolyte balance, respiratory pattern neurological status and response to treatments and medications. Ventilatory management includes monitoring and recording ventilator settings; blood gas values; and ventilator readings for mode, tidal volume, sigh volume, temperature of humidification, inspired gas, measurements for PEEP and tidal volume; compliance, PAO$_2$, Vd/V$_T$ ratio and inspiratory-expiratory ratio.

CHEST PHYSIOTHERAPY

Chest physical therapy includes breathing exercises to increase aeration to the lung tissue. Chest percussion is aimed at loosening secretions and improving aeration. However, it is not done in the presence of chest pain, an acute pulmonary inflammatory process, acute cardiac conditions or hemorrhage.

Mechanical vibrations increase the velocity of expired tidal volume, thereby loosening and moving secretions to larger airways. Postural drainage provides an efficient mechanism for clearing the tracheobronchial tree of secretions by gravity.

INTERMITTENT POSITIVE PRESSURE BREATHING (IPPB)

IPPB provides a greater expansion of lung tissue and an even disbursement of gases; prevents or corrects atelectasis; delivers medications for bronchodilation and decreases respiratory effort.

The indications for IPPB remain controversial. Some indications include chronic or acute hypoventilatory states, retention of secretions, respiratory acidosis, pulmonary edema and carbon dioxide.

IPPB is contraindicated in the presence of pulmonary bleeding and subcutaneous emphysema. Extreme caution must be used in hypovolemia, cardiac diseases, active tuberculosis, and pneumothorax.

Side effects of IPPB include increased intrathoracic pressure, hyperventilation, infection and rupture of alveoli.

CONTINUOUS POSITIVE AIRWAY PRESSURE (CPAP)

CPAP maintains a normal FRC to prevent or treat atelectasis. This technique requires no ventilator. The patient breathes out against a preset water pressure with the aid of a mask and reservoir. When pressures are low, expiration remains passive. As pressure rises, expiratory resistance increases. This allows the patient to inspire low levels of oxygen, but maintains adequate arterial oxygen levels. CPAP is helpful during the weaning process or as an attempt to prevent intubation in nonemergency situations.

HUMIDIFICATION

Humidification of inspired air is important, regardless of the oxygen delivery method. Normally alveolar air is 100 percent humidified at 37°C. Air is warmed to 34°C as it passes through the nose. Air is 80 to 90 percent humidified as it passes through the oral pharynx. By the time air reaches the carina it is 37°C and 100 percent humidified. If this normal process is altered, then water and heat come from the mucosa of the tracheobronchial tree. Ineffective humidification of inspired gases by the upper airway leads to changes in the lower airways. These changes include drying of the tracheobronchial tree, impairment of ciliary action, inflammatory and necrotic changes of ciliated pulmonary epithelium, retention of tenacious secretions, bacterial infiltration of the mucosa, atelectasis and pneumonia.

Humidification devices that increase water content include cold bubble humidifiers, heated cascade and tents. Nebulizer therapy delivers water in particles for deposit along the mucosal lining of the airways. Devices include small hand nebulizers, IPPB devices, ultrasonic nebulizers and continuous aerosol therapy.

OXYGEN THERAPY

The purpose of oxygen therapy is to prevent or treat hypoxia. Hypoxia results from low tissue oxygenation or inadequate oxygen supply. The types of hypoxia include:

Hypoxic: low atmospheric pO_2 hypoventilation diffusion defects and perfusion defects

Stagnant: decreased cardiac output, resulting in prolonged tissue to capillary contact and increased A-V differential

Anemic: low hemoglobin; carbon monoxide poisoning

Histotoxic: disrupted cellular metabolism, resulting in an inability to use oxygen

Oxygen affinity: thyrotoxicosis following massive transfusions

Hypoxemia is a decrease in arterial blood oxygen tension. An acceptable level of pO_2 does not always guarantee adequate oxygenation at tissue level, especially during shock states. Acceptable tissue perfusion and oxygenation are determined indirectly by increased lactic acid production and decreased pH. Clinical symptomatology is seen in the brain, adrenals, heart, kidneys and liver.

Response to acute hypoxia includes tachycardia, hyperventilation, agitation, confusion, cyanosis and hypotension. Severe, acute hypoxia may lead to arrhythmias, bradycardia and cardiac arrest. Chronic hypoxia may result in cor pulmonale secondary to pulmonary vascular constriction and polycythemia.

Long-term oxygen therapy requires monitoring of blood gases. A principle of oxygen therapy is the delivery of the smallest concentration necessary to achieve arterial pO_2 of 60 to 80 mm Hg. The advantage of using the lowest concentration includes avoiding pulmonary intoxication and depressing the hypoxic drive.

Patients with chronic obstructive pulmonary disease have chronically high arterial carbon dioxide levels. Therefore, the respiratory stimulus becomes hypoxemia instead of carbon dioxide. If high flow oxygen concentration is administered to a COPD patient, the patient will develop respiratory depression and eventually apnea due to elimination of the hypoxic drive.

Nursing responsibilities for patients with chronic carbon dioxide retention include administration of oxygen to raise pO_2 to usually 50 to 60 mm Hg, frequent monitoring of arterial blood gases, close observation, oxygenation prior to suctioning and reduction in activity for unstable or cardiac patients.

Complications Associated with Oxygen Therapy

Respiratory depression may result from hypercapnea following oxygenation of the COPD patient. Absorptive atelectasis occurs with high concentrations of oxygen as a result of nitrogen washout. This results in alveoli which contain oxygen, carbon dioxide and water vapor. When oxygen diffuses into pulmonary capillaries, the alveoli collapse, leading to right-to-left shunt. Oxygen therapy dilates pulmonary capillaries. This causes an increase in perfusion around the collapsed alveoli.

Oxygen intoxication is related to the level of FIO_2 and PIO_2. A concentration of 50 percent or more may damage lung tissue, depending on the level of FIO_2 and the length of exposure. Early symptoms include substernal pain, paresthesia of extremities, nausea, vomiting, lethargy, dyspnea and restlessness. Late symptoms include an increase in respiratory distress, cyanosis and asphyxia. Pathological change causes localized intoxication of the pulmonary capillaries, and a change in surfactant, absorptive atelectasis and nitrogen washout. These changes cause a decrease in compliance and an increase in A-a gradient.

ADJUNCTIVE OXYGEN EQUIPMENT

Nasal cannulas are simple and comfortable devices. The range of liter flow is 1 to 6 with potential O_2 delivering oxygen of 24 to 40 percent. Disadvantages include the inability to deliver well-controlled concentrations. The percent of concentration delivered is dependent upon the patient's rate and tidal volume.

Masks are useful for short periods. They have the capability of delivering concentrations from 24 to 100 percent oxygen. The disadvantage includes skin necrosis due to tight fit, inability to control FIO_2 and generalized discomfort. Also, vomiting patients are prone to aspiration. CO_2 retention and hyperventilation may occur if liter flow is too low or mask holes are too small.

Types of masks include simple, partial rebreathing, rebreathing, non-rebreathing and venturi. A ***simple mask*** delivers 35 to 55 percent oxygen. A ***partial rebreathing mask*** delivers 35 to 60 percent oxygen. The flow is adjusted to prevent the reservoir bag from collapsing during inspiration.

Rebreathing masks are used only in the delivery of anesthesia. ***Non-rebreathing masks*** deliver 90 to 100 percent concentration. They have a reservoir bag with a one-way valve. During inspiration, 100 percent oxygen is inspired from the bag. ***Venturi masks*** deliver a precise concentration of oxygen at low levels: 24 percent, 28 percent, 35 percent and 40 percent oxygen. A T-tube is unable to deliver accurate oxygen concentration. It is limited to delivering humidified oxygen.

Nasal catheters deliver below 40 percent oxygen concentration. The disadvantages include gastric distention and nasopharyngeal trauma.

Tracheal masks deliver 35 to 70 percent oxygen concentration and are used with a heated nebulizer.

Hyperbaric oxygenation delivers oxygen under pressure. It is useful in treating gas gangrene, burns, decubiti and CO_2 poisoning.

COMPLICATIONS

Infection: Nosocomial infection may be a serious complication. This results from cross-contamination, unsterile procedures and dirty equipment. Prevention of infection occurs as a result of good basic medical nursing technique, enforcing isolation protocols, routine culturing of equipment, administration of sensitive antibiotics and restriction of visitors.

Emotional impact: Intubated patients are unable to communicate accurately or easily. It is the responsibility of the nurse to provide alternate means for communication. Paper and pencil, magic slates and flash cards offer the patient a means to communicate. Explanations are given prior to procedures and movement. Orientation to time, place and date should be done often. Patients' anxiety levels are extremely high because of unfamiliarity of equipment and the fear of body mutilation.

KEY CONCEPT: Continuous and thorough patient assessment is essential to the management of respiratory problems.

KEY POINT RECOGNITION

Write true or false by each statement. Answers are at the end of this chapter. A score below 80% indicates the need for further study.

1. _____ The most common cause of upper airway obstruction is relaxation of the tongue.
2. _____ Partial airway obstruction is characterized by coughing.
3. _____ Flexing the neck forward corrects airway obstruction.
4. _____ Nursing care of nasopharyngeal airways is aimed at maintaining a patent tube.
5. _____ Effective mouth-to-mouth ventilation delivers 30 to 50 percent oxygen.
6. _____ Demand-positive pressure devices may be used only with nonbreathing patients.
7. _____ The cuff of the esophageal obturator should be located above the level of the carina.
8. _____ Endotracheal tubes without cuffs are used for infants and children.
9. _____ Prior to endotracheal intubation, the patient is well oxygenated with 100 percent oxygen.
10. _____ The distal tip of the endotracheal tube should be 6 to 8 cm above the carina.
11. _____ Complications of endotracheal intubation include perforation and esophageal placement.
12. _____ Nasotracheal intubation may result in bleeding, infection and dislodgment of polyps.

_____13. Slippage of the endotracheal tube into the left main stem bronchus is common.
_____14. An endotracheal tube resting at the level of the carina causes diminished bilateral breath sounds, excessive coughing or difficulty in introducing the catheter.
_____15. A broken endotracheal cuff results in diminished expiratory volume on the ventilator spirometer.
_____16. High-pressure cuffs prevent tracheal damage.
_____17. Low-pressure cuffs require periodic deflation.
_____18. Before extubating, the patient must be alert.
_____19. Complications of a cricothyroidectomy are laryngeal damage and bleeding.
_____20. Tracheostomies are indicated in acute respiratory failure when endotracheal intubation cannot be performed.
_____21. The most common complication of a tracheostomy is kinking.
_____22. Erosion of the tracheal cannula through the posterior wall of the trachea results in a fistula, causing aspiration pneumonia.
_____23. A patient will have an effective cough immediately upon removal of the tracheostomy tube.
_____24. Accumulation of secretions provides a medium for bacterial invasion.
_____25. The iron lung creates negative pressure and is effective for treating respiratory diseases.
_____26. A positive-pressure ventilator adapts to changes in lung compliance and resistance.
_____27. Volume-cycled ventilators provide variable ventilations according to resistance and compliance.
_____28. Excessively high levels of oxygen concentration are never toxic.
_____29. Volume ventilators cause patchy atelectasis.
_____30. Pulmonary pressure dynamics are not altered during mechanical ventilation.
_____31. During mechanical ventilation, expiration is an active process.
_____32. An increase in positive pressure within the pulmonary system increases venous return.
_____33. Humidification by cascade may cause fluid overload and pulmonary edema.
_____34. PEEP is used in disease processes with a decreased FRC.
_____35. As FRC decreases, alveoli collapse causing increased compliance.
_____36. Being out of phase with the respirator causes a decrease in alveolar ventilation.
_____37. Paraldehyde is an effective analgesic.
_____38. Morphine sulfate causes vasoconstriction.
_____39. Valium has muscle relaxant qualities.
_____40. Pavulon induces skeletal relaxation.
_____41. The actual suctioning procedure should take no more than 10 seconds.
_____42. IMV augments spontaneous ventilation.
_____43. IPPB provides an even distribution of gases.
_____44. CPAP maintains a normal FRC to prevent or treat atelectasis.
_____45. Humidification is not important to the tracheobronchial tree.
_____46. Hypoxia may be caused by anemia.

_____ 47. Chronically high arterial carbon dioxide levels are seen in patients with COPD.
_____ 48. Early symptoms of oxygen intoxication include substernal pain, paresthesia, lethargy and restlessness.
_____ 49. The venturi mask delivers O_2 concentration at 100 percent.
_____ 50. T-tubes deliver humidified oxygen.

PASS
PROGRAM ASSESSMENT: SCIENCE AND SITUATION

1. When fat is oxidized in place of glucose, one of the by-products is:
    a. ketones
    b. adipose
    c. glyceraldehyde
    d. fructose

2. The phrase, "mucus or other material in the larger airways" produces which of the following sounds?
    a. wheezes
    b. rhonchi
    c. rales
    d. stridor

3. The normal arterial blood pH is in the range of:
    a. 7.35 to 7.45
    b. 9.35 to 9.45
    c. 7.10 to 7.30
    d. 8.11 to 9.11

4. When checking the neck for tracheal deviation, the trachea will be deviated away from the affected side in:
    a. tension pneumothorax
    b. simple pneumothorax
    c. pneumonia
    d. obstructed bronchus

5. After lifting weights, a 28-year-old male complains of sudden onset of chest pain. On auscultation, breath sounds are diminished on the left side. You should suspect:
    a. hemothorax
    b. acute myocardial infarction
    c. spontaneous hemothorax
    d. asthma

6. A pneumothorax would best be defined as:
    a. air in the peritoneum
    b. air in the periosteum
    c. air in the pleural space
    d. air in the pericardium

7. How many pairs of ribs are attached to the sternum?
    a. 10 pairs
    b. 12 pairs
    c. 14 pairs
    d. 24 pairs

8. What does upper airway obstruction sound like?
    a. wheezing
    b. rales
    c. stridor
    d. rhonchi

9. The carina is:
   a. a layer covering the eye
   b. the base of the lung
   c. the bifurcation of the right and left main stem bronchi
   d. a ring in the inner ear

10. The area between the membranous linings of the lungs and the thoracic cavity is best described as:
    a. diaphragm
    b. visceral space
    c. parietal space
    d. pleural space

11. When a patient with COPD enters an emergency department in obvious respiratory distress, which of the following set of blood gases represent a situation in which giving high concentrations of oxygen would be dangerous?
    a. pO_2 55, pCO_2 36
    b. pO_2 55, pCO_2 62
    c. pO_2 45, pCO_2 28
    d. pO_2 88, pCO_2 32

12. A patient complains of shortness of breath. On examination of the chest, diffuse expiratory wheezing is heard. This may be indicative of:
    a. congestive heart failure
    b. asthma
    c. multiple pulmonary emboli
    d. all the above

13. An 18-year-old asthmatic female arrives in the critical care unit. In the past 24 hours her dyspnea has increased despite frequent use of a nebulizer. On examination, she is extremely anxious, fatigued, has diffuse inspiratory and expiratory wheezing, and cyanosis of the nailbeds. Arterial blood gases may be indicative of:
    a. metabolic acidosis
    b. respiratory alkalosis
    c. metabolic alkalosis
    d. respiratory acidosis

14. Rhythmicity of respiration is controlled by the:
    a. carotid body
    b. apneustic center
    c. medulla
    d. pneumotaxic center

15. Primary hyperventilation will produce all of the following except:
    a. decreased arterial pCO_2
    b. increased HCO_3 excretion by the kidney
    c. increased reabsorption of H ions
    d. decreased HCO_3 excretion by the kidney

16. The action of surfactant on the lungs is to keep the alveoli from collapsing during expiration by:
    a. keeping the alveoli size constant during inspiration and expiration
    b. increasing the surface tension of fluids lining the alveoli
    c. maintaining a negative intrapleural pressure
    d. reducing the surface tension of the fluid lining the alveoli

17. Bag valve mask devices:
    (1) are always effective when used by one person
    (2) are potentially dangerous in the hands of untrained personnel
    (3) frequently provide more ventilation than mouth-to-mouth
    (4) may be modified to deliver 100 percent oxygen for effective resuscitation
    a. 2, 4
    b. 1, 3
    c. 3, 4
    d. 2, 3

18. All of the following are true concerning the aspiration of gastric contents *except* that it:
    a. may follow the removal of endotracheal tubes
    b. may be potentially lethal
    c. may follow removal of an esophageal airway
    d. is always a complication of ventilatory support with a bag-valve device

19. In a normal state, fluid is kept out of the alveoli by the:
    (1) activity of alveolar macrophages
    (2) interstitial osmotic pressure
    (3) low vapor pressure of water
    (4) negative interstitial fluid pressure
    a. 1, 3
    b. 3, 4
    c. 1, 4
    d. 2, 4

20. Total pulmonary compliance is reduced in all of the following conditions except:
    a. chronic obstructive pulmonary disease
    b. multiple fractured ribs
    c. adult respiratory distress syndrome
    d. pulmonary edema

21. Hypoxia causes the pulmonary vasculature to:
    a. vasodilate
    b. spasm
    c. vasoconstrict
    d. spasmodically constrict

22. All of the following are diagnostic signs of pulmonary embolism except:
    a. dyspnea
    b. tachycardia
    c. substernal pressure
    d. all of the above

23. The following blood gas studies were obtained on a patient who is confused and difficult to arouse: pH 7.19, pCO_2 97, pO_2 33, B.E. +12. The correct interpretation of the arterial blood gases is:
    a. respiratory and metabolic acidosis with respiratory insufficiency
    b. metabolic alkalosis with compensating respiratory acidosis and respiratory failure
    c. respiratory acidosis with compensatory metabolic alkalosis and hypoxia
    d. respiratory acidosis with compensatory metabolic alkalosis and respiratory failure

24. The respiratory drive in normal individuals is determined primarily by:
    a. hypoxia
    b. pCO_2
    c. bicarbonate ion concentration
    d. hydrogen ion concentration

25. The most common cause of airway obstruction is:
    a. tongue
    b. dentures
    c. secretions
    d. foreign bodies

26. In which of the following conditions can mediastinal shift toward the left occur?
    a. left pleural effusion
    b. left pulmonary effusion
    c. tension pneumothorax of the right lung
    d. right lung atelectasis

27. Respiratory acidosis is caused by:
    a. hyperventilation
    b. hypoventilation
    c. retention of nonvolatile acid
    d. loss of nonvolatile acid

28. A deficiency of pulmonary surfactant may result in:
    a. pneumonia
    b. asthma
    c. atelectasis
    d. pleural effusion

29. A patient on PEEP should be observed for which of the following complications?
    a. increased cardiac output, pulmonary edema
    b. increased venous return, decreased glomerular filtration rate
    c. decreased cardiac output, pneumothorax
    d. increased cardiac output, interstitial edema

30. The most appropriate oxygen delivery adjunct for a patient with chronic obstructive disease in acute respiratory decompensation is:
    a. face mask
    b. nasal cannula
    c. rebreathing mask with reservoir
    d. venturi mask

31. Ventilation/perfusion (V/Q) inequalities may be exacerbated by:
    a. loss of bicarbonate
    b. sepsis
    c. vomiting
    d. secretions

32. The effect of hypoxemia on pulmonary capillary pressure is:
    a. none
    b. acute decrease
    c. acute increase
    d. a gradual increase followed by a sharp decrease

33. Besides streptococcus, the organism that most frequently causes respiratory infections in patients with chronic bronchitis is:
    a. klebsiella
    b. pseudomonas
    c. seratia
    d. hemophilus influenza

34. When anaerobic metabolism takes place in the body, the following substance is produced by the cells:
    a. ketone bodies
    b. sulfuric acid
    c. lactic acid
    d. increased pCO_2

35. Adult respiratory distress syndrome results in a right-to-left shunt primarily due to:
    a. increased interstitial fluid
    b. pulmonary hypertension
    c. alveolar collapse
    d. pulmonary capillary constriction

36. The primary extreme medical emergency caused by a sucking chest wound is:
    a. shock
    b. tension pneumothorax
    c. respiratory acidosis
    d. bleeding

37. The signs and symptoms of hypoxia include all of the following except:
    a. irritability
    b. confusion
    c. atrial and ventricular arrhythmias
    d. constricted pupils

38. In emphysema, hypercapnia is unusual and
    a. vital capacity is high.
    b. total lung capacity is decreased.
    c. residual volume is decreased.
    d. maximal expiratory flow rates are diminished.

39. Oxygen is carried to the tissues by:
    a. red blood cells
    b. plasma
    c. hemoglobin
    d. leukocytes

40. Normal PAO_2 is:
    a. 50 to 60 mm Hg on room air
    b. 60 to 80 mm Hg on room air
    c. 80 to 100 mm Hg on room air
    d. 100 to 110 mm Hg on room air

41. The physical findings in a patient with emphysema include all except:
    a. distant or absent breath sounds
    b. increased anteroposterior diameter of the chest
    c. dullness to percussion
    d. prolonged breath sounds during expiration

42. The most common cause of hypoxemia is:
    a. decreased pH
    b. decreased tidal volume
    c. pulmonary hypertension
    d. V/Q mismatch

43. Cor pulmonale in patients with chronic obstructive pulmonary disease results primarily from:
    a. high systemic arterial pressure
    b. left ventricular failure
    c. V/Q abnormalities
    d. increased pulmonary capillary pressure

44. Anxiety-produced hyperventilation will produce the following changes in arterial pH and pCO_2:
    a. decreased pH, decreased pCO_2
    b. increased pH, increased pCO_2
    c. decreased pH, increased pCO_2
    d. increased pH, decreased pCO_2

45. The correction of hypoxemia in patients with adult respiratory distress syndrome being mechanically ventilated is:
    a. increased rate
    b. increased inspiratory flow
    c. increased FIO_2
    d. increased tidal volume and PEEP

KEY POINT RECOGNITION ANSWERS

Anatomy and Physiology
1. False—The ultimate goal is the efficient use of the gases at the cellular level.
2. False—Three divisions: nasopharynx, oropharynx and laryngopharynx.
3. True
4. False—The cricoid is the only complete ring of cartilage in the respiratory tract.
5. True
6. True
7. True
8. False—A lobule consists of the terminal bronchioles, respiratory bronchioles, alveolar ducts, alveolar sacs and vessels.
9. False—Respiratory bronchioles participate in gas exchange.
10. True

Lungs, Bony Thorax, Muscles of Respiration
1. True
2. True
3. False—A projection of the left upper lobe
4. True
5. True
6. True
7. False—Inspiration is the active phase.
8. True
9. True
10. True

Pulmonary Circulation
1. False—averages 22 mm Hg
2. True
3. True
4. True
5. True

Ventilation and Regulation of Ventilation
1. False—tidal volume
2. True
3. False—Expiratory reserve volume is the normal volume that can be expired below the tidal volume.
4. True
5. True
6. True
7. True
8. False—CO_2 level
9. True
10. True

Mechanics of Breathing, Compliance, Airway Resistance, Diffusion
1. True
2. True
3. True

4. False—100 ml/cm H_2O
5. True
6. False—Airway resistance is the relationship between pressure and flow.
7. False—The force that causes a gas molecule to enter a liquid is the pressure of the gas.
8. True
9. True
10. False—It increases the A-aDO_2.

Oxygen Transport, CO_2 Transport, Arterial Hypoxemia

1. False—97 percent is bound to Hgb.
2. True
3. True
4. False—O_2 content is the actual amount of O_2 in the blood. O_2 saturation is the actual amount of oxygen in chemical combination with Hgb in relation to the maximal amount of O_2 the Hgb can carry.
5. False—60 to 70 percent is dissolved CO_2.
6. True
7. False—Hypoxemia due to hypoventilation is accompanied by hypercapnea.
8. True
9. True
10. True

Acid-Base

1. True
2. True
3. True
4. True
5. True
6. False—The protein buffer system aids in buffering extracellular fluid.
7. False—Cell metabolism produces and consumes acid.
8. True
9. True
10. False—The respiratory system aids in controlling acid-base balance by increasing or decreasing CO_2 excretion.
11. False—The kidneys play an important role in acid-base balance.
12. False—The cellular response to an acidotic state is for potassium to move out of the cell and hydrogen to move into the cell.
13. True
14. True
15. True
16. True
17. False—The normal anion gap is 8 to 10 meq/L.
18. True
19. True
20. True
21. False—Confusion, hypercalcemia and ventricular fibrillation are signs and symptoms of acidosis.
22. True

Assessment of the Pulmonary System

1. True
2. True
3. True
4. False—The Angle of Louis is a visible angulation about 5 cm below the suprasternal notch.
5. False—The xiphoid process is the lower end of the sternal body.
6. True
7. True
8. True
9. True
10. True
11. False—An increase in fremitus may be seen in lobar pneumonia.
12. False—The point of maximal impulse is located in the fifth intercostal space medial to the midclavicular line.
13. True
14. False—Neck tumors and tension pneumothorax cause tracheal deviation to the opposite side.
15. True
16. True
17. False—Rales are indicative of fluid in the alveoli or airways.
18. True
19. False—In whispered pectoriloquy, the whispered word "99" becomes more audible.
20. False—In egophony, the word "E" is heard as "A."
21. True
22. True
23. True
24. True
25. True
26. True
27. False—Serum protein levels reflect the amount of albumin, globulins, fibrinogen, prothrombin and plasminogen.
28. True
29. True
30. False—The normal arterial $PACO_2$ range is 35 to 45 mm Hg.
31. False—Base excess refers to bicarbonate and other bases in the blood.
32. True
33. True
34. True
35. True

Pathological States and Nursing Management
Respiratory Failure

1. True
2. True
3. False—Respiratory failure can occur without disease.
4. True
5. False—Hypoxia causes an increase in sympathetic nervous system stimulation.

6. True
7. False—In chronic respiratory failure, the arterial pH remains fairly normal.
8. True
9. False—Respiratory insufficiency is diagnosed by a pO_2 less than 50 mm Hg.
10. False—Chronic respiratory insufficiency has a normal pH.
11. True
12. True

Adult Respiratory Distress Syndrome (ARDS)
1. False—ARDS applies to acute and chronic conditions
2. True
3. True
4. True
5. True
6. True
7. True
8. True
9. False—In early ARDS, minimal rales are heard.
10. False—In ARDS, the patient develops a sudden, marked respiratory distress.
11. True

Chronic Obstructive Pulmonary Disease (COPD)
1. True
2. False—Emphysema results in airway narrowing.
3. True
4. True
5. True
6. False—Total lung capacity is often elevated because of loss of elastic recoil and air trapping.
7. True
8. True
9. True
10. True
11. True
12. False—Asthma creates narrowed air passages.
13. False—Asthma may be allergic or idiosyncratic.
14. True
15. False—Asthma increases airway resistance.
16. False—Asthma may alter the ventilation and perfusion ratios.
17. True
18. True
19. True
20. False—The sternodiaphragmatic angle is over 90 degrees.

Status Asthmaticus
1. True
2. True
3. False—In status asthmaticus, severe hypoxemia occurs without a significant rise in carbon dioxide.

4. False—Expiration is usually prolonged.
5. True
6. True
7. True
8. True
9. True
10. True

Pulmonary Embolism
1. True
2. True
3. False—Pulmonary embolism may go undiagnosed because of vague symptoms. It is a combination of predisposing factors, clinical presentation and diagnostic findings that establishes a diagnosis.
4. True
5. True
6. True
7. False—Superficial thrombophlebitis rarely leads to deep vein thrombosis.
8. False—Thromboembolism is the most common cause of pulmonary embolism.
9. False—Oral contraceptives may cause thromboembolism.
10. True
11. False—Diffuse multiple pulmonary emboli present in a manner similar to massive pulmonary embolism.
12. True
13. True
14. True
15. False—Arterial blood gases are important in establishing a diagnosis. Hypoxemia, hypocapnea and respiratory alkalosis are seen.
16. True

Chest Trauma
1. False—Rib fractures may damage the pleura and lung tissue.
2. True
3. True
4. True
5. True
6. True
7. False—Respirations are rapid and shallow.
8. True
9. False—Tension pneumothorax is caused by air leaks into the pleural space.
10. True
11. False—Air passes easily during inspiration, but has difficulty leaving during expiration.
12. False—In pneumothorax, the mediastinum shifts toward the unaffected side.
13. False—Blood does not clot in the pleural space.
14. True
15. True
16. True
17. True

Cardiac Tamponade
1. False—Cardiac tamponade is an accumulation of fluid in the pericardium.
2. True
3. False—Cardiac tamponade decreases cardiac output.
4. True
5. True

Injury to the Diaphragm
1. True
2. True
3. True
4. False—In diaphragmatic injuries, a nasogastric tube does not pass.
5. True

Tracheal or Bronchial Rupture
1. True
2. True
3. False—Radiologic studies do not reveal bronchial rupture.
4. True

Esophageal Rupture
1. True
2. False—Esophageal rupture is seen with fractures of the 1st and 2nd ribs.
3. True
4. True

Care Common to Respiratory Problems
1. True
2. True
3. False—Hyperextension of the head and moving the mandible forward relieves airway obstruction caused by a relaxed tongue.
4. True
5. False—Effective mouth-to-mouth ventilation delivers 17 to 18 percent oxygen.
6. False—Demand positive pressure devices may be used on spontaneously breathing patients.
7. False—The cuff of the esophageal obturator is located below the carina.
8. True
9. True
10. False—The distal tip of the endotracheal tube should be 3 cm above the carina.
11. True
12. True
13. False—It is more common for the endotracheal tube to slip into the right main stem bronchus.
14. True
15. True
16. False—Low pressure cuffs prevent tracheal damage.
17. False—Low pressure cuffs do not require periodic deflation. High pressure cuffs require periodic deflation.
18. True
19. True

20. True
21. False—Infection is the most common complication.
22. True
23. False—Usually, the cough is effective after the incision closes in approximately 72 hours.
24. True
25. False—is effective for neuromuscular diseases
26. True
27. False—Volume-cycled ventilators provide constant ventilation despite changes in resistance and compliance.
28. False—may lead to oxygen intoxication
29. True
30. False—They are altered.
31. False—Expiration remains a passive process.
32. False—An increase in positive pressure within the pulmonary system decreases venous return.
33. True
34. True
35. False—An increase in alveoli collapse causes a decrease in compliance and hypoxemia.
36. True
37. False—Paraldehyde has a hypnotic effect.
38. False—Morphine sulfate causes vasodilation.
39. True
40. True
41. True
42. True
43. True
44. True
45. False—Humidification is important to the tracheobronchial tree in order to prevent complications.
46. True
47. True
48. True
49. False—Deliver low concentration O_2.
50. True

PASS ANSWER SHEET

1. a
2. b
3. a
4. a
5. c
6. c
7. a
8. c
9. c
10. d
11. b
12. d
13. d
14. c
15. d
16. d
17. a
18. d
19. d
20. a
21. c
22. d
23. d
24. b
25. a
26. c
27. b
28. c
29. c
30. d
31. d
32. c
33. d
34. c
35. c
36. b
37. d
38. d
39. c
40. c
41. c
42. d
43. d
44. d
45. d

SURVEY SUMMARY
PULMONARY SYSTEM

I. The Pulmonary System is the system responsible for delivery and removal of respiratory gases at the cellular level.

II. Anatomy
   A. The respiratory tract is divided into the
      1. *Upper airway*
         a. Nasal cavity
         b. Pharynx
      2. *Lower airway*
         a. Larynx
         b. Trachea
         c. Bronchi
         d. Terminal bronchioles
      3. *Alveoli*
         a. Surfactant is a lipoprotein that acts to lower the surface tension in the fluid layer lining the alveoli.
         b. The *acini* is where gas exchange actually takes place.
   B. *Lungs*
      1. The right lung is divided into three lobes and ten bronchopulmonary segments.
      2. The left lung is divided into two lobes and eight bronchopulmonary segments.
      3. *Pleura* cover each lung and are divided into two layers
         a. Parietal
         b. Visceral
   C. The skeletal framework of the thorax consists of
      1. Twelve pairs of ribs and cartilage
      2. Sternum
      3. Twelve vertebrae
   D. Muscles of Respiration
      1. Inspiratory phase is *active* and controlled by the *diaphragm, intercostal,* and *abdominal muscles.*
      2. Expiration is *passive* and caused by the post-inspiratory shortening of the lungs' elastic fibers and surface tension changes.
   E. Pulmonary Circulation
      1. The *pulmonary artery* carries unoxygenated blood from the right ventricle to the lungs.
      2. The four *pulmonary veins* carry oxygenated blood to the left heart.
      3. Blood flow distribution through the lungs varies with need.

III. Physiology
   A. Ventilation is the movement of gas volumes necessary to maintain concentrations of CO_2 and O_2 between the atmosphere and alveoli.
      1. Divisions of *lung volumes*
         a. *Tidal volume*—volume of gas inspired or expired with each breath
         b. *Inspiratory reserve volume*—inspired about tidal volume

c. ***Residual volume***—amount of gas remaining after maximum expiration
2. ***Lung capacities***
   a. ***Total lung capacity***—total lung volume following maximal inspiration
   b. ***Vital capacity***—volume that can be expired following maximal inspiratory effort
   c. ***Functional residual capacity***—volume remaining in lung at resting level
B. ***Regulation of ventilation***
   1. Respiratory Center Medulla
      a. CO_2 powerful respiratory stimulant
      b. CSF sensitivity
   2. Hering Breuer reflex
      a. Stretch receptors in lungs
      b. Activated by inflation
      c. Impulses sent to the medullary centers—inhibits respirations
   3. Hypoxia
      a. Weaker drive
      b. Chemoreceptors in carotid bodies and receptors at arch of aorta
   4. Emotion
      a. increases ventilation
   5. Pain or motion
   6. Sepsis
      a. Endotoxins in CSF
      b. Increased temperature = increased rate, not volume
   7. Medications
      a. Morphine
      b. Decreased respiratory center activity
C. ***Mechanics of breathing***
   1. Intrapleural pressure
      a. Lungs tend to recoil away from chest wall
      b. Chest wall tends to recoil in opposite direction
   2. Atmospheric pressure of -760 mm Hg
      a. Tendency to separate causes negative pressure of 755 mm Hg
      b. Negative intrathoracic pressure of -5 mm Hg
   3. Inspiration
      a. Thoracic volume increases
      b. Pressure falls below atmospheric pressure, gas flows into lungs
      c. End of inspiration alveolar pressure rises above atmospheric pressure to produce expiratory flow
      d. Quiet breathing (-3 to -7 mm Hg)
      e. Maximum effort (-80 mm Hg)
D. ***Compliance***
   1. Relationship between pressure and volume
   2. Decreased by:
      a. Diseases making lungs stiffer
         1. Atelectasis
         2. Pneumonia
         3. Pulmonary fibrosis

b. Processes occupying intrathoracic spaces
　　　　　1. Pleural effusion
　　　　　2. Pneumothorax
　　　c. Factors decreasing chest wall distensibility
　　　　　1. Kyphoscoliosis
　　　　　2. Obesity
　　　　　3. Abdominal distention
　　3. Low compliance equals increased work of breathing
E. *Airway resistance*
　　1. Relationship between pressure and flow
　　2. Normal
　　　a. Highest in nose
　　　b. intermediate in trachea and large bronchi
　　　c. lowest in small bronchi
　　3. Obstructive diseases
　　　a. COPD
　　　　　1. Highest pressure in small bronchioli
　　　　　2. Largest component of airway resistance
　　　b. Other conditions
　　　　　1. Asthma
　　　　　2. Bronchitis
　　　　　3. Retained secretions
F. *Oxygen transport*
　　1. 97% is bound to hemoglobin and three degrees are dissolved in plasma.
　　2. Oxygen saturation $SaO_2 = \frac{O_2 \text{ content}}{O_2 \text{ capacity}} \times 100\%$
　　3. The amount of oxygen combined with hemoglobin is dependent on the partial pressure of O_2.
G. *Carbon dioxide transport*
　　1. Carbon dioxide is carried in the blood by being:
　　　a. Physically dissolved
　　　b. Chemically combined with hemoglobin
　　　c. In the form of bicarbonate
H. *Acid base*
　　1. Acid base components of an acid base balance are:
　　　a. Acid
　　　b. Base
　　　c. pH
　　　d. pO_2
　　　e. pCO_2
　　2. Systems: bicarbonate buffer system and phosphate buffer system
　　　a. Bicarbonate buffer system consists of carbonic acid (H_2CO_2) and sodium bicarbonate ($NaHCO_3$).
　　　　　1. H_2CO_3 dissociates rapidly into CO_2 and H_2O leaving a high concentration of acid
　　　　　2. H_2CO_3 does not dissolve into H and HCO_3 readily
　　　　　3. If HCl and bicarbonate is added then the following occurs: HCl and $NaHCO_3 = H_2CO_3^+$ NaCl.
　　　　　　The pH will drop

4. If sodium hydroxin (NaOH) and H_2CO_2 then the following occurs: $NaOH + H_2CO_3 = NaHCO_3 + H_2O$
     The pH will rise
  b. The phosphate buffer system consists of hydrogen monophosphate (HPO_4) and phosphate (H_2PO_4)
     1. If HCl is added, $HCl + Na_2HPO_4 = NaH_2PO_4 + NaCl$ occurs. The pH will drop.
     2. If NaOH is added, $NaOH + NaH_2PO_4 = Na_2HPO_4 + H_2O$ occurs. The pH will rise.
  c. The protein buffer system consists of proteins of the cells and plasma.
     1. CO_2 can diffuse through the cell membrane changing the pH within the cell.
     2. Aids in buffering extracellular fluid
3. Respiratory Component
  a. Complete combustion of the by-products of metabotism yields $CO_2 + H_2O$
  b. $CO_2 + H_2O = H_2CO_3 = H + HCO_3$
     This equation is reversible and is closely associated with the bicarbonate buffer system.
  c. CO_2 produced by metabolism is excreted by the lungs
  d. Normal PCO_2 level is 40 mm Hg
  e. Henderson-Hasselbalch equation
     1. Is the relationship between the pH level and the concentration of acid and base
     2. The body maintains a ratio of 20:1 at all times
4. Renal component aids in controlling acid base balance by:
  a. Increasing or decreasing CO_2 excretion
  b. Excreting hydrogen ions
  c. Reabsorbing bicarbonate
  d. Synthesis of new bicarbonate
5. Relationship of potassium and acidosis
  a. In ketoacidosis, potassium shifts out of the cell and hydrogen shifts into the cell.
  b. Hydroxyl is formed, and more base is created to neutralize the acids in the plasma.
  c. Then potassium shifts back into the cell which causes a deficiency of potassium in the plasma.
6. Acidosis
  a. Result of primary respiratory disturbance with hypoventilation and an increase in the PCO_2 level
  b. May be result of primary metabolic disturbance causing a lowering of the HCO_3 level
  c. Causes of primary respiratory acidosis
     1. Generalized lung disease
     2. Airway obstructed
     3. Thoracic cage malfunction
     4. Respiratory center depression
     5. Inappropriate mechanical ventilation
  d. Causes of metabolic acidosis
     1. Direct loss of HCO_3

2. Increased acid-loading
3. Drugs
7. Anion Gap
   a. May be due to acid-loading or loss of HCO_3
   b. Unmeasurable anions in the extracellular fluids are sulfates, phosphates, and organic acid ions.
   c. Increased unmeasurable ions may be due to intoxication with salicylates, paraldehyde, methanol and ethylene glycol or in the presence of renal failure, diabetic ketoacidosis and lactic acidosis.
   d. Normal anion gap is 8-10 meq/L
      Normal range is 5-15 meq/L
8. Alkalosis
   a. May be result of a primary respiratory disturbance with hyperventilation and decrease in the pCO_2 level.
   b. May be result of a primary increase in the bicarbonate level.
   c. Causes of respiratory alkalosis
      1. Acute hyperventilation
      2. Chronic hyperventilation
   d. Causes of metabolic alkalosis
      1. Chloride depletion
      2. Severe potassium depletion
      3. Excessive alkali intake
9. Compensation
   a. Body attempts to maintain a 20:1 ratio between acid and base
   b. A reduction of pCO_2 level causes the kidney to excrete HCO_3 to maintain the ratio.
   c. A fall in plasma HCO_3 level will cause the lungs to blow off CO_2 and retain acid to maintain the ratio.
10. Mixed acid base disturbances
    a. Respiratory and renal abnormalities occurring simultaneously
    b. Respiratory acidosis and metabolic alkalosis
    c. Respiratory alkalosis and metabolic acidosis
11. Calcium
    a. Increasing blood pH decreases the amount of ionized calcium and increases the amount of bound calcium.
    b. Decreasing blood pH increases the amount of ionized calcium and decreases the amount of bound calcium.
    c. Increase in ionized calcium causes muscular irritability.
12. Treatment of acid-base imbalance
    a. Respiratory acidosis:
       1. Correction of underlying problem
       2. Support respirations by increasing ventilation
    b. Metabolic acidosis:
       1. Administration of $NaHCO_3$
       2. Avoid severe alkalosis
    c. Respiratory alkalosis:
       1. Elimination of underlying disorder
    d. Metabolic alkalosis:
       1. Potassium chloride administration if caused by diuretics

2. Ammonium chloride or arginine HCl administration of caused by gastric loss
13. Signs and symptoms of acidosis
    a. Confusion to coma
    b. Vascular collapse
    c. Hypercalcemia, hyperkalemia
    d. Ventricular fibrillation
14. Signs and symptoms of alkalosis
    a. Restlessness, irritability
    b. Tetany
    c. Convulsions
    d. Arrhythmias
    e. Hypocalcemia
    f. Hypokalemia

IV. **Assessment of the pulmonary system should include:**
   A. *Patient Assessment*
      1. *Specific signs* of altered functioning
         a. Cough symptoms and productivity
         b. Sputum characteristics
         c. Dyspnea onset and severity
         d. Nasal discharge and bleeding
         e. Sinus pain or tenderness
         f. Chest pain
      2. Assessment of gross cerebral functioning
         a. Consciousness
         b. Orientation
      3. Assessment of specific cerebral functioning
         a. Arousability
         b. Orientation
         c. Ability to follow commands
   B. *Anatomical landmarks*
      1. Anterior thorax
      2. Lateral chest
      3. Posterior thorax
   C. *Lungs*
      1. Apices extend approximately one inch above the medial third of the clavicles on the right.
      2. Diagonal fissure divides the upper and lower lobes.
      3. Horizontal fissure separates the upper and middle lobe.
      4. The left oblique fissure is similar to the fissure of the right lung.
   D. *Inspection*
      1. General appearance
      2. Muscular development
      3. Thorax configuration and movement
      4. Respiratory pattern
   E. *Palpation*
      1. Symmetry of chest
      2. Tenderness
      3. Fremitos

4. Point of maximal impulse (PMI)
5. Subcutaneous crepitus
6. Tracheal deviation

F. *Percussion*

G. *Auscultation*
1. Normal breath sounds
   a. Vesicular
   b. Bronchial
   c. Broncovesicular
2. Abnormal or adventitious breath sounds
   a. Absent
   b. Diminished
   c. Bronchial and Broncovesicular heard over lung fields
   d. *Voice sounds* heard on auscultation

H. *Evaluation of vital signs*
1. Hypertension
2. Respiratory distress

I. *Laboratory and radiologic studies*
1. Sputum
2. Serum protein
3. Blood gas analysis
4. Chest, decubitus, apical lordotic, and anterior oblique films
5. Laminography, tomography, planography
6. Fluoroscopy
7. Bronchography
8. Pulmonary angiography
9. Lung scan
10. Bone scan
11. PPD skin test
12. Endoscopy
13. Laryngoscopy
14. Bronchoscopy
15. Mediastinoscopy
16. Thoracentesis
17. Biopsy
18. Pulmonary function test

V. **Pathological states and nursing management**

A. *Respiratory failure*
1. Failure of the respiratory system to provide for an exchange of oxygen and carbon dioxide and inadequate alveolar ventilation
2. In chronic respiratory failure, the renal system responds to the hypercapnia. Arterial pH remains fairly normal.
3. Acute respiratory failure is detectable by a fall in pH and a sudden rise in arterial pCO_2 level.
4. Respiratory insufficiency is inadequate alveolar ventilation.
   a. The patient presents with:
      1. Hyperventilation
      2. PO_2 less than 50 mm Hg

           b. Acute respiratory insufficiency is alveolar hyperventilation with an increased pH and respiratory alkalosis.
           c. Chronic respiratory insufficiency is alveolar hyperventilation with renal compensation and normal pH.
        5. The patient may present with:
           a. Changes in mentation
           b. Muscular twitching
           c. Asterixis
           d. Papilledema
           e. Skin changes
           f. Hypertension or hypotension
           g. Cardiac arrhythmias
        6. Arterial blood gases are the most important diagnostic aids.
        7. Nursing care includes:
           a. Maintain ventilation
           b. Provide oxygenation
           c. Prevent infection
           d. Monitor arterial blood gases
           e. Maintain nutritional status
           f. Provide meticulous skin care
           g. Monitor hypertensive state
           h. Prevent complications
     B. *Adult respiratory distress syndrome (ARDS)*
        1. Results from injury to the alveolar-capillary unit
        2. An increase in permeability results in leakage of fluid into the interstitial space and alveoli, which produces edema.
        3. The patient presents with dyspnea, cyanosis, hypotension, hypoxia, and rales.
        4. Arterial blood gases, chest x-rays and pulmonary studies are diagnostic aids.
        5. Nursing care includes:
           a. Correct arterial hypoxemia
           b. Monitor ventilators
           c. Maintain PEEP
           d. Restrict fluids
           e. Monitor respiratory status
           f. Administer corticosteroids
           g. Prevent infection
           h. Maintain nutritional status
           i. Provide meticulous skin care
           j. Prevent complications
     C. *Chronic obstructive pulmonary disease*
        1. A chronic obstruction of air flow caused by asthma, chronic bronchitis, or emphysema
        2. Asthma results in an increase in airway resistance, respiratory effort and hyperinflation of lungs.
        3. In emphysema, the most common COPD, the patient may present with:
           a. Scant mucoid sputum
           b. Weight loss

c. Use of accessory muscles with prolonged expiration
d. Pulse-lip breathing
e. Neck vein distention
f. Hyperresonance
g. Rhonchi
4. Chest x-ray, sputum studies, arterial blood gases and spirometry studies are diagnostic aids.
5. Nursing care includes:
   a. Teaching patient
   b. Restrict or remove irritants
   c. Teach chest physiotherapy
   d. Correct arterial hypoxemia
   e. Administer drugs
   f. Maintain adequate hydration
   g. Prevent infection
   h. Prevent complications

D. **Status asthmaticus**
1. A severe asthmatic attack which results in mucosal edema with thickening of the basement membrane
2. The patient may present with:
   a. Hypoxemia
   b. Respiratory distress
   c. Hypercapnia
   d. Wheezing
   e. Rhonchi
   f. Tachycardia
3. Arterial blood gases are the single most important determinant in establishing a diagnosis.
4. Nursing care includes:
   a. Maintain airway
   b. Provide oxygenation
   c. Support ventilation
   d. Reduce stress
   e. Reduce secretions
   f. Maintain fluid and electrolyte balance
   g. Prevent infection
   h. Administer antibiotics
   i. Prevent complications

E. **Pulmonary embolism**
1. A sudden occlusion of the pulmonary artery or one of its branches which is the leading cause of pulmonary complications in the hospitalized patient
2. The patient may present with:
   a. Pain
   b. Shock
   c. Cyanosis
   d. Respiratory distress
   e. Tachypnea
   f. Hemoptysis
   g. Pleural friction rib

3. Chest x-ray, arterial blood gases and lung scan are important determinants in establishing a diagnosis.
4. Nursing care includes:
   a. Prevent thrombosis
   b. Monitor fluid and electrolyte
   c. Correct electrolyte imbalance
   d. Maintain acid-base balance
   e. Maintain oxygenation
   f. Administer anticoagulants
   g. Reduce stress and anxiety
   h. Prevent complications

F. *Chest trauma*
   1. Chest trauma can occur as a result of penetrating, blunt or deceleration injuries.
   2. The patient may present with:
      a. Rib fractures, tenderness/pain, dyspnea, ecchymosis, and self splinting to prevent chest movement
      b. Flail chest: rapid and shallow respirations, paradoxical respirations, cyanosis, hypoxia, hypercapnia, palpable detached rib segment, shock and severe chest pain.
      c. Hemothorax, pneumothorax, tension pneumothorax shock, respiratory distress, cyanosis absent or diminished breath sounds, tracheal deviation, widening of intercostal spaces on the affected side.
   3. Arterial blood gases and chest x-ray are diagnostic aids.
   4. Nursing care includes:
      a. Minimizing pain
      b. Stabilizing chest movement
      c. Restoring adequate cardiopulmonary function
      d. Preventing complications
      e. Monitoring fluid and electrolyte balance
      f. Maintaining correct acid-base balance
      g. Reducing anxiety

G. *Cardiac tamponade*
   1. Cardiac tamponade is the accumulation of fluid in the pericardium.
   2. The patient may present with:
      a. Venous congestion and distended neck veins
      b. Decreased cardiac output
      c. Confusion, restlessness
      d. Muffled or distant heart sounds
      e. Narrowed pulse pressure
      f. Pulsus paradoxus
      g. Shock
   3. Aspiration of pericardial fluid confirms the diagnosis.
   4. Nursing care includes:
      a. Observe for cardiopulmonary changes
      b. Assist with pericardiocentesis
      c. Prepare for surgery; thoracotomy; pericardiotomy
      d. Provide postoperative care

H. *Injury to the diaphragm*
   1. Tearing or herniation of the diaphragm allows abdominal contents to enter the thorax.
   2. The patient may present with:
      a. Respiratory distress
      b. Chest pain
      c. Shock
   3. Radiologic studies reveal an elevated hemidiaphragm and an air-filled viscus in the thorax
   4. Nursing care includes:
      a. Provide ventilatory support
      b. Prepare for surgery
      c. Provide postoperative care

I. *Tracheal or bronchial rupture*
   1. Rupture of the trachea or major bronchi may be associated with blunt trauma or deceleration injury.
   2. The patient may present with:
      a. Hemoptysis
      b. Dyspnea
      c. Subcutaneous—mediastinal emphysema
      d. Shock
   3. The most reliable diagnostic aid is bronchoscopy.
   4. Nursing care includes:
      a. Maintain cardiopulmonary function
      b. Maintain ventilatory support
      c. Prepare for surgery
      d. Provide postoperative care

J. *Esophageal rupture*
   1. Results from rupture or tear of the esophagus from blunt or penetrating trauma or instrumentation.
   2. The patient may present with:
      a. Severe substernal midline chest pain, back pain or upper abdominal pain
      b. Dyspnea
      c. Change in voice tone
      d. Hematemesis
      e. Mediastinitis
      f. Cyanosis
      g. Pleural effusion
      h. Subcutaneous emphysema
   3. Diagnosis is by observation of sudden onset of severe pain and history.
   4. Nursing care includes:
      a. Establish intravenous lines
      b. Maintain fluid balance
      c. Provide oxygenation
      d. Prepare for surgery
      e. Plan postoperative care

VI. Care common to respiratory problems
A. *Airway obstruction*
1. Upper airway obstruction occlusion
   a. Relaxation of the tongue
   b. Mucus, blood, dentures
   c. Laryngeal spasms
2. Lower airway obstruction involving movement of air from the larynx to the alveoli
   a. Foreign bodies
   b. Secretions
   c. Hemorrhage
   d. Pneumonia
   e. Lesions
   f. Tumors
   g. COPD
   h. Bronchospasm
3. Partial airway obstruction
   a. Characterized by snoring, retractions, stridor, wheezing, and coughing
   b. Limited air exchange
   c. Results in hypoxia and hypercapnia

B. *Airway maintenance*
1. Correction may be maintained by:
   a. Hyperextend neck and pull mandible forward
   b. Oropharyngeal airway
   c. Nasopharygeal airway
   d. Mouth-to-mouth ventilation
   e. Mouth-to-nose ventilation
   f. Mouth-to-stoma ventilation
   g. Bag-valve-mask
   h. Demand triggered pressure devices
   i. Positive pressure devices
   j. Esophageal obturator airway
   k. Endotracheal intubation
   l. Nasotracheal intubation
   m. Cricothyroidectomy
   n. Tracheostomy
2. Complications associated with airway intubations
   a. Airway intubation results in damage to pulmonary and mucous membranes
   b. Plastic or metal tubes produce additional mucous secretions
   c. Aphonia is caused by the bypass of the larynx
   d. Ineffective cough is caused by the elmination of pressure below the epiglottis
   e. Oropharyngeal intubation may cause:
      1. tooth damage
2. lacerations or tears of buccal mucous membranes and lips
   f. Nasopharyngeal intubation may cause:
      1. Epistaxis
      2. Rupture of polyp

3. Infection or obstruction by dislodged polyp
  g. Tracheostomy may cause:
    1. Cardiac arrest
    2. Hemorrhage from erosion
    3. Pneumothorax
    4. Damage to neck structures
    5. Mediastinal emphysema
  h. General complications
    1. Obstruction caused by plugging of dried secretions
    2. Herniation of the cuff
    3. Kinking of the tube
    4. Dislodgment or slipping out of the trachea
    5. Lodgment of tube at the level of the carina
    6. Laryngeal edema
    7. Hoarseness
    8. Aspiration of gastric contents
    9. Tracheal stenosis
    10. Tracheoesophageal fistula
    11. Laryngeal stenosis

C. *Continuous ventilatory support*
  1. Cuirass or iron lung is a negative external pressure ventilator.
    a. Not effective for respiratory diseases
    b. Used for neuromuscular diseases
  2. Positive pressure ventilators
    a. Apply positive pressure during the inspiratory cycle
    b. Deliver variable volume
    c. For short term use
  3. Volume-cycled ventilators
    a. Provide constant ventilation despite changes in resistance and compliance.
    b. Major disadvantage is the ability to deliver excessive pressures
    c. Assisted ventilation is synchronized to the patient's inspiratory effort.
  4. Ventilatory Settings
    a. Obtain arterial blood gases
    b. Tidal volume 8 to 10 ml/Kg of body weight
    c. Minute volume 6 to 10 Liters/minute
    d. Respiratory rate varies
    e. Expiratory phase exceeds inspiratory phase by a ratio of 1:2.
    f. Tidal volume rate = minute volume
    g. Sign frequency and volume are preset with an average rate of six per minute.
    h. Alarm settings are designed to trigger as a result of loss in pressure.
  5. Pulmonary pressure dynamics
    a. Are altered during mechanical ventilation
    b. Intrapleural pressure is normally negative, and with chest expansion it becomes more negative.

c. During mechanical ventilation, air is forced into the lungs under pressure, changing intrapulmonary pressure to a positive pressure of +15cm H_2O

6. Complications related to positive pressure ventilators include
   a. Decrease in venous return
   b. Decreased cardiac output
   c. Pneumothorax
   d. Tension pneumothorax
   e. Mediastinal shifts
   f. Atelectasis
   g. Infection
   h. Subcutaneous emphysema
   i. Alkalosis or Acidosis
   j. Hypoventilation
   k. Stress ulcers

7. Positive end-expiratory pressure (PEEP)
   a. PEEP increases FRC
   b. Keeps alveoli from collapsing
   c. Used in disease process caused by decreased FRC: ARDS, acute respiratory failure and pulmonary edema
   d. The hazards of PEEP include barotrauma, reduced cardiac output and decreased venous return.

D. **Drug Therapy**
   1. The goal is keeping the patient in control with the ventilator.
   2. Drugs
      a. Morphine Sulfate
      b. Paraldehyde
      c. Valium
      d. Pavulon

E. **Suctioning**
   1. Strict aseptic technique
   2. Prevent hypoxemia

F. **Weaning**
   1. Requires psychological and physiological readiness
   2. Carefully monitor for complications

G. **Intermittent mandatory ventilation (IMV)**
   1. Allows for spontaneous breaths augmented by mandatory ventilation
   2. IMV dependent upon patient's inherent respirations
   3. Advantages to IMV:
      a. Universally adaptable and technically simple
      b. Prevents uncoordinated movements between chest wall and diaphragm
      c. Requires less sedation
   4. Disadvantages to IMV:
      a. Easily disconnected
      b. Inadequate delivery of humidification
      c. CO_2 build-up
   5. Nursing responsibilities include:
      a. Monitoring patient response

b. Checking concentration levels

c. Checking water levels

d. Monitoring inspiratory rate and minute ventilation

H. *General nursing care*
   1. Observation
   2. Administration of medications
   3. Maintain proper settings of ventilatory equipment
   4. Monitor cardiac and neurological status
   5. Monitor laboratory and pulmonary studies

I. *Chest physiotherapy*
   1. Breathing exercises
   2. Chest percussion
   3. Mechanical vibrations

J. *Intermittent positive pressure breathing (IPPB)*
   1. IPPB provides a greater expansion of lung tissue and an even disbursement of gases.
   2. Prevents or corrects atelectasis
   3. Delivers medication and humidity for bronchodilation
   4. Decreases respiratory effort

K. *Continuous positive airway pressure (CPAP)*
   1. CPAP maintains a normal FRC to prevent or treat atelectasis
   2. Helpful during the weaning process

L. *Humidification*
   1. Important regardless of the oxygen delivery method
   2. Ineffective humidification will cause:
      a. drying of the tracheobronchial tree
      b. impairment of ciliary action
      c. inflammatory and necrotic changes of ciliated pulmonary epithelium
      d. Retention of tenacious secretions
      e. Bacterial infiltration of the mucosa
      f. Atelectasis and pneumonia

M. *Oxygen therapy*
   1. Prevent or treat hypoxia
   2. Long-term oxygen therapy requires monitoring of blood gases
   3. A principle of oxygen therapy is the delivery of the smallest concentration necessary to achieve arterial PO_2 of 60 to 80 mm Hg
   4. Complications associated with oxygen therapy include:
      a. Respiratory depression
      b. Oxygen toxicity

N. *Adjunctive oxygen equipment*
   1. Nasal cannula
   2. Mask
   3. Venti mask
   4. T-Tube
   5. Nasal catheter
   6. Hyperbaric oxygenation

O. *Complications*
   1. Infection
   2. Emotional impact

CHAPTER FIVE
CARDIOVASCULAR SYSTEM

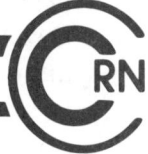

BEHAVIORAL OBJECTIVES

After reading the *Cardiovascular System,* the nurse will be able to:
- Describe the anatomy and physiology of the cardiovascular system
- Relate functions to the major components of the cardiovascular system
- Describe the conduction system
- Describe coronary circulation
- State the components of a physical assessment of the cardiovascular system
- Identify the laboratory and radiologic studies related to cardiovascular disorders
- Describe the pathophysiology of the following states:
    arteriosclerosis
    angina pectoris
    myocardial infarction
    congestive heart failure and pulmonary edema
    pericarditis
    hypertensive crisis
    cardiogenic shock
    pacemakers
- Identify the clinical manifestations and diagnostic findings associated with:
    arteriosclerosis
    angina pectoris
    myocardial infarction
    congestive heart failure and pulmonary edema
    pericarditis
    hypertensive crisis
    cardiogenic shock
    pacemakers
- Develop a nursing care plan for these conditions:
    angina pectoris
    myocardial infarction
    congestive heart failure and pulmonary edema
    pericarditis
    hypertensive crisis
    cardiogenic shock
    pacemakers
    vascular surgery
- List the common problems associated with cardiovascular disorders.

TOPICAL OUTLINE
CARDIOVASCULAR SYSTEM

- I. Cardiovascular System: Overview 235
- II. Anatomy 235
    - Functional and microscopic anatomy 235
    - Coronary chambers, valves, conduction system 238
        - Chambers 238
        - Atria 239
        - Ventricles 240
        - Valves 241
        - Conduction system 241
    - Circulation 243
        - Coronary circulation 243
        - Conduction system blood supply 244
        - Lymph supply 244
        - Vascular anatomy 245
- III. Physiology 246
    - Electrophysiology 246
    - Nervous control of the heart 249
        - Reflex responses 249
    - Factors affecting blood flow and pressure 250
        - Regulation of flow 250
        - Principles of distribution 251
    - Cardiac cycle 252
    - Cardiac output 253
    - Factors affecting cardiac function and output 256
        - Preload 256
        - Central venous pressure (CVP) 257
        - Pulmonary capillary wedge pressure (PCWP) 257
        - Afterload 258
        - Contractility 258
        - Heart rate 259
        - Anemia, ion concentration, hypoxia 259
- IV. Assessment of the Cardiovascular System 260
    - Level of consciousness 261
    - Inspection 261
    - Palpation 262
    - Percussion 262
    - Auscultation 263
    - Heart sounds 263
        - Normal heart sounds 263
        - Physiological splitting 264
        - Fixed splitting 264
        - Gallops 264
        - Order of sounds heard 264
        - Abnormal heart sounds 265
    - Evaluation of vital signs 267

   Laboratory and special studies 267
    Laboratory studies 267
    Special studies 268
    Electrocardiography 269
    Axis-vectors 274
    Axis deviation 276
    Hemiblocks 278
    Electrolytes and EKG changes 282
    Arrhythmia methods 282
    Common methods for rate determination 294
    Invasive assessment methods 295
V. Pathological States and Nursing Management 297
   Arteriosclerosis 297
    Pathophysiology 297
    Clinical presentation 298
    Diagnostic data 298
    Nursing care 298
   Angina pectoris 298
    Pathophysiology 298
    Clinical presentation 298
    Diagnostic data 299
    Nursing care 299
   Myocardial infarction 299
    Pathophysiology 299
    Clinical presentation 299
    Diagnostic data 299
    Nursing care 300
   Congestive heart failure and pulmonary edema 301
    Pathophysiology 301
    Clinical presentation 302
    Diagnostic data 303
    Nursing care 303
   Pericarditis 303
    Pathophysiology 303
    Clinical presentation 303
    Diagnostic data 304
    Nursing care 304
   Hypertensive crisis 304
    Pathophysiology 304
    Clinical presentation 304
    Diagnostic data 305
    Nursing care 305
   Shock 305
    Pathophysiology 305
    Clinical presentation 306
    Diagnostic data 307
    Nursing care 308

      Pacemakers 308
          Pathophysiology 308
          Temporary pacemaker 308
          Clinical presentation 309
          Diagnostic data 309
          Nursing care 309
          Permanent pacemakers 310
          Clinical presentation 311
          Diagnostic data 311
          Nursing care 311
          Types of pacemakers 312
          Electrical complications 314
      Surgical intervention 315
          Nursing care 315
          Vascular surgery 316

VI. Care Common to Cardiovascular Problems 321
      Cardiac circulation 321
      Hemodynamics: monitoring and adjuncts 321
          Central venous pressure 321
          Pulmonary artery wedge pressure monitoring 321
          Intra-aortic balloon pump (IABP) 321
          Nursing care 322

Program Assessment: Science and Situation 327
Key Point Recognition Answers 335
PASS Answer Sheet 311
Survey Summary 345

CARDIOVASCULAR SYSTEM: OVERVIEW

The *cardiovascular system* is composed of the *heart* and *blood vessels.* It is a vital transport system responsible for providing nutrients and oxygen to all body cells and for removing metabolic waste products from the cells. This closed system consists of a major pump and conduit, and may be further subdivided into the *heart, systemic circulation* and *pulmonary circulation.*

The cardiovascular system demonstrates the dynamic equilibrium concept. The mechanical function of the pulsating heart actually maintains the blood flow, but the real phenomenon of the system occurs when, upon demand, the cardiovascular system integrates with the nervous, renal, pulmonary and endocrine systems to adjust blood supply to specific body areas.

KEY CONCEPT: The cardiovascular system supplies oxygen and nutrients to the body cells, removes waste products and actively maintains homeostasis upon demand through continuous adjustments of blood supply to major body organs.

ANATOMY

FUNCTIONAL AND MICROSCOPIC ANATOMY

The *heart,* the central organ of the cardiovascular system, is a bioelectrically driven muscular pump. It lies within the mediastinum, between the sternum and spinal column. It is bordered laterally by the lungs, which overlay most of the heart's anterior surface, and inferiorly by the diaphragm.

The heart approximates the size of the owner's closed fist and is shaped like a blunt cone. The heart great vessels suspend the heart, directing the broader end, or *base,* upward, backward and to the right. The pointed end, or *apex,* points downward, forward and to the left (Fig. 5-1).

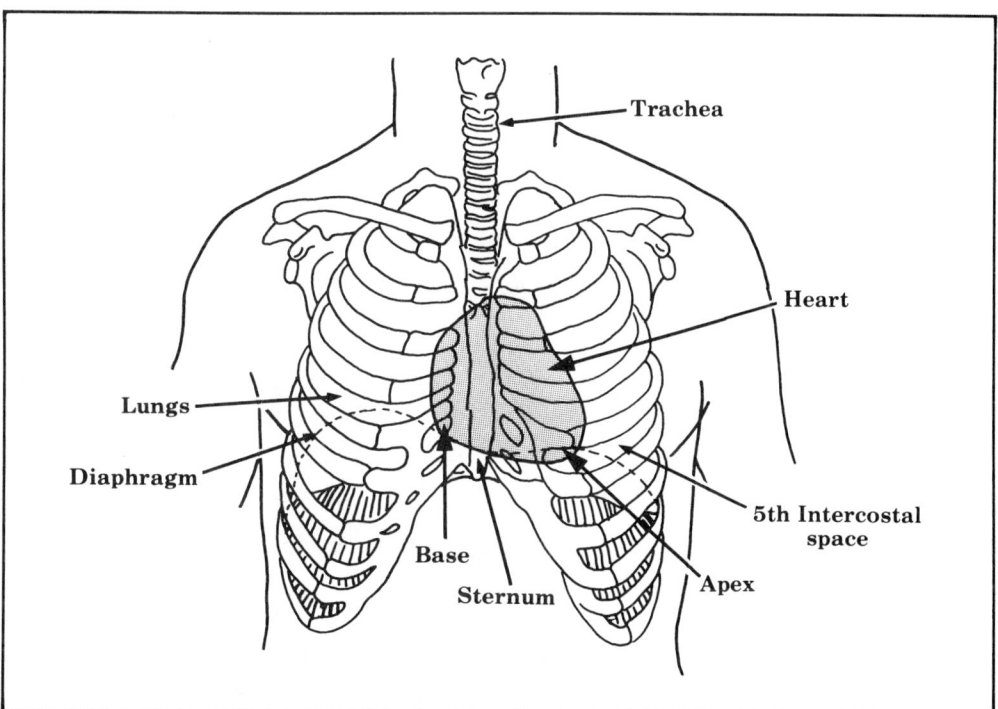

Fig. 5-1. Position of heart

The heart is enclosed in a tough, fibrous sac, the *pericardium,* which is divided into two layers: *fibrous pericardium* (outer layer) and *serous pericardium.* Serous pericardium is further divided into two layers: *parietal* and *visceral.* The visceral pericardium is the outer surface layer of the heart. These two layers are separated by a potential space, which is lubricated by approximately 15 to 20 ml of serous fluid that prevent friction when the two surfaces touch during contraction.

The heart is composed of three layers: the **epicardium, myocardium** and **endocardium.**

The **epicardium** is the surface layer of the heart and is synonymous with the visceral layer of the serous pericardium. In other words, the epicardium is the serous membranous lining of the pericardial sac. Two sulci, the interventricular and coronary, form indentations on the epicardial surface. The coronary arteries traverse within these grooves.

The **myocardium** is the major muscle mass of the heart. It is a mass of individual muscle cells that contains actin and myosin protein myofibrils connected by a tubular system, the sarcoplasmic reticulum, and is enclosed in a membranous sheath or sarcolemma. Cardiac muscle consists of both skeletal and smooth muscle tissue.

The **endocardium** is the innermost layer of the heart. It lines the heart chambers and the valves, and is contiguous with the lining of the major vessels.

KEY CONCEPT: The heart is composed of three layers: epicardium, myocardium and endocardium. It is encased in a fibrous sac, the pericardium, which is composed of two layers: fibrous and serous. The serous is the inner membrane and has a parietal and visceral layer.

Interlacing fibers of specialized cardiac muscle compose the heart. Cardiac muscle cells (Fig. 5-2) differ from skeletal muscle cells in structure and function. The basic cardiac cell forms a functional **syncytium** in which the individual cells are joined together in an irregular complex of bands and spirals. There are no defined attachments for tendons and bony attachments as is characteristic of skeletal muscle. The individual cell consists of a nucleus and mitochondria. Cardiac cells contain more mitochondria than skeletal muscle. Physiologically, this allows cardiac cells to produce more adenosine triphosphate (ATP), which is needed for the high energy requirements of repetitive muscular action specific to the heart (inherent rhythmicity). Each cell is covered by a membrane or **sarcolemma.** From the sarcolemma, a sarcoplasmic reticulum penetrates the cell to form a complex tubular or T-system surrounding each fibril. The electrical activity triggering the contraction of each sarcomere moves through the sarcotubular system as follows: The action potential is transmitted via the T-tubules from the sarcolemma to all the fibrils. Membrane potentials are employed by nerve fibers to transmit nerve impulses. It is by this energy that information signals are transmitted from one part of the nervous system to another. Action potentials are abrupt, pulselike changes in the membrane potential. This action potential causes the calcium-ion-rich sarcoplasmic reticulum to release calcium, and a contraction is sustained.

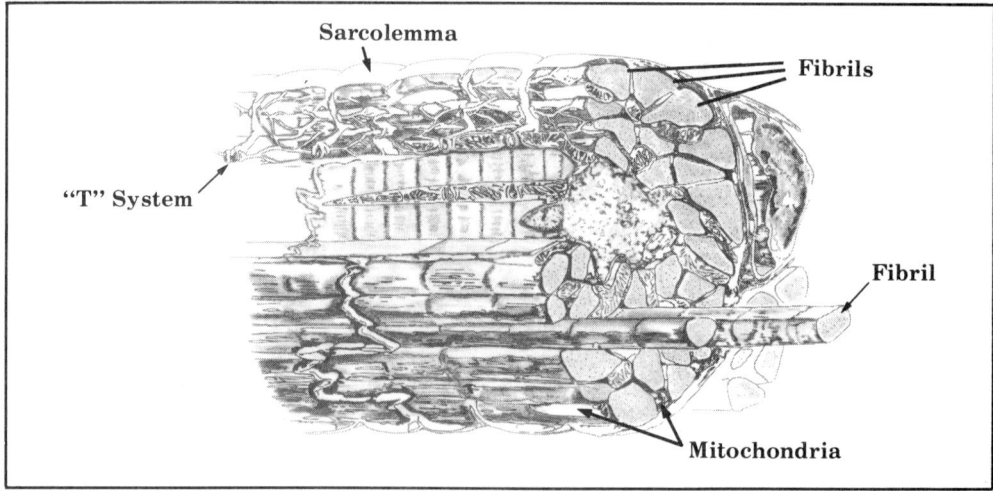

Fig. 5-2. Myocardial cell

Each contractile unit is called a *sarcomere* (Fig. 5-3). This sacromere is made up of many fibrils, which are further made up of filaments. This special protein composition of the filament allows contractility. The two major contractile proteins are **actin** and **myosin.** They overlap and give a striated appearance to the muscle. Myosin is thicker than actin and the two minor proteins, troponin and tropomyosin. The striations are called: *A bands, I bands and Z lines.*

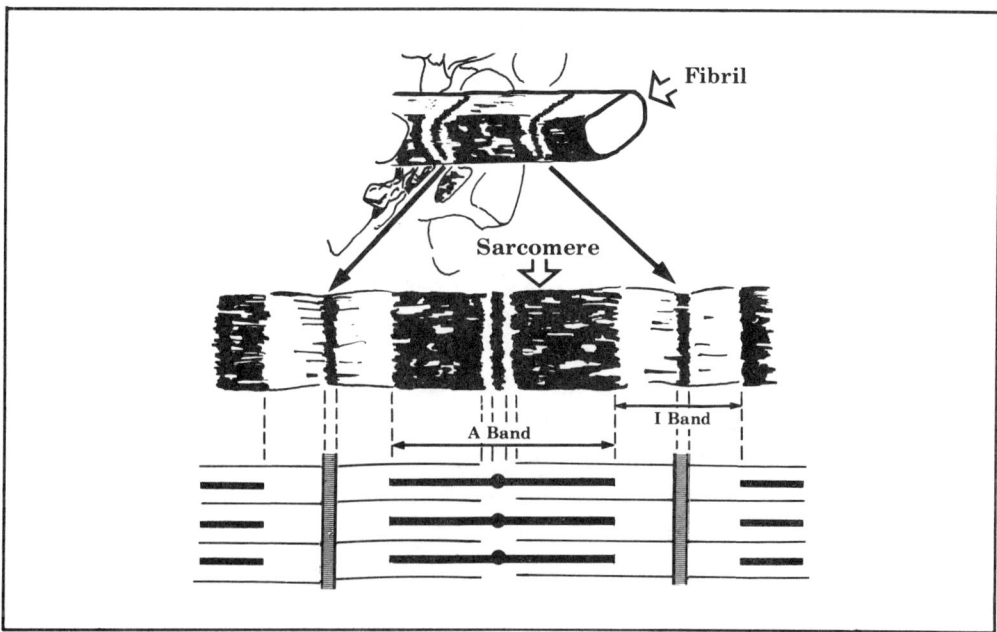

Fig. 5-3. Each sarcomere is a contractile unit.

Wide, dark **A bands** form by myosin overlapping with the lighter actin. **I bands** are lighter and are seen only where actin is present. A **Z line** is actually the end of one sarcomere and the beginning of the next.

Observation with the electron microscope reveals changes in the sarcomere pattern during contraction and relaxation. Upon contraction, the I band shortens, the A band is denser and the Z lines come closer together. Upon relaxation, the overlapping is decreased (Fig. 5-4).

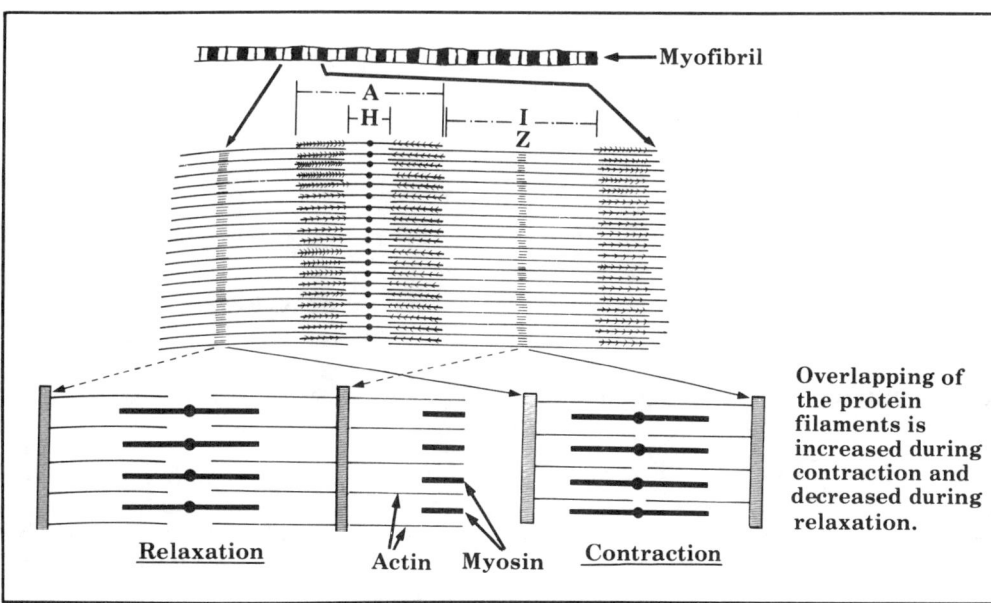

Fig. 5-4. Contraction of myofibril.

KEY CONCEPT: Cardiac muscle differs from skeletal muscle in that it has more mitochondria, can provide more ATP and has inherence rhythmicity. The functional syncytium enhances contractility by allowing an all-or-none fiber response.

KEY POINT RECOGNITION

Write true or false by each statement. Answers are at the end of this chapter. A score below 80% indicates the need for further study.

_____ 1. The heart and blood vessels compose the cardiovascular system.
_____ 2. The heart lies within the mediastinal space.
_____ 3. The lungs overlie most of the heart's posterior surface.
_____ 4. The heart is bordered inferiorly by the diaphragm.
_____ 5. The heart is enclosed in a fibrous sac, the pericardium.
_____ 6. The two layers of the pericardium are the parietal and visceral pericardium.
_____ 7. The serous pericardium is composed of a parietal and visceral layer.
_____ 8. The space between the parietal and visceral pericardium contains 120 to 150 ml of serous fluid.
_____ 9. The heart is composed of three layers.
_____10. The epicardium is the major muscle mass of the heart.
_____11. The myocardium contains actin and myosin protein myofibrils.
_____12. The endocardium is the outermost layer of the heart.
_____13. Cardiac cells have the same properties as skeletal muscle cells.
_____14. A syncytium joins individual cells in an irregular complex of bands and spirals.
_____15. Cardiac cells contain less mitochondria than skeletal muscle.
_____16. Cardiac cells produce more adenosine triphosphate (ATP).
_____17. Each cell is covered by a membrane or sarcolemma.
_____18. The action potential is transmitted via the T-tubules from the sarcolemma to all the fibrils.
_____19. The sarcoplasmic reticulum is rich in sodium ions and is lacking in calcium ions.
_____20. The action potential causes the sarcoplasmic reticulum to release calcium.
_____21. A sarcomere comprises many fibrils which are further made up of filaments.
_____22. The protein make-up of the filament allows for contractility.
_____23. The two major contractile proteins are actin and myosin.
_____24. Actin is thicker than myosin.
_____25. Under the electron microscope, the changes seen during contraction include a lengthening of I bands.
_____26. Under the electron microscope, the changes seen during contraction include a denser appearance to A bands.
_____27. Under the electron microscope, the changes seen during contraction include Z lines coming closer together.

CORONARY CHAMBERS, VALVES, CONDUCTION SYSTEM

Chambers

The heart is divided into right and left halves by a muscular partition called the septum. The septum extends from the base to the apex of the heart. After birth, there is normally no communication between the left and right sides. The septum and trabeculae divide the heart into four chambers: the *right atrium, left atrium, right ventricle* and *left ventricle.*

Atria

The *atria* (Fig. 5-5) are reception chambers for blood entering the heart. Both atria are thin-walled structures located behind, slightly above and to the right of their corresponding ventricles. While the ventricles are contracting, the atria act as reservoirs. The trabeculae divide the atria and ventricles.

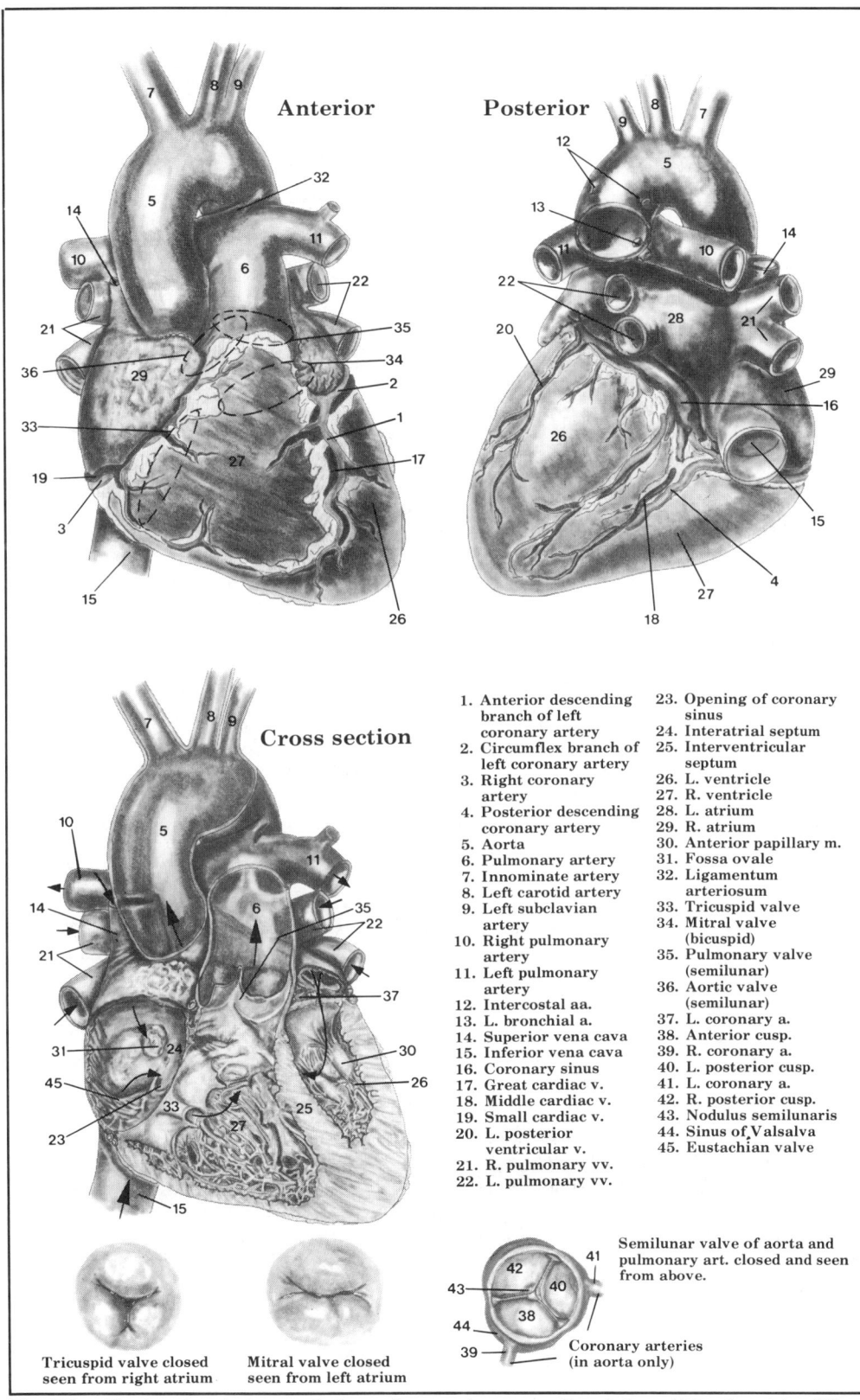

Fig. 5-5. The heart: anterior, posterior and coronal cross-sectional views (After the style of Heart Drawings by The American Heart Association)

In the early phase of ventricular diastole, blood flows passively from the atria to the ventricles; but, during the later phase of ventricular filling, the atria contract in a booster pump effect to give an additional quantity of blood, which accounts for approximately 30 percent of the filling of the ventricles. When atrial systole is lost in an otherwise normal heart, it has a minimal effect on cardiac output and blood pressure. On the other hand, if there is any impediment to filling the left ventricle, as in mitral stenosis, left atrial systole becomes very important and can account for up to 50 percent of the left ventricular filling cycle. Both atria have appendages, referred to as *vestiges* in the fetal heart, that contain pectinate muscle. The right atrial appendage is useful for placement of an atrial pacing catheter, while the left atrial appendage is useful as a surgical approach for a valvotomy.

The *right* atrium receives unoxygenated (venous) blood from the superior and inferior venae cavae and coronory sinus. The venae cavae enter the dorsum of the right atrium. The coronary sinus enters more anteriorly and superiorly to the entrance of the inferior vena cava. Opening into the right atrium above and behind the tricuspid valve is the auricle, a small, ear-shaped appendage. There are also numerous small thebesian veins opening into the right atrium which drain some of the venous blood from the myocardium directly into the right heart.

The *left* atrium receives oxygenated (arterial) blood from the lungs via four pulmonary veins. In contrast to the right atrium, which comprises multiple prominent bands on its inner surface, the interior of the left atrium is smooth, except within its auricle. The left atrium might be more appropriately titled the posterior atrium. When it becomes dilated, as in mitral valve disease, it extends to the right and upward, and may put significant pressure on and elevate the left lower-lobe bronchus. When the left atrium becomes greatly engorged, it may form the right border of the heart on x-ray. If it elevates the left lower lobe bronchus, it occasionally causes some left lower-lobe atelectasis.

Ventricles

The *ventricles* are the pressurizing chambers of the heart that force the blood to circulate. The left ventricle squeezes out blood as it contracts, whereas the right ventricle has a pumping action similar to a bellows pump. Each ventricle ejects about 75 ml of blood with each contraction, approximately 60 percent of the 120 ml each normally contains at the end of diastole.

The *right ventricle* is a thin-walled, crescent-shaped musculature, approximately 3 to 4 mm thick. The inflow tract directs blood to the apex, where it is routed, during contraction, to the outflow tract and through the pulmonic valve. Right ventricular pressure is 25/0 to 5 mm Hg, which is reflected in jugular venous and central venous pressure (CVP). It is a low-pressure system and pumps blood into the low-pressure pulmonary system. However, in the presence of tricuspid valve or pericardial pathology, the right ventricular pressure (reflected through the CVP) rises. Trabeculated muscle at the apex stabilizes a ventricular pacing catheter.

The *left ventricle* is a thick-walled musculature, approximately 8 to 14 mm thick. It contains approximately three times more muscle mass than the right ventricle. It is cone-shaped and is positioned posteriorly and laterally to the left. The left ventricle is a high-pressure chamber and pumps blood into a high-pressure systemic circulation. Left ventricular pressure ranges from 90/4 to 140/12 mm Hg and is reflected in *pulmonary capillary wedge pressure* (PCWP or PWP). In the presence of mitral insufficiency* and increased pulmonary vascular resistance, left ventricular pressure is increased. The normal left ventricle must push against a *systemic vascular resistance* (SVR) mean pressure of approximately 90 mm Hg, which is normally about five to six times that of the pulmonary circuit.

$$SVR = \frac{MAP\text{-}MVP}{CO\ (L/min)}$$

*Pure mitral stenosis→LVEDP↓+PCW↑

KEY CONCEPT: The four chambers of the heart are the right and left atria and the right and left ventricles. The left ventricle is a high pressure chamber.

Valves

The main purpose of the cardiac valves is to maintain a unidirectional blood flow through the heart chambers. Cardiac valves are classified as: ***atrioventricular valves*** (AV) and ***semilunar valves*** (Fig. 5-5).

The valves open and close in response to changes in volume and pressure within the heart. AV valves separate the atria from the ventricles. There are two AV valves: ***Tricuspid*** (between right atrium and right ventricle) and ***mitral*** (between left atrium and left venticle).

The tricuspid is formed by three cusps and the mitral by two cusps, which in diameter have greater surface areas than their apertures. Thus during closing, there is an overlapping of tissue surfaces. The cusps have tendinous attachments called ***chordae tendinae,*** which are inserted into thick muscle bodies called ***papillary*** muscles (Fig. 5-5). Papillary muscles are attached to the ventricular walls and the interventricular septum. During contraction, these muscles shorten and pull down on the cusps to prevent valvular eversion into the atria.

The AV valves open and close as follows: Valve cusps open on ventricular diastole; valve cusps close as ventricular pressure increases during systole.

There are two ***semilunar valves*** that direct circulation into the pulmonic and systemic circulations: the ***pulmonary valve*** (between the right ventricle and pulmonary artery) and the ***aortic valve*** (between the left ventricle and aorta).

Each valve has three thin, delicate leaflets that are somewhat thickened along their edges. These cusps are attached at the base to a thick fibrous ring. The semilunar valves open and close as follows: Semilunar valves open when the ventricle contracts; semilunar valves close after ventricular systole, when pressure in the outflow tract is greater than in the ventricle.

KEY CONCEPT: The cardiac valves, AV and semilunar, maintain unidirectional flow through the heart and the pulmonary and systemic circulations.

Conduction System

The heart depends on a specific sequence of electrical activation of all myocardial cells during each beat. This necessary rhythmic excitation is accomplished by a specialized pathway called the ***conduction system.*** The specialized conduction tissue has the following properties: ***automaticity, rhythmicity, conductivity*** and ***excitability.***

It is through this electrical activation that the pump, via muscular contraction, is effected. The conduction system (Fig. 5-6) is composed of the: ***sinoatrial (SA) node, internodal atrial pathways, atrioventricular (AV) node, bundle of His, right and left bundle branches*** and ***Purkinje system.***

The SA node lies at the junction of the superior vena cava and the right atrium. It contains 1.5 cm of conducting tissue that discharges an impulse about 80 to 100 times per minute. The SA node is referred to as the pacemaker of the heart because it discharges the fastest and strongest impulse of all the pacemakers. The impulse spreads through both atria via three ***internodal pathways,*** Bachmann's, Wenckebach's and Thorel's, to the ***atrioventricular (AV) node.***

The AV node is located in the right posterior portion of the interatrial septum near the base of the tricuspid valve, and is continuous with the ***bundle of His.*** It discharges 40 to 60 times per minute. The AV node delays impulses for .08 to .12 seconds to allow for ventricular filling. The impulse then spreads from the AV node to the ***bundle of His.***

The bundle of His, a thick bundle of fibers, runs down the right side of the interventricular septum. At the muscular portion of the septum, it divides into ***right*** and ***left*** bundle branches. The right continues as a single branch; but the left divides into a long, thin branch anteriorly and into a short, thick branch posteriorly. Both branches parallel the septum subendocardially and are continuous with the ***Purkinje system.***

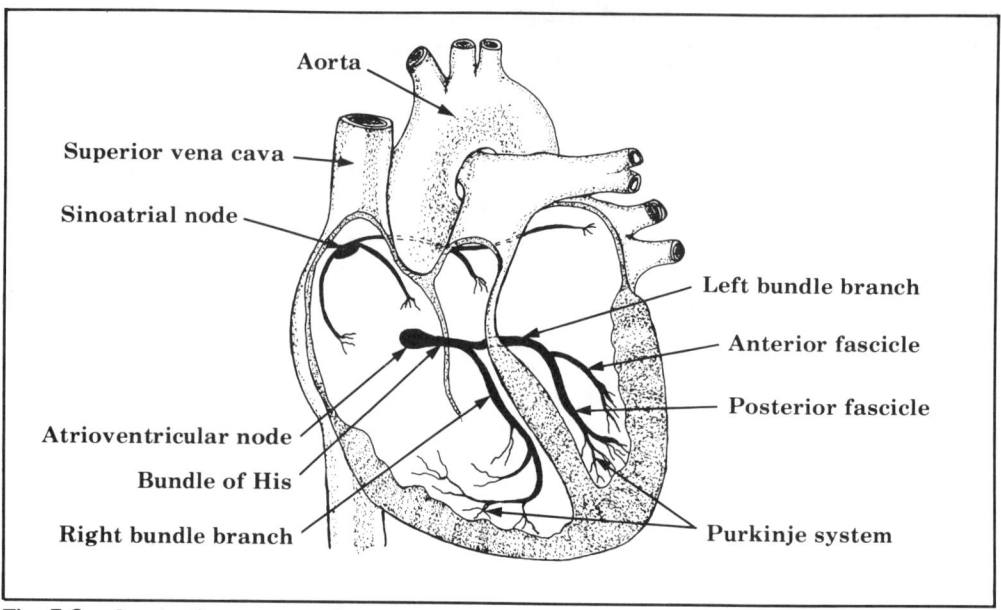

Fig. 5-6. Conduction system (illustration © Anna Seroka)

The Purkinje system is responsible for transmitting impulses subendocardially into the ventricles. These fibers can function as an intrinsic pacemaker in the presence of AV block or the absence of AV nodal impulses. The firing rate is 20 to 30 times per minute.

KEY CONCEPT: The conduction pathway: SA→interatrial nodal pathways (3)→AV→ bundle of His→right and left bundle branches→Purkinje fibers→ventricular musculature.

KEY POINT RECOGNITION
Write true or false by each statement. Answers are at the end of this chapter. A score below 80% indicates the need for further study.

_____ 1. The septum divides the heart into right and left halves.

_____ 2. The trabeculae divide the atria and ventricles.

_____ 3. In the early phase of ventricular diastole, atrial contraction initiates blood flow from the atria to the ventricles.

_____ 4. When atrial systole is lost in normal heart, it has a devastating effect on cardiac output.

_____ 5. The left atrial appendage is useful as a surgical approach for valvotomy.

_____ 6. The right atrium receives oxygenated blood from the coronary sinus.

_____ 7. An engorged left atrium may cause left lower lobe atelectasis.

_____ 8. Each ventricle ejects about 5 to 10 ml of blood with each contraction.

_____ 9. Right ventricular pressure is 25/0 to 5 mm Hg.

_____10. Right ventricular pressure is reflected in jugular venous and central venous pressure.

_____11. The left ventricle is located anteriorly and laterally to the left.

_____12. Left ventricular pressure is 90/4 to 140/2 mm Hg.

_____13. Left ventricular pressure may be decreased in the presence of mitral valve pathology and increased pulmonary vascular resistance.

_____14. The normal left ventricle must push against a systemic vascular resistance mean pressure of approximately 50 to 60 mm Hg.

_____15. The cardiac valves maintain blood flow in one direction through the heart.

_____16. The tricuspid and mitral valves are atrioventricular valves.

___17. The AV valve cusps have tendinous attachments called chordae tendinae.
___18. Chordae tendinae insert muscle bodies called papillary muscles.
___19. AV valve cusps close during ventricular diastole.
___20. The semilunar valve cusps are attached at the base to a thick fibrous ring.
___21. Semilunar valves close when the ventricle contracts.
___22. The conduction system causes electrical activation of myocardial cells.
___23. The SA node lies at the junction of the inferior vena cava and the right atrium.
___24. The three artrial internodal pathways are Bachmann, Wenckebach and Thorel.
___25. The AV node is located in the right portion of the interatrial system near the base of the tricuspid valve.
___26. **The AV node is not continuous with the bundle of His.**
___27. The bundle of His runs down the right side of the interventricular system.
___28. The Purkinje system is responsible for transmitting impulses subendocardially into the ventricles.

CIRCULATION
Coronary Circulation

Coronary circulation is responsible for the nourishment of the heart muscle. The coronary arteries are more variable in anatomical pattern than any part of the cardiac anatomy (Fig. 5-7). Large branches traverse the epicardium, with subbranches penetrating through to myocardial and subendocardial tissue layers. Coronary artery perfusion is primarily dependent on pressure in the root of the aorta during diastole. The three major coronary arteries are: the *right, left* and *circumflex.*

The right coronary artery (RCA) arises from the right aortic sinus of Valsalva and runs between the right atrium and ventricle. It then runs back to the posterior interventricular groove, where it becomes the posterior descending artery. It supplies the right atrium and posterior walls of the right and left ventricles. An anterior right atrial branch frequently arises near the origin of the right coronary artery. A branch of the right coronary artery that arises from the posterior descending branch commonly supplies the atrioventricular node (AV node).

The *left coronary artery* arises from the left aortic sinus of Valsalva and generally divides within 1 to 2 cm into the left anterior descending and left circumflex coronary arteries. The left anterior descending artery travels down the anterior surface of the heart in the interventricular sulcus and a few centimeters up the posterior surface of the same groove. Blood is supplied to the anterior aspects of the right and left ventricles, the interventricular septum, which contains the ventricular conduction system, and a small posterior part of both ventricles. The left *circumflex* runs laterally and then posteriorly between the left atrium and ventricle; the obtuse marginal branch breaks off before it descends on the posterior surface of the left ventricle. It supplies the lateral and posterior portions of the left ventricle.

The majority of the *coronary* veins drain into the *coronary sinus.* Some veins, such as the *thebesian veins,* drain directly into the cardiac chambers. The anterior cardiac veins drain the right ventricle.

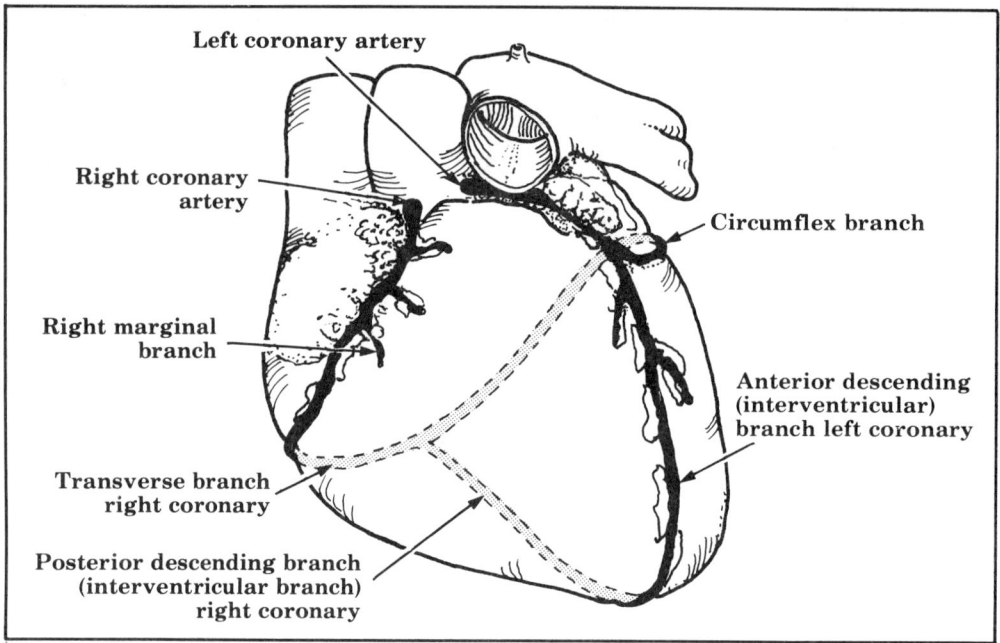

Fig. 5-7. Coronary arteries

Conduction System Blood Supply

Knowing the coronary arteries that supply specific areas of the conduction system enables the nurse to understand postmyocardial infarction arrhythmias. The artery that supplies the sinus node commonly arises from the right coronary artery, although it may branch off the circumflex artery. The posterior descending branch of the right coronary artery usually supplies the AV node and the upper portion of the bundle of His. This blood supply can come from the posterior circumflex.

Coronary blood flow in an adult male at rest is approximately 5 percent of the total cardiac output (about 300 ml). Ventricular contraction (systole) compresses the coronary vessels and decreases myocardial perfusion. During diastole, the ventricular muscle relaxes, the coronary vessels dilate and myocardial blood flow increases.

The myocardium of the left ventricle is thicker and contracts with greater force than the myocardium of the right ventricle. Since the left ventricle contracts more forcibly, the left myocardium experiences a greater decrease in perfusion during systole. Coronary artery blood flow is controlled almost entirely by local autoregulation.

In response to the metabolic needs of the cardiac musculature, blood flow through the coronary arteries is determined almost entirely by local autoregulation. It works equally well whether the nerves to the heart are intact or severed.

Oxygen extracted by the myocardium usually is greater than in any other tissue. In a resting state, approximately 70 percent of the oxygen in the arterial blood is removed as it passes through the heart. If the heart requires more oxygen, it can only be supplied by increasing coronary blood flow.

Lymph Supply

The heart is richly supplied with lymph capillaries, which form a continuous network from the endocardium through the muscle layers to the epicardium. There is a superficial set that arises from the areolar tissue of the heart's surface and a set that arises from the deeper tissues of the heart. They traverse the course of the coronary vessels. The right-sided lymph capillaries form a trunk at the root of the aorta which then communicates with the cardiac glands. This lymph system then passes backward and ascends the trachea, terminating at the root of the neck in the right lymphatic duct.

The left-sided lymph capillaries form a single vessel at the base of the heart. This vessel follows the pulmonary artery and ascends the trachea, terminating in the thoracic duct. Few valves can be found in the cardiac lymphatics. The force that drives the lymphatic flow from the heart appears to be the cardiac cycle of contraction. The role the cardiac lymphatic system plays in the disease process has not been established. After the cardiac lymphatics are severed, as is done during cardiac transplants, regeneration occurs in approximately two weeks.

Vascular Anatomy

The *arteries* are composed of three tissue layers:

Tunica Intima

This inner layer consists of three cell layers: a layer of endothelial cells, a layer of delicate connective tissue that is found only in the larger vessels and an elastic layer consisting of a membrane or network of elastic fibers.

Tunica Media

This middle layer contains mostly smooth muscle fibers and various amounts of elastic and collagenous tissue. In larger arteries, elastic fibers form layers that alternate with the layers of muscle fibers. Some of the larger arteries contain white connective tissue fibers.

Tunica Externia or Adventitia

This external layer comprises loose connective tissue.

The structure of the middle layer makes the arteries elastic and extensile, two properties that determine the arteries' proper functioning. The degree of arterial extensibility and elasticity enables the arteries to receive the increased blood volume forced into them with each cardiac contraction. If the arteries lacked extensibility and elasticity, as in arteriosclerosis, the systolic blood pressure would be markedly increased.

The body's arteries vary in size. The largest arteries in the body are the *aorta* and the *pulmonary* artery. These vessels adapt to large volumes of blood.

As the arteries decrease in size, they are called *arterioles.* Arterioles are vital to the maintenance of arterial blood pressure. A precapillary sphincter is located on the arteriole just before it enters the capillary network. Arterioles are well supplied with vasoconstrictor fibers. The autonomic nervous system and autoregulation control arteriolar constriction and dilation.

The *capillaries* are exceedingly minute perfusion vessels. They connect the arterioles (smallest arteries) to the venules (smallest veins). The capillary walls consist of a layer of endothelial cells continuous with the layer that lines the arteries, veins and the heart. Approximately 5 percent of the total blood volume lies at rest in the systemic capillary bed.

Veins carry unoxygenated blood to the heart. The venous structure is very similar to that of the arteries. The veins are composed of three layers: an inner endothelial lining, a middle muscular layer and an external layer of connective tissue. The walls of the veins have a less developed middle coat and therefore are not as elastic as arteries. The walls of veins are much thinner than those of arteries, and tend to collapse when not filled with blood.

Many veins contain valves. These *valves* are semilunar folds of the vessel's inner layer and usually consist of two flaps. The valve's convex border is attached to the side of the vein and the free edge points toward the heart. Valves prevent reflux of the blood and keep it flowing toward the heart. The valves are more numerous in the veins of the extremities, where reflux is most likely to occur. In an upright individual, gravity alone can cause high pressures in the lower extremities, resulting in edematous tissue; but, normally, pressure in the lower extremities is 25 mm Hg or less.

KEY POINT RECOGNITION

Write true or false by each statement. Answers are at the end of this chapter. A score below 80% indicates the need for further study.

1. _____ Coronary artery perfusion is dependent on pressure in the root of the aorta during diastole.
2. _____ The right coronary artery arises from the right aortic sinus of Valsalva.
3. _____ The right coronary artery supplies the posterior walls of the right and left ventricles.
4. _____ A branch of the right coronary artery commonly supplies the AV node.
5. _____ The right coronary artery divides into the anterior descending and circumflex.
6. _____ The left coronary artery supplies blood to the anterior aspects of the right and left ventricles.
7. _____ The thebesian veins drain into the coronary sinus.
8. _____ Capillary blood flow in the left ventricular muscle rises during systole.
9. _____ Coronary artery blood flow is controlled by local autoregulation.
10. _____ Superficial cardiac lymph vessels arise from the areolar tissue of the heart's surface.
11. _____ Cardiac contraction drives the lymphatic flow from the heart.
12. _____ The tunica intima is the inner layer of arteries.
13. _____ The tunica adventitia layer of the artery is responsible for elasticity and extensibility.
14. _____ Arterioles are well supplied with vasoconstrictor fibers.
15. _____ Veins are totally different in structure than arteries.
16. _____ All veins have valves.

PHYSIOLOGY

ELECTROPHYSIOLOGY

Myocardial fibers can be compared to electrical wires. Consider the cell membrane as an insulator that is wrapped around the intracellular contents on the conducting core. The low-resistance connections between cells, called nexus or tight junctions, allow intercellular current flow.

A voltage can be measured across the cell membrane during the cardiac cycle. This voltage is called the *resting membrane potential (RMP)*. RMP represents an electrochemical equilibrium that results from selective permeability. Potassium has the ability to cross the cell membrane, but other ions are much less permeable. It is thought that RMP is determined primarily by potassium. Therefore, its value should vary with the concentration of potassium in the extracellular fluid.

When an appropriate amount of current is applied to the heart, the cell membrane reaches threshold potential at the site of application. When the cell membrane reaches this threshold potential, a sudden change in permeability occurs. This change results in the transmembrane potential called the *action potential* (Fig. 5-8).

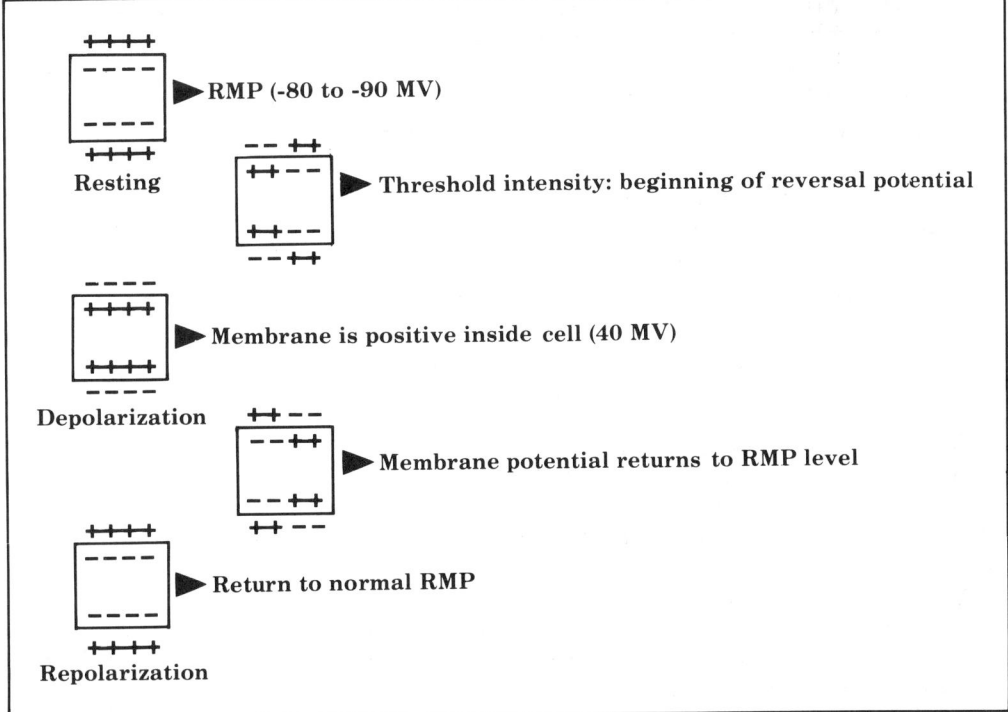

Fig. 5-8. Cardiac electrical events leading to depolarization

The **action potential** (Fig. 5-9) is divided into five phases: 0, 1, 2, 3, 4. Phase **zero** (0) is a rapid-rising phase called depolarization. This phase is thought to be caused by sodium moving rapidly across the cell membrane into the cell. During phase zero, calcium also moves into the cell carrying positive charges. Unlike sodium, calcium moves much slower, causing a longer-lasting positive charge on the cell membrane. This slower movement of positive ions begins at membrane potentials less negative than threshold potentials, approximately -35 mV. This can usually be seen in cells where sodium currents are inactivated or where depolarization is slow. These slow response action potentials are usually found in the SA node, AV node and AV valve area. How rapidly this phase develops is dependent upon (1) the resting membrane potential (RMP), and (2) in fast response, the equilibrium potential for sodium, and in the slow response for calcium.

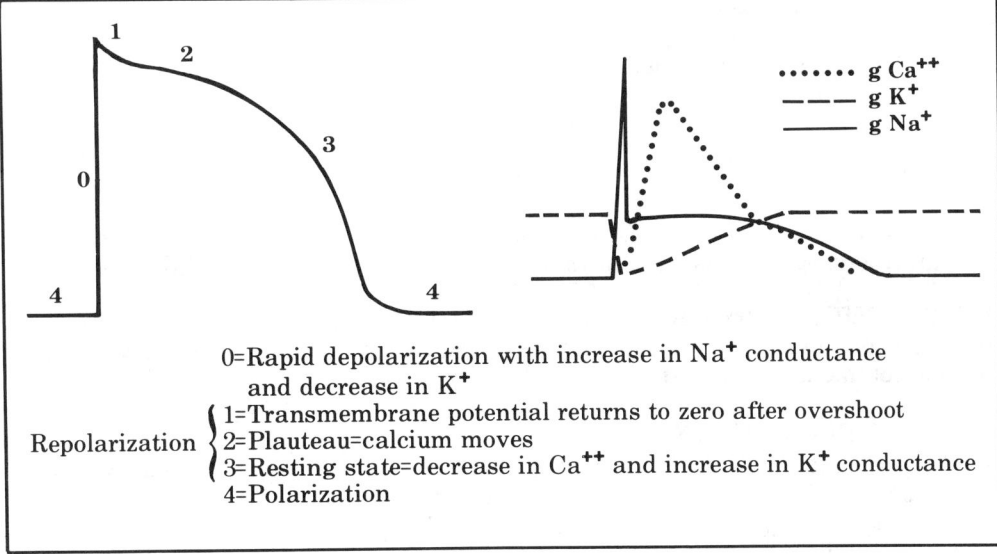

Fig. 5-9. Five phases: action potential

Phases 1 through 3 are the *repolarization* phases. Phase 1 occurs because the transmembrane potential is influenced by the sodium equilibrium, the inside of the cell being positive in relation to the outside. This phenomenon is referred to as overshoot and is not seen in slow response potentials.

Calcium may be the ion that helps bring the transmembrane potential to zero following the overshoot.

The plateau, or phase 2, slowly develops an inward movement of positive charge carried largely by calcium, which peaks and begins to inactivate. Potassium, which falls in phase 0, begins to return.

Phase 3 results from inactivation of transmembrane calcium and an increase in potassium conductance.

Phase 4 is called *polarization*. This potential is not associated with any current or ionic flow. Characteristic of all automatic cells, the Purkinje fibers demonstrate automaticity and slow diastolic depolarization during this phase. This is thought to be related to the constant inward diastolic movement of sodium and a time-dependent decrease in the permeability of potassium. Other pacemaker fibers may not share this mechanism of phase 4. This change may be mediated by a time-dependent increase in the slow inward current carried mainly by calcium.

When the membrane is depolarized, it is almost impossible to elicit an immediate action potential. The membrane is refractory to stimulation. This time period is referred to as the ***absolute refractory period (ARP)***. The ***relative refractory period (RRP)*** follows with a voltage and time-dependent recovery of excitability. Increased current is required to elicit a response. This period ends when excitability reaches a stable value in phase 4 (Fig. 5-10).

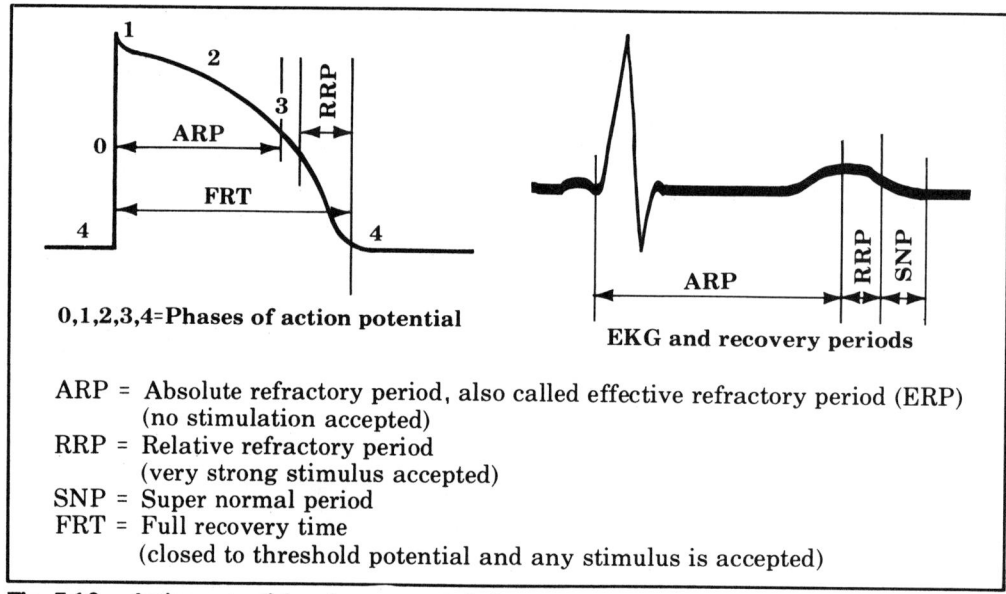

Fig. 5-10. Action potential and recovery periods

Impulse conduction depends on the current-conduction properties of the myocardial fibers, as well as the characteristics of the action potential.

KEY CONCEPT: Electrical activity of the myocardium initiates mechanical activity. Repolarization (potassium) and depolarization (sodium) are electrical activity necessary for muscle contraction (calcium).

KEY POINT RECOGNITION
Write true or false by each statement. Answers are at the end of this chapter. A score below 80% indicates the need for further study.

_____ 1. Resting membrane potential represents an electrochemical equilibrium resulting from selective permeability.

_____ 2. Resting membrane potential is determined by calcium.

_____ 3. When large amounts of current are applied, the cell membrane reaches threshold potential at the site of application.

_____ 4. When a sudden change in permeability results in the transmembrane potential, this is called action potential.

_____ 5. Phases 1 through 3 of the action potential are the repolarization phase.

_____ 6. Phase 1 of the action potential is influenced by the chloride equilibrium.

_____ 7. Phase 2 of the action potential slowly develops an inward movement of positive charges carried largely by calcium.

_____ 8. Phase 4 of the action potential is considered polarization.

_____ 9. Phase 4 of the action potential is associated with current and ionic flow.

_____ 10. When the membrane is depolarized, the membrane is refractory to stimulation.

NERVOUS CONTROL OF THE HEART

Autonomic innervation is extensive in the heart. *Sympathetic* nerve fibers are found throughout the atria and ventricles, including both the SA and AV nodes. *Parasympathetic* fibers are found primarily in the atria, including the SA and AV nodes, but also extend into the ventricles. Regulation of impulse and conduction of the excitation impulse through the heart are controlled by the autonomic nervous system.

The ANS is divided into the sympathetic and parasympathetic systems. *Sympathetic* innervation arises in the upper thoracic spinal cord and approaches the heart via cervical ganglia. These fibers, composed mostly of adrenergic fibers, possess the dominant influence on ventricular function. *Norepinephrine* is the sympathetic neurohormone transmitter. It is a vasoconstrictor and has little effect on cardiac function. The effects of sympathetic stimulation are:

Positive chronotropy—increase in heart rate

Positive inotropy—increase in contractility

Positive dromotropy—increase in atrioventricular conduction

The sympathetic response is also referred to as the *adrenergic* response. Alpha and beta receptors within the heart and blood vessels are stimulated by the sympathetic system and result in:

Alpha stimulation—vasoconstriction

Beta stimulation—increased heart rate, increased contractility, increased irritability, vasodilation

Parasympathetic innervation originates in the medulla oblongata and approaches the heart via the vagus nerve, joining sympathetic fibers in the cardiac plexus. These fibers are the dominant influence on heart rate. The neurohormone transmitter released is acetylcholine. The parasympathetic system stimulates the beta receptors in the heart. The cardiac effects of parasympathetic (vagal) stimulation are:

Negative chronotropy—decrease in heart rate

Negative dromotropy—decrease in atrioventricular conduction

The parasympathetic response is also called the *cholinergic* response. It is the dynamic interplay of the ANS divisions, which helps to maintain heart function.

Reflex Responses

Afferent pain fibers travel from the pericardium and walls of the heart to the lower cervical and upper thoracic ganglia of the spinal cord. These impulses then ascend the ventral spinal-thalamic tract and terminate in the posteroventral nucleus of the thalamus. These fibers are responsible for reflex responses of the heart to ischemia and injury.

KEY CONCEPT: The ANS is divided into the sympathetic and parasympathetic systems. The sympathetic stimulation increases heart rate, contractility and conduction, which increases cardiac output during body stress. Parasympathetic stimulation decreases heart rate, which may or may not decrease cardiac output, depending on how slow the rate becomes. The parasympathetic system modifies the sympathetic effect of the heart.

KEY POINT RECOGNITION

Write true or false by each statement. Answers are at the end of this chapter. A score below 80% indicates the need for further study.

_____ 1. Sympathetic nerve fibers are found throughout the atria and ventricles.

_____ 2. Parasympathetic fibers are found primarily in the atria.

_____ 3. Norepinephrine is the sympathetic neurotransmitter.

_____ 4. Sympathetic stimulation results in an increased heart rate, increased contractility and an increase in AV conduction.

_____ 5. Alpha stimulation results in vasoconstriction.

_____ 6. Vagal stimulation results in a decreased heart rate.

_____ 7. The parasympathetic response is also called the cholinergic response.

FACTORS AFFECTING BLOOD FLOW AND PRESSURE

Regulation of Flow

Blood flow is regulated by *nervous control, hormones* and *autoregulation.*

The *nervous system* plays a key role in maintaining homeostasis whenever there is a massive alteration of the circulation. The sympathetic division of the autonomic nervous system immediately responds to the body's need for increased blood supply. Sympathetic stimulation increases cardiac output and causes vasoconstriction of peripheral vessels, increasing blood pressure and directing blood supply toward major body organs. The sympathetic nervous system dictates major organ vessels, increasing blood flow to the brain, heart and muscles. The parasympathetic division has little effect on blood flow, but acts as a moderator to prevent over response of the sympathetic system. ANS regulation is effected through intact neural pathways and specialized sensor tissue. This specialized sensor tissue may be divided into two groups: *pressoreceptors* (baroreceptors) and *chemoreceptors.*

Pressoreceptors are located in the walls of the aortic arch and at the origin of the internal carotid (carotid sinuses). These sensors respond to stretching of the vessel walls. An increase in blood pressure stretches arterial walls and stimulates these receptors. When stimulated, the pressoreceptors inhibit the vasomotor center and the pressure returns to normal.

Pressure exerted on the carotid sinuses in a normal individual will inhibit sympathetic activity and result in a drop in heart rate and blood pressure (approximately 15 mm Hg).

Chemoreceptors are found in the bifurcation of the carotid arteries and along the aortic arch. These receptors (carotid and aortic bodies) are sensitive to changes in arterial oxygen (PaO_2), carbon dioxide ($PaCO_2$) and hydrogen ion concentrations. The carotid bodies send impulses along a tract of nerves called Herings. The vagus nerve transmits impulses from the aortic bodies. A decrease in PaO_2, an increase in $PaCO_2$ or a decrease in the pH stimulates these chemoreceptors and results in sympathetic excitation, stimulation of the vasomotor center and increased cardiovascular activity (pulse and B.P.).

An increase in the hydrogen ion concentration (acidosis) can cause acidosis and may indirectly increase vascular tone. Mild alkalosis (decrease in hydrogen ion concentration) may cause arteriolar constriction, while severe alkalosis tends to cause dilatation.

Local vasodilation is also affected by hypercarbia. Carbon dioxide is a powerful vasoconstrictor that overrides the local effect in all tissues except the brain.

Another set of receptors, *osmoreceptors*, regulates cardiovascular activity by reflex response. When blood volume is increased, these receptors act by signalling for increased heart rate and diuresis.

Cushing's reflex is another central nervous system response that affects blood pressure. This reflex is stimulated by an ischemic response in the central nervous system. Increased cerebrospinal pressure compresses arteries and reduces blood flow. This produces the Cushing's reflex, which results in increased blood pressure.

A hormonal response occurs when the following hormones enter the circulatory system to compensate for a cardiovascular imbalance. Each hormone has a specific effect on cardiovascular activity.

Hormone	Action
Epinephrine/Norepinephrine	Systemic vasoconstriction
	Increased B.P.
	Increased heart rate
Aldosterone	Na and H_2O retention
	Increased B.P.
Angiotensin	Peripheral vasoconstriction
	Increased B.P.
Vasopressin	Arteriole vasoconstriction
	(Plays a minor role in regulation of peripheral circulation)

Autoregulation causes the body to respond to local tissue changes by regulating local blood flow. This process is independent of ANS regulation. Autoregulation causes local dilation, increased blood supply, and increased capillary permeability.

Blood flow depends upon *resistance* and *pressure.*

Resistance to flow depends on blood vessel length and radius, and blood viscosity. The smooth muscle of the arteriole is the dominant site of resistance.

Pressure gradients are responsible for blood flow through the cardiovascular system. Very simply, a high-pressure gradient increases blood flow. Therefore, a change in cardiac output or peripheral resistance causes alterations in the mean arterial pressure, which then cause changes in pressure gradients and result in changes in blood flow. Changes in right atrial pressure can also effect pressure gradient changes, resulting in changes in blood flow.

Principles of Distribution

Blood is distributed according to metabolic need. This is accomplished by two controls: *extrinsic* and *intrinsic.*

Extrinsic control increases blood flow to an organ by increasing cardiac output or by shunting blood from other areas. The sympathetic nervous system effects this process through selective stimulation of alpha and beta receptors.

Intrinsic control increases blood flow to an organ by vasodilation. Tissue ischemia stimulates vasodilation.

KEY CONCEPT: Blood flow is regulated by nervous control, hormones and autoregulation. Blood flow is dependent upon resistance and pressure. Blood is distributed, extrinsically and intrinsically, according to metabolic need.

KEY POINT RECOGNITION
Write true or false by each statement. Answers are at the end of this chapter. A score below 80% indicates the need for further study.

_____ 1. Blood flow is regulated by nervous control, hormones and autoregulation.

_____ 2. Baroreceptors respond to vasoconstriction.

_____ 3. Increased atrial pressure stimulates the pressoreceptors and results in inhibition of the vasomotor center.

_____ 4. Pressure on the carotid sinus stimulates sympathetic activity.

_____ 5. Chemoreceptors are sensitive to changes in PaO_2.

_____ 6. Stimulation of chemoreceptors results in decreased cardiovascular activity.

_____ 7. Carbon dioxide is a powerful vasodilator.

_____ 8. Cushing's reflex is a CNS response that results in increased blood pressure.

_____ 9. Norepinephrine and epinephrine cause generalized systemic vasodilation.

_____ 10. Autoregulation is a local response that causes vasodilation and increased capillary permeability, resulting in an increased blood supply.

_____ 11. Resistance to blood flow is determined by vessel length, radius and blood viscosity.

_____ 12. The pressure gradient has a direct effect on the blood flow.

_____ 13. Changes in pressure gradients may be caused by changes in C.O. or peripheral resistance.

_____ 14. The sympathetic nervous system extrinsically controls blood flow through selective stimulation of alpha and beta receptors.

_____ 15. Intrinsic blood flow control causes local vasodilation.

CARDIAC CYCLE

The cardiac cycle is the time period from the beginning of one heartbeat to the beginning of the next beat. A normal cardiac cycle lasts 0.8 second.

The cardiac cycle involves both electrical and mechanical events of the heart (Fig. 5-11). As electrical excitation (depolarization) begins, it stimulates the mechanical event (systole). Electrical recovery (repolarization) is followed by muscular relaxation (diastole).

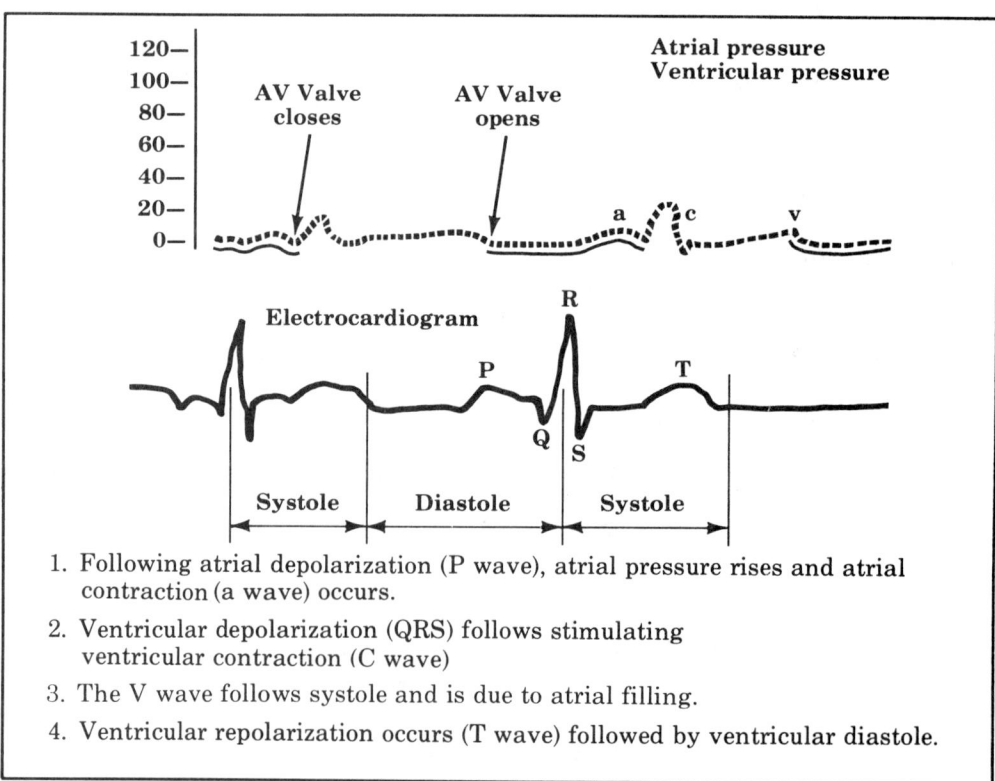

1. Following atrial depolarization (P wave), atrial pressure rises and atrial contraction (a wave) occurs.
2. Ventricular depolarization (QRS) follows stimulating ventricular contraction (C wave)
3. The V wave follows systole and is due to atrial filling.
4. Ventricular repolarization occurs (T wave) followed by ventricular diastole.

Fig. 5-11. Electrical and mechanical events in the cardiac cycle

Electrical events are recorded on the electrocardiogram. The waves that represent electrical activity are:

P wave = atrial depolarization

QRS complex = ventricular depolarization

T wave = ventricular repolarization

A, c, v waves = mechanical events

The cardiac cycle can be divided into two phases: *systole* and *diastole.*

Systole can further be divided into *early* and *late systole. Early* systole is the period when depolarization spreads to the ventricular musculature and contraction begins. Pressure rises in the ventricles and the AV valves close. Pressure within the aorta and pulmonary artery is higher than ventricular pressure, keeping the semilunar valves closed. *Late* systole is the period when ventricular pressure becomes higher than aortic or pulmonary artery pressure. The semilunar valves open and blood is ejected.

Diastole can be divided into *early, mid* and *late diastole. Early* diastole is the period when the ventricles relax. Ventricular pressure drops; the semilunar valves close; the AV valves open and rapid ventricular filling begins. *Mid* diastole is the period when both atria and ventricles are relaxed. Slow ventricular filling occurs. *Late* diastole is the period when the atria depolarize and contract. Ventricular volume is increased.

Maintenance of systolic and diastolic pressures is necessary for efficiency of the cardiac system. *Systolic* pressure is the peak pressure occurring with each heartbeat.

Diastolic pressure is the lowest pressure occurring during diastole. It is largely determined by the degree of vasoconstriction within the arteries.

Pulse pressure is the difference between systolic and diastolic pressures. It is determined by stroke volume and the compliance of the aorta and its branches.

Mean pressure is the average of the *systolic* and *diastolic* pressures.

KEY CONCEPT: The cardiac cycle is made up of closely related mechanical and electrical events that extend from the beginning of one heartbeat to the beginning of the next beat. Systolic and diastolic pressures occur during the cardiac cycle.

KEY POINT RECOGNITION

Write true or false by each statement. Answers are at the end of this chapter. A score below 80% indicates the need for further study.

_____ 1. Electrical recovery is followed by diastole.

_____ 2. In early systole, pressure rises in the ventricles and the AV valves open.

_____ 3. In late systole, the semilunar valves are closed.

_____ 4. In early diastole, the semilunar valves close and the AV valves open.

_____ 5. In late diastole, the ventricular volume is increased.

_____ 6. Systolic pressure is the lowest pressure occurring during systole.

_____ 7. **Diastolic pressure is largely determined by the degree of vasoconstriction within the arteries.**

_____ 8. Mean pressure is the average of the systolic and diastolic pressures.

CARDIAC OUTPUT

Cardiac output (C.O.) is the amount of blood ejected by the heart per unit of time and is recorded as liters per minute. The output of both ventricles is usually the same. However, C.O. measures the volume of blood the left ventricle ejects into the aorta. Normal C.O. is approximately 5 L/minute in the average 70 kg male.

A more specific parameter is the *cardiac index* (CI), the cardiac output in relation to *body surface area (BSA).* BSA is determined from a simple table by using the patient's height and weight. Once the BSA is determined, the CI is calculated using the following formula: $CI = \dfrac{C.O.}{BSA}$

A 70 kg male would have a normal CI of 3 L/minute.

Cardiac output is determined from the product of heart rate (HR) and stroke volume (SV):

$$C.O. = HR \times SV$$

Stroke volume is the amount of blood ejected with each heartbeat. It is the difference between the volume of the left ventricle at end diastole (the end of the filling cycle) and the volume remaining in the ventricle at end systole (the end of ejection). The amount of blood ejected with each contraction is approximately 75 cc. This is commonly referred to as the ejection fraction and composes about 70 percent of the 100 cc normally contained in the ventricle. Diastolic filling and systolic ejection are the major determinants of stroke volume. For example, if the heart's pumping ability is decreased, as in heart failure, the ejection fraction is reduced. If there is a larger amount of blood in the heart with a less forward flow at the end of systole, a marked reduction in the ejection fraction occurs. The pressure during diastole at the end of the filling period is increased as the pump decompensates or as volume increases.

Diastolic filling occurs rapidly early in diastole and is dependent upon ventricular compliance and filling pressures. Systolic ejection occurs during contraction of the ventricle and is dependent upon the degree of muscle fiber shortened in the ventricular myocardium while working against the arterial blood pressure.

In summary, C.O. is influenced by five major factors:

Arterial blood pressure
Heart rate
Ventricular distensibility
Ventricular filling
Myocardial contractile properties

Three methods commonly used to determine C.O. are the:

Fick method
Indicator-dilution method
Thermodilution method (Fig. 5-12)

Method	Formula	Advantage	Disadvantage
Fick	C.O. (ml/min) = $\dfrac{O_2 \text{ consumption (ml/min)}}{\text{arterial } O_2 \text{ content vol. \%} - \text{venous content vol. \%}}$	Indicates pulmonary status reliable in low output states, cardiac shunts, valvular insufficiencies	Arterial and blood venous samples needed; patient cooperation essential; requires two nurses; administraton of O_2 changes results
Indicator-dilution	C.O.(L/min) = $\dfrac{I}{Cxt} \times 60$ (calculations can be computerized)	O_2 administration does not affect result; faster than Fick method	Calculations are extensive; recording device may not be accurate; arterial blood needed; arterial and venous catheters needed
Thermo-dilution	C.O. is calculated from temperature curve	No blood samples Rapid O_2 administration does not affect result One catheter, inserted at bedside	Requires computer; not always accurate in low cardiac output states; possible hazards: damaged thermistor

Fig. 5-12. Methods to determine C.O.

The ***Fick*** principle states that blood flow through an organ can be determined if a substance is removed from or added to the blood during its flow to that organ. When applied to the lung, this principle is used to calculate the volume of blood required to transport the oxygen taken up from the alveoli per unit of time. Because of its accuracy, it gives an indication of pulmonary status and is relatively reliable in the presence of low output states, cardiac shunts and valvular insufficiencies. However, it requires a cooperative patient and a 20 cc sample from both the arterial and venous blood. The administration of oxygen affects the results. It is a time-consuming process, as it requires at least two people for simultaneous collection of expired air and blood samples.

The formula to calculate C.O. is:

$$\text{C.O. (ml/min)} = \frac{O_2 \text{ consumption (ml/min)}}{\text{Arterial } O_2 \text{ content (vol. \%)} - \text{Venous } O_2 \text{ content (vol. \%)}}$$

Oxygen consumption in a normal individual is approximately 250 ml/min. The pulmonary arterial (mixed venous) blood O_2 content is about 150 ml/L. The arterial oxygen content is about 200 ml/L. Therefore, the cardiac output is 250/50 or 5 L/min. Body surface area, mentioned earlier, has to be taken into consideration when obtaining a C.O. Thus, on an individual basis, the cardiac index is more meaningful. The normal is about 3 to 4 L/min/m^2.

The *indicator-dilution* method is accomplished by injecting dye into the venous system while arterial blood is steadily withdrawn through an instrument called a densitometer. A time-concentration curve is recorded as the dye passes once through the circulatory system.

After injection, the concentration of dye peaks and then returns to a baseline until the downward course is interrupted by the recirculated dye. Recirculation refers to the reappearance of dye that has made a complete circuit by way of the shortest path that blood follows through the systemic circulation.

The formula to calculate C.O. using this method is:

$$\text{C.O. (L/min)} = \frac{I}{C \times t} \times 60$$

I = Known amount of dye injected

C = Average concentration of dye under the curve for the first circulation

t = time of total curve duration in seconds

To obtain I, the amount of injected dye must be known. The total area under the curve must be calculated. There are several ways to do this. An important factor to consider in determining the total area under the curve is the fact that recirculation of the dye prevents the curve from returning to the baseline. You must extrapolate or extend the curve down toward the baseline by "eyeballing" to eliminate the effect of the recirculated dye. The T is the time of total curve duration measured in seconds.

You must judge exactly where to begin extrapolation. Two different people may arrive at two different conclusions, resulting in vastly different measurements. Therefore, the greatest source of error arises in faulty standardization techniques.

The *thermodilution method* is an application of the indicator-dilution theory. It requires no blood samples. If a solution with a known temperature is injected into the bloodstream, a temperature change is recorded at a point downstream. The temperature changes are placed on a curve and C.O. is calculated. Popular acceptance was gained after the introduction of the pulmonary, flow-directed catheter, designed by Drs. Swann and Ganz. Its results compare favorably with the other methods for determining blood flow.

Reproducibility is relatively constant because of its rapidity and minimal recirculation. Readings may be made as frequently as every minute.

An important factor is the proper positioning of the pulmonary catheter. Cold fluid flows from the CVP line port into the right atrium, through valves and chambers, and is detected by the thermistor located in the main pulmonary artery. This is considered adequate time for mixing. Thermodilution is minimally changed by recirculation and can be performed quickly with relative safety. It is easily performed at the bedside by one person.

KEY POINT RECOGNITION
Write true or false by each statement. Answers are at the end of this chapter. A score below 80% indicates the need for further study.

_____ 1. C.O. measures the amount of blood that the left ventricle ejects into the aorta.

_____ 2. Normal C.O. is 10 to 12 L/min.

_____ 3. BSA is obtained from a table using the patient's height and weight.

_____ 4. $C.O. = \dfrac{HR}{SV}$

_____ 5. Stroke volume is the amount of blood ejected from the heart each minute.

_____ 6. The ejection fraction composes about 70 percent of the 100 cc of blood normally contained in the ventricle.

_____ 7. Heart rate and ventricular distensibility influence C.O.

_____ 8. The administration of oxygen affects C.O. results when using the Fick method.

_____ 9. When using the indicator-dilution method, the greatest source of error is in faulty standardization techniques.

_____ 10. The disadvantage of the thermodilution method is that it requires two persons and 20 cc of blood for each sampling.

FACTORS AFFECTING CARDIAC FUNCTION AND OUTPUT

The main factors affecting cardiac function and output are: ***preload, afterload, contractility*** and ***heart rate.***

Preload

Preload is the amount of tension or load on the muscle prior to contraction. It influences systolic performance. Specifically, preload describes the pressure or quantity of blood in the ventricle at the end of diastole. Contractility of the left heart is evaluated by cardiac function curves. The stroke-work index is often plotted against the left ventricular **end-diastolic pressure** (LVEDP), which represents the preload. Remember that diastole is the time cycle when the heart is at rest. End-diastole is the point of greatest rest. Therefore, there is an end-diastolic pressure for each chamber; but since the left ventricle is the major chamber, it is that pressure (LVEDP) which is most frequently referred to.

The heart has an intrinsic ability to adapt to increasing loads of inflowing blood. This ability is known as the Frank-Starling law, which states that the degree of cardiac muscle stretch during diastole (preload) determines the force during systole. In the uncompromised heart, the pressure, volume and stretch are directly proportional to each other. This form of autoregulation in which the ventricular size varies is called ***heterometric autoregulation.*** Other forms of autoregulation exist in the body system. Homeometric autoregulation (Bowditch's effect) demonstrates changes in ventricular activity due to increased heart rate. Changes in aortic pressure without any change in ventricular fiber length during diastole are called Anrep's effect. Both an increased heart rate and aortic pressure, without any change in the filling of the heart, tend to increase myocardial contractility.

Bainbridge's reflex refers to an increased filling of the heart that results in an increase in the resting heart rate. This reflex may be initiated primarily by receptors in the right atrium that transmit via the vagal afferent fibers.

A sudden increase in blood volume of about 25 percent may double the cardiac output. This effect usually lasts only a few minutes. When a person first lies down, blood quickly leaves the legs and returns to the thorax. This sudden surge of blood volume returning to the heart quickens the pulse and increases the cardiac output.

Cardiac output gradually returns to normal because (1) the increase of cardiac output increases the hydrostatic pressure in the capillaries; the fluid flows out of the capillaries into the tissues, decreasing the blood volume; and (2) increased pressure in the venous system causes the veins to distend, producing increased vascular capacity and reduced venous return.

Central Venous Pressure (CVP)

The CVP provides information concerning the filling of the right heart. CVP is the amount of pressure in the central systemic veins of the chest, including the innominate veins, subclavian veins, superior vena cava and right atrium. The CVP reflects the diastolic pressure of the right ventricle. The CVP, which also reflects the filling pressure of the right heart, tends to rise if: (1) blood volume increases, (2) there is peripheral vasoconstriction or (3) the right heart fails.

The normal CVP is usually 0 to 5 mm Hg. In healthy adults, it may only reach 2 mm Hg. In hospitalized patients, the normal range is higher (4 to 6 mm Hg or 6 to 8 cm H_2O).

Always remember that most CVPs are read with water manometers (cm H_2O). Some CVPs may be read with transducers (mm Hg). They are *not* equal!

$$1 \text{ mm Hg} = 1.36 \text{ cm } H_2O$$

Always state the appropriate measurement you are using.

An increase in blood volume tends to increase venous return to the right heart *(preload),* and thereby increase the CVP. If large amounts of fluid are delivered rapidly to a hypovolemic patient, they may have little effect on the CVP. However, if the same delivery is made to a patient who is already hydrated, a sharp rise in the CVP may occur.

Distended neck veins are the classic sign of right heart failure. Right-sided failure is usually secondary to or follows left heart failure. Pulmonary artery pressure tends to increase when left atrial and left ventricular end-diastolic pressure rise.

If vascular capacity is reduced, it tends to produce relative hypervolemia and increased venous return. If the compromised heart has to pump against any increase in resistance, the cardiac output may be reduced, and the blood volume in the heart increases. When this occurs, the ventricular end-diastolic pressure and the atrial pressure may rise.

In the critically ill or injured patient, correlation between the blood volume and CVP level is often very poor. More important and reliable is the response of the CVP to fluid delivered.

Respiratory failure, cardiac tamponade, massive pulmonary embolism and acute respiratory distress syndrome are examples of conditions that may result in CVP of 25 cm H_2O or above. This is true even if hypovolemia is present because of increased pulmonary vascular resistance and right heart failure.

"Pressure" is visualized in wave forms. Venous pressure waves are symbolized by three letters: a, c, v. The *a* wave is caused by the contraction of the atria. The *c* wave is caused by the elevation of the bulging AV valves into the atria and by pressure waves from adjacent large arteries. The rapid flow of blood into the atrium during early ventricular systole causes a fall in the venous pressure. This fall is called the *x* descent. A *v* wave demonstrates increased pressure in the atria as they fill during ventricular systole. Rapid emptying of the atria immediately after the AV valves open causes the y descent. Collectively, these waves may be called right atrial (RA) wave forms.

A combined c-v wave may be extremely high if the AV valve is incompetent.

The RA wave form has a normal range of 5 mm Hg and offers a poor wave form to view. For this reason, most CVP lines are not connected to transducers.

Pulmonary Capillary Wedge Pressure (PCWP)

The *pulmonary capillary wedge pressure* (PCWP) is measured in the pulmonary artery beyond the pulmonary and tricuspid valves. Since there are no valves between the pulmonary capillaries and the left atrium, the PCWP is a reflection of the *left atrial pressure* (LAP). A normal pulmonary bed offers low resistance to this pressure reflection. During diastole, the mitral valve opens, and the PCWP directly reflects the left ventricular end-diastolic pressure (LVEDP).

When the pulmonary catheter balloon tip is inflated, it occludes or wedges the pulmonary artery. With the balloon inflated, the pressure readings are coming from the area in front of the catheter tip. This explains how a catheter in the right side of the heart can evaluate the left side.

NORMAL PRESSURES: (mm Hg)

SVC (superior vena cava) 0 to 5

IVC (inferior vena cava) 0 to 5

RA (right atrium) 0 to 5

RV (right ventricle) 25/0 to 5

PA (pulmonary artery) 25/10 (15 mean pressure)

P. CAPILLARIES 5 to 10

LA (left atrium) 5 to 10

LV (left ventricle) 120/0 to 5

AORTA 120/80 (90 mean pressure)

Prior to developing the pulmonary catheter, measurements were obtained through catheters inserted into the left atrium during intrathoracic surgery.

Significance of preload in relation to PCWP:

Clinical Status	PCWP
Onset of pulmonary congestion	18 to 20 mm Hg
Moderate pulmonary congestion	20 to 25 mm Hg
Severe pulmonary congestion	25 to 30 mm Hg
Pulmonary edema	30 mm Hg

The above table is an approximate range of pressures used to evaluate status. It depends upon the individual patient's vascular status and degree and chronicity of heart failure. Therefore, it is possible for a patient to be in pulmonary edema prior to a pressure of 30 mm Hg.

Pulmonary artery catheters contribute a great deal of information about the cardiovascular system. In general, complications during their use are minimal. However, complications that can occur include arrhythmias, sepsis, clotting and intracardiac knotting (rare).

KEY CONCEPT: Preload (1) directly affects left ventricular stroke volume, (2) cannot be measured directly in the left ventricle and (3) is measured in the pulmonary artery by obtaining a pulmonary capillary wedge pressure (PCWP).

Afterload

Afterload is the impedance to ejection of blood from the ventricle. Afterload is the most sensitive clinical measure of systemic vascular resistance (SVR). Afterload, input impedance or wall stress can be calculated using appropriate instrumentation during a cardiac catheterization. However, this information is not available at the bedside.

When evaluating vasopressor therapy at the bedside, measurements of arterial or left ventricular systolic pressure are usually relied upon. If a cardiac output measurement is available, it will help determine the systemic vascular resistance (SVR) and reflect changes in afterload on the left ventricle.

Vasopressor agents are used to correct hypotension. They increase the peripheral vascular resistance and raise the blood pressure.

Contractility

Contractility is the muscle function of the heart. This function is independent of preload and afterload. Contractility is affected by inotropic agents such as epinephrine or norepinephrine. Cardiac contractility is an inherent property of the myocardium. Independent of the Starling mechanism, contractility allows the heart to increase its effect and force of shortenings. Contractility is not directly measureable. However, if the stroke volume (SV) increases without a change in preload or afterload, an increase in contractility can be assumed. The large reserve capacity of the heart makes is difficult to detect impaired cardiac function in its early stages. Contractility deteriorates in individuals with a sedentary lifestyle and with the aging process. The heart has the capability of pumping larger than normal quantities of blood with the usual amount of resistance. This may be due to a strong sympathetic impulse or hypertrophied cardiac muscle. Hypertrophy may result as a response to a chronic increase in the amount of blood received and may be seen in patients with hypertension or aortic stenosis, or in athletes.

When treating cardiogenic shock patients, afterload reduction alone may not be sufficient. The administration of a positive inotropic agent (dopamine or dobutamine) may be needed to improve cardiac output and maintain arterial pressures high enough for adequate tissue perfusion (B.P. = C.O. x SVR). This improved myocardial contractility increases myocardial oxygen demands. Therefore, care must be employed to balance the effects in order to achieve the desired goal.

A counterpulsation device called the intra-aortic balloon pump may assist the decompensated heart.

The intra-aortic balloon pump assists the heart by (1) increasing diastole, which enhances coronary perfusion; (2) decreasing resistance (afterload) to ventricular flow during systoles, allowing the ventricle to eject more blood per beat; (3) reducing myocardial oxygen demands as less work is required to eject stroke volume.

The increase in stroke volume and cardiac output improves systemic circulation. The reduction in myocardial oxygen demands improves myocardial perfusion.

The normal systemic vascular resistance (SVR) ranges between 750 to 1500 dynes-sec cm.

An increase in afterload usually increases the SVR and the systolic or mean arterial pressure. A decrease in afterload is reflected by a decrease in the SVR and systolic or mean arterial pressure.

Heart Rate

The most effective method of altering cardiac output is changing the heart rate. The cardiac output may triple in a healthy individual who can increase his rate to approximately 175 beats per minute.

The sino-atrial (SA) node is influenced by both adrenergic and cholinergic fibers. The autonomic nervous system may transmit efferent impulses to the SA node.

Average heart rates in the adult range from 60 to 100 beats per minute (bpm). In the normal heart, maximal C.O. is reached at approximately 130 bpm. As the rate continues to increase, the C.O. progressively decreases because of a shortening ventricular diastolic filling time.

As the heart rate decreases to less than 120 bpm, the C.O. also decreases. However, the decrease in C.O. is not proportional to the heart rate, because the degree of filling of the ventricle is enhanced during the prolonged diastolic filling. This increases stroke volume, offsetting the decrease in heart rate.

If the heart rate falls below 40 bpm, the C.O. drops drastically in relation to the drop in rate. The ventricles have reached the maximum stroke volume and compensation.

Given a constant SV the output can be increased by increasing the HR.

Anemia, Ion Concentration, Hypoxia

Other criteria that may affect cardiac output and function are *anemia, ion concentration* and *hypoxia.*

In *anemia,* the red cell composition of blood decreases, resulting in decreased blood flow resistance. Tissue hypoxia may develop, and a further decrease in resistance occurs because of dilation of the peripheral vessels. As the hematocrit falls, the cardiac output tends to rise in a linear mode. The cardiac output may not be sufficient to maintain tissue perfusion when the hematocrit falls about 15 percent because the blood has lost considerable oxygen-carrying capabilities.

Ion concentration plays an important role in cardiac function. For example, atrioventricular blocks and cardiac standstill may be produced if potassium rises above 7 meq/L. Excessive potassium decreases the action potential. The heart becomes progressively weaker and slower. Myocardial function may increase as potassium concentrations are decreased.

Myocardial force and contraction increase as calcium ions oppose the action of potassium. The heart becomes more sensitive to digitalis as the amount of calcium increases and potassium decreases.

Mild *hypoxia* may stimulate the sympathetic system, increasing blood pressure and cardiac output. In severe hypoxia, blood pressure and cardiac output fall because of impaired muscle function. In some hypoxic situations, such as cardiac failure, cardiac output may increase because hypoxia leads to peripheral vasodilation, reducing afterload.

KEY POINT RECOGNITION

Write true or false by each statement. Answers are at the end of this chapter. A score below 80% indicates the need for further study.

1. Preload refers to the pressure of blood in the ventricle at the end of systole.
2. The degree of stretch during diastole determines the force during systole.
3. A sudden increase in blood volume may more than double the C.O.
4. The CVP rises if blood volume increases or if there is peripheral vasoconstriction.
5. Distended neck veins are the classic sign of left heart failure.
6. CVP measures left ventricular preload.
7. PCWP reflects left atrial pressure.
8. The onset of pulmonary congestion may be evidenced by a PCWP of 25 to 30 mm Hg.
9. Afterload is the most sensitive clinical measure of systemic vascular resistance.
10. Vasopressor agents increase blood pressure.
11. Inotropic agents affect contractility.
12. If SV is increased and preload is decreased, contractility is increased.
13. The IABP reduces myocardial oxygen demands, decreases diastole and increases resistance to forward flow from the ventricle.
14. An increase in afterload usually increases the systemic vascular resistance.
15. Maximal C.O. is reached at about 180 bpm.
16. Given a constant SV, the output can be increased by increasing heart rate.
17. When the hematocrit falls below 15 percent, C.O. may not be sufficient to maintain tissue oxygenation.
18. Sensitivity to digitalis increases as the amount of potassium decreases.
19. Mild hypoxia stimulates the sympathetic nervous system.
20. Hypoxia causes peripheral vasodilation and increases afterload.

ASSESSMENT OF THE CARDIOVASCULAR SYSTEM

Physical assessment of the patient experiencing cardiovascular disorders is not very different from the assessment of any other patient. Significant medical problems, current therapies, family history and review of systems are all included. Particular attention must be paid to the presenting complaint, its duration, character and circumstances surrounding exacerbations and remissions. The following symptoms require further investigation: weakness, pain, fatigue, dyspnea, edema, weight changes, nausea, vomiting, clubbing, hypertension or hemoptysis.

Specific signs of altered cardiovascular function may include dysrhythmias, chest pain, cyanosis (circumoral, peripheral, mucosal, conjunctival), palpitations, dyspnea (exertional, orthopnea) and intermittent claudication.

LEVEL OF CONSCIOUSNESS

Under any condition, the *level of consciousness* is the single most important determinant of neurological status. To assess level of consciousness, the following must be determined:

Arousability

Orientation

Ability to follow commands

Gross cerebral function—consciousness, awareness, orientation, memory, judgment

Specific cerebral function—conversational ability, attention span, ability to follow commands

INSPECTION

Observe for apparent health: handshake, personal appearance, gross deformity, nutrition, posture and gait. Determine awareness and cooperation.

Inspect skin for moisture, temperature, texture, turgor, elasticity, thickness, color, edema, lesions and superficial vascularity.

Observe nails for color, size, shape and clubbing.

Inspect for precordial pulsations; check apical pulse for character and location of point of maximal intensity (PMI).

Check for heaves, thrusts, systolic retractions and vibrations.

Note any depression, flattening or bulging of the precordium.

Observe for jugular vein distention by positioning the patient at a 45° angle. The center of the right atrium lies approximately 5 cm below the sternal angle. Therefore, the distance of the column above the sternal angle plus 5 cm equals the central venous pressure (Fig. 5-13).

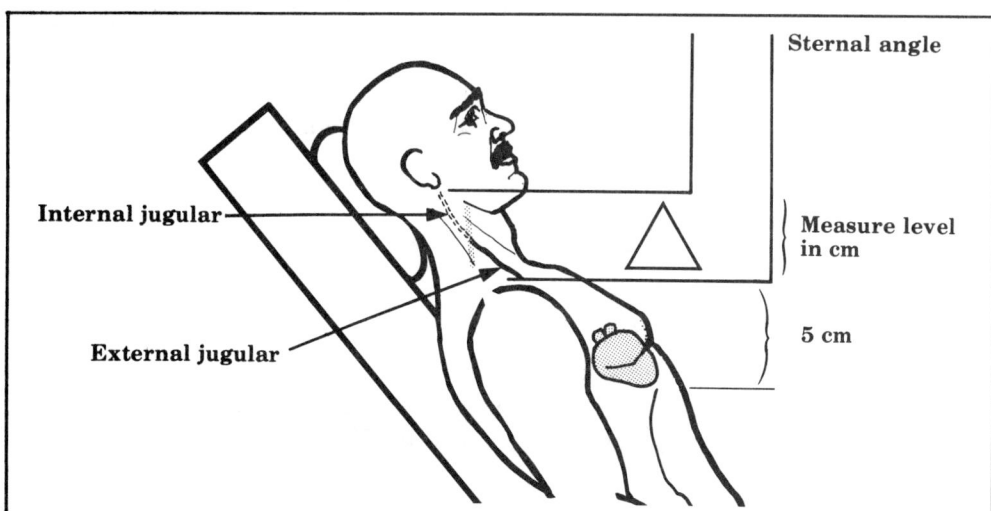

Fig. 5-13. Observing for jugular vein distention

Check for hepatojugular reflex (HJR) by adjusting the patient so that the highest level of palpation is detectable in the middle of the neck. Place your hand over the patient's right upper quadrant and apply firm pressure for 60 seconds. A rise of more than 1 cm in the jugular venous pressure is abnormal.

PALPATION

Palpate *pulses:* carotid, radial, brachial, femoral, popliteal, dorsalis pedis and posterior tibialis.

Note type of pulses:

Pulsus magnus—felt as rapid, strong upstroke and downstroke

Pulsus parvous—felt as a delayed upstroke and a prolonged downstroke

Pulsus alternans—felt as a regular beat alternating with a weak beat

Pulsus paradoxus—a physiological response to inspiration; 10 mm Hg or greater drop in arterial pressure on inspiration

Pulsus bisferiens—felt as two impulses during systole

Note the rate and rhythm.

Note intensity:

0 absent

+1 palpable

+2 normal

+3 full

+4 full and bounding

Palpate the following areas:

Precordium—for thrills, precordial friction rubs and tenderness

Sternoclavicular area—suprasternal notch; if pulsation, rule out aneurysm

Aortic Arch—felt at second right intercostal space; check for slight thrill—may be indicative of dilatation of the aorta

Pulmonic area—felt at the second left intercostal space which includes the pulmonary artery and valve. A thrill may be indicative of pulmonary artery stenosis. Other causes of a thrill include anemia, fever, pregnancy, and thin chest walls. Thrills are often felt in children.

Anterior precordium—xyphoid process, tip of the sternum. This is the area of the right ventricle. Abnormalities include right ventricular hypertrophy or atrial-septal defects.

Apical area—apex and pulse of maximal intensity (PMI). The PMI is found in the fifth intercostal space, medial midclavicular line, covering an area about the size of a nickel. If enlarged, it may be indicative of ventricular hypertrophy.

Epigastric area—inferior to the tip of the xiphoid. The abdominal aorta comes through the diaphragm. If vigorous pulsations are noted, this may be indicative of an aneurysm.

Ectopic area—lies halfway between the pulmonary and apical area. This area is frequently affected with myocardial infarctions.

PERCUSSION

Air is less dense than bone.

The sounds most frequently associated with percussion are:

Tympany—very low density

Dullness—felt over tissue

Flatness—can be felt over tissue or bone

Hyperresonance—heard over tissue filled with air (emphysema)

Resonance—decrease in density as normally heard in most of the lung

Impaired resonance—slightly more dense

In the cardiovascular system, percussion can be used to determine the size of the cardiac silhouette:

Left border cardiac dullness (LBCD): note most lateral space

Right border cardiac dullness (RBCD): usually not percussed due to surrounding cartilage

Abnormalities that may cause changes in the LBCD, other than cardiac enlargement, are tumor, pleural effusion and mediastinal shift.

AUSCULTATION

Auscultation is performed in four major areas. The sites are named according to the underlying valves. Major characteristics of sound are frequency and pitch. ***High frequency*** vibrations produce high-pitched sounds that are best heard with the diaphragm of the stethoscope. Common high-pitched sounds are S_1, S_2, opening snaps, ejection clicks and murmurs due to stenosis. ***Low frequency*** vibrations are produced by low-pitched sounds that are best heard with the bell of the stethoscope. Common low-pitched sounds are S_3, S_4, and ventricular filling murmurs.

The intensity or loudness is directly proportional to the amount of energy producing the vibration. The quality of sound depends on the loudness and pitch. The duration is directly proportional to the length of time the sound lasts. If the vibrations increase, the sound lasts longer.

KEY POINT RECOGNITION

Write true or false by each statement. Answers are at the end of this chapter. A score below 80% indicates the need for further study.

1. Dysrhythmias and palpitations may indicate cardiovascular dysfunction.
2. Cardiovascular assessment includes checking the extremities for peripheral pulses, edema and ulcerations.
3. When performing a cardiovascular assessment, evaluate the point of maximal intensity (PMI) for character and location.
4. Evaluate the PMI for heaves, thrusts and systolic retractions.
5. A negative hepatojugular reflex is evaluated by applying pressure over the right upper quadrant and observing for a rise of 1 cm or more in the neck veins.
6. Pulsus parvous is recognized by a delay in the upstroke and a prolonged downstroke.
7. Pulsus paradoxus indicates inspiratory exaggeration of a normal event.
8. A +1 pulse is normal.
9. The palpation of a sternoclavicular pulsation may indicate an aneurysm.
10. Resonance heard over most of the lung fields indicates an increase in density.
11. Low-frequency vibrations are best heard using the diaphragm of the stethoscope.
12. Common high-pitched sounds are ejection clicks and murmurs caused by stenosis.

HEART SOUNDS

Heart sounds are divided into two general categories: normal sounds and abnormal sounds.

Normal Heart Sounds

S_1 and S_2 are the normal heart sounds.

At normal and slow rates, S_1 is the first part of the sound (lub). S_1 occurs at the beginning of ventricular systole and is produced by the closing of the mitral and tricuspid valves. The S_1 sound precedes the upstroke of the carotid pulse and coincides with the radial pulse. It is characterized by a low-pitched lub sound. When auscultating S_1, place the diaphragm of the stethoscope at the apex of the heart.

S_2 (dub) is the second part of the heart sound and occurs at the end of ventricular systole. It is produced by the closing of the pulmonic and aortic valves. S_2

follows the carotid pulse. It is characterized by a high-pitched dub, which is louder and shorter than S_1. When auscultating S_2, place the diaphragm of the stethoscope at the base of the heart.

Physiological Splitting

Slight splitting of normal heart sounds is often heard during inspiration. Called physiological splitting, S_1 splitting occurs because the tricuspid valve closes late. Pathology such as right bundle branch block causes the triscupid valve to close late. A delay in pulmonary valve closure causes a normal split in S_2 during inspiration. During expiration, the split diminishes or disappears.

Fixed Splitting

Splitting of S_2, which is constant during inspiration and expiration, is abnormal. It usually indicates atrial septal defects.

Gallops

A gallop is an abnormal diastolic event in which the sound resembles the sound of a galloping horse.

S_3, the third heart sound, is a ventricular diastolic gallop that occurs during congestive heart failure. An unusually large diastolic blood flow into a normal ventricle, or a normal blood flow filling an abnormal ventricle, causes the sound. S_3, which is dull and low-pitched, is best heard by using the bell of the stethoscope. The patient should be on the left side and the bell should be placed at the apical area. The sound increases on expiration. A loud S_3 may be caused by an increase in cardiac output due to anemia, hyperthyroidism, ventricular-septal defects, exercise, mitral regurgitation, left-to-right shunts or tricuspid insufficiency.

Physiological S_3 heard in children and young adults is considered normal. It is caused by the normal increase in filling velocity.

S_4, the fourth heart sound, is an atrial or presystolic gallop and therefore, occurs before S_1. It may be heard in ventricular failure, postmyocardial infarction, pulmonary hypertension, aortic or pulmonary stenosis and hyperthyroidism. It is heard just before S_1 and is caused by increased resistance to ventricular filling following atrial contraction. S_4 is a low-pitched sound and is best heard by placing the bell of the stethoscope medial to the right apex or at the third or fourth intercostal space of the left sternal border. S_4 may be heard in ventricular hypertrophy.

In distinguishing S_4 from S_1, remember that S_4 is low-pitched and heard using the bell of the stethoscope. Split S_1 is high-pitched and heard using the diaphragm of the stethoscope.

Order of Sounds Heard

Physiological contraction and filling of the heart create the order in which the sounds are heard. S_4 and S_1 are presystolic and systolic sounds. S_2 and S_3 are prediastolic and diastolic sounds. Therefore, S_4 is heard just before S_1, and S_3 is heard just after S_2 (Fig. 5-14).

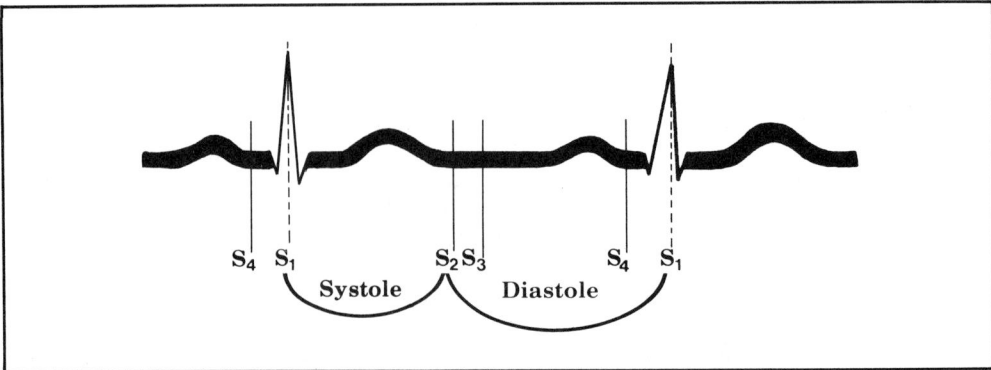

Fig. 5-14. Heart sounds correlated with systole and diastole

KEY CONCEPT: S_1 and S_2 are normal heart sounds. S_3 indicates heart failure due to a distended left ventricular myocardium and an increase in left ventricular end diastolic filling pressure. S_4 indicates a decrease in left ventricular compliance (stiff myocardium) and an increase in left ventricular end diastolic pressure.

Abnormal Heart Sounds

A *gallop* rhythm is characterized by a cadence of the extra sounds of S_3 and S_4. If the sound is presystolic, it may be difficult to discern the rhythm from a split first sound or an ejection click following S_1. The cadence for each gallop rhythm is distinct. The presystolic gallop cadence is described as "TENNESSEE." The diastolic gallop cadence is described as "KENTUCKY" (Fig 5-15). In some clinical situations, the third and fourth sounds are simultaneously audible in heart rates greater than 100 beats per minute. When this occurs, the sound is called a summation gallop. Summation gallops are usually mid-diastolic and are louder than S_1 or S_2. They are commonly found in advanced heart failure.

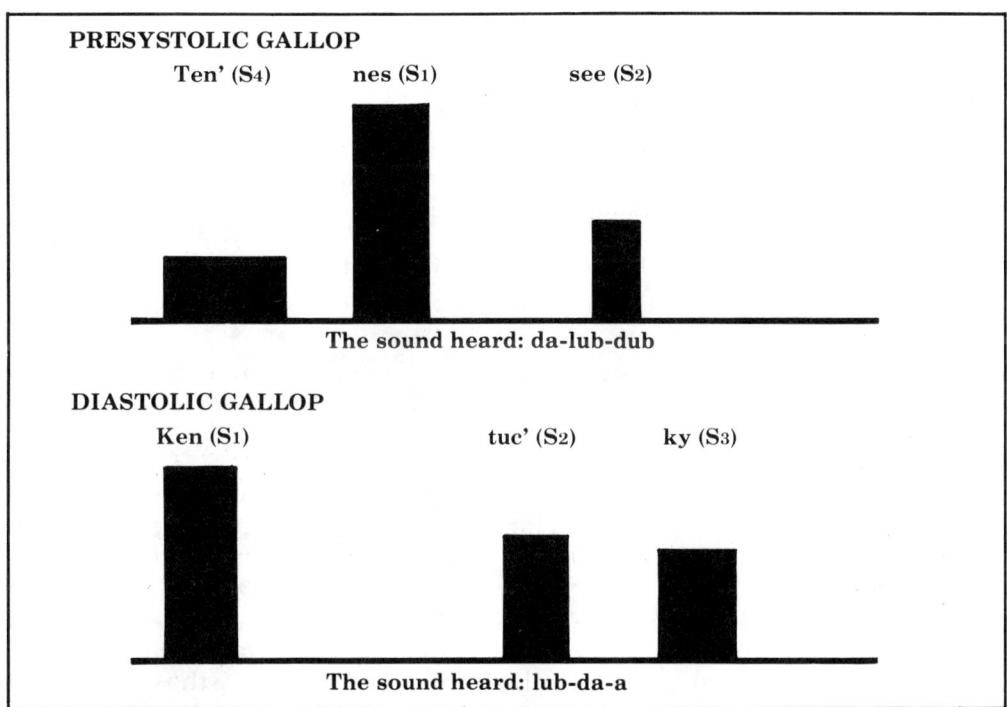

Fig. 5-15. Gallop: cadence

A *snap* is a sound that occurs in rheumatic valvular disease. The sound is the opening snap of the atrioventricular valve. It is heard approximately .10 second after the second heart sound. A snap is heard best between the third or fourth left intercostal space and may be the loudest and most widely heard sound in the entire cardiac cycle. A snap is earlier, sharper and higher in pitch than an S_3.

A *click* is a sound heard during systole. The sound arises from the valves. The most common click is the systolic ejection click which usually precedes a systolic ejection murmur. It usually occurs very early in systole—approximately .02 second after S_1. Ejection clicks occur with pulmonary artery dilation or with increased aortic blood flow. Clicks are louder on expiration. They are common in patients with minimal stenosis of the valve, but may be heard with normal valves.

A *rub* is a grating, harsh sound heard over the precordium during systole. Rubs sound similar to hair rubbing against the diaphragm of the stethoscope. The time and phase of respiration and posture affect the sound of a rub. Use a bell when listening for a rub, but remember, the degree of pressure exerted on the bell alters the intensity of the sound.

A *murmur* is a vibration within the heart. Heart murmurs result from turbulent blood flow around the valve and through abnormal valvular openings. Turbulent blood flow heard through a vessel is called a ***bruit.*** Turbulent blood flow felt in a vessel is called a ***thrill.*** Murmurs are heard over the auscultatory area of their origin. Murmurs are classified according to where they occur in the cardiac cycle.

They are classified as ***systolic, diastolic*** or ***continuous.***

Assessment of murmurs includes eliciting the following:

Grading: A murmur is graded on an intensity scale from 1 to 6.

Timing: Timing describes the phase of the cardiac cycle in which the murmur occurs (systolic, diastolic).

Location: Auscultatory location is described as *interspace* and *centimeters* from midsternum, midclavicle and axillary lines.

Radiation: Radiation describes transmission of the sound to another area of the body, such as the neck.

Pitch: Pitch describes high-, medium- or low-frequency sounds.

Intensity: Intensity is classified in six grades: Grade I—very faint, may not be heard in all positions; Grade II—quiet, heard immediately with the stethoscope; Grade III—moderately loud, not associated with a thrill; Grade V—very loud, with a thrill, heard with stethoscope partly off the chest; Grade VI—very loud, with a thrill, heard with stethoscope off the chest.

Quality: The quality describes the sound as blowing, harsh, rumbling or musical.

Systolic murmurs are less significant than diastolic murmurs and may occur in patients with no evidence of heart disease. Most systolic murmurs are early or midsystolic. The two main types of systolic murmurs are ***ejection*** and ***regurgitant.***

Blood flow from the high-pressured ventricle into a vessel with lower pressure causes ***ejection*** murmurs. Ejection murmurs are heard in aortic and pulmonic stenosis. Intensity and duration depend upon the stroke volume and the severity of the stenosis. Ejection murmurs are harsh and medium-pitched, and can be heard using the diaphragm of the stethoscope.

Mitral and tricuspid incompetence produce ***regurgitant*** murmurs. High-pitched, they are heard best with the diaphragm of the stethoscope. These murmurs are pansystolic or continuous systolic murmurs.

Diastolic murmurs are commonly classified as early, mid, late and presystolic. Early or immediate diastolic murmurs are sounds caused by an incompetent pulmonic or aortic valve. Although high-pitched, they decrease in intensity during diastole and are often difficult to hear.

Delayed or mid-diastolic murmurs are sounds that occur when ventricular pressure falls below the level of atrial pressure. This sound is low-pitched and rumbling, and can be heard using the bell of the diaphragm. The severity of the stenosis and amount of stroke volume determine the time span of the murmur.

A presystolic murmur indicates the presence of mitral stenosis. This sound is best heard after exercise, with the patient positioned on the left side. The murmur may be accentuated in severe aortic incompetence and is called an Austin Flint murmur.

Continuous murmurs are sounds heard when a pressure discrepancy is present between two chambers throughout the cardiac cycle. Patent ductus arteriosus, with a left-to-right shunt, is the most common cause of a continuous murmur. This murmur also occurs with a shunt surgically created for relief of tetralogy of Fallott and aortopulmonary fistulas.

KEY CONCEPT: Stenotic valves do not open adequately to allow free flow of blood from one chamber to another. Incompetent, insufficient or regurgitant valves allow a backflow of blood into the heart chambers.

Common causes of murmurs:
Systolic murmurs:
  aortic stenosis, pulmonic stenosis, tricuspid insufficiency, mitral insufficiency
Diastolic murmurs:
  tricuspid stenosis, mitral stenosis, aortic insufficiency, pulmonic insufficiency

EVALUATION OF VITAL SIGNS

Alterations in blood pressure are *hypotension* and *hypertension.* Hypotension indicates low cardiac output. Hypertension may be a compensatory mechanism to ensure perfusion.

Alterations in heart rate are *bradycardia* and *tachycardia.* Bradycardia is a slow rate often seen with cardiac dysrhythmia, such as heart block. Tachycardia is usually a compensatory response to injury of the myocardium.

Alterations in body temperature are *hyperthermia* and *hypothermia.*

Hyperthermia may be seen in response to an infectious or inflammatory process. These elevated temperatures are usually accompanied by tachycardia. *Hypothermia* is rarely observed, although it may be seen in profound shock, resulting in brain death.

Alterations in respiration are *bradypnea* and *tachypnea. Tachypnea* is more commonly seen with cardiovascular disease as a compensatory mechanism to bring more oxygen into the body. Cheyne-Stokes respirations are rhythmic hypo- and hyperventilations alternating with periods of apnea. The entire sequence is a crescendo-decrescendo response to alternations in pCO_2 levels.

KEY CONCEPT: Physical assessment of the patient with a cardiovascular problem includes assessment of: gross and specific cerebral functions, inspection, palpation, percussion, and auscultation.

LABORATORY AND SPECIAL STUDIES
Laboratory Studies

Enzymes are valuable diagnostic tools. They are proteins that alter the speed of chemical reactions and provide for coagulation. Most enzymes are found in the intracellular compartment; however, small amounts of cellular enzymes leak through normal membrane pores. Elevated serum enzyme levels indicate damage to the cell membrane. The major cardiac enzymes are ***CPK*** (creatinine phosphokinase), ***LDH*** (lactic dehydrogenase), ***HBD*** (hydroxybutyrate dehydrogenase) and ***SGOT*** (serum glutamic oxalacetic transaminase).

Enzymes are used for diagnosing a myocardial infarction (estimation of infarction size is usually done by serial CPK levels); determining prognosis following a myocardial infarction; and evaluating therapeutic interventions designed to reduce the infarction (Fig. 5-16).

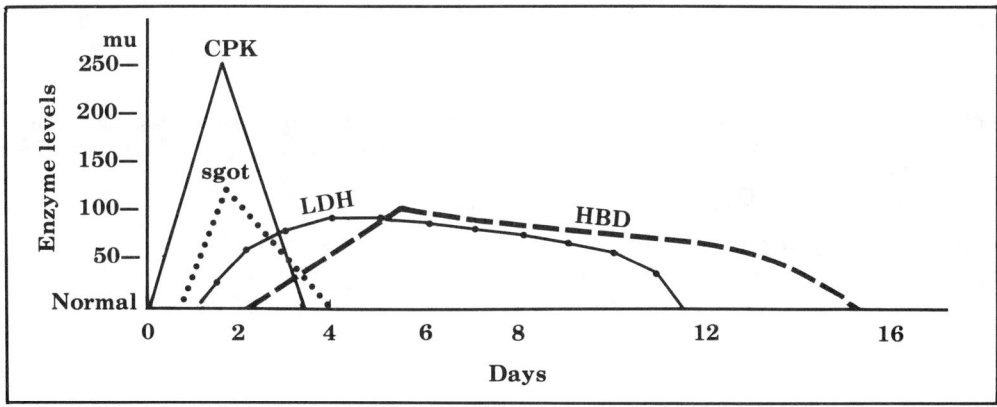

Fig. 5-16. Cardiac enzymes: onset and duration

Enzymes generally start to rise four to six hours postmyocardial infarction. The CPK rises first; the SGOT rises next. All enzymes are significantly elevated by the third day.

The CPK is the most sensitive enzyme. The smallest amount of injury causes an elevated CPK. The CPK can be more specific for cardiac damage if brain or skeletal muscle abnormalities are ruled out.

The *isoenzymes* are the most specific diagnostic aid. Isoenzymes are different forms of a particular enzyme. Each of the routinely measured enzymes actually reflects a group of enzymes, with slight molecular differences, that influence the same metabolic reactions.

CPK isoenzyme (CPK-MB) is normally slight to none in the serum. Levels, specifically CPK-MB, greater than 3.5 percent indicate a myocardial infarction. CPK-MB is released in other situations, such as cardiac trauma and cardiac surgery. LDH_2 isoenzyme is usually greater than LDH_1. In acute myocardial infarction, this pattern is reversed with LDH_1 being greater than LDH_2.

HBD is equivalent to LDH_1 and LDH_2, but it does not show a reversed pattern.

Other serum findings include:

Lipids: Cholesterol, triglycerides and phospholipids circulate in plasma and are bound to protein. A patient who has large amounts of these lipids in the bloodstream experiences hyperlipidemia. Hyperlipidemia predisposes to coronary artery disease.

Glucose: A chronically elevated glucose level is a risk factor to the patient with coronary artery disease. The normal range is 80 to 120.

CBC: Changes in CBC values may give clues for diagnosing coronary artery disease. Anemia may precipitate angina.

WBC: An elevated WBC may represent bacterial endocarditis or myocardial infarction.

Sedimentation rate: An elevated sedimentation rate may indicate myocardial infarction, bacterial endocarditis or Dressler's syndrome. A low sedimentation rate may indicate congestive heart failure.

Prothrombin time: Prothrombin time (PT) is used to determine anticoagulation status during anticoagulant drug therapy. Usually, the prothrombin time is within 2 to 2½ times of normal. Partial prothrombin time (PTT) is used to determine anticoagulation status during heparin therapy.

Urinalysis: The presence of RBCs may indicate infectious endocarditis or embolic disease of the kidneys. Mild proteinuria may occur in congestive heart failure. Massive proteinuria may indicate an elevated venous pressure in constrictive pericarditis or tricuspid insufficiency. Myoglobulinuria may occur in the diagnosis of myocardial infarction.

Special Studies

Noninvasive diagnostic procedures are specific and tailored to the presumptive diagnosis at hand. Nurses should be aware of these when making nursing assessments.

Apex cardiography determines the displacement of the chest wall produced by the left ventricle. It is a graphic recording that diagnoses aortic valve stenosis and mitral valve disease.

Radioisotope scanning, or myocardial scanning, determines the size and extent of myocardial ischemia or infarction, diagnoses coronary artery disease and evaluates patency of venous bypass grafts. Other uses include the evaluation of left ventricular contraction and ejection, and left ventricular aneurysms.

Echocardiography reflects ultrasound echoes which identify mitral stenosis, tricuspid stenosis, pericardial effusion, atrial-septal defects, prolapsing mitral leaflet, hypertropic cardiomyopathy, atrial tumors and congenital defects.

Vectorcardiography determines the balance of electrical forces of the heart and identifies ventricular hypertrophy, left and right bundle block, posterior and anterior fasicular blocks, myocardial ischemia and infarctions, atrial hypertrophy and atrial-septal defects.

Electrocardiography

The electrocardiogram (EKG) is a graphic representation of the electrical activity of the heart. These electrical forces are recorded on graph paper. The graph paper has a horizontal time scale and vertical voltage scale. Each horizontal space represents a time interval of .04 second. A heavier line is seen every fifth line, both horizontally and vertically. The time interval between the two heavier lines is .20 second (.04 x 5 = .20 second). Voltage or amplitude between the two heavy lines is 0.5 mv (Fig. 5-17).

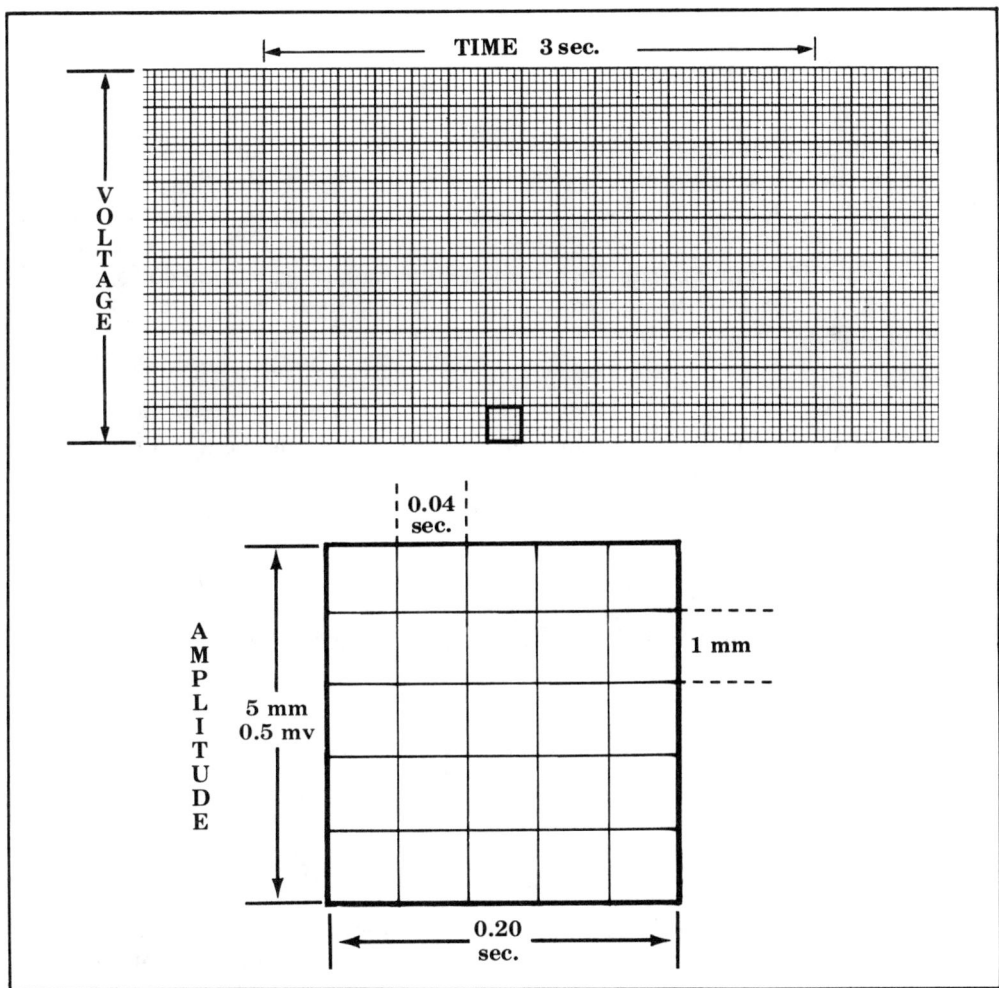

Fig. 5-17. EKG paper

The typical EKG represents a cardiac cycle designated by the following PQRST wave forms and intervals (Fig. 5-18).

P—The P wave is the first positive deflection and represents atrial depolarization. It normally appears smoothly rounded and precedes each QRS complex at a specific interval.

P-R interval—The P-R interval represents impulse conduction through the atria and into the AV node. It extends from the beginning of the P wave to the onset of the Q wave. This interval should be no longer than .20 second (5 small squares or 1 large square on the EKG paper).

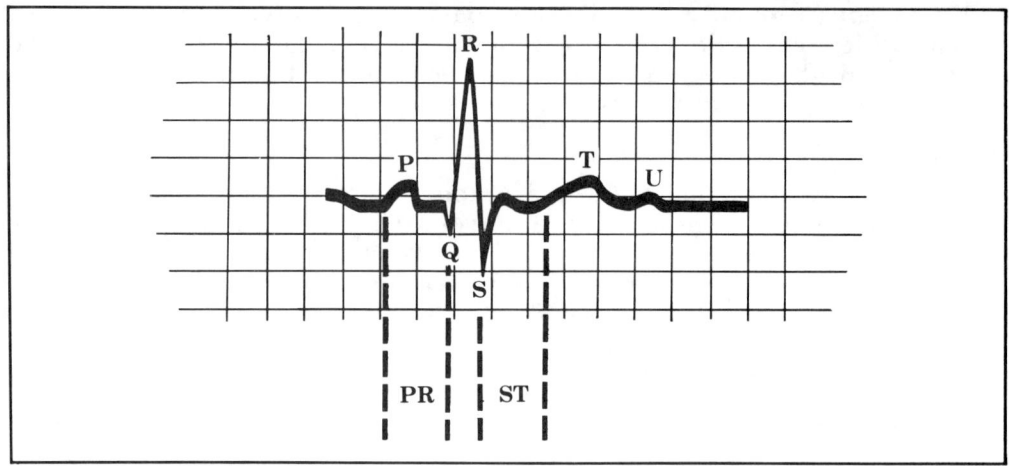

Fig. 5-18. Normal wave pattern

QRS complex—The QRS complex represents ventricular depolarization. It consists of three deflections:

Q wave: The Q wave is the first negative deflection after the P wave. It results from the initial left-to-right septal depolarization. An abnormal Q wave indicates an acute or old myocardial infarction. However, there are exceptions to this rule; conduction defects that alter pathways may influence the appearance and course of this wave.

R wave: The R wave is the first positive deflection after the P wave.

S wave: The S wave is the negative deflection following the R wave.

Although specific Q R and S waves may not be present in each complex, it is still called the QRS complex.

Q waves followed by a positive deflection have greater diagnostic value, when abnormal, than ST-T abnormalities.

ST segment: The ST segment extends from the end of the S wave to the beginning of the T wave. A normal ST segment is .32 second. ST changes are usually transitory, but indicate cardiac abnormalities. The following are some causes of ST segment changes:

Change	Cause
1. Elevation	Acute MI aneurysm or pericardial muscle injury, ventricular hypertrophy
2. Depression	Angina, coronary insufficiency
3. Sag	Digitalis effect
4. Prolonged	Hypocalcemia

T wave: The T wave represents ventricular repolarization. Normally, this wave is positive and symmetrical. Drugs, change of position, electrolyte imbalance and food intake may alter the T wave. This phase is the most vulnerable time in the cycle.

QT interval: The QT interval extends from the beginning of the QRS complex to the end of the T wave. It represents ventricular depolarization and repolarization.

U wave: The U wave is a small positive deflection after the T wave. It reflects repolarization of the Purkinje fibers. This wave is not usually visible on the EKG. Some causes of a positive U wave are hypokalemia, thyrotoxicosis, bradycardia and exercise. Drugs that may cause a prominent U wave are digitalis, quinidine and epinephrine. An MI coronary insufficiency and left ventricular hypertrophy may cause a negative U wave. A U wave can be separated from the T wave by providing carotid sinus pressure. It is during this supernormal phase that PVCs frequently occur.

The electrical forces are transmitted through skin electrodes and wires. One must understand basic principles of 12-lead electrocardiography to understand EKG monitoring techniques.

An equilateral triangle, Einthoven's triangle, is used as a reference for the standard bipolar leads (I, II, III). The heart is the electrical center of Einthoven's triangle. A second reference is created by positioning leads that radiate from the triangle's center. These are the **augmented limb leads** (aVR, aVL and aVF). The remaining six leads are **unipolar chest leads** (V1 through V6) (Fig. 5-19).

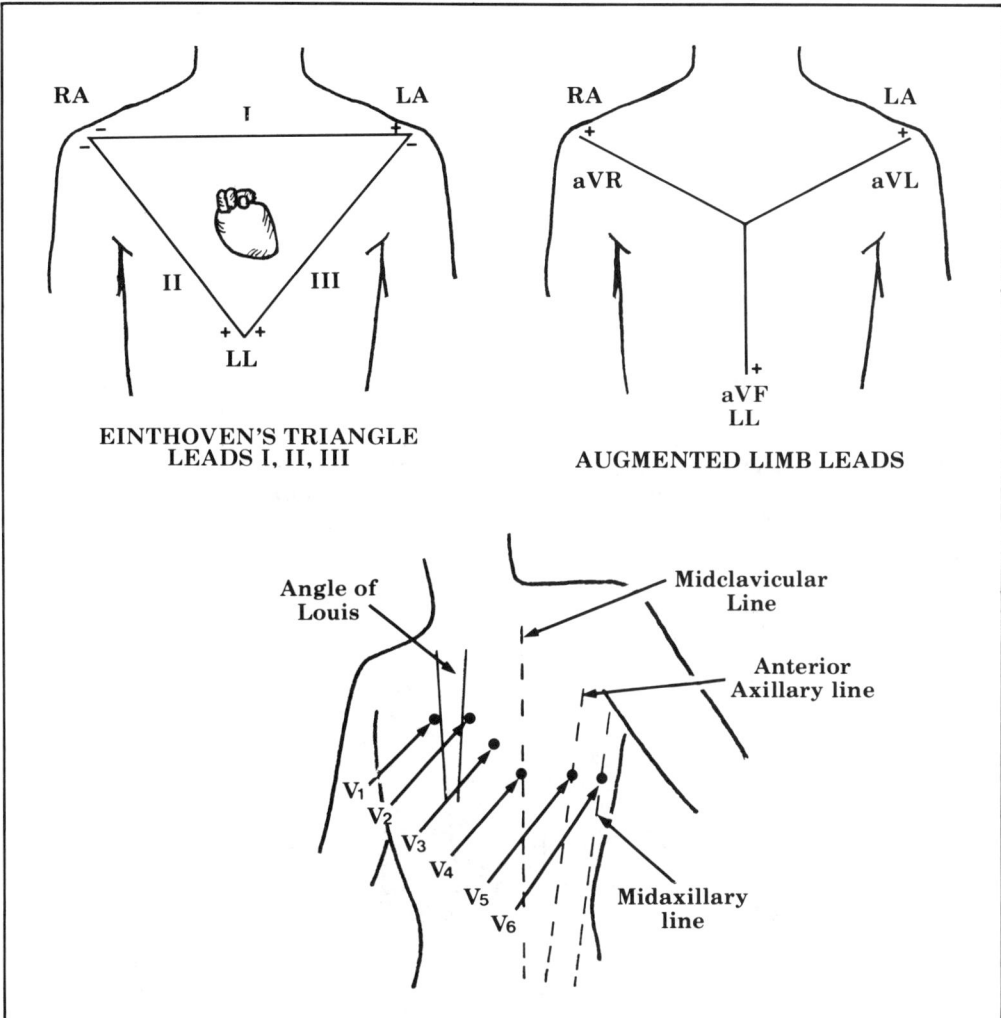

Fig. 5-19. 12 Lead EKG: electrode placement

The AV node of the heart is actually the focal point for Einthoven's center. The right arm, left arm and left leg are the three points of the equilateral triangle. The right leg is called the ground and is used to prevent electrical interference.

The **standard bipolar leads** have both a positive and negative electrode on the body surface. The electrodes are usually placed on two extremities or on the chest.

Bipolar chest leads have a positive electrode on the precordial area and a negative electrode going away from the heart. The positive electrode is close to the heart's apex.

The negative electrode is usually on an extremity. P wave deflections are produced by the movement of electrically charged particles across the myocardial cell membrane, which creates a measurable flow of current. The electrical field extends to the surface of the body. As the current flows to a positive electrode, it creates an upright deflection on the graph paper. Current flowing to a negative electrode results in a downward deflection.

Electrode position in relation to the heart's apex causes configuration of the complex. Thus, for diagnostic purposes, single lead changes are inaccurate.

Unipolar leads and the **augmented leads** represent the voltage of the heart in a specific area. In augmented leads a VR, a VL and a VF, the negative electrode is formed by combining two of the three leads. The positive electrode is perched on either side of the right arm (aVR), left arm or left leg.

The V leads are unipolar precordial leads. They are created by positive lead placement on the precordium. The common precordial positions are:

V1—4th intercostal space at the right sternal border

V2—4th intercostal space at the left sternal border

V3—equal distances between V2 and V4

V4—5th intercostal space in the left midclavicular line

V5—anterior axillary line

V6—midaxillary line

Bedside monitors, excluding telemetry, either have a three-, four-, or five-lead system.

In the **three-lead system** (I, II, III), the reference or ground lead is the electrode not being used. For example, on lead II, the electrodes on the right arm and left leg are being used. The left arm electrode becomes the reference lead (Fig. 5-20). The flow of current is negative to positive. The monitor does not know where a specific electrode is located; it only knows where the electrode or lead wire is plugged into the cable. Consequently, it works on polarity and not color coding.

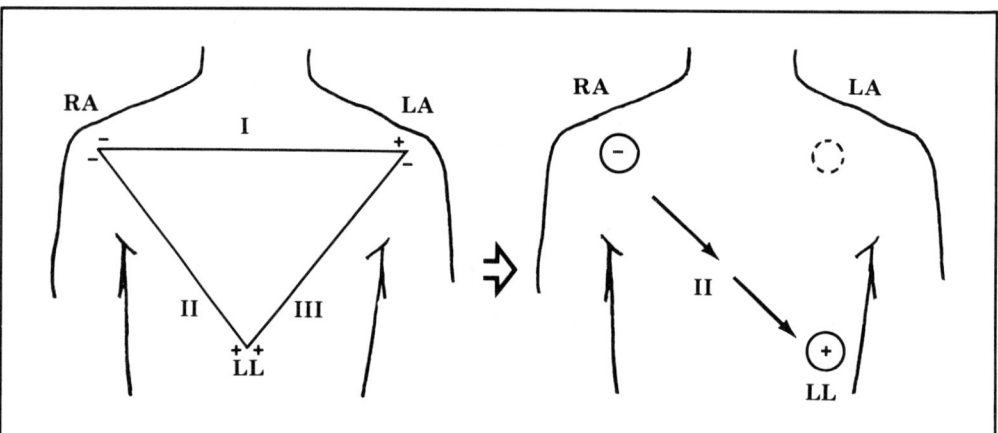

Fig. 5-20. Electrode placement: 3-lead monitoring system

Most equipment has separate modes for diagnosis and monitoring. The monitoring mode is used routinely. This mode filters out interference. When switching from one mode to the other, a change in baseline or ST segment may be noted. The term *diagnostic* refers to an unfiltered mode. It is electrically described as the specific bandwidth of the signal.

The **four-lead system** has an added electrode with no polarity. It is assigned to the right leg.

The *five-lead system* adds a positive electrode, usually attached to the chest (Fig. 5-21). When a five-lead cable is available, but only four leads are being used, the chest lead should be plugged in to prevent electrical interference.

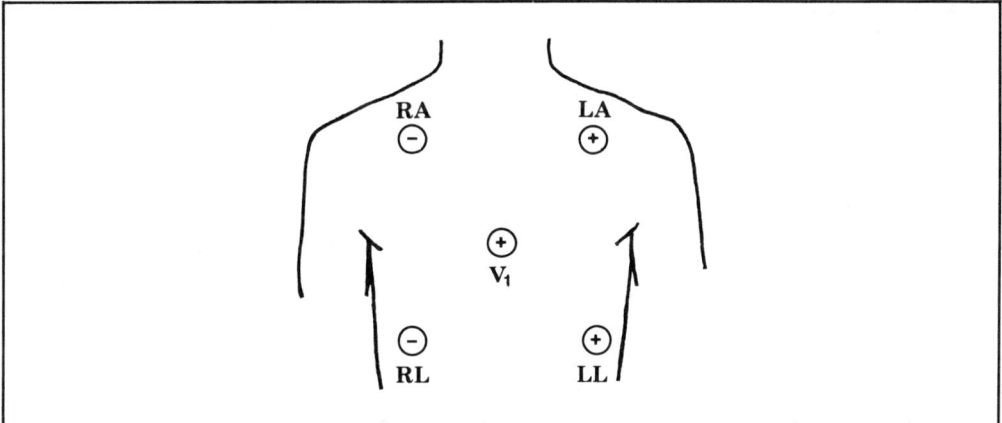

Fig. 5-21. Electrode placement: 5-lead monitoring system

A three-lead system is usually used when displaying a modified chest lead (MCL). The electrode position is physically changed to V1 and allows for closer scrutiny of ventricular aberrations. By using the appropriate monitor switch, the nurse may observe the monitored complexes as follows (Fig. 5-22):

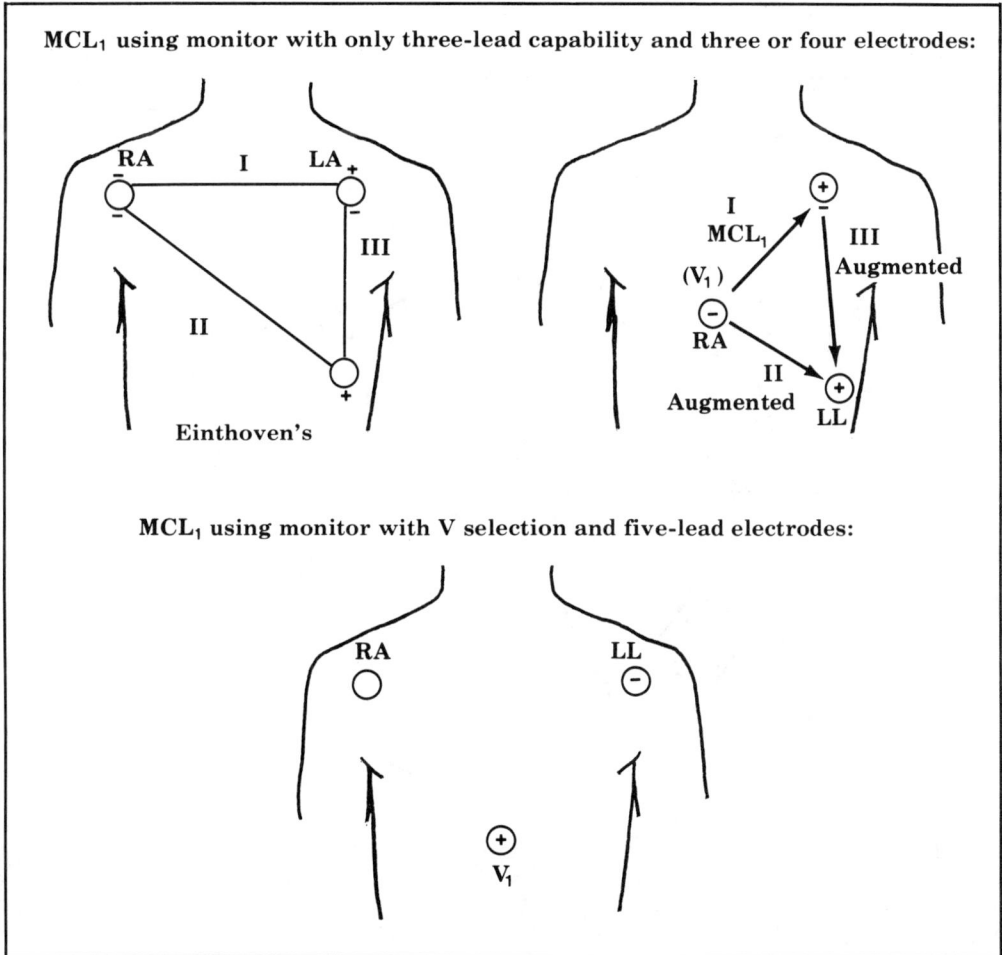

Fig. 5-22. Electrode placement: modified chest lead

Monitor selector	Patient	Polarity of complex
Lead I RA LA	MCL	Negative
Lead II RA LL	Augmented limb Lead III	Bifasic
Lead III LA LL	Augmented limb Lead II	Positive

MCL usually displays a negative complex, but some monitors may have an external switch to make the complex positive. On newer equipment, polarity is internalized. The polarity switch senses the complex to count heart rate. It may not synchronize. Therefore, in cardioversion situations, the nurse must ensure a positive complex (R) by adjusting lead selector or turning the polarity switch to positive. Check with your manufacturer for the monitor's capabilities.

KEY CONCEPT: The 12-lead EKG is the most accurate diagnostic method of monitoring. The three-lead monitoring system is most commonly used at the bedside to detect arrhythmias. MCL is used to identify ventricular rhythms. Review manual instructions to ensure proper use of monitoring equipment.

Axis-Vectors

Electrical *axis* is the direction in which electrical current flows through the heart. Normally, it flows from the base to apex and right-to-left through the heart. The neutral axis of the heart lies halfway between the vertical and left horizontal axis (Fig. 5-23).

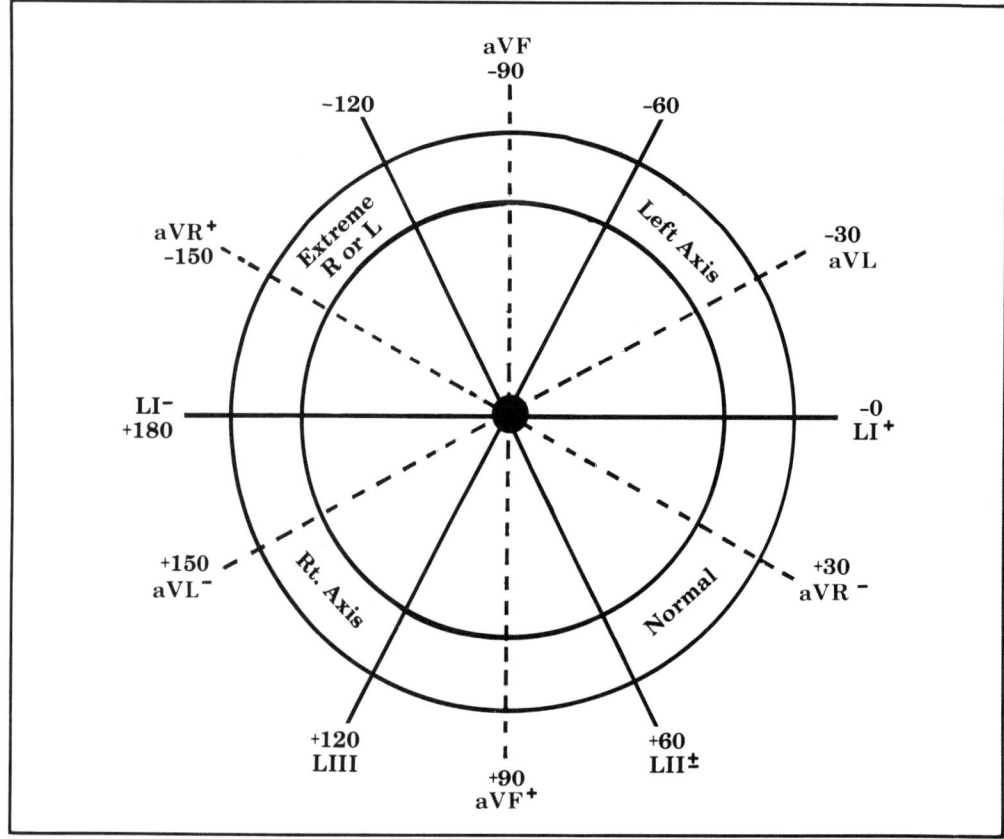

Fig. 5-23. Axis

Deviations occur with anatomical changes caused by pathophysiological processes.

A vector is a physical force having both magnitude and direction. Vectors are used to represent electrical activity of the heart. They can be shown for an entire cardiac cycle. When the direction of the force moves toward the positive pole of the lead, the EKG wave deflects upward. Conversely, when the force moves toward the negative pole, the wave deflects downward. The vector resulting from all the forces represents the electrical axis of the heart. For example, a QRS vector represents ventricular force (Fig. 5-24). When plotting a vector graphically, the length of the line represents *magnitude* of the force, and its position indicates *direction.*

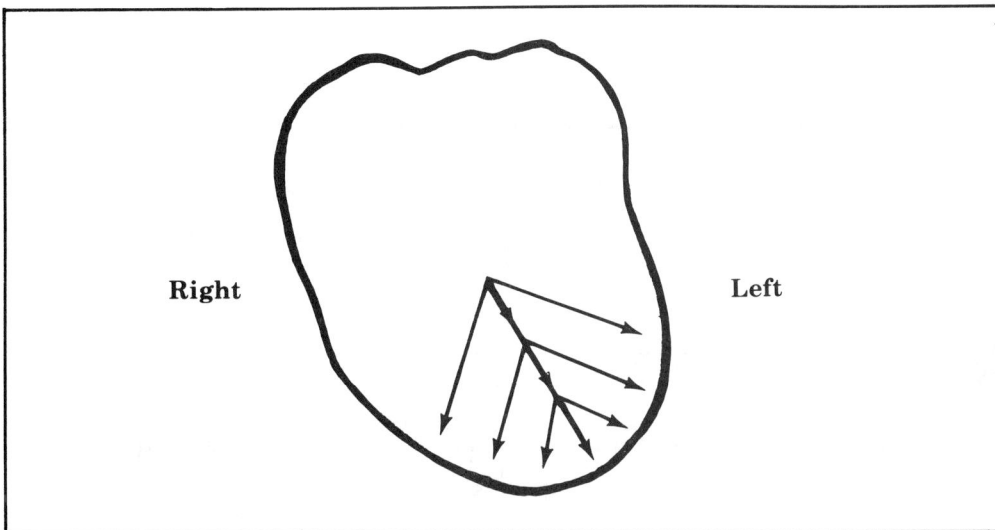

Fig. 5-24. QRS—Vector = Ventricular force

KEY CONCEPT: The sum of all electrical forces travelling through the heart is referred to as the mean vector. The direction that the mean vector takes is the electrical axis of the heart. Vector plotting helps determine MI, hypertrophy and abnormal conduction pathways.

In the frontal plane, electrical axis is determined by referring to Einthoven's triangle. The QRS complex in each bipolar lead approximates the general direction of the ventricular depolarization vectors (Fig. 5-25). In Lead I, the QRS complex is positive, indicating the ventricular force is to the left shoulder. Lead III reveals a negative complex indicating the vector is away from the left leg.

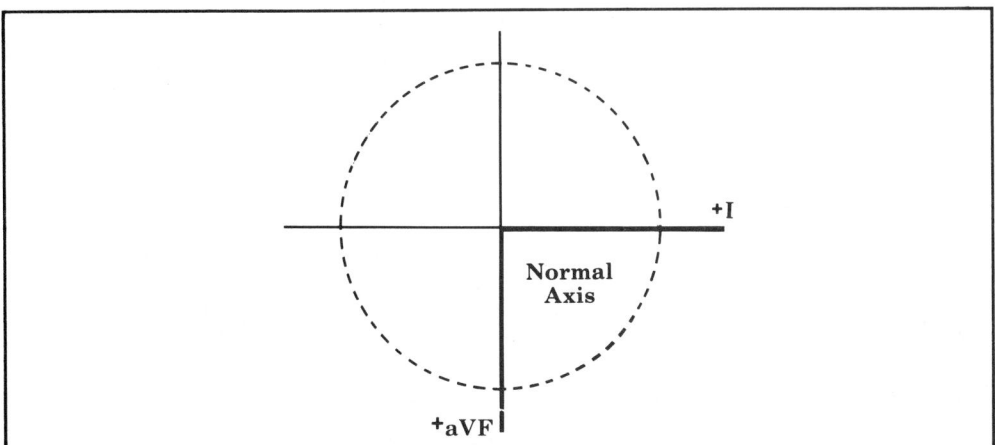

Fig. 5-25. Normal axis

Axis Deviation

Normal axis: toward the positive pole of Lead I and aVF (Fig. 5-25)

Right axis deviation: away from the positive pole of Lead I; toward the positive pole of aVF; into the lower right quadrant; seen in anteriolateral MI, left posterior hemiblock and right ventricular hypertrophy (Fig. 5-26)

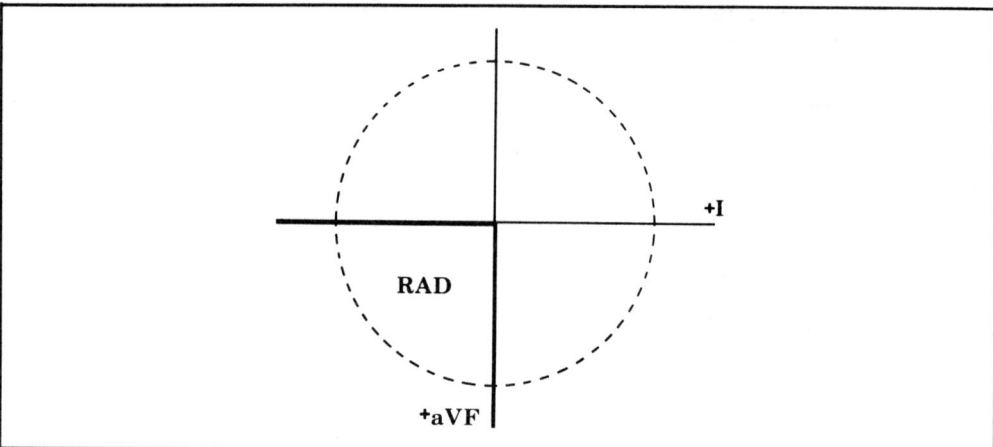

Fig. 5-26. Right axis deviation

Left axis deviation: toward the positive pole of Lead I; away from the positive pole of aVF; deviates to upper left quadrant (Fig. 5-27)

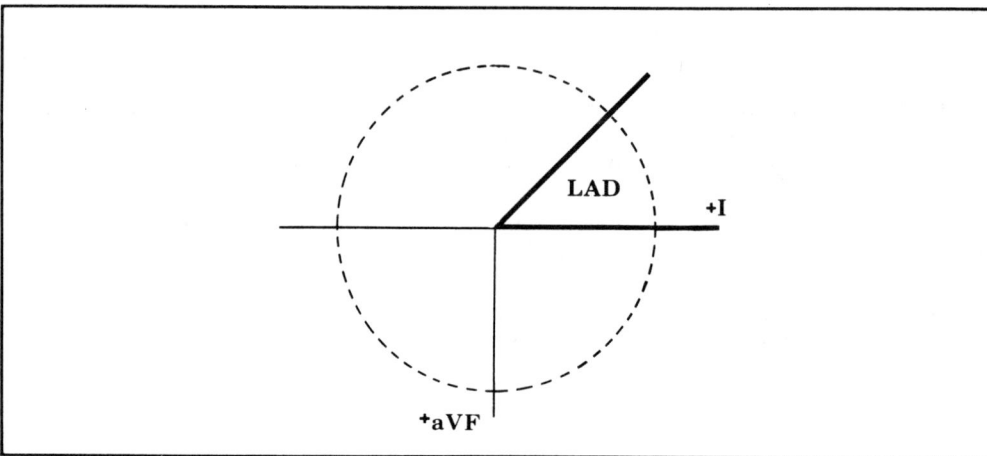

Fig. 5-27. Left axis deviation

Abnormal left axis deviation: toward the positive pole of Lead I; away from the positive pole of an aVF and Lead II; clinically seen in inferior wall MI, left anterior hemiblock and right ventricular pacing; deviates farther to left and LAD (Fig. 5-28).

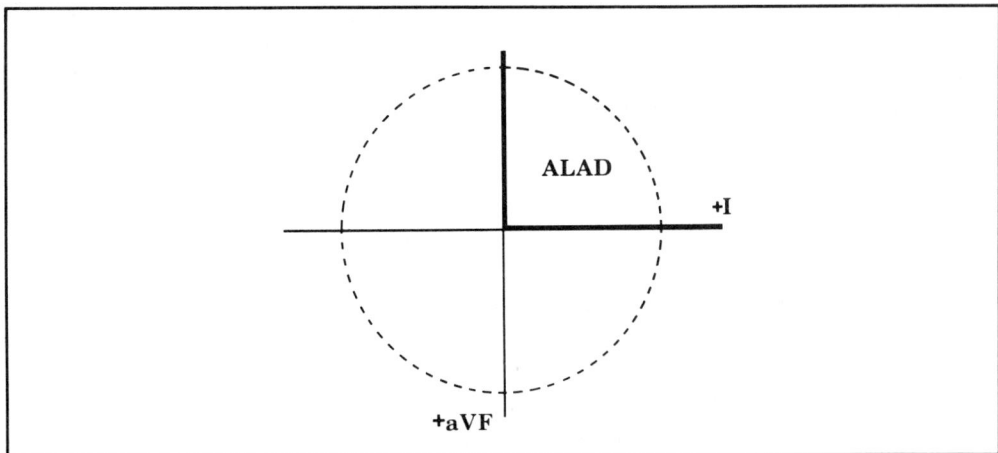

Fig. 5-28. Abnormal left axis deviation

Indeterminate axis: away from the positive pole of Lead I and aVF; deviates to upper right quadrant; seen in ventricular tachycardia (Fig. 5-29)

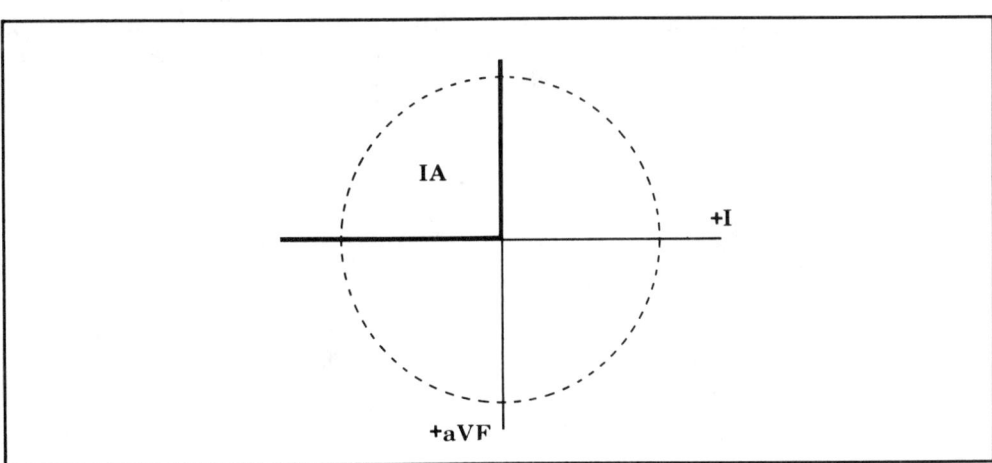

Fig. 5-29. Indeterminate axis

KEY CONCEPT: QRS complex change can give clues to axis deviations and clinical problems.

	I	II	aVF
Normal axis	⊥	⊥	⊥
Right axis	⊤	⊥	⊥
Left axis	⊥	⊤	⊤
Abnormal left axis	⊥	⊤	⊤
Indeterminate axis	⊤	⊤	⊤

Hemiblocks

Bundle branch blocks and hemiblocks are clinically significant. They may be precursors of symptomatic Mobitz II and third degree AV block. These blocks may indicate left coronary artery pathology. They are commonly associated with fibrosis of the conduction system and anterior wall myocardial infarctions.

The three fascicles that conduct stimuli to the ventricles are supplied by the left coronary artery. The left inferior posterior division is supplied by the right and left coronary artery. There are three types of fascicular blocks (hemiblocks):

Monofascicular: This type occurs in one fascicle, such as the right bundle branch, the left anterior division or fascicle, or the left posterior division or fascicle.

Bifascicular block: This type occurs in the two fascicles, such as the right bundle branch block and the left anterior division, or the right bundle branch block and left posterior division.

Trifascicular block: This type occurs in three fascicles, such as the right bundle branch block, the left anterior division and the left posterior division, causing complete heart block. This may occur intermittently or may be constant:

Intermittent—Mobitz II

Constant—complete heart block

Symptomatic second and third degree blocks are often preceded by bundle branch blocks and hemiblocks. Studies show that pathology in two of the three fascicles increases the likelihood of trifascicular block.

Right bundle branch blocks result from left coronary artery pathology. Diagnosis is made by changes in V1 and V6. EKG changes that indicate right bundle branch block are: slurring and widening of the S wave in Lead I and V6; an RSR or QR configuration in V1; the ST segment and T wave opposite in direction to the terminal QRS deflection (Fig. 5-30).

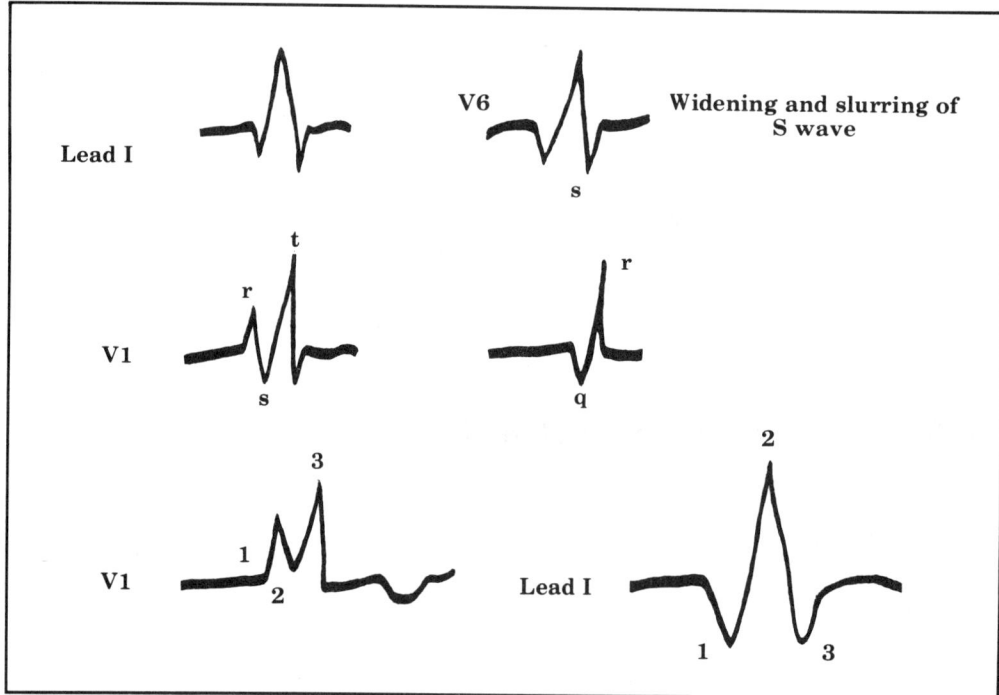

Fig. 5-30. EKG changes: right bundle branch block

Right bundle branch block patterns occur with an anterior wall myocardial infarction (AWMI) and acute pulmonary embolism. They may be transient and reverse after the acute phase.

Right bundle branch block may be diagnosed in the presence of an acute myocardial infarction. Right bundle branch block does not alter the initial deflection, but causes the development of R1 in V1 and a terminally shirred S wave in V6 (Fig. 5-31).

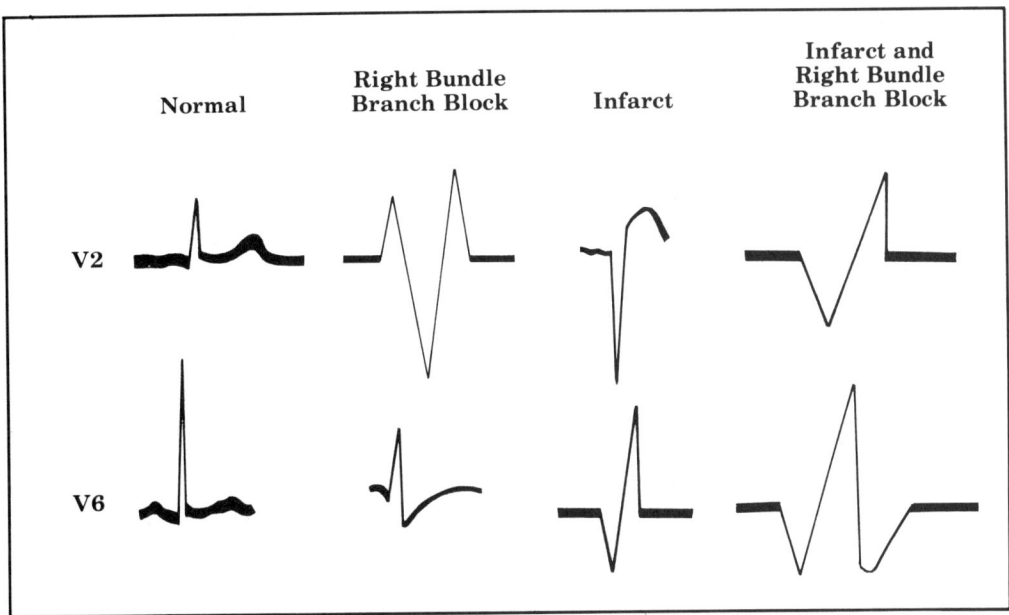

Fig. 5-31. Bundle branch block in acute MI

KEY CONCEPT: The anterior division of the left bundle is supplied by the left coronary artery. Left bundle branch blocks may be associated with anterior wall myocardial infarction and fibrosis of the conduction system. Left anterior hemiblock accompanies right bundle branch block. EKG diagnosis of left anterior hemiblock includes a positive deflection in Lead I and a negative deflection in II and aVF.

The left bundle branch arises from the bundle of His and lies next to the septum. Septal depolarization is initiated from left to right through the left bundle branch. The right and left coronary arteries supply the left bundle branch.

Left bundle branch block is diagnosed in V1 and V6, Lead I and, occasionally, aVL. The criteria for diagnosing includes: (1) QRS duration greater than .12; (2) septal depolarization from right to left instead of left to right; (3) loss of small r in V1 and small q in V6; (4) medial delay in QRS and wide and notched QRS in leads facing the left ventricle—Lead I, aVL, V5 and V6; and (5) wide and notched QS complex in leads facing the right ventricle (Fig. 5-32).

The ST segment and T wave are opposite in direction to the terminal QRS complex.

Complete left bundle branch block may be associated with valvular or coronary artery disease and hypertensive heart disease.

Left bundle block conduction defect alters the initial QRS vector and obscures normal EKG signs in the presence of an acute myocardial infarction.

Left anterior hemiblock results from blocked impulse conduction in the left anterior division of the left bundle branch. The left anterior division is the most vulnerable part of the conduction system.

Left anterior hemiblock is diagnosed by axis shift. The QRS does not widen. A left anterior hemiblock causes ALAD and is seen in Leads II, III and aVF.

During left anterior hemiblock, the left posterior division activates and causes the initial vector to be directed inferiorly and to the right. Initially, a Q wave develops in Lead I and a smaller wave occurs in aVF. Therefore, the main forces center around the blocked area. Later, a large R wave occurs in Lead I and a deep

S wave occurs in aVF and Lead II. The main vector shifts to the left and superiorly (Fig. 5-33).

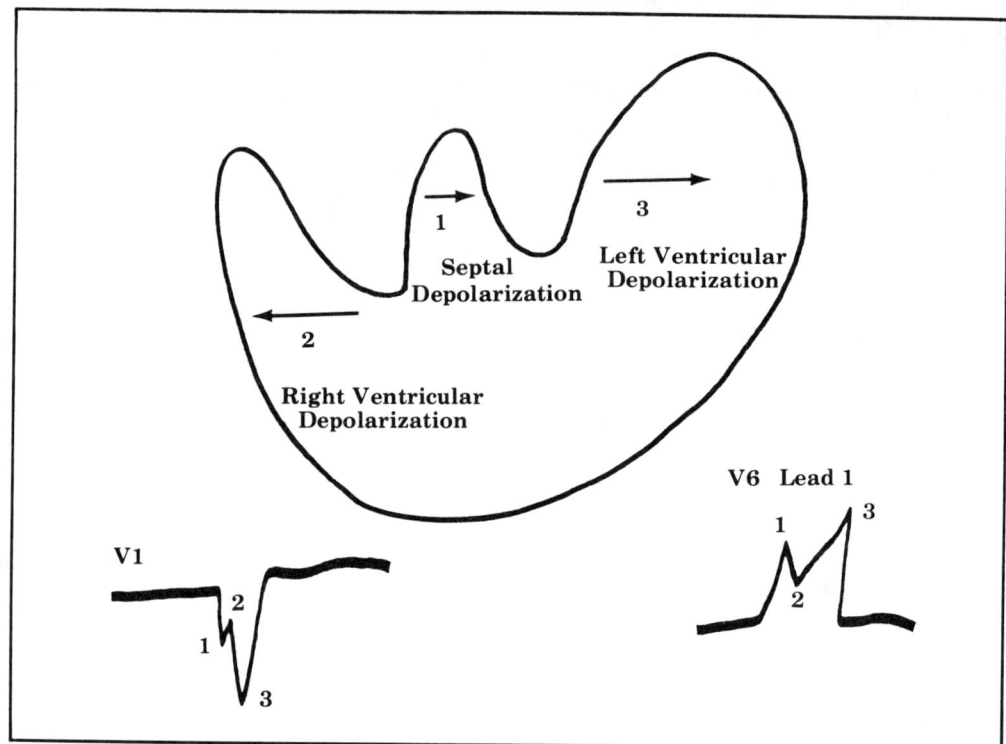

Fig. 5-32. EKG changes: left bundle branch block

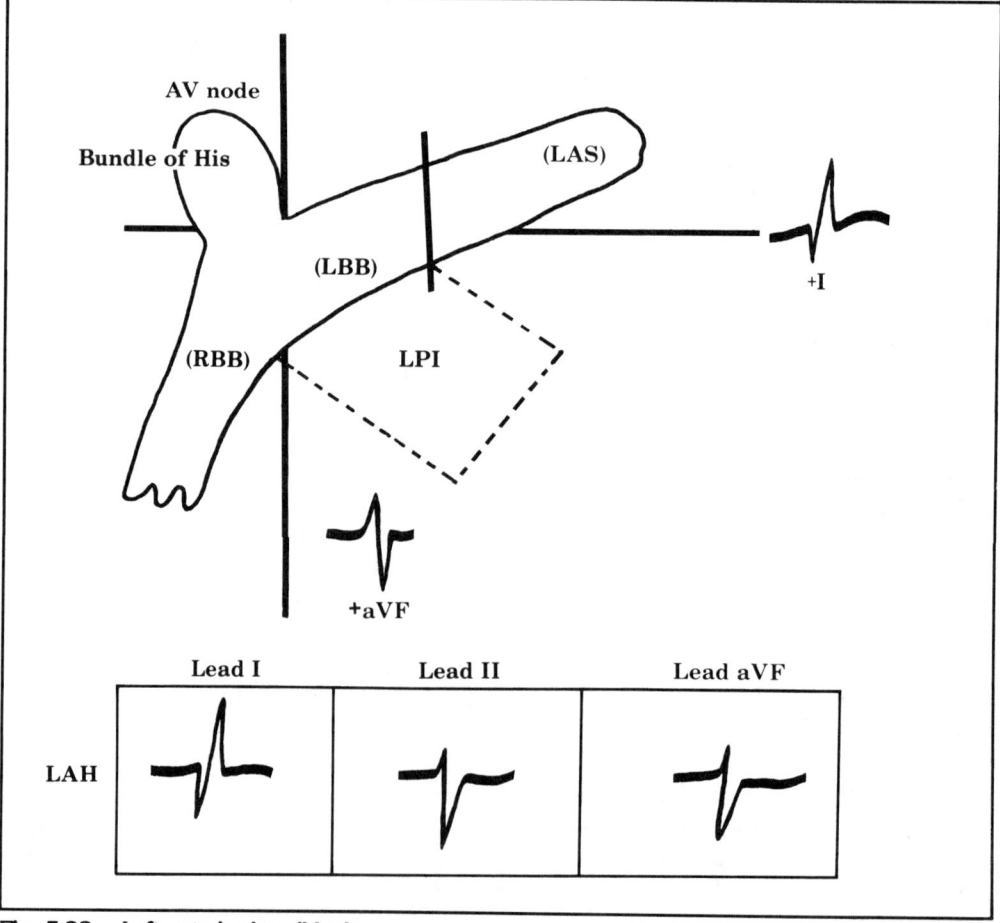

Fig. 5-33. Left anterior hemiblock

Inferior wall myocardial infarction (IWMI) may also cause LAD. Thus it is necessary to differentiate left axis deviation EKG changes of LAH from IWMI. IWMI changes include a positive deflection in Lead I and a negative deflection in Lead II and aVF. Lead II and aVF develop large Q waves which represent necrosis (Fig. 5-34).

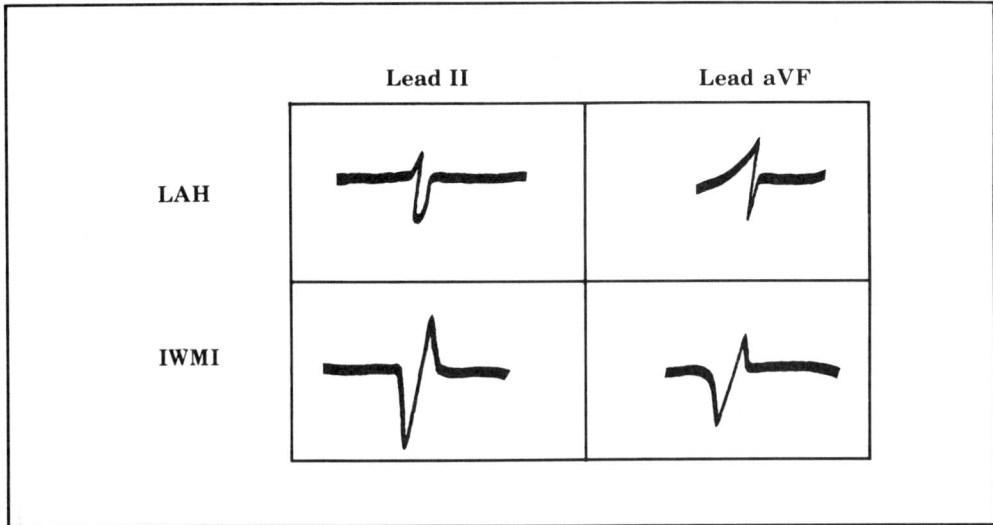

Fig. 5-34. EKG changes: LAH and IWMI

Left posterior hemiblock (LPH) occurs when the posterior division of the left bundle branch blocks. It is the least vulnerable structure. The right and left coronary artery provide blood supply to the left posterior division. Right axis deviations seen in Lead I and aVF confirm a left posterior hemiblock diagram. The QRS does not widen significantly. When a left posterior hemiblock first occurs, the vectors move superiorly and to the left. Then the main forces move inferiorly and to the right toward the blocked area. Lateral wall myocardial infarction (LWMI) may also cause right axis deviation.

In right axis deviation, Lead I is predominantly negative, and Lead II and aVF are predominantly positive. Lateral wall myocardial infarction may also cause RAD. Lead I displays a QR configuration. Lead II and aVF are positive and display a QR configuration. The large Q wave represents lateral wall necrosis (Fig. 5-35).

KEY CONCEPT: The posterior division is supplied by the right and left coronary artery. Left posterior hemiblock is usually associated with right bundle branch block. Left posterior hemiblock is suggested by right axis deviation.

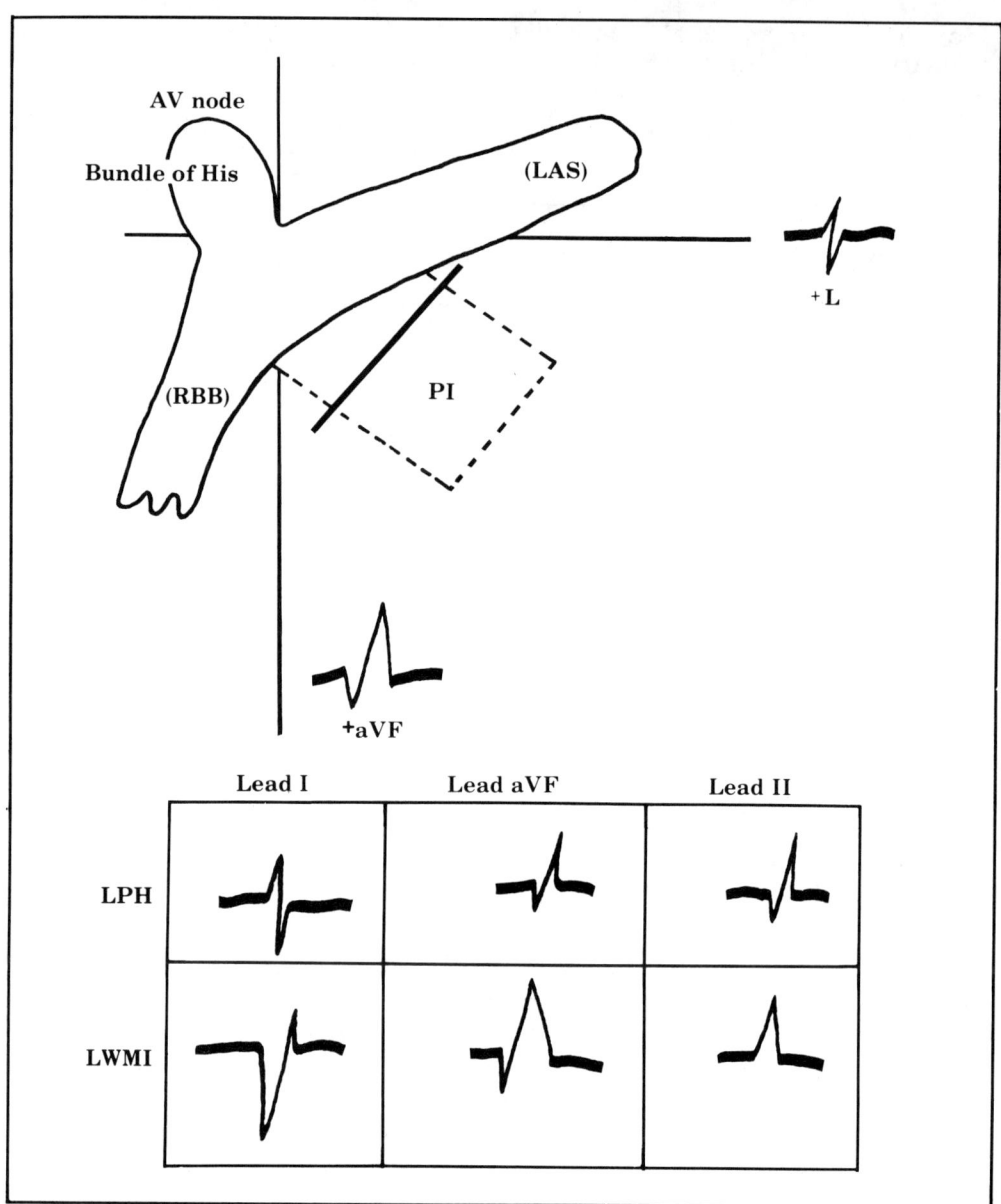

Fig. 5-35. Left posterior hemiblock

Electrolytes and EKG Changes

The following electrolyte disturbances may cause EKG changes:

Hypokalemia: prolonged P-R interval, ST depression, U waves, small T waves

Hyperkalemia: peaked T waves, small P waves, prolonged P-R interval, widened QRS

Hypocalcemia: prolonged Q-T interval

Hypercalcemia: shortened Q-T interval

Arrhythmia Methods

Arrhythmia recognition plays a vital role in the nursing assessment of the patient with cardiovascular problems. Arrhythmias may be classified by origin: *sinus rhythms, atrial rhythms, atrioventricular rhythms, AV blocks* and *ventricular rhythms.*

Rhythms originating from the sinus (SA) node are:

Normal sinus rhythm (NSR) (Fig. 5-36)

QRS:	Normal, less than .12 second duration
Rate:	60 to 100 bpm
P waves:	Normal (upright, smoothly rounded)
Conduction:	Each QRS is preceded by a P; each P is followed by one QRS.
Rhythm:	Regular
Rx:	None (This is a normal rhythm.)

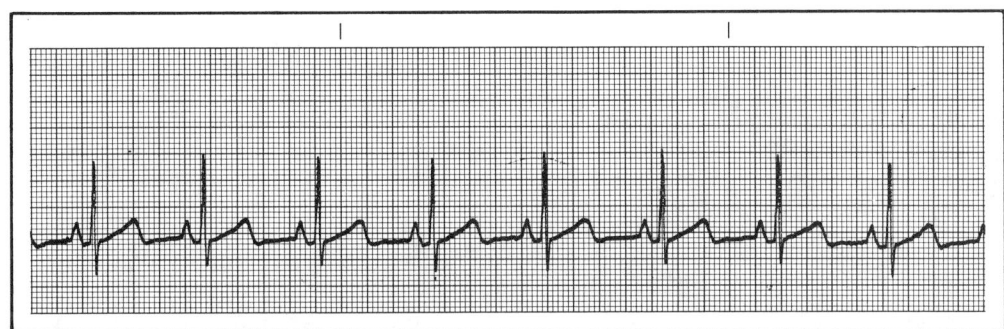

Fig. 5-36. Normal sinus rhythm

Sinus bradycardia (Fig. 5-37)
All criteria for NSR except:

Rate:	Less than 60 bpm; seldom below 45
Causes:	Common during sleep and in athletes. Drugs used to slow the conduction system may produce this rhythm.
Treatment:	In the presence of deteriorating clinical states, atropine is treatment of choice.

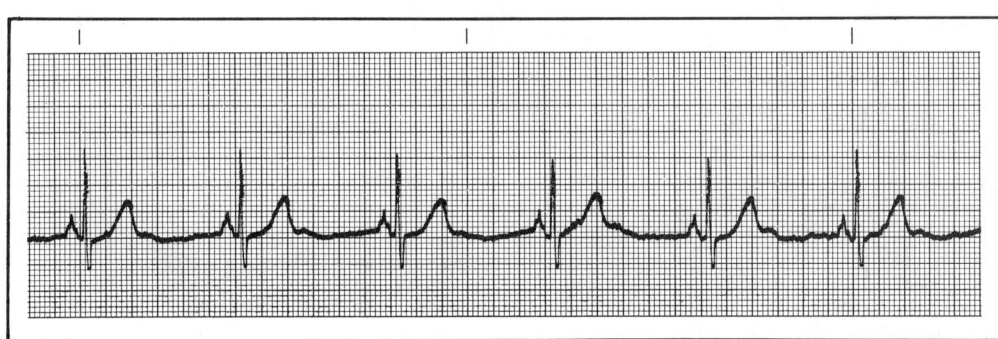

Fig. 5-37. Sinus bradycardia

Sinus tachycardia (Fig. 5-38)
All criteria for NSR except:

Rate:	Greater than 100 bpm, but not greater than 160
Cause:	Usually secondary to sympathetic stimulation; may be caused by fear, caffeine, fever, decreased C.O. or increased metabolic demand
Treatment:	Treat the underlying problem.

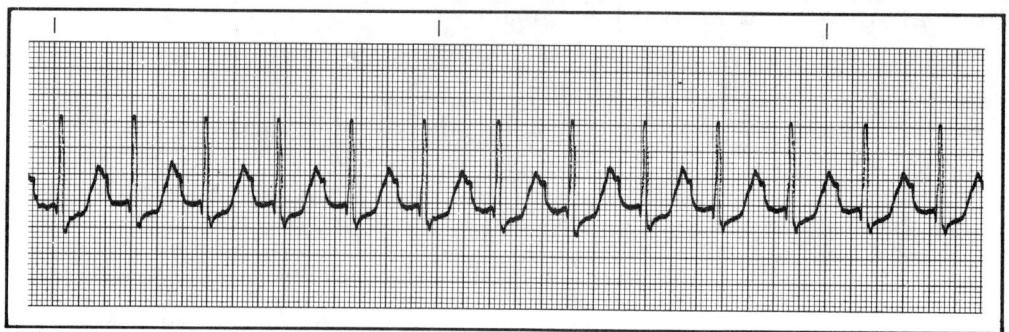

Fig. 5-38. Sinus tachycardia

Sinus arrhythmia (Fig. 5-39)

All criteria for NSR except:

Rhythm:	Regularly irregular
Cause:	Respirations are the controlling factor; rate increases on inspiration and decreases on expiration; common in children and young men
Treatment:	No treatment is needed. This is a benign rhythm that does not decrease C.O.

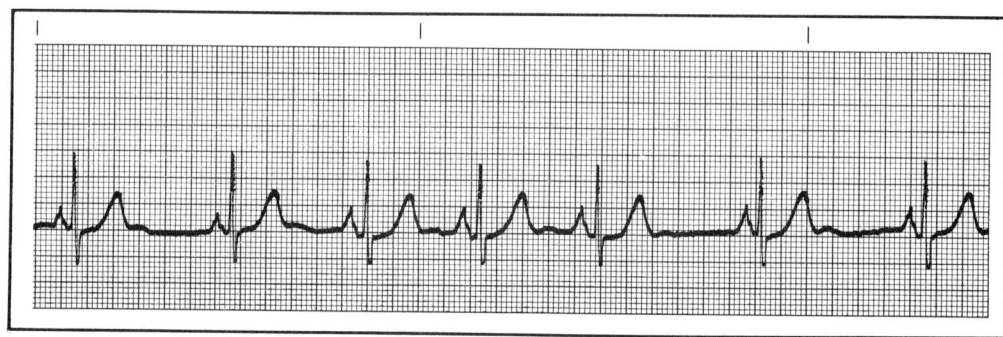

Fig. 5-39. Sinus arrhythmia

Sinus block (Fig. 5-40)

All criteria for NSR except:

Rhythm:	During a sinus rhythm, one complete P, QRS, T-cycle is dropped. There is no interruption in the timing cycle.
Cause:	Vagal stimulation; digitalis intoxication
Treatment:	If clinical symptoms are present, treat with atropine, isuprel or pacemaker.

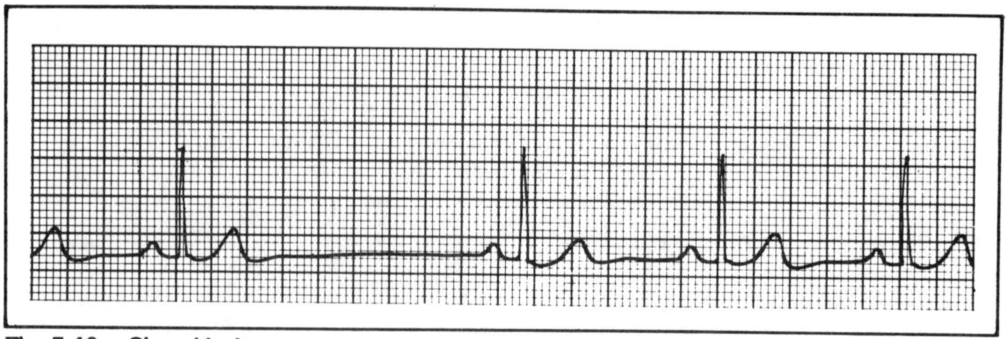

Fig. 5-40. Sinus block

Sinus arrest (Fig. 5-41)

All criteria for NSR except:

Rhythm:	During a sinus rhythm, more than one complex is dropped. The timing cycle is interrupted.
Cause:	Same as sinus block
Treatment:	Treat the same as in sinus block.
Note:	Some cardiologists classify sinus block and sinus arrest as *one* arrhythmia, referring to them collectively as *sinus arrest.*

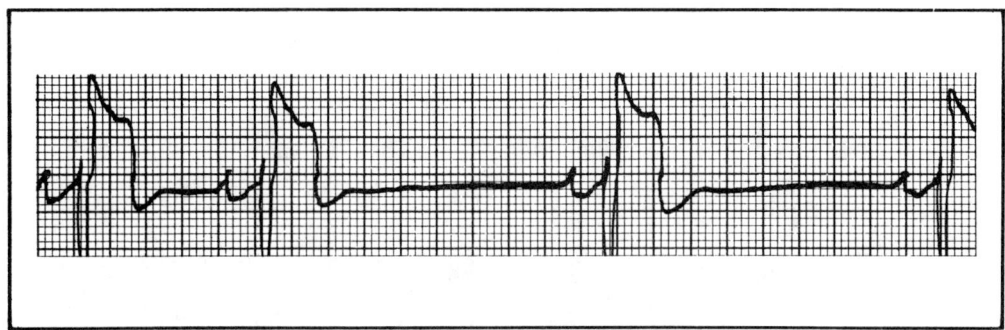

Fig. 5-41. Sinus arrest

When the atrial rate exceeds the SA node, it becomes the dominant pacemaker. Rhythms originating from the atria are:

Premature atrial contractions (PAC) (Fig. 5-42)

QRS:	Usually normal; may be conducted with abberation
Rate:	Varies
P waves:	The morphology is different from normally conducted P waves.
Conduction:	Normal QRS follows the premature P wave.
Rhythm:	Regular except for PACs
Cause:	Irritability of atrial tissue; may be warning of more serious atrial arrhythmias
Treatment:	Quinidine is the drug of choice. Mild sedation may be needed for anxiety.

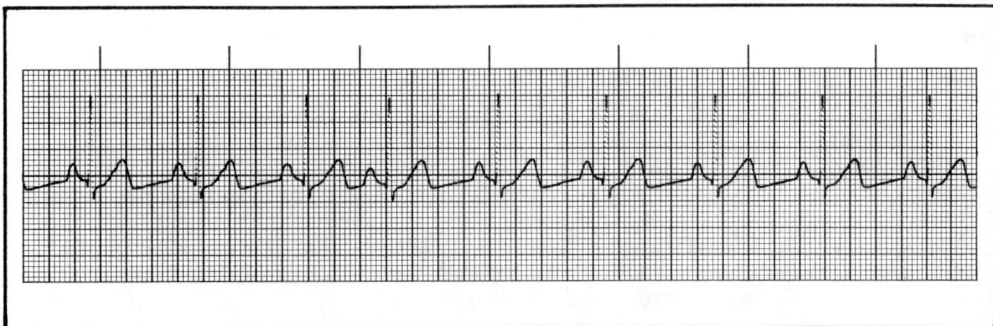

Fig. 5-42. Premature atrial contractions

PACs with block (Fig. 5-43)

QRS:	See PAC
Rate:	Varies
P waves:	See PAC
Conduction:	This is usually seen during an NSR. An ectopic focus originates from the atria, but it is *not* conducted through the AV node. Consequently, there will be a premature P wave of different morphology with no ventricular response.
Rhythm:	Regular, except for PACs
Cause:	Same as PAC
Treatment:	Same as PACs

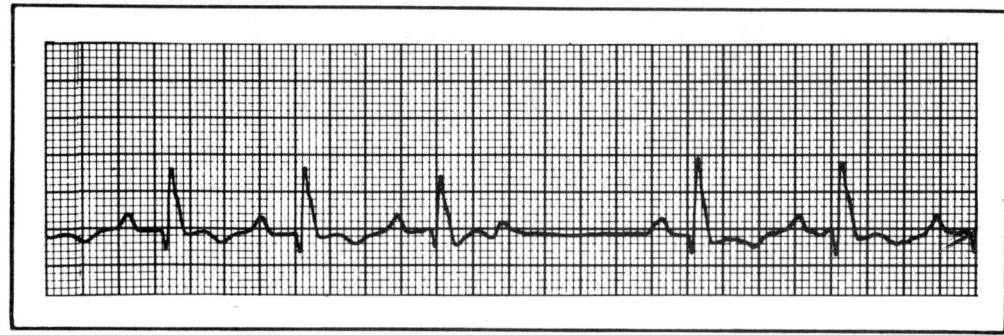

Fig. 5-43. PACs with block

Aberrant PACs

QRS:	Greater than .12 seconds when aberrantly conducted
Rate:	Varies
P waves:	Aberrant Ps have different morphology.
Conduction:	Conducted abnormally (not through the normal conduction system) through the ventricles
Rhythm:	Regular, except for PACs
Cause:	Aberrant focus originating from atria
Treatment:	Same as PACs

Paroxysmal atrial tachycardia (PAT) (Fig. 5-44)

QRS:	Normal
Rate:	Regular 150 to 250 bpm
P waves:	Usually hidden in previous T waves
Conduction:	Sudden onset of rapid atrial discharge. The atrial rate may be so rapid that some atrial impulses are blocked at the AV node.
Rhythm:	Usually regular, may continue or suddenly terminate
Cause:	Common in young adults
Treatment:	In compromised hearts, treat with vagal stimulation. A Valsalva manuever increases intrathoracic pressure and decreases venous return, which raises blood pressure and slows the pulse. Stimulating the vagal nerve may produce dangerous slowing or even cardiac arrest. Always monitor and have advanced life support equipment available.

Clinical cardioversion using conduction-depressing drugs, such as digitalis, Pronestyl and Inderal, may be used. If these fail and CHF is imminent, electrical cardioversion may be necessary.

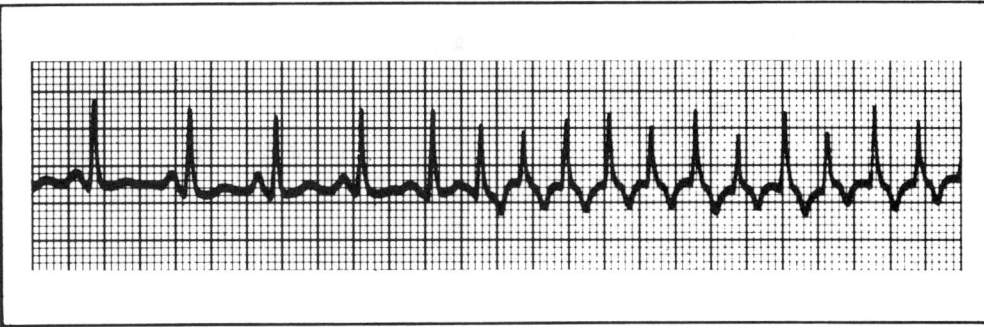

Fig. 5-44. Paroxysmal atrial tachycardia

PAT with block (Fig. 5-45)

QRS:	Normal
Rate:	Atrial—150 to 250; ventricular—slower, often half of atrial
P waves:	Conducted P waves are normal. Nonconducted P waves have a different morphology.
Conduction:	Premature beats are not conducted to the ventricles.
Rhythm:	Usually irregular
Cause:	Digitalis intoxication
Treatment:	Treat as PAT. PAT with block must be differentiated from second degree Mobitz II. Check the atrial rate. A rapid atrial rate diagnoses PAT with block.

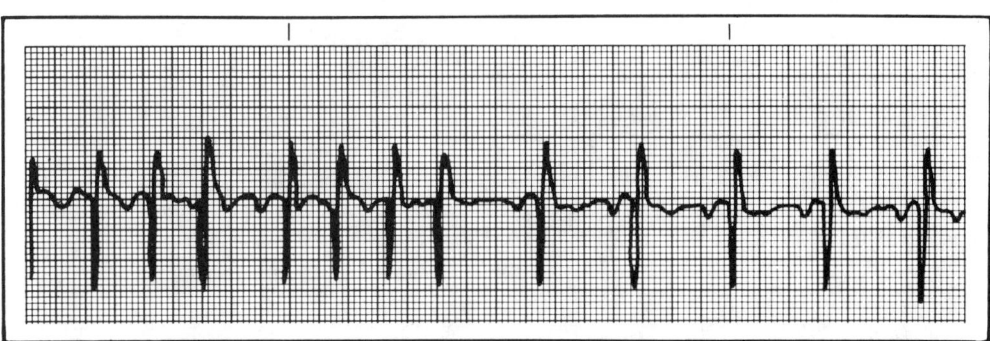

Fig. 5-45. PAT with block

Atrial flutter (Fig. 5-46)

QRS:	Normal; flutter waves may distort T wave
Rate:	Ventricular rate is 60 to 300, depending on the degree of AV block.
P waves:	Regular, sawtoothed waves, 250 to 350/min; some may be hidden in QRS
Conduction:	The AV node cannot conduct each wave. Therefore, either one out of 1, 2, 3, 4 or more of the flutter waves reaches the ventricle. This is described as 2:1, 3:1, 4:1 conduction.
Rhythm:	Regular or irregular, depending on the regularity of blocked P waves

Cause: Digitalis intoxication
Treatment: Treat with digitalis, quinidine or cardioversion in severe clinical states.

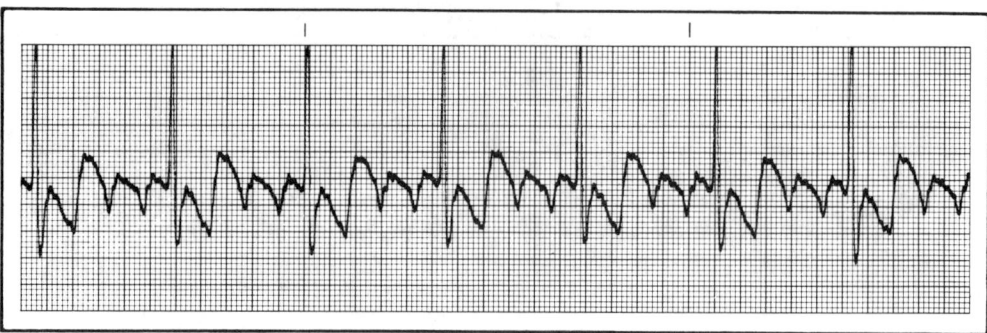

Fig. 5-46. Atrial flutter

Atrial fibrillation (AF) (Fig. 5-47)

QRS: Normal shape and duration; occurs without a preceding P wave. Therefore, the rate is irregularly irregular.
Rate: Varies according to ventricular response from very slow to very fast
P waves: No true P waves; many small, fibrillatory waves
Conduction: The conduction from the atria to the AV junction is bizarre, but becomes normal past the AV junction. There is no P-R interval.
Rhythm: Irregularly irregular
Cause: Drug-induced or chronic in mitral valve disease
Treatment: Treat with digitalis, quinidine or cardioversion, de-depending on the patient's clinical state and ventricular rate.

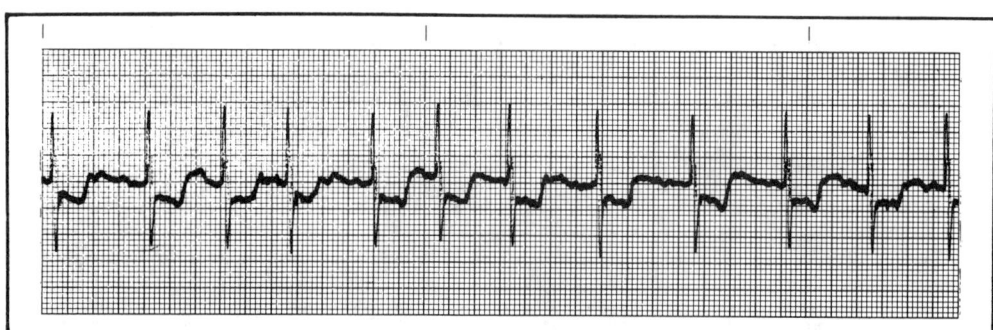

Fig. 5-47. Atrial fibrillation

Chaotic atrial rhythm

This rhythm can mimic AF. Ventricular rhythm appears irregularly irregular. Although multiple foci are present, there is one P wave for every R wave.

The AV node acts as a delay station for impulses originating in the SA node or atria. It delays the impulse briefly before conducting it to the bundle of His. The area of the AV node (junctional area) has pacemaker capabilities firing at 45 to 60 bpm.

When the AV node area (junctional area) initiates an impulse, the atria are stimulated retrogradely. This causes inverted P waves in normally positive leads. The inverted P waves occur prior to, buried within or after the QRS complex. The P wave location is dependent upon the order of atrial and ventricular stimulation.

Rhythms originating from the AV node are:

Premature junctional contraction (Fig. 5-48)

QRS:	Usually normal
Rate:	Irregular
P waves:	Normal, except for premature bests; may be upright or inverted. P waves may precede, follow or be hidden in the QRS.
Conduction:	Premature ectopic discharge occurs at the AV junction. Conduction through the ventricles is normal. Retrograde conduction occurs through the atria
Rhythm:	Regular except for PJCs
Cause:	Irritable AV nodal tissue
Treatment:	Usually no treatment is necessary. If irritability increases, treat with quinidine.

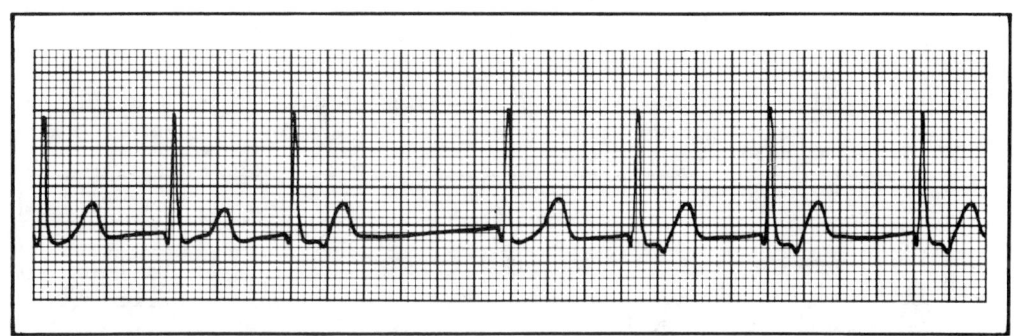

Fig. 5-48. Premature junctional contraction

AV junctional rhythm

QRS:	Usually normal
Rate:	Regular, usually 40 to 60/min.
P waves:	May be upright or inverted; closely precede (short P-R interval), follow or are hidden in the QRS
Conduction:	Normal into ventricles; retrograde into the atria.
Rhythm:	Usually regular
Cause:	Compensates for bradycardia
Treatment:	If symptomatic, treat with atropine, Isuprel or a temporary pacemaker.

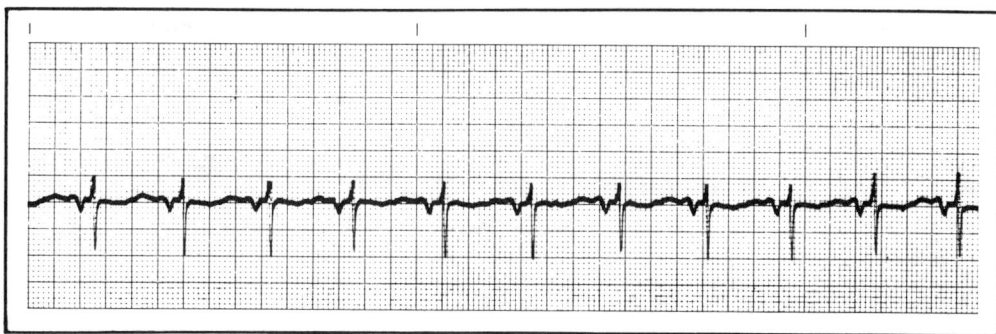

Fig. 5-49. AV junctional tachycardia

AV junctional tachycardia (Fig. 5-49)
Same as junctional rhythm except for the following:
Rate: Junctional rates of 60-120 bpm

Supraventricular tachycardia
Any tachycardia that originates above the ventricles is called supraventricular tachycardia. This term is used when it is difficult to distinguish whether the rhythm originates in the SA node, atria or AV nodal area.

Rhythms originating from AV blocks are:

First degree block (1° degree block) (Fig. 5-50)
QRS:	Usually normal
Rate:	Varies
P waves:	Normal and regular
Conduction:	The sinus impulse is delayed at the AV node, resulting in a P-R interval greater than .20 second.
Rhythm:	Regular
Cause:	Digitalis intoxication
Treatment:	Usually clinically asymptomatic and no treatment is needed

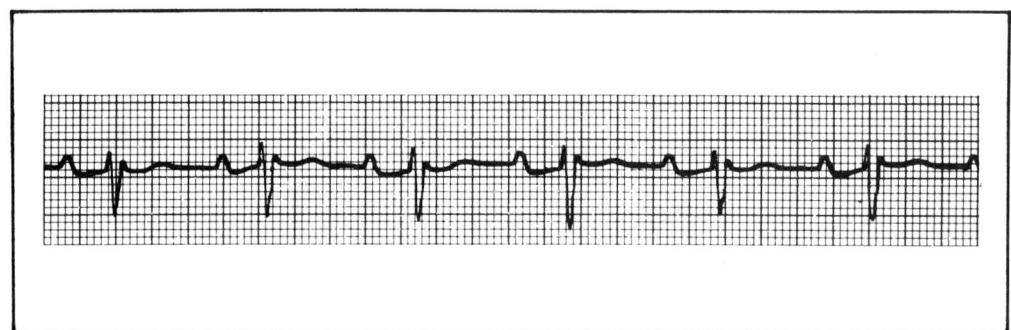

Fig. 5-50. First degree AV block

Second degree AV block
Mobitz Type I (Wenckebach) (Fig. 5-51)
QRS:	Usually normal
Rate:	Varies
P waves:	Usually normal, regular
Conduction:	A progressively prolonged impulse at the AV junction results in a gradual lengthening P-R interval until a P wave is dropped in the refractory period of the ventricle. Therefore, there is no QRS or ventricular depolarization.
Rhythm:	P-P regular; R-R irregular
Cause:	Inferior wall MI, digitalis intoxication; usually self-limiting
Treatment:	If symptomatic, treat with atropine, Isuprel or a pacemaker.

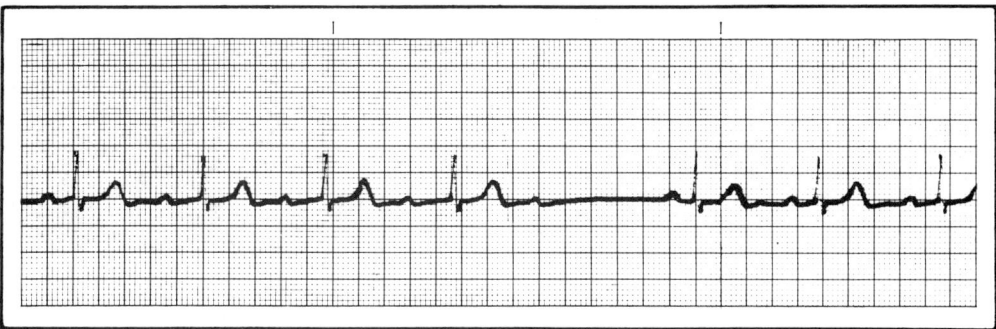

Fig. 5-51. Second degree AV block Mobitz I

Second degree AV block
Mobitz II (Fig. 5-52)

QRS:	Usually normal; may be wide
Rate:	Varies
P waves:	Usually normal and regular
Conduction:	Sudden block at or below the AV junction; P-R interval is constant for conducted beats
Rhythm:	P-P regular; R-R is regular or irregular; nonconducted QRS may occur in a cyclic pattern; 2:1 block 3:1 block
Cause:	Acute MI, digitalis intoxication
Treatment:	May progress to complete heart block. If symptomatic, treat with atropine, Isuprel or pacemaker.

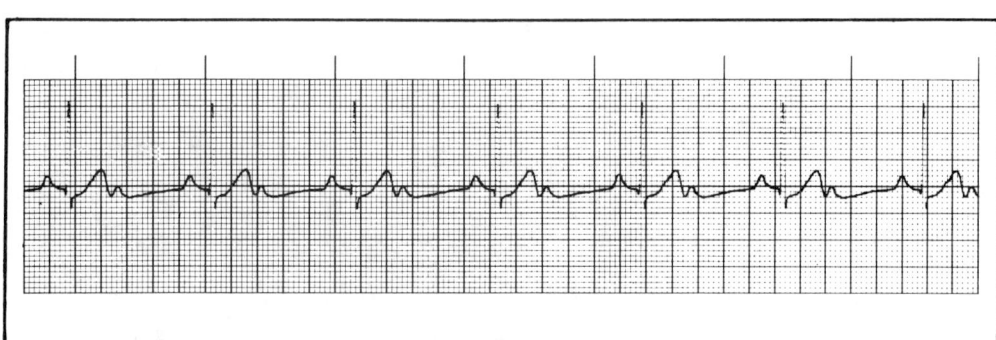

Fig. 5-52. Second degree AV block Mobitz II

Third degree AV block (complete heart block) (Fig. 5-53)

QRS:	Normal or wide
Rate:	Usually regular
P waves:	Usually normal and regular
Conduction:	Atrial impulses are completely blocked at the AV junction or below. The ventricles are paced independently of the atria by an ectopic focus in the AV junction or Purkinje's cells. The P-R interval varies.
Rhythm:	P-P regular, R-R regular. The P waves and R waves are completely independent of one another.
Cause:	MI, inflammation or fibrosis in the conduction system; digitalis intoxication
Treatment:	Treat with atropine and Isuprel. If symptoms persist, treat with a pacemaker.

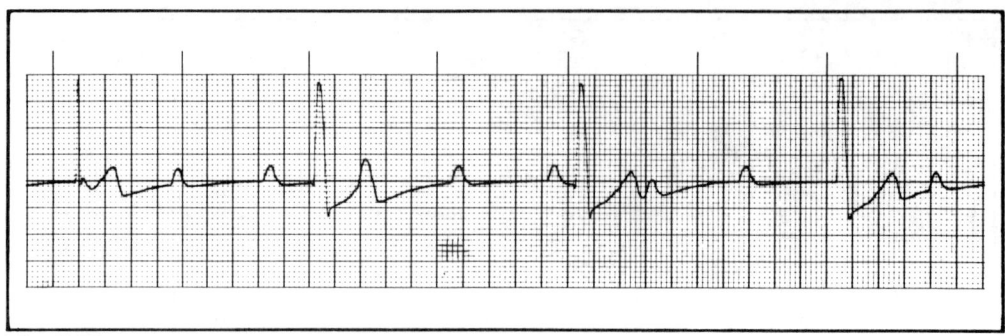

Fig. 5-53. Third degree AV block

Ventricular rhythms require quick, accurate assessment and intervention to avoid serious complications and death.

Rhythms originating from the ventricles are:

Idioventricular (Fig. 5-54)

QRS:	Wide, bizarre, different from normal QRS
Rate:	20 to 60/min.; may increase to 60 to 100; called accelerated idioventricular rhythm
P waves:	Absent or not related
Conduction:	The stimulus occurs from an ectopic focus in ventricles.
Rhythm:	Regular
Cause:	Compensatory rhythm for an extreme bradycardia
Treatment:	If symptomatic, treat with atropine, Isuprel or pacemaker. Try to maintain a rhythm.

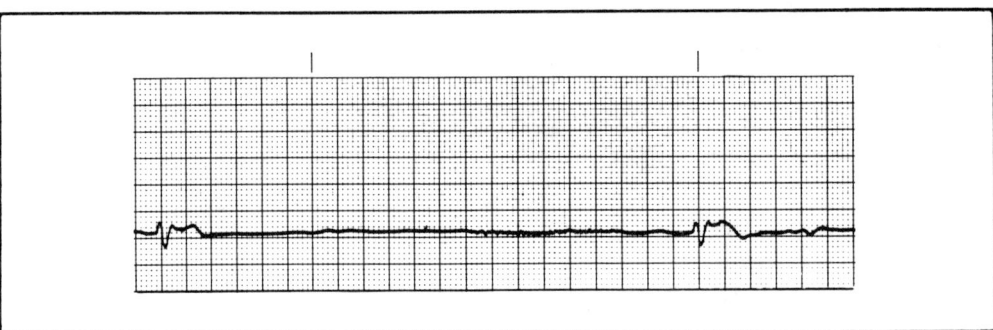

Fig. 5-54. Idioventricular

Premature ventricular contraction (PVC) (Fig. 5-55)

QRS:	Wide, bizarre and different than normal QRS; duration usually beyond .12 second; T wave is usually opposite the deflection of the QRS
Rate:	Varies
P waves:	Absent, may be hidden in QRS
Conduction:	No conduction between atrium and ventricle
Rhythm:	Irregular—A full compensatory pause is usually observed after a PVC. A compensatory pause means the time between the beat preceding and the beat subsequent to the PVC equals two R-R cycles.

Types of PVCs:

Unifocal PVC: Originates from one focus; all look alike on the rhythm strip

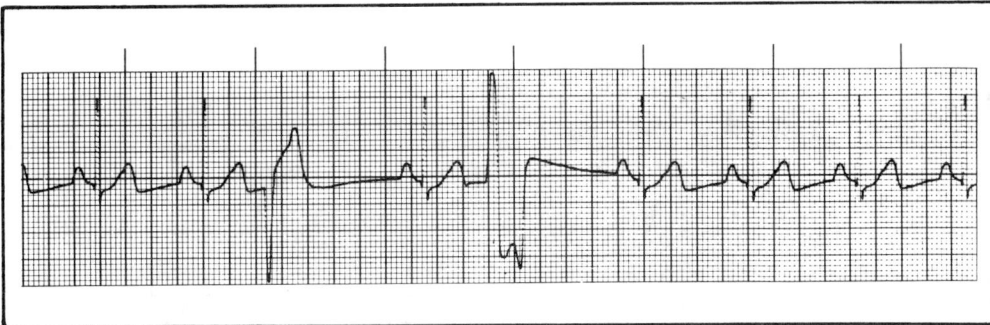

Fig. 5-55. Premature ventricular contraction

Multifocal PVC: Originates from more than one focus; all look different on the rhythm strip

Malignant PVC: Occurs close to or on the T wave (R on T phenomenon); likely to initiate ventricular fibrillation

Ventricular bigeminy: Occurs with every other beat

Ventricular trigeminy: Occurs with every third beat

Ventricular Quadrageminy: Occurs with every fourth beat

Note: Bigeminy, trigeminy and quadrageminy refer to frequency. Always state whether it is atrial or ventricular.

Interpolated PVC: Occurs between normal beats—Normal rhythm is not interrupted; no compensatory pause exists.

Salvo of PVCs: More than two PVCs in a row; burst of ventricular tachycardia.

Causes: Fatigue, caffeine, alcohol, anxiety; irritability caused by heart disease is more serious.

Treatment: Treatment is indicated for the following:

More than six per minute

Coupled or salvo PVCs

Multifocal

Ventricular bigeminy

Ventricular trigeminy

Malignant—R on T

Treatment of choice is lidocaine:

100mg I.V. push followed by an I.V. drip of 1 to 2 gm in 250 to 500 D₅W titrated to control PVCs (14 mg/min.).

Pronestyl is used if the patient is allergic to lidocaine or if the condition warrants its use. If PVCs occur with bradycardia, they are compensatory in nature and should not be eliminated with lidocaine. Treat with atropine or a pacemaker to increase the heart rate.

Ventricular trachycardia (Fig. 5-56)

QRS: Run of PVCs

Rate: Usually between 140 to 300/min.

P waves: Buried within the QRS complex

Conduction: An ectopic focus stimulates the ventricles independently of the atria.

Rhythm: Regular
Causes: Damage from MI, electrical shock
Treatment: If the patient is conscious, treat with Xylocaine (lidocaine), O₂, Dilantin. If the patient is unconscious, treat with cardioversion and Xylocaine.

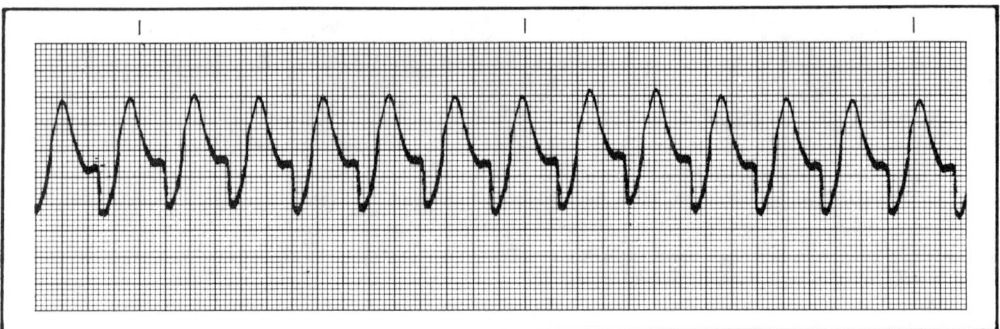

Fig. 5-56. Ventricular tachycardia

Ventricular fibrillation (Fig. 5-57)

QRS: None
Rate: None
P waves: None
Conduction: None
Rhythm: Chaotic; no effective ventricular conduction; rapid, chaotic twitching or waves originating in ventricles; bizarre morphology
Causes: MI, electrical shock
Treatment: Treat with CPR, defibrillation and drug therapy per ACLS standards.

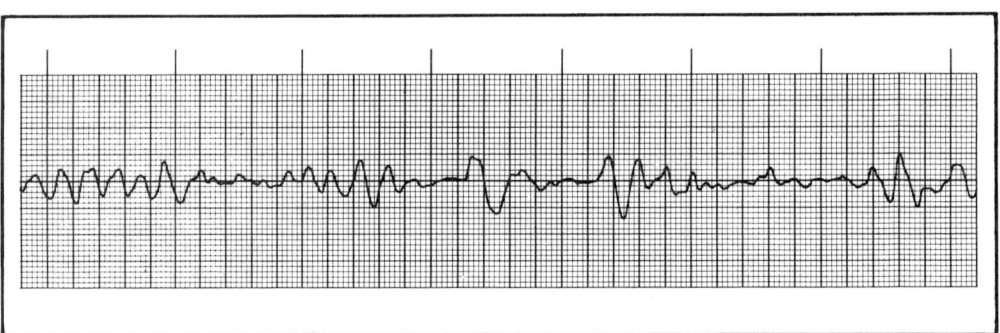

Fig. 5-57. Ventricular fibrillation

Common Methods for Rate Determination

In *regular* rhythms, calculate the ventricular rate by finding an R wave that falls on a heavy dark line. Use this as a reference point. The next R wave determines the rate. Each block line after the reference point has a given value: 300, 150, 100, 75, 60, 50, 43, 37, 33 (**Fig. 5-58**)

In *regular* or *irregular* rhythms, the six-second method is the easiest to use. EKG paper is divided along the border into three sectioned segments. Two segments equal six seconds. Count the number of complexes within the six seconds and multiply by 10.

6 seconds x 10 = 60 seconds

Number of QRS complexes x 10 = heart rate/min.

10 complexes x 10 = 100 bpm

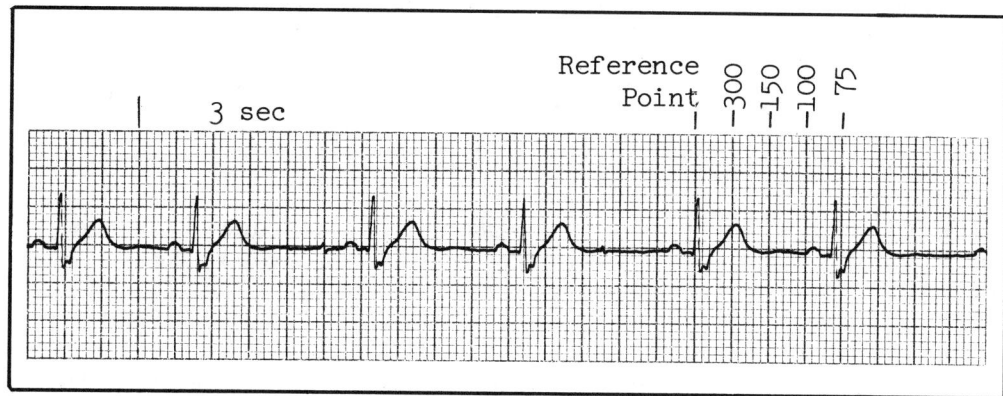

Fig. 5-58. Determining rate when rhythm is regular

It should be noted that this method only "ballparks" the rate. However, the patient's clinical response to the rate is more important than whether the rate is 130 or 140.

Rate rulers are a common aid. They are an accurate way to measure rate, but it is best to know the basics in case the ruler is not available.

KEY CONCEPT: Rhythm interpretation is an essential part of the nursing assessment. Note clinical symptoms in respect to rhythm interpretation. Use the following guide for interpreting rhythms.

- Check QRS complex
- Check P wave
- Check PR interval
- Check rate
- Check rhythm

Invasive Assessment Methods

Invasive methods are used to confirm, evaluate, assess, measure and provide valuable information regarding the heart and its activities.

Cardiac Catheterization

Cardiac catheterization is performed to determine heart function, coronary artery patency and to obtain blood samples and pressure readings. Radiographic studies evaluate the heart chambers and the pulmonary arterial circulation.

Swan-Ganz insertion allows direct measure of the right heart pressures, pulmonary artery pressure and pulmonary capillary wedge pressure. Measurement of these pressures helps diagnose right and left heart failures, pulmonary hypertension, valvular abnormalities, intracardiac shunting, intrapulmonary shunting and cardiac output. The pulmonary artery (PA) pressures of the left heart are:

Systolic PA: Right ventricular pressure: 20 to 30 mm Hg

Diastolic PA: Diastolic PA pressure usually equals LVEDP, therefore giving an indirect measurement of left ventricular function. Pressure is usually less than 10 mm Hg.

PA mean: An average of the PA systolic and PA diastolic—The mean is usually less than 20 mm Hg.

Pulmonary catheter wedge pressure: The pressure obtained by wedging the inflated balloon in a small branch of the PA—Wedge pressure equals left atrial pressure and left ventricular end diastolic pressure, except in mitral stenosis (4 to 12 mm Hg).

Changes in pressures may indicate complications or may be used in differentiating types of shock: hypovolemic, cardiogenic and sepsis.

His bundle electrocardiography determines electrical activity of the AV conducting system, such as AV junction, bundle of His and bundle branches.

Intracardiac phonocardiography detects murmurs and sounds associated with heart disease.

Coronary arteriography determines the extent of coronary artery disease and locates areas of infarction.

Ventriculography determines ventricular function by measuring end diastolic volume, end systolic volume, stroke volume and ejection fraction.

Aortography determines the size of the aortic lumen and aortic valve, and detects coarctation of the aorta.

KEY CONCEPT: Nursing assessment of the patient with a cardiovascular disorder includes taking an accurate history and evaluating level of consciousness, heart sounds, vital signs, laboratory studies, the electrocardiogram and diagnostic studies.

KEY POINT RECOGNITION

Write true or false by each statement. Answers are at the end of this chapter. A score below 80% indicates the need for further study.

1. _____ S_1 is heard at the beginning of ventricular systole.
2. _____ S_1 follows the carotid pulse.
3. _____ S_2 occurs at the end of systole.
4. _____ S_2 is low-pitched and longer than S_1.
5. _____ A constant splitting of S_1 and S_2 during inspiration and expiration may indicate septal defects.
6. _____ S_3 is a normal ventricular gallop sound.
7. _____ The presence of S_3 is an early sign of congestive heart failure.
8. _____ Anemia, hyperthyroidism, ventricular-septal defects or left-to-right shunts may cause an S_3.
9. _____ S_4 is a normal atrial gallop sound.
10. _____ Aortic or pulmonic stenosis causes an S_4.
11. _____ A summation gallop indicates advanced heart failure.
12. _____ Heart murmurs are heard over the auscultatory area of their origin.
13. _____ Enzymes help diagnose myocardial infarction.
14. _____ CPK, LDH, HBD, and SGOT are cardiac enzymes.
15. _____ CPK-MB and LDH_1 and LDH_2 are isoenzymes specific to certain muscle tissue.
16. _____ Prothrombin time determines anticoagulation with oral anticoagulants.
17. _____ Normal partial prothrombin time is four to six times the normal clotting time.
18. _____ Mild proteinuria may indicate congestive heart failure.
19. _____ Echocardiography is the recording of ultrasound vibrations.
20. _____ Apexcardiography determines the electrical forces of the heart.
21. _____ An electrocardiogram represents the mechanical activity of the heart.
22. _____ Regurgitant murmurs are high-pitched and are heard best using the diaphragm of the stethoscope.
23. _____ Bedside monitors are used only for diagnosis.
24. _____ A four-lead system usually adds the right leg, which has a positive polarity.
25. _____ A five-lead system adds the chest lead, which has a positive polarity.
26. _____ The P wave represents atrial depolarization.
27. _____ Normal P-R interval is .04 to .12 second.
28. _____ A Q wave is a positive deflection.

_____29. An abnormal Q wave indicates a myocardial infarction and conduction defects.
_____30. Normal ST segment time is .32 second.
_____31. Prolonged ST segment indicates hypercalcemia.
_____32. T waves represent ventricular repolarization.
_____33. A QT segment represents electrical asystole.
_____34. A U wave represents repolarization of the Purkinje's fibers.
_____35. A prominent positive U wave indicates hypokalemia, thyrotoxicosis, bradycardia and exercise.
_____36. Myocardial infarction, coronary insufficiency and left ventricular hypertrophy may cause a negative U wave.
_____37. The physiological pacemaker of the heart is the AV node.
_____38. Normal sinus rhythm has a regular R-R interval and P-R interval greater than .20 second.
_____39. In sinus arrhythmias, respirations cause the irregular rhythm.
_____40. An atrial ectopic focus causes a premature atrial contraction.
_____41. Premature atrial contraction with block is characterized by a P wave with different morphology and followed by a ventricular response.
_____42. Paroxysmal atrial tachycardia increases the heart rate and decreases the demand for oxygen.
_____43. In atrial fibrillation, the rhythm is usually irregularly irregular.
_____44. Digitalis intoxication may cause paroxysmal atrial tachycardia with block.
_____45. Atrial flutter always produces a regular ventricular rhythm.
_____46. Mobitz I is a regular rhythm.
_____47. In Mobitz II, all beats conduct through the AV node.
_____48. Premature ventricular contractions may be benign or malignant.
_____49. Interpolated premature ventricular contractions do not interrupt the cycle or rhythm.
_____50. The clinical result of ventricular tachycardia is an unconscious patient with no cardiac output.
_____51. Hypokalemia may produce a depressed ST segment.
_____52. Hyperkalemia may produce a prolonged P-R interval and a widened QRS.
_____53. Normal systolic pulmonary artery pressure is 50 to 60 mm Hg mercury.

PATHOLOGICAL STATES AND NURSING MANAGEMENT

ARTERIOSCLEROSIS

Pathophysiology

Arteriosclerosis is a chronic thickening and hardening of the walls of the arteries. A major effect is loss of elasticity. Arteriosclerosis is divided into three types: ***atherosclerosis, medial sclerosis*** and ***arteriolar sclerosis.***

In ***atherosclerosis,*** the inner muscle layer (tunica intima) becomes thickened, resulting in an obstruction or partial obstruction of the lumen. The aorta, cerebral and coronary blood vessels are usually involved.

In ***medial sclerosis,*** the middle layer of the artery (tunica media) becomes calcified and hypertrophies, causing narrowing of the lumen.

Arteriolar sclerosis occludes mainly smaller arteries because of hypertrophy of the tunica intima and tunica media.

Precipitating factors of arteriosclerosis include heredity, arterial hypertension, diabetes mellitus in persons over the age of 55, women in menopause, race

(Caucasian), competitive personality, smoking, obesity, aggressive behavior, sedentary lifestyle, elevated blood lipids and gout.

Clinical Presentation

The clinical presentation is extremely variable and dependent on the degree of sclerotic involvement. Angina pectoris, ischemic heart disease, myocardial infarction, congestive heart failure and death can result from arteriosclerosis. The most common preceding symptom of arteriosclerosis is pain. Elevated blood pressure, cyanosis, dyspnea, intermittent claudication, diaphoresis, weakness, reduced or absent pulses, and coolness of the skin may be present.

Diagnostic Data

Arteriography or angiography are excellent diagnostic aids used to visualize the involved vasculature. A complete history and physical will aid in determining the extent of pathology. Electrocardiographic and laboratory studies are valuable in determining the overall patient condition and providing baseline guides to involvement of the disease process.

Nursing Care

(1) Provide warmth of extremities.
(2) Administer vasodilating drugs and antihypertensive agents.
(3) Provide exercise to maintain circulation and prevent embolic formation.
(4) Prevent infection and shock.
(5) Avoid unnecessary injury.
(6) Educate the patient and family about the precipitating factors of arteriosclerosis and the need to modify lifestyle.

KEY CONCEPT: Nursing care involves teaching the patient to understand the disease process, encouraging the patient and family to live within the established limitations of the illness, and carrying out medical instructions in an effort to control the disease.

ANGINA PECTORIS

Pathophysiology

Angina pectoris is usually caused by several etiologic factors: atherosclerosis, hypertension, aortic valvular disease, anemia, shock and thyrotoxicosis. In angina, the decrease blood flow causes decreased oxygen to the myocardial tissue. The resulting ischemia leads to chest pain. Since enough oxygen is received to maintain tissue life, the functional ability of the ischemic cell is not permanently lost.

Precipitating factors of angina are increased physical activity, emotional stress, overeating, smoking and lying flat. A change in position from sitting to lying decreases cardiac output and coronary perfusion, and leads to angina.

Clinical Presentation

The patient with angina complains of chest pain. The description of the pain varies and depends on the individual. Pain may locate over the precordium, middle or lower sternal areas, or retrosternally. It often radiates to the shoulders, arms, neck, jaw and epigastrium. Burning, squeezing, an aching pressure on the chest and a smothering feeling are typical descriptions associated with the pain. There are different types of angina. Preinfarction or **unstable angina** is not a common indicator for infarction. **Crescendo angina** occurs at rest or during sleep. The pain may be of different duration, or may radiate or worsen over a period of days. An increased need for nitroglycerin is needed to relieve the pain. If allowed to progress, myocardial infarction occurs. **Angina decubitus** occurs during sleep. This indicates the patient's need for additional rest. It offers a great potential for sudden death, probably due to ventricular fibrillation. **Prinzmetal's** or **variant angina** is a spasm of the large coronary arteries. The introduction of a catheter, coldness or drugs precipitates Prinzmetal's angina. It occurs with arrhythmias causing conduction defects and ST segment depression. The patient may have a history of previous myocardial infarction.

Diagnostic Data

History and physical may reveal angina. History alone may not be sufficient to diagnose angina. The patient presents with chest pain. An electrocardiogram definitely diagnoses angina if taken during the episode of pain. A positive stress test enables the physician to begin treatment. Coronary angiograms may confirm the presence of coronary arteriosclerosis.

Nursing Care

(1) Prevent pain-inducing activity.

(2) Prevent complications or further extension.

(3) Avoid emotional and physical stress.

(4) Provide bedrest and a quiet environment.

(5) Use nitroglycerine, long-term nitrates or propranolol to manage pain.

KEY CONCEPT: Management of angina is aimed at providing relief by restoring the oxygen supply and demand balance and reducing the frequency of episodes.

MYOCARDIAL INFARCTION
Pathophysiology

Myocardial infarction is the complete occlusion of an artery with resultant myocardial death. The most common cause of a myocardial infarction is arteriosclerosis. Emboli, trauma and complications of collagen disease are less common causes.

Infarctions are classified according to the amount of myocardium involved. *Transmural* involves the full thickness of the myocardial wall. *Subendocardial* involves the inner thickness of the myocardium. Infarctions are also classified according to the location of the infarction on the ventricular wall: *anterior, posterior, inferior, lateral* and *septal.*

Clinical Presentation

The patient with a myocardial infarction generally complains of pain in the back, chest, epigastrium, arms, neck, jaw or even the teeth. The pain usually lasts longer than thirty minutes and is unrelieved by rest, oxygen or nitrates. Nausea, vomiting, dyspnea, orthopnea, anxiety, diaphoresis, rales, cyanosis, dysrhythmias and weakness may also be present. A narcotic is generally indicated for relief of pain.

Diagnostic Data

History and physical may reveal myocardial infarction. The patient complains of chest pain. Physical examination reveals a variety of the above mentioned signs. Laboratory studies show an increase in the serum sedimentation rate, leukocyte count and enzymes. History, enzymes and electrocardiographic changes definitively diagnose an MI.

Enzyme elevation begins within two to five hours after onset and may not return to normal for up to three weeks. The enzymes include CPK, SGOT, LDH, HBD, CPK-MB and LHD-1. The CPK is the first enzyme to elevate.

Ischemia, injury and infarction may be seen on the electrocardiogram (Fig. 5-59). Rarely, the electrocardiogram is the only evidence that a myocardial infarction has occurred. ST and T wave changes may not specifically diagnose a myocardial infarction since medication, ischemia and electrolyte levels may cause the changes.

Abnormal Q waves or altered R wave voltage and morphology are diagnostic. T wave abnormalities may be delayed two to ten days following an infarction. There are "silent" areas in the left ventricles that include the endocardium papillary muscles, septum, the right ventricle and atria, and the back of the left ventricle. Silent areas may reveal little or no electrocardiographic change or significant damage. In a patient with a previous myocardial infarction, diagnosis by electrocardiogram may be very difficult, if not impossible. T wave inversion may not appear for 24 hours, but may persist for years. ST segment

Pattern		Tracing	Leads	Return to Normal
Normal				
Ischemia-reversible	ST depression T wave inversion		1, aVL, aVF V 4-6	Within minutes or hours
Injury-reversible	ST elevation T elevation		Varies	Returns to isolectric line after a few days
Infarction	Abnormal Q wave Wider than 0.04 or 25% of R wave ST segment elevated over in- farcted region ST depression in reciprical leads T wave changes later ST elevation leads to T wave inversion ST depression T waves become tall and symmetrical		Varies according to infarction	T wave changes may return to normal or remain inverted

Fig. 5-59. MI: EKG injury patterns

elevation appears immediately and may remain elevated from half a day to 14 days. If the elevation persists, the possibility of a ventricular aneurysm should be considered. As the ST segment finally returns to the baseline, the T wave inversion deepens. A deep, wide Q wave may be present and an R wave may be absent indefinitely in some leads (Fig. 5-60)

Area of Infarction	Electrocardiographic Findings
Anteroseptal MI	Usually persistent QS, the usual progression increase in voltage of the R wave will be absent from V, through V3 or V4.
Anterolateral MI	Mainly localized to the anterolateral portion of the left ventricle; the greatest EKG changes will be present in leads I, aVL, V5 and V6; reciprocal changes may be noted in aVR.
Inferior (diaphragmatic) MI	Most changes are in limb leads. Minimal changes may appear in (V1 to V6). Abnormal Q waves are seen in II, III and aVF. A prominent R wave is seen in 1 and aVL.
Inferoposterior MI	Q wave in II, III and aVF, and prominent R waves in I and aVL; in V1 through V4 a tall R and upright T is noted. The usual R/S ratio is reversed.
Posterior MI	If small infarct, little or no EKG changes. If a large area is involved, a tall R and upright T waves are seen in V1-V4, with a small R in V6. A Q wave may or may not be present and the T wave inversion is noted in V5 and V6. In II, III and aVF little or no changes noted.
Inferolateral MI	May produce changes characteristic of anterolateral and inferior infarctions. The greatest change will be noted in II, III and aVF. There may be only T wave inversions and possibly abnormalities in V5 and V6.

Fig. 5-60. EKG: area of infarction

Nursing Care

Complications are the most common cause of severe morbidity and death. Dysrhythmias often occur immediately following the myocardial infarction. The first two hours postinfarction may result in life-threatening dysrhythmias. Other serious complications include congestive heart failure, pulmonary edema, cardiogenic shock, conduction defects, thromboembolism, mitral insufficiency, pericarditis, ventricular aneurysm and ventricular rupture (Fig. 5-61).

Arrhythmias	Approximately 90% of all patients with acute MI will have some degree of disruptive rhythm. The cause should be corrected as soon as possible. Some potential causes are: hypotension, hypoxia, increased automaticity.
Cardiogenic shock	As the left ventricle fails, the mortality rate increases. Approximately 90% will die.
Pulmonary edema	In the presence of MI, approximately 65% will die within 2-3 years.
Persistent pain	Implies persistent ischemia around the infarcted muscle; usually 2 or 3 coronary arteries will be involved. Prognosis is poor. This pain should be treated aggresively with sedation.
Conduction defects	Prophylactic cardiac pacing has greatly reduced the incidence of complete heart block and sudden death. Evidence reveals involvement of the left anterior descending coronary artery in loss of two or three main conduction fascicles, right bundle and/or left anterior posterior bundle.
Thromboemboli	Predisposition to venous thrombosis with resultant pulmonary emboli includes bedridden patients, CHF and ventricular aneurysm. Anticoagulants will not reduce or prevent an infarction but may reduce the formation of emboli.
Ventricular aneurysm	Is a gradually ballooning in the fibrotic ventricular wall; stroke volume is reduced as a result of inferior contractions. Thrombi may form because of the stasis of blood.

Fig. 5-61. MI: complications

For proper nursing care:
(1) Manage airway, oxygenation and circulation using advanced cardiac life-support guidelines.
(2) Prevent complications by cardiac monitoring and early recognition of dysrhythmias.
(3) Provide complete bedrest and a quiet environment.
(4) Provide pain relief by administering intravenous narcotics (morphine SO_4 is usually the drug of choice).
(5) Limit sodium intake to avoid fluid retention.
(6) Eliminate bowel straining and administer stool softeners or gentle laxatives.
(7) Prevent venous stasis by providing range of motion exercises and an antiembolic stocking.
(8) Maintain fluid and electrolyte balance by measuring intake and output, and by recording daily weights.
(9) Monitor hemodynamic lines. The data provide valuable information in a relatively short period of time, leading to better assessment and nursing intervention.

KEY CONCEPT: The complications following myocardial infarction account for the high mortality rate of MIs. Early recognition, treatment and intervention are essential for survival.

CONGESTIVE HEART FAILURE AND PULMONARY EDEMA
Pathophysiology
Congestive heart failure involves the left, right or both sides of the heart. In left-sided heart failure, the diseased myocardium fails to pump blood from the lungs into the systemic circulation. This results in increased pulmonary venous pressure, left atrial pressure and left ventricular diastolic pressure. Cardiac output is decreased. An accumulation of blood increases lung pressure, engorging pulmonary capillaries. If pulmonary capillary hydrostatic pressure is allowed to exceed 30 mm of mercury, fluid leaks into the pulmonary interstitial spaces. This leads to pulmonary edema and impedes oxygen-carbon dioxide exchange.

Right-sided heart failure is a direct result of an increase in lung pressure. The right side fails to pump blood to the lungs and impedes venous return. As pressure continues to build, fluid accumulates in organs, producing engorgement of the liver and spleen, neck vein distention and edema of the extremities.

Precipitating factors leading to left-sided failure include atherosclerotic heart disease, acute myocardial infarction, myocarditis, fluid overload and valvular disease. Precipitating factors leading to right-sided failure are left-sided heart failure, atherosclerotic heart disease, acute myocardial infarction, pulmonary emboli, fluid overload, chronic obstructive pulmonary disease, cor pulmonale, tachyarrhythmias, bradyarrhythmias and valvular disease (Fig. 5-62).

Primary:
  myocardial failure
  myocardial infarction
  cardiomyopathy
  hypothyroidism
  interference with diastolic filling
    pericardial tamponade
    pericardial effusion
    constrictive pericarditis
  arrhythmias
  electrolyte and acid-base abnormalities
    severe potassium or calcium abnormalities
    severe acidosis or alkalosis

Inadequate venous return:
  hypovolemia
  vasodilators
  spinal or general anesthesia

Circulatory overload:
  increased blood volume
  increased venous return
  (high output failure)
    anemia
    cirrhosis
    arteriovenous fistulas
    thyrotoxicosis

Fig. 5-62. Causes of heart failure

Clinical Presentation

The clinical presentation depends on the side and extent of involvement.

Left heart failure:

(1) *Dyspnea:* Breathing becomes difficult as the lungs become stiffer. Dyspnea first occurs on exertion and then eventually occurs at rest. Fluid in the alveolar spaces causes a cough on exertion. Symptoms usually occur slowly.

(2) *Orthopnea:* Shortness of breath while lying is relieved by a mid- or high Fowler's position. As venous return from the lower extremities increases, a greater force of contraction is needed.

Consequently, increased contractility cannot compensate for the greater venous return.

(3) *Paroxysmal nocturnal dyspnea* (PND): A cough usually develops with dyspnea on exertion, but can occur at any time. This is an exaggerated form of orthopnea and may occur with expiratory and inspiratory wheezing due to bronchospasm. The amount of fluid present may be enough to cause the patient to waken from sleep. It dissipates when the patient sits or stands, or it may progress to acute pulmonary edema.

(4) *Acute pulmonary edema:* Rising capillary pressure causes a massive exchange of fluid into the alveoli. The patient presents with cold, pale skin, anxiety and diaphoresis, and gasps for breath. The patient is extremely fearful of dying as air hunger increases. The expectorated sputum is white or pink-tinged.

(5) *Fatigue:* Fatigue on exertion and moderate to severe weakness from reduced cardiac output are usually late symptoms. Fatigue may disappear with rest. Patients with mitral stenosis, low cardiac output and pulmonary hypertension often complain of extreme fatigue.

(6) *Nocturia:* The excretion of fluid that accumulates during the day reflects the decreased work of the heart at rest. Nocturia may also occur in the absence of cardiac disease.

(7) *Elevated pulmonary artery diastolic pressure* and *pulmonary capillary wedge pressure* are symptomatic.

Right heart failure

Right heart failure can occur alone, but usually it is secondary to left heart failure. Some common causes are cor pulmonale from chronic lung disease, pulmonary valve stenosis, mitral stenosis with pulmonary hypertension and atrial-septal defects. The prime symptom is systemic venous congestion. Pulmonary symptoms are rare unless left heart failure is present.

(1) *Fatigue:* As cardiac output decreases, the patient complains of weakness and fatigue.

(2) *Edema:* Edema of the lower extremities and ankles occurs when the patient ambulates. If the patient is on bedrest, fluid accumulates in the sacrum, flank and thighs.

(3) *Liver engorgement:* The capsule around the liver becomes engorged. Right upper quadrant pain is often misdiagnosed as cholecystitis.

(4) *Anorexia:* Gastrointestinal symptoms such as anorexia, bloating and other nonspecific symptoms occur as hepatic and visceral engorgement raise the venous pressure.

(5) *Hepatomegaly:* Dependent edema and jugular neck distention are common symptoms of right heart failure.

Diagnostic Data

Chest x-ray, history and physical are excellent diagnostic aids to determine interstitial density and hypertrophy of the cardiac silhouette. Liver function tests reveal abnormal findings in the presence of hepatomegaly. Swan-Ganz findings determine the degree of failure.

Nursing Care

(1) Establish and maintain a patent airway. Provide ventilation and suction as needed. Administer humidified oxygen or intermittent positive pressure breathing. Position to provide maximum lung inflation. Check arterial blood gases. Administer drugs such as theophylline as ordered.

(2) Reduce venous congestion and blood volume by administering diuretics as ordered. Keep accurate intake and output records. Apply rotating tourniquets. Assess and maintain fluid and electrolyte balance. Administer inotropic agents as ordered.

(4) Observe for complications of fluid and electrolyte imbalance, digitalis intoxication, oxygen intoxication, pulmonary emboli and venous stasis.

(5) Monitor and assess changes in cardiopulmonary status and the development of dysrhythmias.

KEY CONCEPT: Nursing care is aimed at airway maintenance and assessment and prevention of further complications.

PERICARDITIS
Pathophysiology

Pericarditis is an inflammation of the pericardium. Pericardial constriction may result from fibrotic changes and calcification. The most common agents causing pericarditis are bacteria, virus or fungus. Precipitating factors leading to pericarditis are acute myocardial infarcton, trauma, collagen diseases, lesions, dissecting aortic aneurysms and uremia. Procainamide, hydralazine, diphenylhydantoin and Adriamycin may cause pericarditis. Thoracotomy, cardiotomy, radiation and tuberculosis may also cause pericarditis.

Clinical Presentation

The clinical presentation depends on the extent of constriction. Cough, pleuritic chest pain, hemoptysis, changes in mentation, fever, cyanosis and pallor may be present. Accentuated S_2, pulsus paradoxus, dysrhythmias and friction rub are more specific clinical indications. Chest pain decreases upon sitting upright or leaning forward. The chest pain increases when the patient lies down or inspires deeply.

Diagnostic Data

A differential diagnosis must be made between pericarditis and myocardial infarction. At the onset of pericarditis pain, fever and electrocardiographic changes are present. In pericarditis, no Q waves are present on the EKG. Upon breath-holding, a pericardial friction rub is heard. Routine serum tests reflect an increase in white blood cells. The physical findings are auscultatory: friction rub and pulsus paradoxus. Echocardiography may reveal pericardial effusion. Cardiac catheterization determines severity and differentiates pericarditis from restrictive cardiomyopathies.

Nursing Care

The major nursing responsibilities are to prevent complications and relieve pain.

(1) Recognize cardiac tamponade: muffled heart sounds, pulsus paradoxus and distended neck veins.

(2) Observe for dysrhythmias.

(3) Relieve pain; administer steroids and aspirin.

(4) Monitor and assess hemodynamic changes, electrocardiographic changes and bleeding.

(5) Administer antipyretic measures.

KEY CONCEPT: Differential diagnosis is the most important factor in the institution of treatment for pericarditis. The nurse should observe for signs of cardiac tamponade so it is treated as early as possible.

HYPERTENSIVE CRISIS

Pathophysiology

Hypertensive crisis is a significant rise in the blood pressure, producing a crisis situation. Systemic vascular resistance times the mean cardiac output equals mean arterial pressure (SVR x C.O. = Mean AP). Therefore, a rise in cardiac output or a rise in systemic vascular resistance leads to an increase in the blood pressure.

Several etiologic factors cause hypertensive crisis: necrotizing arteriolites appearing on the arterial walls; the release of renin and angiotensin; and encephalopathy due to edema and hemorrhage.

Precipitating factors leading to hypertensive crisis are untreated hypertension, renal disease, toxemia of pregnancy, polycythemia, pheochromocytoma, pituitary tumors, coarction of the aorta, adrenocortical dysfunction, acromegaly and Cushing's syndrome. The administration of catecholamine precursors and monoamine oxidase inhibitors together may cause a hypertensive crisis.

Clinical Presentation

The clinical presentation depends on the cause. Malignant hypertensive symptoms include: diastolic pressure greater than 120 mm Hg; impaired renal function; severe retinopathy with exudate, hemorrhage and papilledema; restlessness; headache; and epistaxis. Symptoms of hypertensive encephalopathy include: malignant hypertension associated with renal disease; a sudden increase in pressure; nausea; vomiting; headache; convulsions; nystagmus and visual disturbances; localized weakness; and confusion, stupor and coma.

Be aware of the following signs when assessing the degree of involvement on organs affected by hypertension:

Eye: The retina, narrowing of arterioles, circular hemorrhages or the presence of papilledema with blurring of the temporal edge of the optic disk may be present.

Cardiovascular: Evidence of left ventricular hypertrophy may be noted by a left ventricular heave. This does not displace to the left unless cardiac failure is present. The thickness of the left ventricle produces an S_4, indicating decreased left ventricular compliance. S_4 and heave are signs of long-standing disease.

Bruits over the carotids are caused by arteriosclerotic changes. Check all pulses and bruits for symmetry, weakness or delays. The presence of weak or delayed femoral pulses compared to radial pulses is a strong indication of coarctation of the aorta.

Central nervous system: A positive Babinski, hemiplegia, hemiparesis or hemianopsia may be present.

Renal: Large, easily palpated, polycystic kidneys are present.

Endocrine: Cushing's syndrome presents with central trunk obesity, acne, moon face and hirsutism.

Diagnostic Data

Until renal impairment occurs, the urinalysis will be normal. With renal dysfunction, the specific gravity may be low and protein may be present. A culture and sensitivity test should be done and repeated as chronic pyelonephritis may develop. A 24-hour urine study may be conducted to rule out Cushing's syndrome. In all types of ACTH-dependent syndromes, 17-hydroxycorticosteroids or serum cortisol is elevated. If pheochromocytoma is suspected, then studies for catecholamines and their metabolic products should be done.

Renal parenchymal disease is suspected when serum creatinine and blood urea nitrogen (BUN) are elevated. When the creatinine is greater than 1.5 mg/dl, a creatinine clearance is indicated to determine glomerular filtration rate.

Electrocardiographic findings are sensitive to left ventricular hypertrophy.

Excretory urography diagnoses renal vascular disorders. If the clinical picture indicates renovascular hypertension with bruits, a renal angiogram is needed to confirm stenosis.

Radiologic studies include renal arteriography to detect renal arterial stenosis. An intravenous pyelogram confirms kidney disease. A chest x-ray confirms cardiomegaly.

Nursing Care

The major nursing goal is aimed at reducing the blood pressure.

(1) Administer antihypertensive drugs.
(2) Prevent complications: untreated malignant hypertension results in cerebral infarcts, myocardial infarctions, renal disease and dissecting aortic aneurysm. If treated, the prognosis is reversed and long-term survival is possible.

KEY CONCEPT: Hypertension is a serious and chronic elevation of blood pressure interfering with the function of major body functions. With proper treatment, good prognosis is possible. Without treatment, death may occur.

SHOCK

Pathophysiology

Shock is a severe pathophysiological disturbance characterized by poor tissue perfusion. Shock is generally caused by one of two factors: a decrease in venous return or a decrease in the heart's ability to pump. Decreased venous return is due to decreased blood flow as a result of diminished blood volume, vasodilatation, or vasoconstriction. Pump failure produces a deficit caused by inadequate filling and emptying. Hemodynamically, shock can reduce effective circulating volume; decrease venous return; decrease cardiac output; reduce perfusion; reduce tissue oxygenation; and cause tissue death. The body's physiological response to shock can be analogized to the body's ability to compensate for a change in environment. When a sudden change occurs; as in blood loss or shifting of fluids, there is a marked sympathomimetic response. Baroreceptor response increases peripheral resistance by stimulating constriction of the capillary network. This constriction enhances cardiac output by increasing the rate and force of contraction. In addition, adrenal response increases the circulating catecholamine, epinephrine and norepinephrine. These catecholamines are alpha and beta stimulators, which further sympathetic vasoconstriction and aid the perfusion of the heart and brain. A drop in mean arterial pressure below 50 mm Hg stimulates a central nervous system response. This response leads to an elevation in carbon dioxide levels and further development of ischemia. Renal constriction causes a decrease in glomerular filtration and renal plasma flow, and results in decreased urine output and sodium retention. A reduction in afferent arteriolar pressure stimulates the baroreceptors to activate the renin-angiotension mechanism. This mechanism causes an elevation of arterial pressure by arteriolar vasoconstriction, stimulation of aldosterone and reabsorption of sodium and water. Sodium is retained and extracellular fluid volume increases. Failure of the body to activate compensatory mechanisms or failure to correct the underlying disorder leads to myocardial ischemia, severe cerebral hypoxia, vascular collapse, thrombosis of minute vessels, release of endotoxins, cellular deterioration, acidosis and anaerobic metabolism.

Types of shock include **cardiogenic, hypovolemic, septic** and **neurogenic**. **Cardiogenic shock** occurs when the heart fails as a pump. The major causes include acute myocardial infarction, pulmonary emboli, cardiac tamponade, postcardiac surgery, tension pneumothorax, arrhythmias, dissecting aortic aneurysm and myocarditis. The patient displays cold and clammy skin, hypotension, cyanosis, oliguria, cerebral hypoxia and hypothermia.

Physiologically, there is low cardiac output, increased heart rate, increased peripheral vascular resistance and a normal or increased filling pressure in the heart. Approximately 15 percent of patients with a myocardial infarction develop cardiogenic shock. **Hypovolemic shock** occurs as a direct result of a decrease between the intravascular volume and the vascular capacitance. There is usually a blood volume deficit of 20 percent and an even greater interstitial deficit. Common causes include hemorrhage, severe dehydration, excessive vomiting, diarrhea, burns, diabetes mellitus, trauma, surgery, diuretic therapy, peritonitis, cirrhosis and hemothorax. There is significant tissue damage in shock due to trauma. Traumatic injuries result in the pooling of large amounts of fluid in and around injured cells. Lysosomal enzymes and vasoactive substances are released, causing vasodilation and loss of fluids from the vascular spaces that potentiates the shock state. The shock state persists if inadequate fluids are administered. **Septic shock** can be divided into two categories: hyperdynamic and hypodynamic. With increased administration of fluid, the cardiac output can be normal or high. Hyperdynamic septic shock is a normal or increased cardiac output state. It may occur because of improper utilization of the tissues' glucose and oxygen. A hyperdynamic state may occur with an increase in arteriovenous shunting. Hypodynamic refers to a low cardiac output state. This is called an absolute hypovolemia. Increased capillary leak surrounding the infected area is the primary cause. Common causes include an overt infection, urinary tract infection, postpartum or abortion infection and immunosuppressant therapy. **Neurogenic shock** occurs as a result of damage to or chemical blockage of the sympathetic nervous system. In the affected body areas vasodilation of the arterioles and an increased vascular capacitance occurs. This is an uncommon phenomenon. Consequently, a relative hypovolemia ensues, cardiac output remains normal, but peripheral vascular resistance is reduced. In spite of the hypovolemic state, the skin usually remains warm and dry. This usually occurs because the sympathetic nervous system is blocked. Trauma to the brain seldom causes shock; therefore, shock in the presence of a head injury should be further assessed. Common causes of neurogenic shock are general and spinal anesthesia, spinal cord injuries, antihypertensive drugs and anaphylaxis. The use of fluids or vasopressors is self-limiting. Other causes include barbiturate or phenothiazene overdose, vasovagal syncope and direct damage to the vasomotor center of the medulla.

Clinical Presentation

The criteria most often used to determine shock is systolic blood pressure less than 80 mm Hg, metabolic acidosis and oliguria or anuria. Although these signs are useful, they are rather late signs and are not always reliable.

The pulse pressure, the difference between the systolic and diastolic pressure, provides a clinical indication of the increase or decrease in stroke volume. As the aging process occurs, cardiac output and stroke volume decrease. The pulse pressure increases because the blood vessels lose elasticity.

Drastic decreases in stroke volume and pulse pressure may be noted long before a significant fall occurs in the systolic pressure. This often occurs in hypovolemic shock. In severe sympathoadrenal stimulation with hemorrhage, the diastolic pressure rises. The pulse pressure and stoke volume decrease, but the systolic pressure remains relatively stable. As compensatory vasoconstriction fails, the systolic and diastolic pressure fall. A rapid, weak, thready pulse is present.

The correlation of renal blood flow and urine output is relatively dependable, but both rely on the cardiac output. In the hypovolemic state, it is important to maintain accurate intake and output. Arterioles constrict when renal blood flow decreases, and renal arterioles constrict and reduce glomerular filtration.

Shock states usually produce a classic metabolic acidosis. In early shock and sepsis, respiratory alkalosis and metabolic alkalosis may be present. Shock, trauma and sepsis powerfully affect ventilations. Initial blood gases reveal an elevated pH, a low $PaCO_2$ and a normal bicarbonate. This occurrence leads to hyperventilation. A valuable sign that a stable patient is deteriorating is the onset of tachypnea.

As the condition deteriorates, metabolic acidosis occurs at the cellular level. A useful indicator of the potential prognosis is blood lactate levels. Clinically, the acidotic patient presents with apathy, lethargy, confusion and, eventually, coma.

If the underlying cause of shock is not treated, the compensatory mechanism begins to fail. If the arterial pressure cannot maintain coronary blood flow, myocardial ischemia occurs and cardiac output falls. With depression of sympathetic stimulation, blood pools in the periphery, reducing cardiac output. A decrease in vessel nutrition during shock results in arterial and venous dilation. This reduces blood flow to vital organs. Blood pools in the venous bed and minute vessels thrombose because of sluggish blood flow. The following factors precipitate agglutination of leukocytes, erythrocytes and platelets: platelet aggregation by catecholamines; deposition of fibrin and accumulation of microthrombi; hypoxia increasing the rigidity of red blood cells; and complement activation causing the release of vasoactive peptides and anaphylatoxins. Common complications of shock include:

Cardiac failure: usually caused by myocardial damage. Myocardial contractility may decrease further because of acidosis. Cardiac failure is evaluated by the increase in left ventricular end diastolic pressure.

Adult respiratory distress syndrome (ARDS): a shock state affecting the capillary bed of the lungs. An increase in blood flow resistance, interstitial pulmonary edema and systemic hypoxia is seen in ARDS.

Inadequate renal perfusion: Hypoperfusion over a prolonged period of time results in acute tubular necrosis and causes renal failure.

Liver damage: The shock state damages reticuloendothelial cells and increases the probability of massive infection.

Gastrointestinal bleeding: occurs most often during septic shock. This may be related to the reduction in blood flow to the gastric mucosa and to the stimulation of the sympathetic nervous system.

Disseminated intravascular coagulation (DIC): occurs following multiple trauma or any shock state in which a major portion of clotting factors are consumed or are absorbed. This is caused by the activation of the clotting system by the Hageman factor (factor XII).

Diagnostic Data

The best diagnostic aid is laboratory data. Arterial blood gases (ABG), urinalysis and serum analysis results document shock. Arterial blood gases may show respiratory alkalosis or metabolic acidosis. Serum analysis reveals elevated BUN and creatinine, and hyperkalemia. Urinalysis reveals elevated osmolarity and specific gravity. A decrease in urine creatinine clearance is seen. Septic shock reveals leukocytosis, thrombocytopenia, abnormal prothrombin time, partial prothrombin time and positive blood cultures.

Nursing Care

The major nursing responsibilities include:

(1) Provide oxygenation; patients in shock derive some benefit from oxygen therapy. Administer 100 percent oxygen in most cases. After stabilization, titrate the oxygen concentration according to the blood gases.

(2) Maintain fluid and electrolyte balance. Patients in shock require aggressive intravenous therapy. Volume replacement in an injured patient in the first hour ranges from 3 to 4 liters. If no response is noted, consider further assessment of injuries. Blood, plasma, plasmanates or albumin are administered. Consider the following factors in determining fluid replacement: blood pressure, pulse, urinary output, rales, skin perfusion and pulmonary wedge pressure.

(3) Maintain acid-base balance. If adequate ventilation and tissue perfusion are properly treated, the acid-base problem will improve. There exists some controversy over the treatment of acidosis, unless the pH is less than 7.20. Half the base deficit is corrected at one time, not exceeding 5/meq of sodium bicarbonate per minute. A combined acidosis may be noted in the terminal stages of shock and treatment is ineffective.

(4) Provide drug therapy. In hypovolemic shock, the normal sympathetic response is contraindicated. In cardiogenic shock, vasoactive therapy is recommended. Levophed (norepinephrine) is a peripheral vasoconstrictor that has a positive inotropic effect and increases afterload. This drug is an alpha-adrenergic stimulator. Dopamine (Intropin) and isoproterenol (Isuprel) are beta-adrenergic stimulators. Dopamine has both inotropic and chronotropic effects in low doses. In large doses, it becomes a positive inotropic agent similar to Levophed. Isuprel increases the myocardial oxygen demand through its positive inotropic effect. It also dilates the coronary arteries, thereby improving coronary perfusion. Vasodilators such as Nipride (sodium nitropresside) and intravenous nitroglycerine reduce the arterial pressure by reducing preload and afterload.

KEY CONCEPT: Shock is the lack of tissue perfusion. The types of shock are hypovolemic, neurogenic, cardiogenic and septic. Decreased circulating volume, loss of vascular tone, or cardiac pump failure cause shock. Nursing care is aimed at early recognition and treatment to prevent further deterioration.

PACEMAKERS

Pathophysiology

Pacemakers consist of a pulse generator, a lead and electrodes. They are external *(temporary)* or implantable *(permanent)*. Two types of electrodes exist. A *unipolar* electrode is connected to another (indifferent) electrode located elsewhere. This produces a large pacemaker spike on the EKG. *Bipolar* means two electrodes are used. This is more common. Both the positive and negative electrodes are placed on the anterior surface of the heart or within the chamber. If one electrode fails, it can become a unipolar system by adding a skin electrode. A small pacemaker spike appears on the EKG.

Temporary Pacemaker

The patient who develops a sudden severe dysfunction requiring emergency intervention needs temporary rather than permanent pacing. One of three techniques are used for insertion of a temporary pacemaker: transvenous endocardial, epicardial and transthoracic.

Transvenous endocardial is the most common technique. The catheter inserts via a percutaneous route or venous cutdown. Subclavian, antecubital, femoral or jugular veins are common sites. Electrocardiogram or fluoroscopy monitors insertion. In ventricular pacing, the catheter tip lodges in the trabeculae of the right ventricular apex. The proper site for atrial pacing is the atrial appendage or coronary sinus.

The electrodes attach to the battery unit or external pulse generator. The unit's functional ability depends on battery output, pacing threshold, and sensitivity threshold.

Pacing threshold is the stimulation threshold necessary to obtain measurement that maintains continuous capture. It is the amount of current used to capture at a 1:1 ratio. A setting in excess of 1.5 milliamps (MA) is undesirable, and adjustments of lead position may be necessary. Confirmation and stability of the catheter tip may be ascertained by changing position and creating pressure changes within the thorax. Intrathoracic pressure changes are accomplished by deep breathing and coughing.

Sensitivity threshold is the measurement that confirms adequate sensing of intrinsic activity for demand pacing. Move the sense-pace indicator to the sense mode. Turn the demand pacemaker rate below the patient's rate and the sensitivity dial to maximum. If the R wave is not sensed, repositioning of the catheter is necessary.

Epicardial pacing is routinely used following heart surgery. If an emergency arises, atrial and ventricular leads may be attached to a pulse generator. Following stabilization, the wires are easily removed.

Emergency pacing is the least effective method. This may be accomplished by inserting electrodes into the ventricle or by using an external pacemaker. Electrodes inserted via a needle have inherent dangers. Possible complications include coronary artery laceration, cardiac tamponade and dysrhythmias. However, it is more effective than external pacing. External pacing is accomplished by delivering 50 to 150 volts of electricity to the chest wall. Complications include pain and burns.

Clinical Presentation

Stokes-Adams syndrome is a serious condition caused by a disturbance in the heart's electrical system. The patient generally complains of dizziness, fainting or feeling light-headed. Cardiac output decreases and central nervous system hypoxia may exist.

Symptomatic bradycardia, atrioventricular blocks, sino-atrial block or digitalis-induced arrhythmias may be present. Other clinical indications for a temporary pacemaker are congestive heart failure with slow ventricular rates that are unresponsive to medical intervention; complete atrioventricular block following heart surgery, or preceding or during implantation of a permanent pacemaker; or while changing a pulse generator.

Diagnostic Data

History and physical provide the objective data and may elicit therapeutic indications for a pacemaker. A useful diagnostic test for conduction system disease is an electrocardiogram. This provides the data that determines the need for a temporary pacemaker. Atrial pacing is done during His bundle studies. It determines the effect of heart rate changes on the conduction system and examines the intrinsic function of the SA node. Atrial pacing may be used to increase the heart rate during stress testing in patients with coronary artery disease. A temporary pacemaker produces premature stimuli during episodes of tachycardia. If this causes re-entry, automaticity is ruled out as the cause of the tachycardia.

Nursing Care

The goals of nursing care are supportive and restorative. Certain basics are essential when dealing with the temporary pacemaker patient. Preoperative care includes careful and concise explanation of the pacemaker's indications, use and risks. It is necessary to briefly explain these in the emergency situation as well. The nurse should obtain consent, administer sedation, establish intravenous lines and prepare equipment.

Postoperative care includes:
(1) Accurately document insertion date, site, settings and type of pacer.
(2) Protect dial settings.
(3) Immobilize arm, catheter and pacer.
(4) Avoid electrical hazards by covering pacemaker terminals with rubber. Wear rubber gloves to connect, disconnect or adjust battery pack or terminals when necessary. Have engineering check the safety of radio equipment, electric shavers or other unnecessary electrical items when necessary.
(5) Continuously monitor and assess: serial electrocardiographic tracings for rate; rhythm, pacing current, sense-pace indicator; pacemaker function for proper stimulus release, capture and sensing; vital signs.
(6) Control infection: Use aseptic technique for dressing changes and observe the patient for signs of infection or inflammation.
(7) Treat cardiac arrest: If the pacemaker is off, immediately turn it on, increase milliamps two increments, increase rate to above 60 and observe electrocardiogram, pulse and sense-pace indicator. Check and compare the patient's pulse to the electrocardiographic reading. If the pacemaker is on and defibrillation becomes necessary, turn the pacemaker off by disconnecting wires from the pacemaker's terminal. This prevents the defibrillator's current from bypassing the cardiac muscle and prevents damage to the pacemaker.
(8) Provide emotional support to the patient and family.

Permanent Pacemakers

Permanent pacemakers are generally used in the long-term treatment of symptomatic chronic heart block. The particular pathology of heart block depends upon the etiology, but the most common problems are nonspecific, degenerative, fibrotic and sclerotic changes. Acute myocardial infarction and heart block due to rheumatic heart disease, cardiomyopathies, surgery, trauma, sarcoidosis and unusual lesions may require insertion of a permanent pacer. Heart block falls into several categories: complete heart block, atrioventricular block, bifascicular blocks and bilateral bundle branch blocks. Conditions other than heart block that may require a permanent pacemaker include: congestive heart failure with bradycardia refractory to medical management; improved cerebral or renal blood flow as a result of temporary pacing; sinus bradycardia unresponsive to atropine or exercise; sinoatrial block or sinus arrest with long periods of ventricular asystole; alternating episodes of bradycardia with tachycardia; hypersensitive carotid sinus syndrome; and refractory tachyarrhythmias improved by temporary pacing.

Permanent pacemakers are inserted by one of three methods: (1) transvenous endocardial, (2) thoractomy epicardial, and (3) subxiphoid, transxiphoid or transmediastinal epicardial pacing.

Transvenous endocardial pacing may be indicated for the poor surgical risk since a thoracotomy is not required. It requires only a minor surgical set up. Catheter displacement, ventricular perforation, diaphragmatic stimulation, air embolism, infection, and pulmonary embolism are complications. Transvenous endocardial pacing of the right ventricle produces an EKG pattern similar to left bundle branch block. If a right bundle branch block pattern develops, suspect septal perforation or catheter lip displacement into the coronary sinus.

Thoracotomy epicardial pacing is the most reliable pacing method. A synchronous atrial pacemaker requires this insertion method. It is the best approach for young people and reduces the risk of bacterial endocarditis and embolisms. Complications such as postoperative infection may develop. Epicardial transthoracic pacing of the left ventricle produces an EKG pattern that simulates right bundle branch block.

Epicardial pacing uses the subxiphoid, transxiphoid or transmediastinal method and offers a shortened postoperative period, no chest tubes and stabilization of electrodes by screws. The risk of complications, such as bacterial endocarditis and embolism, are greatly reduced.

Clinical Presentation

The patient generally complains of syncopal episodes, dizziness, weakness and, occasionally, seizures. If bradycardia or failure of the idioventricular pacemaker occurs, the patient may experience decreased cardiac output and central nervous system hypoxia.

Diagnostic Data

The electrocardiogram, along with a history and physical, is the best diagnostic aid to determine the cause and extent of heart disease. Coronary angiograms may be useful. Routine laboratory tests are valuable to determine overall patient condition. A temporary pacemaker may confirm the need to implant a permanent pacemaker.

Nursing Care

The major responsibilities divide into three phases: preoperative, postoperative and rehabilitative. Preoperative care includes monitoring the temporary pacemaker, providing emotional support to the patient and family, and explaining the advantages, risks, discomforts, skin changes and postoperative period to the patient and family.

Postoperative care follows surgical insertion method. The thoracotomy approach carries additional risk factors and complications. The postoperative nurse must:

(1) Maintain accurate documentation of site and type of pacemaker.
(2) Record pacemaker function: escape interval, spontaneous and magnet-induced discharging intervals, refractory period, sensed P to QRS for synchronous atrial pace; sensed QRS for demand ventricular pacing; current or voltage, artifact, size and threshold.
(3) Obtain electrocardiogram and chest radiograph following insertion for baseline information.
(4) Monitor and assess. Observe cardiac rhythm for competition with fixed rate pacemakers caused by the pre-set high energy level. Usually in six to ten days, the energy level lowers as a result of fibrosis occurring around the electrodes. Catheter stiffness may produce myocardial injury or irritability, resulting in premature ventricular contractions.
(5) Evaluate the stimulation threshold in demand or synchronous ventricular pacemakers.
(6) Limit patient activity following insertion of a transvenous pacemaker to prevent catheter displacement.
(7) Watch for infection. Use aseptic technique and observe operative site for pain, infection, bleeding and edema. Administer antibiotics if ordered.
(8) Prevent complications by providing range-of-motion exercises to extremities nearest the operative site.

The rehabilitative phase includes psychological intervention and patient teaching. Psychological factors result from the patient's attitude toward the pacemaker, dependency, exercise and pacemaker failure and function. Encourage the patient and family to discuss these fears with professional staff, as well as with another pacemaker wearer. Use principles of adult education when teaching the patient. A sample teaching program should provide the following information:

(1) A simple statement of function with emphasis on the implanted pacemaker's function

(2) The importance of follow-up care, daily pulse counts, unusual symptoms, pacemaker clinics, telephone monitoring, pulse generator replacement indications, battery failure and replacement procedure

(3) The need for identification, including name, address, physician's name, address and phone number; and type of pacemaker

(4) Information that should be reported to the physician: pulse changes after counting twice for a full minute, dizziness, edema of extremities, chest pain, dyspnea, fever or changes in operative site

(5) Nutrition and diet

(6) Medication: use, dose, side effects, toward effects and contraindications

(7) An understanding of lifestyle and changes: working, traveling, driving, exercise and sexual relations

(8) Hazards in the use of certain electrical equipment: magnetic tape erasers, tool demagnetizers, large transformers, driven devices, arc-welding machines, diathermy over a pacemaker site and electroconvulsive therapy. Encourage pacemaker recipients to use electrical devices in good repair. Explain that these electrical devices should not be repeatedly turned on and off. Recipients should never work directly over an ignition system. Theft-prevention devices, microwave ovens, cautery and cutting instruments may intererfere with permanent pacemakers. Always inform dentists, physicians and physical therapists about the pacemaker.

Types of Pacemakers

There are two basic types of pacemakers: **fixed-** and **demand-rate.** The fixed-rate or asynchronous pacer is set to fire at a fixed rate and does not respond to alterations in physiological needs. It functions independently of the intrinsic activity of the heart and may compete with spontaneous ventricular activity. The electrode stimulates the atrium or ventricle. The demand or programmable pacer avoids generating competitive rhythms because spontaneous cardiac activity is sensed. It also stimulates the atrium or ventricle.

Atrial Pacemakers

Atrial pacemakers stimulate the atria when the atrioventricular conduction is functioning properly. A consistent atrial rhythm must be present. Atrial pacemakers provide the hemodynamic benefits (atrial kick) of a normal contraction and reduce the dangers of ventricular competition. Atrial pacemakers produce an artifact or spike that differs in morphology from the normal P wave.

A fixed-rate or asynchronous atrial pacemaker delivers continuous stimuli to the atria regardless of atrial beats.

P wave inhibited or demand atrial pacemakers sense atrial depolarization and inhibit the stimulus. When the rate falls below the preset interval, the pacemaker initiates atrial depolarization.

P wave-triggered atrial pacemakers fire during the natural formation of a P wave and prevent the natural rate from overriding the pacemaker rate. Following a preset escape interval, the pacemaker fires, initiating atrial depolarization. If the natural rate falls, the pacemaker acts as a fixed-rate pacemaker.

A QRS inhibited atrial pacemaker provides atrial escape beats when the QRS fails to respond. This occurs at a preset interval.

Ventricular Pacemaker

A fixed-rate or asynchronous pacemaker is rarely used. Its stimulating mechanism delivers continuous stimuli to the ventricles. The clinical situation determines the discharge rate, but the pacemaker remains unaffected by spontaneous contractions. Disadvantages include formation of a fusion beat, which is the simultaneous occurrence of a natural and pacemaker beat. If the stimulus falls during the vulnerable period (on the T wave), consecutive ventricular beats or ventricular fibrillation may occur. Also, the system lacks the booster pump effect of atrial input.

A demand QRS-inhibited ventricular pacemaker can both stimulate and sense. If a natural contraction is sensed, the pacemaker inhibits formation of a stimulus. The advantage is twofold: the pacer eliminates competition, and, as the heart rate falls, the pacer fires at a preset rate.

A demand QRS-triggered ventricular pacemaker delivers a stimulus during the natural formation of the QRS complex. When the heart rate falls, the pacer will fire at a preset rate. A disadvantage is the distorted morphology of the QRS complex, which makes it difficult to identify arrhythmias.

P wave-triggered ventricular pacemakers (P wave synchronous) have separate electrodes for atrial sensing and ventricular stimulating circuits. The P wave triggers the release of the ventricular stimulus. If no P wave forms, the ventricular rate fires at a preset rate. This type of pacemaker reduces competition by allowing the atria to vary ventricular rate according to physiological needs. Another advantage is that the atrial kick is not lost. A major disadvantage is the frequency of thoracotomies needed to achieve sensing and capture. This pacer type has very complex circuitry with a short battery life and may precipitate dysrhythmias.

Artrial and Ventricular Pacemakers

Two electrodes provide stimulation within the atria and ventricle. It sequentially delivers a stimulus to the atria and ventricles. A sequential delay occurs between the two stimuli, corresponding to the normal P-R interval. The disadvantage of this pacemaker is the likelihood of developing a competitive rhythm.

QRS-inhibited sequential atrial and ventricular pacemakers are called AV-sequential or bifocal-demand pacemakers. They combine the advantages of atrial, sequential and demand pacing. Patient needs are automatically met, while the natural sequence of depolarization is preserved. In bradycardia-related heart failure, this pacemaker improves cardiac output by providing the atrial kick. It does not compete with spontaneous ventricular activity. A noninvasive, programmable, AV-sequential demand pacemaker is the only pacing concept that has potential use for every patient requiring a pacemaker.

The transvenous approach uses two bipolar leads. Sensing, which occurs only in the ventricles, inhibits spontaneous intracardiac potentials. The intrinsic atrial activity has no effect on the operation of the pulse generator (Fig. 5-63).

P Wave Triggered	AV Sequential	Bifocal Demand
Normal atrial activity with AV block	Atrial bradycardia with AV block	Atrial bradycardia with or without AV block
Monitors P waves	No monitoring	Monitors QRS complexes
P waves control ventricular stimulation; no atrial stimulation available	Continuous atrial and ventricular stimulation	QRS complexes control atrial and ventricular stimulation
Stimulation delivered continuously to ventricles	Stimulation delivered continuously to atria and ventricles	Stimulation may be: absent delivered only to atria delivered to atria and ventricles

Fig. 5-63. AV pacing

Pacemaker complications are generally due to either pacemaker malfunctions or electrical leakage (Fig. 5-64). Failure of a stimulus release, failure to capture, or failure to sense may cause pacemaker malfunctions.

Battery failure, disconnection, sensing problems and interference in the electromagnetic field may cause failure to release a stimulus. The electrocardiogram reveals pacemaker problems such as the intermittent or absent pacing stimulus. Occasionally, a runaway pacemaker develops. This emergency requires disconnection of the pacing unit. Low voltage, faulty connections, improper catheter position, broken catheter wire, or fibrosis of a catheter tip may cause failure to capture or stimulate. The electrocardiogram confirms the problem by showing a

	Causes	Effects
Body	Rejection	Infection, edema, migration
Leads	Displacement of atrial lead Broken Myocardial irritability on insertion Transvenous insertion	Increased ventricular rate, ventricular output inhibited; asynchronous, loss of capture or sensing; fibrillation; air embolism
Battery	Early depletion as a result of high internal losses	Decreased output voltage; increased pulse width; decreased rate; loss of capture
Connector	Poor connection	Intermittent or continuous loss of capture, improper sensing
Circuitry	Electromagnetic interference	Inhibits output; reverts to asynchronous mode
Components	Electrical changes due to shorts, opens or shifts	No output; rate increase, rate decrease; reverts to asynchronous mode; loss of capture; increase or decrease of AV delay; programming function lost

Fig. 5-64. Pacemaker complications

slowing atrial or ventricular rate and the pacing artifact's failure to produce a P or QRS. Chest x-ray confirms displacement of the catheter tip.

Nursing Care

The major nursing responsibilities include checking for faulty connections, repositioning of the limb, increasing milliamp or volts, recording electrocardiograms and ordering chest films for catheter placement.

QRS-inhibited ventricular pacemakers may fail to sense because of faulty sensing of the pacemaker unit, improper location of the catheter, or battery failure and poor signals within the cavity. The electrocardiogram reveals competition which leads to ventricular tachycardia or ventricular fibrillation, especially in the presence of an acute myocardial infarction, electrolyte imbalance, hypoxia or increased catecholamine release. Frequently, the patient complains of palpitations, angina or lightheadedness. The major nursing responsibilities are: in the presence of an adequate rate, turn the pacemaker off; if an inadequate rate is present, several measures are possible:

(1) Increase the rate of the pacemaker.
(2) Administer lidocaine for unsensed ventricular beats.
(3) Increase the sensitivity.
(4) Change the position of the patient.
(5) Convert a bipolar to a unipolar system.
(6) Replace the battery pack.

Electrical Complications

Electrical leakage from line-powered (AC-60 cycle) equipment occurs when equipment comes in contact with the myocardial pacing lead. This is always a threat when electrodes transverse the skin, and may lead to ventricular fibrillation. Precautions include: remove any equipment that causes tingling sensations; ground all equipment; wear rubber gloves to adjust a temporary pacemaker's electrodes; use battery-powered pacemakers with myocardial electrodes; connect the intracavitary lead to the V lead of the electrocardiogram machine.

Depending upon the type of pacemaker, there may be a wide range of sensitivity to electrical fields. Strong alternating currents or magnetic fields can convert a demand to a fixed-rate pacemaker. Low conducted currents and magnetic fields can cause a lower than normal stimulation rate or complete inhibition.

KEY CONCEPT: Pacemakers are energy-emitting, artificial devices that produce artifacts known as spikes on electrocardiograms. Electrodes are either unipolar or bipolar. Pacemakers may be temporary or permanent depending on patient need.

SURGICAL INTERVENTION

Surgery for valvular disease: The most common valve to be replaced is the mitral valve. Rheumatic stenosis, mitral insufficiency and regurgitation often require replacement. Aortic stenosis and aortic regurgitation due to dissection of the aorta (Marfans syndrome) require aortic valve replacement.

Surgery for coronary artery disease: Both partial and complete coronary obstruction from atherosclerotic placques require direct revascularization or coronary artery bypass.

Precipitating factors that lead to cardiac surgery include acute myocardial infarction, congestive heart failure, rheumatic fever, syphilis and congenital anomalies.

Clinical symptoms differ with each anomaly. Mitral valve disease presents with dyspnea on exertion, orthopnea, paroxysmal nocturnal dyspnea, easy fatigability and peripheral edema. Deterioration is slow and gradual. Aortic valve disease presents with external dyspnea, angina, fainting spells and syncopal episodes. It occurs rapidly. Sudden death is not uncommon.

Nursing Care

The major nursing responsibilities include the following:

(1) Establish and maintain a patent airway and adequate ventilation. Prevent pneumonia, atelectasis, embolism, pulmonary edema and pneumothorax.

(2) Watch for the development of arrhythmias; treat it aggressively. Common arrhythmias include supraventricular rhythms (especially after mitral valve), congenital defects and coronary artery surgery. Nodal rhythms and block frequently occur with aortic valve and ventricular septal defect repairs. Ventricular irritability occurs with coronary artery surgery.

(3) Differentiate tamponade from myocardial dysfunction of a low cardiac output. Distinguishing signs include: sudden decrease in chest tube drainage, narrowing pulse pressure, widened mediastinum on chest radiograph without signs of failure and pulsus paradoxus.

(4) Observe for low cardiac output states that prevent the heart from maintaining adequate output as a result of anesthesia, hypoxemia and medication. The treatment includes drugs to improve contractility, increase preload and reduce afterload.

(5) Coagulation problems may cause bleeding following cardiopulmonary bypass surgery. Other causes include heparin rebound, decreased clotting factors and depressed function of platelets. A causative factor often overlooked is medications such as Coumadin or aspirin taken preoperatively. Intravascular coagulation may occur in a patient with multiple postoperative complications disseminated.

(6) Maintain acid-base balance. Observe ABGs for imbalances.

(7) Maintain renal perfusion. Observe urinary output for volume (at least 30 cc/hr) and concentration.

(8) Maintain and accurately measure fluid and electrolyte balance. Observe for signs of electrolyte imbalance, especially K, which is lost from damaged red cells during surgery.

(9) Provide emotional support to the patient and family.

KEY CONCEPT: Surgical intervention is dependent upon the pathology present. Nursing care is extremely tailored to the surgical intervention.

Vascular Surgery

Carotid occlusive disease is described as an extracranial blood supply by two internal carotid arteries and two vertebral arteries-basilar. These patients tend to have atherosclerotic lesions that progress to thrombus formation on an ulcerated area.

This can be diagnosed symptomatically by a bruit or thrill over the carotids, and four-vessel angiography to include the aortic area internal carotids and vertebrals.

The surgical procedure is a carotid endarterectomy. Intraoperative risks include stroke and MI, making it imperative to maintain the blood pressure, cardiac output and adequate oxygenation.

A major complication postoperatively is decreased cerebral function from micro emboli. Approximately 10 percent of the patients suffer from severe hypertension. Arrhythmias are a common complication. Hematomas may occur due to leaks.

In *occlusive disease* of the terminal aorta and iliac, the patient usually presents with symptoms of claudication in the thigh and hip areas, and decreased or absent femoral pulses. The male patient may be impotent. This disease type is usually diagnosed by arteriography.

The corrective surgery commonly performed is aorto-iliac thromboendarterectomy or bypass. A good preoperative evaluation is essential. With early thrombosis, poor outflow and hypotension leading to MI or hypovolemia is noted. If hemorrhage occurs, surgical intervention will be necessary.

Postoperative complications may include placques that lead to an embolus. Aneurysm at the suture line and ureteral obstruction occur less commonly.

The patient with diseases of the femoral and popliteal arteries displays intermittent claudication in the lower leg. This is also diagnosed by arteriography.

Indications for surgery are pain at rest, alteration of lifestyle and potential gangrenous or frank gangrene state.

Some operative problems may include placques which lead to emboli and an incompetent popliteal vein, which results in a reduction of venous return.

Postoperative Complications

Thrombosis may occur in aortoiliac because of poor outflow, and in femoral popliteal due to poor distal runoff. Hypotension from decreased volume may lead to an MI. The loss of the limb may be an early complication.

Infection is the most serious complication. False aneurysms may also occur.

Aneurysm

An aneurysm is a dilatation or ballooning of the vessel, which results in weakness of the vessel wall. Hypertension and a continuous pulsatile pressure lead to dilatation, thinning of the vessel wall and eventual rupture. The types of aneurysms are:

True: This type involves all layers of the arterial wall. It is usually saccular, arising from a distinct portion of the wall, and possesses a "mouth and neck." An "outpocketing" effect also describes a true aneurysm. Survival rate is approximately 90 percent.

Fusiform: Another type of true aneurysm is fusiform. It involves the total circumference of the artery with diffuse dilatation. Abdominal aneurysms and thoracic aneurysms are true aneurysms. An abdominal aneurysm is a weaking in the vessel wall in the presence of hypertension or a normal blood pressure with an increased pulse wave. Arteriosclerosis, trauma, Marfan's syndrome, infection, syphillis and cystic medial necrosis, also cause true aneurysms.

Clinically, they may be asymptomatic, and may be found during a routine physical examination by discovering a pulsatile abdominal mass.

Symptoms may vary greatly, from vague epigastric discomfort to excruciating pain. Severe pain in the back or flanks which radiates into the testicles may indicate leakage or rupture.

If leakage and rupture occur, look for usual signs of blood loss and sudden vascular collapse. This emergency requires immediate surgical intervention.

Complications include arrhythmias, respiratory insufficiency, renal failure, pancreatitis, ischemia to the left colon, sepsis and an infected graft (uncommon).

Within one year, 20 percent of all aneurysms will rupture; in five years, 50 percent will rupture. If the patient is asymptomatic and the aneurysm is less than approximately 6 cm, 50 percent will survive without surgery and 7 percent will survive with surgery over a five-year period. If surgery is elective, only a 3 percent mortality is noted.

If the aneurysm is greater than 6 cm, over a five-year period, 5 percent will survive without surgery and 50 percent with surgery. If surgery is elective, 10 to 15 percent mortality rate is noted.

If the patient is symptomatic, it is an acute medical emergency and surgical intervention is indicated. Approximately 80 percent of these aneurysms will rupture within one year.

Common causes of thoracic aneurysms include congenital, arteriosclerotic, syphilitic, dissecting and traumatic. An aortogram is valuable in diagnosis. A widening mediastinum seen on x-ray may confirm the diagnosis.

The typical patient is middle-aged and black, with known hypertension.

Clinical presentation may consist of a sudden excruciating knifelike pain that does not radiate. It usually presents in the anterior chest or between the shoulder blades. The patient may appear "shocky," but the blood pressure is normal or elevated.

Surgical intervention may be required. Complications in 10 to 20 percent of these cases may consist of bleeding.

Prognosis

3 percent die immediately.

60 percent die within two weeks.

90 percent die within three months.

The primary cause of death is usually extension of the dissection, with eventual rupture and death due to hemorrhage and/or tamponade.

Traumatic aneurysm usually occurs during a deceleration injury or blunt trauma. This occurs because the aortic arch is fixed by the great vessels, while the heart and descending thoracic aorta are mobile. A sudden deceleration occurs in the intima, media or entire wall. Prehospital survival depends on the continuity of adventitia.

Diagnosis is determined through history of injury, x-ray and aortogram. 90 percent of these patients die of exsanguination, making this a true emergency. Of the 10 percent surviving, 80 percent die within a month because of delayed rupture.

Nursing Care

Nursing care in vascular surgery aims at maintaining the graft.

(1) Administer medications as ordered.

(2) Maintain blood pressure.

(3) Observe color and temperature of extremities.

(4) Prevent emboli by using anti-emboli techniques.

(5) Check pulses bilaterally distal to site.

(6) Do not allow the patient to bend the knees.

(7) IPPB is contraindicated for 48 hours following carotid endarterectomy.

KEY CONCEPT: Complications of vascular surgery include clotting of grafts with loss of extremity, bleeding from graft site, hypertension, infection and cerebrovascular accident. Nursing care aims at maintaining vessels or grafts by close observation and assessment.

KEY POINT RECOGNITION

Write true or false by each statement. Answers are at the end of this chapter. A score below 80% indicates the need for further study.

_____ 1. Arterosclerosis is an acute condition, causing vessel wall thickening.

_____ 2. In atherosclerosis, the tunica intima becomes thickened, resulting in partial or total obstruction of the lumen.

_____ 3. In medial sclerosis, there is narrowing of the lumen due to calcification and hypertrophy of the vessel.

_____ 4. Conditions resulting from arteriosclerosis are angina pectoris and congestive heart failure.

_____ 5. There is no preceding symptom of arteriosclerosis.

_____ 6. Nursing care for arteriosclerosis involves teaching the patient about the disease process.

_____ 7. Anemia and thyrotoxicosis may cause angina pectoris.

_____ 8. Angina results in anoxia to myocardial tissue.

_____ 9. In angina, functional ability is permanently lost.

_____ 10. Overeating, emotional stress and overexercising may precipitate angina.

_____ 11. Anginal pain is always described as retrosternal and squeezing in nature.

_____ 12. There is no diagnostic aid for determining angina.

_____ 13. Preinfarction or unstable angina is a common indicator of an impending infarction.

_____ 14. A patient with crescendo angina complains of pain at rest or pain worsening over a period of days.

_____ 15. Myocardial infarction is an incomplete occlusion of an artery, causing myocardial ischemia.

_____ 16. Emboli, trauma and complications of collagen diseases cause myocardial infarction.

_____ 17. The patient experiencing a myocardial infarction always complains of pain lasting longer than two hours.

_____ 18. Pain caused by myocardial infarction is relieved by rest, oxygen or nitrates.

_____ 19. The diagnostic data for a myocardial infarction reveals decreased sedimentation rate and elevated cardiac enzymes.

_____ 20. Changes in the electrocardiogram are the only evidence that a myocardial infarction has occurred.

_____ 21. ST and T wave changes only occur in myocardial infarction.

_____ 22. Development of Q waves and an alteration in R wave voltage morphology are diagnostic changes indicating a myocardial infarction.

_____ 23. The most serious complication of a myocardial infarction is dysrhythmia occurrence.

_____ 24. An acute exacerbation of congestive heart failure may occur with a myocardial infarction.

_____ 25. Potential causes of dysrhythmias are hypotension, hypoxia and increased automaticity of the heart.

_____ 26. Anticoagulants reduce or prevent an infarction.

_____ 27. Early recognition of complications associated with myocardial infarctions reduce the mortality rate.

_____ 28. Pacemakers consist of a pulse generator and a battery.

_____ 29. In a bipolar lead setup, one lead is placed on the anterior surface of the heart and the other is located outside the body.

_____30. The patient with chronic heart dysfunction needs a temporary pacemaker.

_____31. Temporary pacemakers are only inserted using the transvenous endocardial technique.

_____32. Stokes-Adams syndrome is a serious condition caused by a disturbance in the heart's electrical system.

_____33. A temporary pacemaker may be inserted prior to or during implantation of a permanent pacemaker.

_____34. Atrial pacing may be used during stress testing in patients with coronary artery disease.

_____35. The nurse must record rate, site, settings and type of pacer and the patient's tolerance to the procedure.

_____36. Rubber gloves should be worn when converting or disconnecting the battery pack or terminals.

_____37. Following pacemaker insertion, serial electrocardiograms reveal rate, rhythm, pacing current, capture and sensing.

_____38. If ventricular fibrillation occurs while the temporary pacemaker is on, immediately turn the pacemaker up.

_____39. Permanent pacemakers are generally used for long-term treatment of asymptomatic acute heart block.

_____40. The best method for the poor surgical risk requiring a permanent pacemaker is the transvenous endocardial technique.

_____41. Transvenous endocardial pacing has no complications.

_____42. Transvenous endocardial pacing of the right ventricle produces a right bundle branch block pattern.

_____43. If bradycardia or failure of the idioventricular pacer occurs, there will be a profound decrease in cardiac output and central nervous system hypoxia.

_____44. Catheter wire stiffness may produce myocardial injury or irritability, resulting in premature ventricular contractions.

_____45. Microwave ovens, cautery instruments and tool demagnetizers may interfere with the pacemaker's function.

_____46. A fixed-rate pacemaker fires at a set rate and does not respond to alterations in physiologic needs.

_____47. Fixed-rate pacemakers depend on the intrinsic activity of the heart.

_____48. Atrial pacemakers reduce the danger of ventricular competition by providing the atrial kick of a normal contraction.

_____49. P wave or demand atrial pacemakers sense atrial depolarization and inhibit the stimulus.

_____50. A QRS-inhibited atrial pacemaker fires during natural formation of the P wave.

_____51. A fixed-rate pacer delivers continuous stimuli to the ventricles.

_____52. A demand QRS-inhibited ventricular pacemaker stimulates and senses through an atrial electrode at a preset rate.

_____53. A demand QRS-triggered ventricular pacemaker delivers the stimulus during the natural formation of the QRS complex.

_____54. A demand QRS-triggered ventricular pacemaker stimulus closely resembles the morphology of the inherent beat.

_____55. P wave-triggered ventricular pacemakers increase competition.

_____56. AV-sequential or bifocal demand pacemakers automatically adapt to the patient's needs and preserve the natural sequence of depolarization.

_____57. Pacemaker complications include malfunction and electrical leakage.

_____58. Failure to capture or stimulate a pacer artifact may indicate low voltage, faulty connections, improper catheter position or broken catheter wire.

_____59. Pacemaker competition in a patient with a myocardial infarction may lead to ventricular fibrillation or ventricular tachycardia.

_____60. Leakage from line-powered equipment will never have an effect on a pacemaker.

_____61. Congestive heart failure involves only the left side of the heart.

_____62. Left-sided heart failure is a direct result of increase in lung pressure.

_____63. The most common presenting symptom of congestive heart failure is dyspnea.

_____64. Pulmonary edema develops as a result of congestive heart failure because of rapidly rising pulmonary pressure.

_____65. Cor pulmonale, pulmonary valve stenosis and atrial-septal defects may cause right-sided heart failure.

_____66. The major nursing responsibilities in caring for a patient with congestive heart failure are airway management and prevention of further deterioration.

_____67. Bacterial agents are the only cause of pericarditis.

_____68. Procainamide, hydralazine and diphenylhydantoin administration may cause pericarditis.

_____69. S_2, pulsus paradoxus and friction rub are specific clinical indicators of pericarditis.

_____70. Hypertension occurs from a rise in cardiac output or a rise in systemic vascular resistance.

_____71. Release of renin and angiotensin is the only cause of hypertensive crisis.

_____72. Precipitating factors causing hypertensive crisis include toxemia, polycythemia and pituitary tumors.

_____73. A symptom of malignant hypertensive crisis is a diastolic pressure greater than 150 mm Hg.

_____74. Poor tissue perfusion characterizes shock.

_____75. Failure of compensatory mechanisms to activate during shock leads to aerobic metabolism.

_____76. Baroreceptor response increases peripheral resistance by stimulating vasoconstriction.

_____77. A decrease between intravascular volume and vascular capacitance causes hypovolemic shock.

_____78. Causes of hypovolemic shock may be hemorrhage, vomiting or diarrhea.

_____79. Hyperdynamic septic shock creates a low cardiac output state.

_____80. Damage to or chemical blockage of the sympathetic nervous system causes neurogenic shock.

_____81. Adult respiratory distress syndrome affects the capillary bed of the lungs by decreased blood flow resistance, intracellular edema and hypoxia.

_____82. In shock states, thrombosis of minute vessels may form from a sluggish blood flow.

_____83. Thrombocytopenia, leukocytosis, abnormal prothrombin time and partial prothrombin time may indicate septic shock.

_____84. Vascular disease may cause accumulation of plaque in the vessel walls, which partially or completely occludes the lumen.

_____85. Mitral valve disease displays dyspnea on exertion, orthopnea, paroxysmal noctural dyspnea, easy fatigability and peripheral edema.

_____86. Aortic valve disease displays the same symptoms as mitral valve disease.

CARE COMMON TO CARDIOVASCULAR PROBLEMS

CARDIAC CIRCULATION

Changes in vital signs, neurological status or electrocardiographic pattern are the most sensitive signs of changes in the cardiovascular system. Cardiac pressure changes may develop and reflect in the pulmonary artery pressure, pulmonary capillary wedge pressure, cardiac output, and central venous pressure. Subjective signs include changes in pulse rate, rhythm and quality; jugular vein distention; confusion; cyanosis and dysrhythmias.

HEMODYNAMICS: MONITORING AND ADJUNCTS

Types of hemodynamic monitoring are:

Central Venous Pressure

A catheter is inserted in the superior vena cava or right atrium, usually via the subclavian vein. This measures the central venous pressure, which reflects right heart function. Complications of this procedure include thrombophlebitis, endocarditis and obstruction of flow because of clot formation and inaccurate readings.

Pulmonary Artery Wedge Pressure Monitoring

A catheter is placed in the pulmonary artery, usually via the subclavian vein. This measures pulmonary artery pressure and PCWP, which may reflect left ventricular function. This type of monitoring has a higher risk of infection, ventricular irritability, electrically-induced ventricular fibrillation, pulmonary hemorrhage, pulmonary infarction and thrombi formation.

Intra-Aortic Balloon Pump (IABP)

The IABP is an adjunctive device inserted surgically or percutaneously into the aorta to reduce afterload, reduce myocardial oxygen consumption and increase coronary perfusion. Ultimately, the IABP reduces the work of the left ventricle by decreasing systemic resistance to ventricular systole. It also augments diastole, increasing coronary artery perfusion. The balloon is deflated prior to the opening of the aortic valve. Deflation of the balloon lessens aortic pressure and blood rushes out with ease during ventricular systole. The balloon inflates during diastole, increases aortic pressures and forces blood through the coronary arteries.

The IABP is indicated in the following conditions: cardiogenic shock secondary to myocardial infarction, cardiopulmonary bypass surgery, intractable angina pectoris, intractable left ventricular failure and low cardiac output states such as burns and major trauma.

Criteria for the use of the IABP in cardiogenic shock includes:
(1) Diagnosis of myocardial infarction, with low cardiac output
(2) Systolic arterial pressure below 80 mm Hg
(3) Pulmonary capillary wedge pressure or diastolic pulmonary artery pressure greater than 18 mm Hg
(4) Apical pulse rate greater than 100 bpm
(5) Decreased cardiac output with poor peripheral perfusion
(6) Cerebral impairment or decreased urinary output
(7) Unresponsiveness to drug management

Criteria for IABP after cardiac surgery includes:
(1) Inability to wean from bypass within 30 minutes

(2) Persistent vasopressor dependence or decreased cardiac output with hypotension

(3) Left ventricular end diastolic pressure greater than 20 mm Hg after ineffective drug therapy

Contraindications for the IABP include aortic aneurysm, aortic insufficiency, irreversible brain damage, severely sclerotic iliac and femoral arteries, and patients who cannot receive heparin.

Complications associated with IABP include clotting of the femoral artery; ischemia of the foot distal to the balloon insertion site; inguinal wound infection; renal failure; trauma to the aorta, iliac or femoral arteries; thrombocytopenia; azotemia or palsy.

The hemodynamic effects of balloon pumping are:

(1) Marked increase in diastolic pressure coupled with a marked decrease in presystolic pressure

(2) Decreased pulmonary capillary wedge pressure with increased mean aortic pressure, thus improving cardiac output

(3) Increased coronary artery blood flow with maintenance of peripheral perfusion

Nursing Care

Nursing interventions include:

(1) Keep the head of the bed below 45 degrees.

(2) Evaluate pulses, temperature, skin color and vital signs hourly.

(3) Prevent leg flexion at the groin.

(4) Inspect balloon catheter for signs of kinking, cracking, disconnection or blood in tubing (ruptured balloon).

Humidified oxygen, reducing anxiety, restful environment and prevention of bowel straining further decrease the heart's workload.

When caring for the patient with hemodynamic monitoring equipment at the bedside, the nurse must be familiar with waveforms. Size and shape of pressure waves depend on the part of the arterial tree from which the wave is obtained. For example, as the aortic valve closes at the end of systole, a sharp pressure drop occurs. This is displayed on the descending limb of the pressure curve as a notch, the dicrotic notch. As the aortic valve closes, an upward deflection is observed. As the wave moves to the periphery, the ascending portion of the wave becomes steeper. And as systolic pressure rises and the AV valves open, a notch is again observed, the anacrotic notch.

Systolic pressure in peripheral arteries may range up to 40 mm Hg higher, and diastolic pressure may range up to 20 mm Hg lower than in the proximal aorta. When blood is ejected into the aorta, a rapidly moving wave occurs as it moves toward the periphery. It may move as much as 15 times faster than the actual blood flow. The velocity of a pressure wave along the aorta is approximately 5 meters/second. On reaching the periphery, it may increase as much as 35 meters/second or about 100 times faster than the actual blood flow.

This factor can be responsible for peaking of waveforms, which may be called "overshoot."

Waveforms on a monitor do not always look like textbook waveforms. By thinking in terms of heart rate and comparing waveforms to the EKG waves, the difference in forms is easier to understand. As the rate increases, the P and T tend to merge and make specific diagnosis difficult. A similar phenomenon happens to the waveform. It becomes steeper and narrower as the heart rate increases. As the heart rate slows, the P and T separate and become easier to identify. The waveform is also likely to become wider and smoother with a slower rate.

Know your monitor detection capabilities. Some manufacturers with fixed-sized waveforms have "filtered" the waveform to make it look more "textbook." Using an adjunctive filtering device may be disastrous with this type of monitor. Other manufacturers have flexible scopes which produce diagnostic (unfiltered) waveforms. Of this type, most have filtered digits and unfiltered recorders, which usually means "overshoot" is present on the scope. The waveform appears peaked. Pressures read quickly from the scope appear higher. Pressures should be read from calibrated scopes or recorders. It is the consecutive readings which are pertinent. Readings from scope to digits may provide the nurse with incorrect information. Be consistent in order to reflect the patient's response to therapy.

Each waveform is individual to the patient being monitored. Medications, increased vascular tone, hypothermia and artifacts may cause variations in the waveform. Evaluate each patient's waveform to determine actual systolic and diastolic values for that particular patient.

From a calibrated scope, a rule of thumb is, "The scope pressure is higher than digital readings (because of filtering), and digits are higher than cuff pressure (because of quality of vessels, stethoscope, clinician, etc.)."

If the cuff pressure is higher than the digits, the problem is usually in the setup. The monitor is only as good as the clinician using it!

Arterial Waveforms

True waveform (Fig. 5-65)
Damped waveform (Fig. 5-65)
Systolic overshoot (Fig. 5-65)

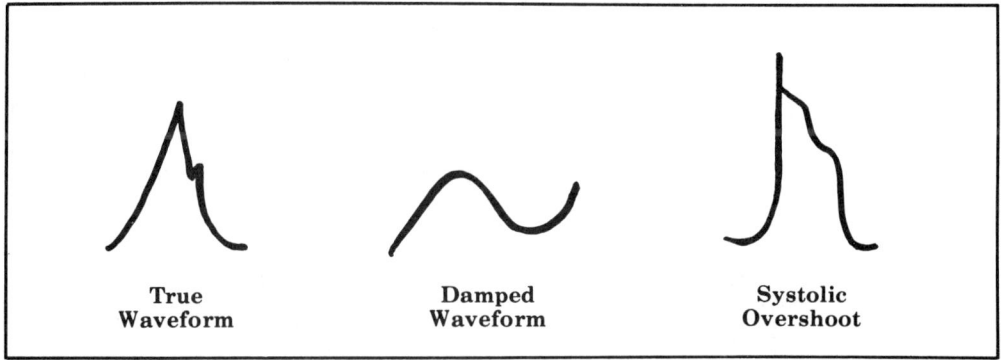

Fig. 5-65. Waveforms

Pulsus Alternans—Every other waveform alternates in amplitude. Rhythm must be regular (Fig. 5-66).

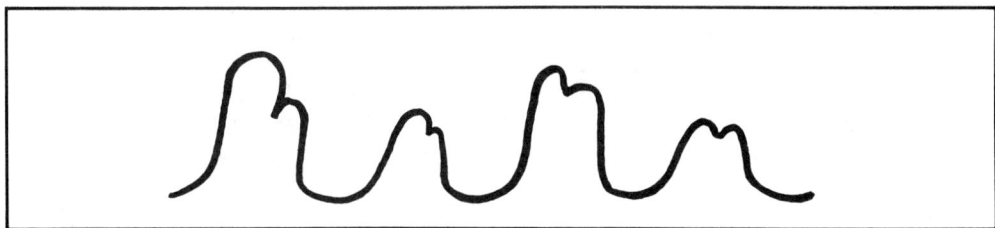

Fig. 5-66. Pulsus alternans

Bigeminal pulse—waveforms of alternating rhythm; irregular rhythm (Fig. 5-67)

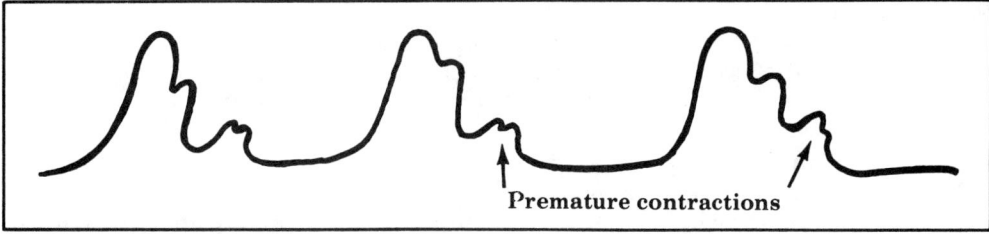

Fig. 5-67. Bigeminal pulse

Pulsus paradoxus—pulse diminishes in amplitude on inspiration (Fig. 5-68)

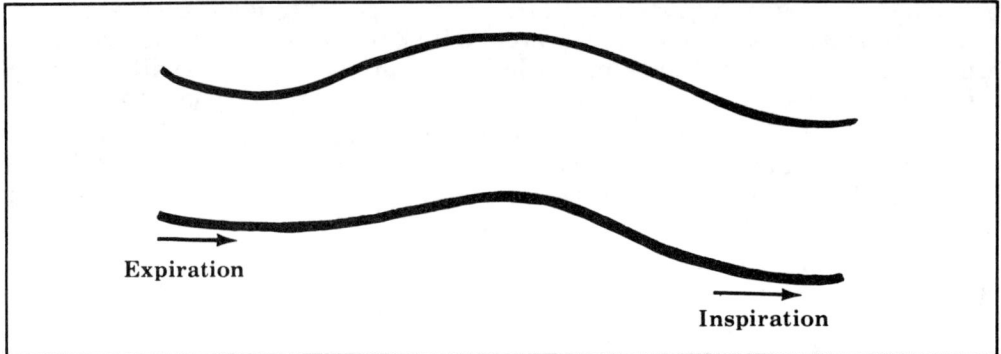

Fig. 5-68. Pulsus paradoxus

Water-hammer pulse—an extremely high, strong, bounding pressure which almost completely collapses during diastole (Fig. 5-69)

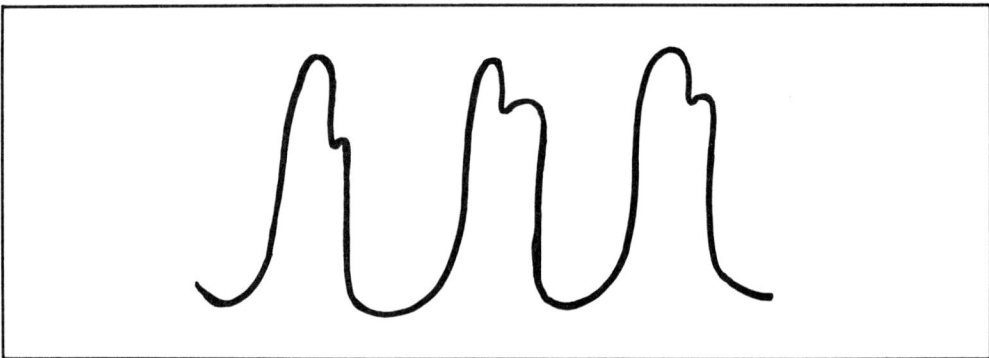

Fig. 5-69. Water-hammer pulse

Peripheral Circulation

Sufficient peripheral circulation can be measured by color, temperature and pulses of the extremities. Passive and active range-of-motion, deep breathing and anticoagulant therapy promotes peripheral circulation.

Maintenance of Fluid and Electrolyte Balance

Many factors influence electrolyte balance. Conditions that cause an imbalance include nausea, vomiting, and retention of sodium and water. Monitoring of fluid and electrolyte balance includes proper administration of intravenous solutions, accurate record of intake and output, assessment of renal ability, assessment of laboratory data, observation for edema, skin turgor and weight changes.

Provide Rest: Emotional and Physical

Promote rest by planning for periods of rest, providing for pain relief, observing facial expressions for pain, and providing emotional support to both the patient and family. Plan for and provide patient teaching.

Prevent Infection

Prevent infection by observing for signs of infection, culturing catheter tips, administering antibiotics, using aseptic techniques, changing position, observing urinary output and reporting abnormal laboratory findings.

Maintain Nutrition

Maintain nutritional status by providing a diet sufficient to meet the needs of the body. The diet may be low caloric, sodium restricted or cholesterol restricted.

Rehabilitate

Patient rehabilitation includes allowing the patient to participate in routine care when possible, as well as preparing for discharge from the critical care setting. Use an individualized nursing care plan to plan for and coordinate all aspects of care, including discharge and social service referrals.

KEY CONCEPT: Continuous assessment for changes is essential to the management of cardiovascular problems.

KEY POINT RECOGNITION

Write true or false by each statement. Answers are at the end of this chapter. A score below 80% indicates the need for further study.

　　　　1. Changes in the vital signs and electrocardiographic patterns may indicate cardiovascular problems.

　　　　2. A central venous pressure catheter is inserted into the left ventricle.

　　　　3. Pulmonary artery pressure reading reflects left ventricular function.

　　　　4. The intra-aortic balloon pump increases afterload.

　　　　5. An anxious state causes an increase in the workload of the heart.

PASS
Program Assessment: Science and Situation

1. The phrase "less than .20 second" best describes the following:
   a. abnormal P-R interval
   b. normal QRS interval
   c. normal Q-T interval
   d. normal P-R interval
   e. abnormal QRS interval

2. The physiological pacemaker of the heart describes the
   a. AV node.
   b. SA node.
   c. bundle of His.
   d. Purkinje's fibers.
   e. bundle of Kent.

3. The artery that carries unoxygenated blood is the
   a. aorta.
   b. radial.
   c. pulmonary.
   d. brachial.
   e. femoral.

4. An EKG strip displays a ventricular rate of 30 to 40 bpm, a regular rhythm, a regular P-P, a P-R interval that is not constant, an atrial rate of 70. You are most likely looking at which of the following?
   a. idioventricular rhythm
   b. complete heart block
   c. Mobitz I
   d. Mobitz II
   e. first degree block

5. The heart rate is 150 to 300 uncoordinated beats per minute. Rhythm is very irregular, P waves may be present, but are unrecognizable. No P-R interval exists; QRS complexes are absent. Multiple ectopic pacemaker sites produce waves of varying amplitude and shapes. You are most likely looking at an EKG strip of
   a. idioventricular rhythm.
   b. atrial fibrillation.
   c. ventricular fibrillation.
   d. "dying heart."

6. Distended jugular veins in an upright position are a probable indication of
   a. low blood pressure.
   b. left heart failure.
   c. right heart failure.
   d. intraseptal rupture.
   e. hypertension.

7. To obtain cardiac output, which of the following equations should be used?
    a. C.O. = SV + HR
    b. C.O. = SV x HR
    c. C.O. = SV - HR
    d. C.O. = SV + HR - BP
    e. C.O. = HR + BP - SV

8. With regard to blood pressure, cardiac tamponade would clinically manifest itself in which of the following ways?
    a. increased systolic; decreased diastolic
    b. increased diastolic; increased systolic
    c. decreased diastolic; decreased systolic
    d. increased diastolic; decreased systolic

9. The pharmacological treatment of choice for rate-dependent PVCs would be which of the following?
    a. lidocaine 50 to 100 gm I.V.P.
    b. lidocaine 1 to 2 mg in 500 cc 5% D/W
    c. atropine .5 gm I.V.P. x 2
    d. atropine .5 mg I.V.P. x 2

10. The coronary arteries fill during
    a. atrial contraction.
    b. systole.
    c. formation of the P wave.
    d. diastole.

11. The coronary circulation has a rather unique ability to compensate for blocked or damaged vessels, helping the heart to mend itself. This feature is known as
    a. unilateral circulation.
    b. bilateral circulation.
    c. collateral circulation.
    d. trilateral circulation.

12. Electrical cardioversion may be dangerous in the presence of which of the following drugs?
    a. Lasix
    b. digitalis
    c. Valium
    d. morphine

13. In a patient with an acute myocardial infarct who is having PVCs, which of the following would be a cause for concern (treatment)?
    a. two or more consecutive PVCs
    2. PVCs coming close to the preceding QRS complex
    3. Multifocal PVCs
    4. 10 PVCs per minute
    5. salvos
    a. 1, 4, 5
    b. 1, 2, 5
    c. 1, 2, 3, 5

d. 1, 2, 4, 5
e. 1, 2, 3, 4, 5

14. The rhythm below is an indication of
    a. complete heart block.
    b. idioventricular rhythm.
    c. nodal rhythm.
    d. sinus bradycardia.

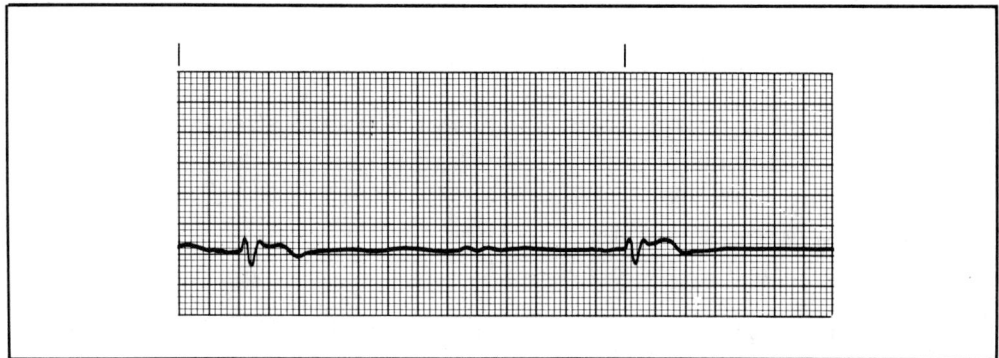

15. On seeing the above strip on your monitor, you should first
    a. check a pulse and initiate CPR, if necessary.
    b. administer atropine .5 mg I.V.
    c. administer Isuprel 1 mg I.V.
    d. give M.S. 5 mg, oxygen.

16. A cause of sinus block is
    a. irritability of atrial tissue.
    b. digitalis intoxication.
    c. increased metabolic demand.
    d. irritability of AV nodal tissue.

17. For sinus bradycardia, the treatment of choice would be which of the following?
    a. atropine
    b. epinephrine
    c. observe the patient and treat symptomatically
    d. Isuprel

18. Irritable AV nodal tissue is a cause of
    a. supraventricular tachycardia.
    b. ventricular fibrillation.
    c. atrial fibrillation.
    d. premature junctional contraction.

19. The treatment for atrial fibrillation can include all of the following *except*
    a. lidocaine.
    b. digitalis.
    c. quinidine.
    d. cardioversion.

20. Which of the following phrases best describes shock?
    a. the inability of the body to meet its metabolic needs
    b. the collapse of the central nervous system
    c. the inability of the body to excrete waste products
    d. the collapse of the respiratory system

21. The most common cause of cardiogenic shock is
    a. failure of the heart.
    b. failure of the lungs.
    c. failure of the brain.
    d. failure of the kidney.

22. Stimulation of the parasympathetic nervous system affects the heart by
    a. increasing the heart rate.
    b. increasing contractility.
    c. decreasing the heart rate.
    d. It has no effect on the heart rate.

23. Ventricular systole best refers to which of the following?
    a. relaxation
    b. contraction
    c. filling
    d. pressure

24. The pain associated with an MI can best be described as
    a. pressure lasting longer than 20 minutes; fear of death.
    b. pressure lasting less than 20 minutes; relieved with NTG.
    c. relieved with NTG, rest and oxygen; fear of death.
    d. nonradiating pain, low in intensity; fear of death.

25. There are two major classifications for angina. The predictable angina is referred to as
    a. postinfarction.
    b. unstable.
    c. stable.
    d. preinfarction.
    e. hiatus.

26. Of the following pathological states, which is due to mechanical failure of the heart?
    a. arteriosclerosis
    b. congestive heart failure
    c. angina
    d. myocardial infarction

27. In the presence of ventricular fibrillation, ineffective countershock attempts might be caused by
    a. presence of metabolic acidosis.
    b. ventricular irritability.
    c. inadequate oxygenation.
    d. all of the above

28. Asystole represents the lack of electrical and mechanical activity in the heart. The initial treatment should consist of
    a. CPR.
    b. defibrillation.
    c. calcium chloride.
    d. sodium bicarbonate.

29. The electrical events in the cardiac cycle are referred to as the action potential. The absolute refractory period (ARP) refers to
    a. the time in the cycle when the muscle will not respond to any stimuli.
    b. the time in the cycle when the muscle will respond to minimal stimuli.
    c. the time in the cycle when the muscle will respond to strong stimuli.
    d. none of the above

30. The circumflex artery branches off the
    a. right coronary artery.
    b. left coronary artery.
    c. pulmonary artery.
    d. aorta.

31. Inderal (propranolol) is contraindicated in which of the following?
    1. hypotension
    2. asthma
    3. cardiogenic shock
    4. sinus bradycardia with a first degree block
    5. right heart failure due to pulmonary hypertension
    a. 1, 2
    b. 2, 5
    c. 1, 2, 5
    d. 1, 3, 4
    e. 1, 2, 3, 4, 5

32. A patient is most likely to rupture a necrotic area following MI
    a. within the first two hours.
    b. within 24 hours.
    c. within the first week.
    d. after the second week.

33. On teaching a cardiac patient how to take nitroglycerin at home, which of the following points are pertinent?
    1. Take it in a sitting or lying position.
    2. Acquire a new supply approximately every three months.
    3. Remove cotton from the container, as it absorbs the drug.
    4. Store it in a cool, dark place.
    5. Avoid taking it with alcohol.
    a. 1, 4
    b. 1, 4, 5
    c. 1, 2, 4
    d. 1, 2, 4, 5
    e. all of the above

34. On a standard 12-lead EKG, a Q wave is prominent in 2, 3 and aVF. Where is the area of the infarct?
    a. posterior
    b. anterior
    c. inferior
    d. septal
    e. lateral

35. An EKG change that would indicate right or left atrial enlargement would be
    a. positive P waves.
    b. bifasic P waves.
    c. prolonged P-R intervals.
    d. widened QRS complexes.

36. Which of the following may be complications of pulmonary catheters?
    1. infection
    2. intracardiac knotting
    3. pulmonary emboli
    4. pulmonary infarction
    5. wedging of the catheter with balloon deflation
    a. 1, 4
    b. 1, 3, 4
    c. 1, 2, 4
    d. 1, 3, 4, 5
    e. all of the above

37. An intracardiac injection should be given in which chamber?
    a. right atrium
    b. left atrium
    c. right ventricle
    d. left ventricle

38. Blunt trauma to the left side of the chest would result in injury to which chamber of the heart?
    a. left atrium
    b. left ventricle
    c. right atrium
    d. right ventricle

39. If blunt trauma is delivered to the right side of the chest, the most common arrhythmias to be expected would be
    a. atrial.
    b. nodal.
    c. ventricular.
    d. There would be no effect on rhythm.

40. In the heart, the anatomical location for the SA node is
    a. anterior and superior in the left atrium.
    b. posterior and lateral in the right atrium.
    c. anterior and superior in the right atrium.
    d. anterior and superior in the right ventricle.

41. Which area of the heart depolarizes the fastest?
    a. septum—left to right
    b. septum—right to left
    c. septum—top to bottom
    d. septum—bottom to top

42. Other than ventricular rhythms, the most significant arrhythmias seen in an MI are
    a. sinus.
    b. atrial.
    c. blocks.
    d. tachycardias.

43. Mobitz II is considered to be what type of rhythm?
    a. first degree block
    b. second degree block
    c. third degree block
    d. complete heart block

44. Which of the following signs and symptoms are not associated with atrial fibrillation?
    a. decreased urine output
    b. complaints of weakness
    c. complaints of palpitations
    d. irregularly irregular pulse
    e. increased cardiac output

45. Which of the following would you attempt to cardiovert?
    a. paroxysmal atrial tachycardia
    b. sinus tachycardia
    c. complete heart block
    d. Mobitz II

46. Digitalis' effect on the heart is primarily
    a. increased force of contraction; primarily decreased HR.
    b. increased force of contraction; secondarily decreased HR.
    c. decreased force of contraction; increased heart rate.
    d. decreased force of contraction; decreased heart rate.

47. Atrial depolarization on the EKG complex is represented by
    a. P wave.
    b. QRS complex.
    c. T wave.
    d. U wave.

48. Capillary filling adequacy is demonstrated by the Allen test in the absence of
    a. pedal circulation.
    b. ulnar circulation.
    c. tibial circulation.
    d. radial circulation.

49. Administration of oxygen in a myocardial infarction may
    a. enhance the formation of scar tissue.
    b. cause the necrotic area to completely resolve.
    c. prevent the expansion of necrosis.
    d. prevent scar tissue formation.

50. The *major* determinants of myocardial oxygen demands include all of the following except:
    a. heart rate
    b. ventricular wall tension
    c. myocardial contractility
    d. cardiac output

KEY POINT RECOGNITION ANSWERS

Functional and Microscopic Anatomy
1. True
2. True
3. False—The lungs overlie most of the heart's anterior surface.
4. True
5. True
6. False—The pericardium is composed of two layers—the fibrous pericardium and serous pericardium.
7. True
8. False—The space contains 15 to 20 ml of serous fluid.
9. True
10. False—The myocardium is the major muscle mass of the heart.
11. True
12. False—The endocardium is the innermost layer of the heart.
13. False—Cardiac cells differ from skeletal muscle in structure and ability for inherent rhythmicity.
14. True
15. False—Cardiac cells contain more mitochondria than skeletal muscle.
16. True
17. True
18. True
19. False—Sarcoplasmic reticulum is rich in calcium ions.
20. True
21. True
22. True
23. True
24. False—Myosin is thicker than actin.
25. False—I-bands shorten.
26. True
27. True

Coronary Chambers, Valves, Conduction System
1. True
2. True
3. False—In the early phase of ventricular diastole, blood flows passively from the atria to the ventricles.
4. False—When atrial systole is lost in a normal heart, it has minimal effect on cardiac output.
5. True
6. False—The right atrium receives unoxygenated blood from the superior and inferior vena cava and coronary sinus.
7. True
8. False—Each ventricle ejects about 75 ml of blood with each contraction.
9. True
10. True
11. False—The left ventricle is located posteriorly and laterally to the left.
12. True
13. False—Left ventricular pressure is increased in the presence of mitral valve pathology and increased pulmonary vascular resistance.

14. False—The mean pressure is approximately 90 mm Hg.
15. True
16. True
17. True
18. True
19. False—Valve cusps open on ventricular diastole.
20. True
21. False—Semilunar valves open when the ventricle contracts.
22. True
23. False—The SA node lies at the junction of the superior vena cava.
24. True
25. True
26. False—The AV node is continuous with the bundle of His.
27. True
28. True

Circulation
1. True
2. True
3. True
4. True
5. False—The left coronary artery divides into the left anterior descending and left circumflex.
6. True
7. False—The Thebesian veins drain directly into the cardiac chambers.
8. False—Blood flow through capillaries during systole in the left ventricular myocardium falls to low levels.
9. True
10. True
11. True
12. True
13. False—The tunica media layer of the artery is responsible for elasticity and extensibility.
14. True
15. False—Veins are very similar in structure to arteries.
16. False—Many veins have valves.

Electrophysiology
1. True
2. False—Resting membrane potential is determined primarily by potassium.
3. True
4. True
5. True
6. False—Phase 1 of the action potential is influenced by the sodium equilibrium.
7. True
8. True
9. False—Phase 4 of the action potential is not associated with current and ionic flow.
10. True

Nervous Control of the Heart
1. True
2. True
3. True
4. True
5. True
6. True
7. True

Factors Affecting Blood Flow and Pressure
1. True
2. False—Baroreceptors respond to stretching of the vessel walls.
3. True
4. False—It will inhibit sympathetic activity with a resultant drop in heart rate and blood pressure.
5. True
6. False—It results in increased cardiovascular activity.
7. False—CO_2 is a powerful vasoconstrictor.
8. True
9. False—They cause generalized systemic vasoconstriction.
10. True
11. True
12. True
13. True
14. True
15. True

Cardiac Cycle
1. True
2. False—The AV valves close.
3. False—The semilunar valves open and blood is ejected.
4. True
5. True
6. False—Systolic pressure is the peak pressure occurring during the cardiac cycle.
7. True
8. True

Cardiac Output
1. True
2. False—4 to 8 L/minute
3. True
4. False—C.O. = HR x SV
5. False—SV is the amount of blood ejected with each heart beat.
6. True
7. True
8. True
9. True
10. False—Its advantage: no blood samples are needed and it only requires one person at the bedside.

Factors Affecting Cardiac Function and Output
1. False—at the end of diastole
2. True
3. True
4. True
5. False—right heart failure
6. False—CVP is not a good measure of left ventricular preload.
7. True
8. False—onset of pumonary congestion—18 to 20 mm Hg.
9. True
10. True
11. True
12. True
13. False—The IABP reduces O_2 demand, shortens systolic ejection, increases diastole and decreases resistance to forward flow.
14. True
15. False—130 bpm
16. True
17. True
18. True
19. True
20. False—Hypoxia leads to peripheral vasodilation, reducing afterload.

Assessment of the Cardiovascular System
1. True
2. True
3. True
4. True
5. False—A rise of 1 cm or more is indicative of hepatojugular reflex.
6. True
7. True
8. False—A +1 is indicative of a palpable pulse; +2 is normal.
9. True
10. False—Resonance heard over most of the lung fields is indicative of a decrease in density.
11. False—Low frequency vibrations are best heard with the bell of the stethoscope.
12. True

Assessment: Cardiovascular
1. True
2. False—S_1 precedes the carotid pulse.
3. True
4. False—S_2 is high-pitched and shorter than S_1.
5. True
6. False—S_3 is an abnormal ventricular gallop sound.
7. True
8. True
9. False—S_4 is an abnormal atrial gallop sound.
10. True
11. True

12. True
13. True
14. True
15. True
16. True
17. False—Normal partial prothrombin time is 2 to 2½ times the normal.
18. True
19. True
20. False—Apexcardiography determines the displacement of the chest wall by an enlarged left ventricle.
21. False—An electrocardiogram represents the electrical activity of the heart.
22. True
23. False—Bedside monitors are for arrhythmia detection.
24. False—A 4-lead system adds the right leg, but it has no polarity. It is for reference.
25. True
26. True
27. False—Normal P-R interval is .12 to .20 second.
28. False—A Q wave is the first negative deflection after the P wave.
29. True
30. True
31. False—Prolonged ST segment is indicative of hypocalcemia.
32. True
33. True
34. True
35. True
36. True
37. False—The physiological pacemaker of the heart is the SA node.
38. False—NSR has a regular R-R interval and a P-R interval of .12 to 20 seconds.
39. True
40. True
41. False—Premature atrial contraction with block is characterized by early P waves of different morphology, with no QRS complex.
42. False—Paroxysmal atrial tachycardia increases both the heart rate and oxygen consumption.
43. True
44. True
45. False—Atrial flutter is usually a regular rhythm; but if the number of P waves changes, the rhythm becomes irregular.
46. False—Mobitz 1 is an irregular rhythm. There are more P waves than QRS complexes.
47. False—In Mobitz II, some beats are conducted, while other beats are blocked.
48. True
49. True
50. True
51. True
52. True
53. False—Normal systolic pulmonary artery pressure is 20 to 30 mm Hg.

Pathological States and Nursing Management

1. False—Arteriosclerosis is a chronic thickening and hardening of the walls of the arteries.
2. True
3. True
4. True
5. False—Pain is the most common preceding symptom of arteriosclerosis.
6. True
7. True
8. False—Angina causes ischemia of the myocardial tissue.
9. False—The functional ability of the ischemic cell is not permanently lost, and it gradually returns.
10. True
11. False—The description varies and is dependent on the individual.
12. False—An electrocardiogram during the episode of pain reveals ST depression. A positive stress test enables the physician to begin presumptive treatment.
13. False—Preinfarction or unstable angina is not a common indicator of infarction.
14. True
15. False—Myocardial infarction is the complete occlusion of an artery, causing myocardial death.
16. True
17. False—The patient experiencing a myocardial infarction complains of pain lasting longer than 30 minutes.
18. False—A narcotic is indicated for relief of pain.
19. False—To diagnose a myocardial infarction, the diagnostic data reveals an elevation in the serum sedimentation rate, leukocyte count and enzymes.
20. False—Diagnosis of a myocardial infarction is made by history, laboratory data and electrocardiographic changes.
21. False—ST and T wave changes may be altered by medication, ischemia, necrosis and electrolyte levels.
22. True
23. True
24. True
25. True
26. False—Anticoagulants will not reduce or prevent an infarction, but may reduce the formation of emboli.
27. True
28. False—The components of a pacemaker are a pulse generator, lead and electrodes.
29. False—In a bipolar lead system, both leads are placed on the anterior surface of the heart or within the chamber.
30. False—The patient requiring a temporary pacemaker develops a sudden severe dysfunction of the heart.
31. False—Temporary pacemakers may be inserted by transvenous endocardial method, epicardial pacing or emergency pacing directly over the ventricles.
32. True
33. False—It represents ventricular depolarization and repolarization.
34. True
35. True

36. True
37. True
38. False—The temporary pacemaker is turned off and the terminal wires disconnected for defibrillation.
39. False—Permanent pacemakers are generally used in the long-term treatment of symptomatic chronic heart block and congestive heart failure with bradycardia.
40. True
41. False—Complications are catheter displacement, ventricular perforation, diaphragmatic stimulation, air embolism infection and pulmonary embolism.
42. False—Temporary pacing produces a left bundle branch block pattern. Right bundle branch block pattern usually means perforation or displacement of the catheter tip into the coronary sinus.
43. True
44. True
45. True
46. True
47. False—A fixed-rate pacemaker is independent of the intrinsic activity of the heart.
48. True
49. True
50. False—QRS-inhibited atrial pacemakers provide atrial escape beats when the QRS fails to respond at a preset interval.
51. True
52. False—A demand QRS-inhibited ventricular pacemaker stimulates and senses through a ventricular electrode. If a natural contraction is sensed, the pacemaker inhibits formation, eliminating competition. If the heart rate falls, the pacer fires at a preset rate.
53. True
54. False—QRS morphology is distorted.
55. False—P wave-triggered ventricular pacemakers reduce competition by allowing the atria to vary the ventricular rate.
56. True
57. True
58. True
59. True
60. False—Leakage from line-powered equipment coming in contact with a myocardial pacing lead may cause ventricular fibrillation.
61. False—Congestive heart failure may involve the right, left or both sides.
62. False—Right-sided heart failure is a direct result of an increase in lung pressure.
63. True
64. True
65. True
66. True
67. False—Pericarditis may be caused by bacterial, viral or fungal agents.
68. True
69. True
70. True
71. False—Hypertensive crisis may be caused by necrotizing arterioles, release of renin and angiotensin, cerebral edema or cerebral hemorrhage.

72. True
73. False—A symptom of malignant hypertensive crisis is a diastolic pressure greater than 120 mm Hg.
74. True
75. False—Failure of the compensatory mechanism to activate during shock leads to anaerobic metabolism.
76. True
77. True
78. True
79. False—Hyperdynamic septic shock is a normal or increased cardiac output state.
80. True
81. False—Adult respiratory distress syndrome affects the capillary bed of the lungs by increased resistance to blood flow, interstitial pulmonary edema and systemic hypoxia.
82. True
83. True
84. True
85. True
86. False—Aortic valve disease may present with exertional dyspnea, angina, fainting spells and syncopal episodes.

Care Common to Cardiovascular Problems

1. True
2. False—A central venous pressure catheter is inserted into the right ventricle.
3. True
4. False—IABP reduces afterload.
5. True

PASS ANSWER SHEET

1.	d	26.	b
2.	b	27.	d
3.	c	28.	a
4.	b	29.	a
5.	c	30.	b
6.	c	31.	e
7.	b	32.	c
8.	d	33.	e
9.	d	34.	c
10.	d	35.	b
11.	c	36.	e
12.	b	37.	d
13.	e	38.	b
14.	b	39.	a
15.	a	40.	c
16.	b	41.	a
17.	a	42.	c
18.	d	43.	b
19.	a	44.	e
20.	a	45.	a
21.	a	46.	b
22.	c	47.	a
23.	b	48.	d
24.	a	49.	c
25.	c	50.	d

SURVEY SUMMARY
CARDIOVASCULAR SYSTEM

I. **The cardiovascular system: an overview**
   A. The cardiovascular system comprises the heart and blood vessels.
   B. Circulation is divided into the heart, systemic and pulmonic system.
   C. The mechanical function of the heart maintains the blood flow.
   D. The cardiovascular system supplies oxygen and nutrients to body cells, removes waste products and maintains homeostasis.

II. **Anatomy**
   A. The heart is a muscular pump.
      1. It is located within the mediastinal space.
      2. It is bordered laterally by the lungs.
      3. It is bordered inferiorly by the diaphragm.
      4. The apex points downward.
      5. The base is directed upward.
      6. The pericardium encloses the heart and is composed of layers:
         a. *fibrous pericardium*
         b. *serous pericardium*
            1. Parietal
            2. Visceral
      7. The heart is composed of three layers:
         a. *Epicardium*—surface layer
         b. *Myocardium*—major muscle mass
         c. *Endocardium*—innermost layer
   B. Cardiac cells differ from skeletal muscle in structure and ability for rhythmicity.
      1. Individual cells join to form a *syncytium*.
      2. They contain more mitochondria than skeletal muscle.
      3. Cells are covered by *sarcolemma*.
      4. Electrical activity of the cell moves through the *sarcotubular system*.
      5. The contractile unit of the cardiac cell is a *sarcomere*.
         a. The major contractile proteins are *actin* and *myosin*.
         b. Striations form bands.
   C. *Coronary chambers, valves, conduction system*
      1. The heart is divided into right and left halves by the *septum*.
      2. The heart has four chambers:
         a. *Right atrium*
         b. *Left atrium*
         c. *Right ventricle*
         d. *Left ventricle*
      3. Atria accept blood entering the heart.
         a. The right atrium receives unoxygenated blood from the body.
         b. The left atrium receives oxygenated blood from the lungs.
      4. Ventricles are pressurizing chambers.
         a. The right ventricle is a thin-walled musculature.
         b. The left ventricle is thick-walled and is under a high pressure.
      5. Cardiac valves maintain unidirectional flow.
         a. They are classified as:

1. *Atrioventricular*
   a. *Tricuspid*
   b. *Mitral*
2. *Semilunar*
   a. *Pulmonary*
   b. *Aortic*

6. The **conduction system** is the electrical system of the heart.
   a. The properties of the conduction system include:
      1. *Automaticity*
      2. *Rhythmicity*
      3. *Conductivity*
      4. *Excitability*
   b. The conduction pathway includes the:
      1. *SA node*
      2. *Internodal atrial pathways*
      3. *AV node*
      4. *Bundle of His*
      5. *Right and left bundle branches*
      6. *Purkinje's system*

D. *Coronary circulation* is vital to the nourishment of the heart.
   1. The *coronary arteries* include:
      a. *Right coronary artery*
      b. *Left coronary artery*
         1. *Left anterior descending*
         2. *Left circumflex*
   2. Coronary venous drainage is mainly into the coronary sinus.
   3. The heart is richly supplied with lymph tissue.
   4. Arteries are composed of three layers:
      a. *Tunica intima* (inner)
      b. *Tunica media* (middle)
      c. *Tunica externa* (outer)
   5. Arterioles are vital to maintenance of arterial blood pressure.
   6. Capillaries are perfusion vessels.
   7. Veins carry unoxygenated blood to the heart.

III. Physiology
A. *Electrophysiology*
   1. *Resting membrane potential* is the voltage that can be measured across the cell membrane and represents an electrochemical equilibrium.
   2. *Action potential* is the threshold potential.
      a. The five phases are:
         1. 0 = depolarization
         2. 1, 2, 3 = repolarization
         3. 4 = polarization
         4. 5

B. *Nervous control of the heart*
   1. Autonomic innervation is extensive in the heart.
   2. The ANS is divided into two divisions:
      a. *Parasympathetic*

1. Effects: negative chronotropy and dromotropy
2. Produces a cholinergic response
3. Acetylcholine: neurotransmitter
  b. **Sympathetic**
   1. Effects: positive chronotropy, inotropy and dromotropy
   2. Produces an adrenergic response
   3. Norepinephrine: neurotransmitter
C. **Factors affecting blood flow and pressure**
 1. Blood flow is regulated by **nervous control, hormones** and **autoregulation.**
 2. The ANS has a key role in maintaining homeostasis when there has been a massive alteration in circulation.
  a. Specialized sensors effect ANS regulation.
   1. **Pressoreceptors** respond to arterial stretching by inhibition of the vasomotor center.
   2. **Chemoreceptors** are sensitive to changes in arterial oxygen concentration.
  b. Parasympathetic has little effect on blood flow.
 3. The **hormones** epinephrine and norepinephrine cause generalized systemic vasoconstriction and increased heart rate.
 4. **Autoregulation** is a local response to tissue changes and is independent of the ANS.
 5. Blood flow is dependent upon **resistance** and **pressure** gradients.
 6. Blood is distributed according to metabolic needs and is controlled by two means: **extrinsic** and **intrinsic.**
D. The **cardiac cycle** is the time period from the beginning of one heart beat to the beginning of the next.
 1. It lasts 0.8 second.
 2. It involves electrical and mechanical events.
 3. It is divided into two phases:
  a. **Systole**
  b. **Diastole**
E. **Cardiac output** (C.O.) is the amount of blood ejected by the heart per unit of time.
 1. C.O. is 4 to 8 L/minute.
 2. **Cardiac index** is C.O. in relation to body surface area:
  $$CI = \frac{CO}{BSA}$$
 3. C.O. = HR x SV
 4. C.O. is influenced by:
  a. **Arterial blood pressure**
  b. **Heart rate**
  c. **Ventricular distensibility**
  d. **Ventricular filling**
  e. **Myocardial contractile properties**
 5. Three methods to determine C.O. are:
  a. **Fick method**
  b. **Indicator-dilution method**
  c. **Thermodilution method**
F. The main factors affecting **cardiac function** and **output** are:

1. **Preload** (the amount of load on the muscle prior to contraction)
   a. LVEDP represents the preload.
   b. The degree of stretch during diastole (preload) determines the force during systole.
   c. CVP is the amount of pressure in the central systemic veins of the chest. CVP reflects the diastolic pressure of the right ventricle.
      1. Normal CVP is 0 to 5 mm Hg. Most CVPs read with cm H_2O. (1 mm Hg = 1.36 cm H_2O.)
      2. CVP responds to fluid changes.
   d. PCWP is a reflection of left atrial pressure. During diastole, when the mitral valve is open, the PCWP reflects the LVEDP.
2. **Afterload** is the impedence to ejection of blood from the ventricles. Afterload is most significant and a clinical measure of SVR.
3. **Contractility** (muscle function) is an inherent property of cardiac cells.
4. Changing the **heart rate** is the most effective method of altering C.O. Average heart rate = 60 to 100 bpm.
5. In **anemia,** the composition of blood is decreased, thereby decreasing resistance. Hypoxia develops.
6. **Ion concentration** is an important factor in cardiac function.
7. **Hypoxia**

III. **Assessment of the Cardiovascular System**
   A. **Level of consciousness** and **gross cerebral** functioning
      1. Arousability
      2. Orientation
      3. Ability to follow commands
      4. Memory
      5. Orientation
      6. Judgment
   B. **Inspection**
      1. Apparent health
      2. Skin
      3. Nails
      4. Precordial pulsations and PMI
      5. Heaves, thrusts, systolic retractions
      6. Jugular vein distention
   C. **Palpation**
      1. Temperature of skin
      2. Pulses for rate and rhythm
      3. Precordium for thrills, friction rubs and tenderness
      4. Epigastric area for pulsations
   D. **Percussion**
      1. Cardiac silhouette
   E. **Auscultation**
      1. Perform over the underlying valves
      2. Check for **heart sounds**
         a. Normal sounds
            1. S_1
            2. S_2

b. Abnormal sounds
   1. *Fixed splitting*
   2. *Gallops* (abnormal diastolic event: S_3, S_4)
      a. Cadence
         1. Presystolic: *Tennessee*
         2. Diastolic: *Kentucky*
      b. Summation gallops are mid-diastolic and louder than S_1 or S_2.
   3. *Snaps* (opening of AV valve)
   4. *Clicks* (systolic sounds)
   5. *Rubs* (systolic, grating sounds)
   6. *Murmurs* (vibration due to turbulent flow around valve or due to abnormal valvular opening)
      a. Assess murmurs by
         1. Grading
            a. I
            b. II
            c. III
            d. IV
            e. V
            f. VI
         2. Timing
         3. Location
         4. Radiation
         5. Pitch
         6. Intensity
         7. Quality
      b. Murmurs are classified as:
         1. *Systolic*
            a. Ejection
            b. Regurgitant
         2. *Diastolic*
            a. Early
            b. Mid
            c. Late
            d. Pansystolic
         3. *Continuous*

F. *Vital signs*
   1. Blood pressure
   2. Heart rate and quality
   3. Temperature
   4. Respiratory changes
   5. *Specific signs* to check for:
      a. Dysrhythmias
      b. Chest pain
      c. Cyanosis
      d. Palpitations
      e. Dyspnea
      f. Intermittent claudication

G. *Laboratory and special studies*
  1. Cardiac enzymes
     a. CPK—rise within 4 to 6 hours post-MI
     b. LDH
     c. HBD
     d. SGOT—rise within 4 to 6 hours post-MI
  2. Isoenzymes
     a. CPK-MB isoenzyme levels above 3.5% indicate MI
     b. LDH_2 isoenzyme is usually greater than LDH_1
  3. Other studies include:
     a. Lipids
     b. Glucose
     c. CBC
     d. Prothrombin time, PPT
     e. Urinalysis
  4. Noninvasive procedures for cardiac assessment include:
     a. Apex cardiography (displacement of chest wall by left ventricle)
     b. Radioisotope scanning (determines cardiovascular disorders)
     c. Echocardiography (ultrasound to determine disorders)
     d. Vectorcardiography (determines balance of electrical forces of the heart)
     e. Electrocardiography (graphic representation of electrical activity of heart)
        1. Waves:
           a. P = atrial depolarization
           b. QRS = ventricular depolarization
           c. T = ventricular repolarization
           d. U = repolarization of Purkinje's fibers
        2. 12-lead EKG
           a. Einthoven's triangle is used as reference for lead placement I, II, III; AV node is the focal point for triangle's center.
           b. Augmented limb leads (aVR, aVL, aVF) radiate from triangle's center.
           c. Six unipolar chest leads, V_1-V_6
        3. Bedside monitoring for arrhythmia detection; use 3-lead, 4-lead, or 5-lead system.
        4. Electrical axis is the direction in which electrical current flows through the heart.
           a. Normal flow: base to apex
           b. *Vectors* are used to represent electrical activity of the heart.
              1. When direction of the force is toward the positive pole of the lead, the EKG wave will be upward.
              2. The vector that is the result of all the forces represents the electrical axis of the heart.
        5. **Bundle branch blocks** and **hemiblocks** are precursors of symptomatic *Mobitz II* and third-degree AV block.
           a. These blocks are indicative of left coronary artery pathology and associated with anterior wall myocardial infarctions.

b. Left anterior hemiblock is the blockage of impulse conduction in the left anterior superior division of the left bundle branch.

c. Left posterior hemiblock is a blockage of the posterior inferior division of the left bundle branch.

6. Electrolyte disturbances may cause EKG changes.
7. Arrythmias may be classified by origin:
    a. *Sinus* (SA)
        1. Sinus bradycardia
        2. Sinus tachycardia
        3. Sinus arrhythmia
        4. Sinus block
        5. Sinus arrest
    b. *Atrial*
        1. Premature atrial contractions (PAC)
        2. Aberrant PACs
        3. Paroxysmal atrial tachycardia (PAT)
        4. PAT with block
        5. Atrial flutter
        6. Atrial fibrillation
        7. Chaotic atrial rhythm
    c. *AV node*
        1. Premature junctional contractions (PTC)
        2. AV junctional
        3. AV junctional tachycardia
    d. *Supraventricular tachycardia*
    e. *AV blocks*
        1. First degree AV block
        2. Second degree AV block
            a. Mobitz I
            b. Mobitz II
        3. Third degree AV block
    f. *Ventricular*
        1. Idioventricular
        2. Premature ventricular contraction (PVC)
        3. Ventricular tachycardia (VT)
        4. Ventricular fibrillation (VF)

5. *Invasive assessment methods*
    a. Cardiac catheterization (determines heart function)
    b. Swann-Ganz insertion (direct measurement of right and left heart)
    c. His bundle electrocardiography (determines electrical activity of AV junction, bundle of His and bundle branches)
    d. Intracardiac phonocardiography (detects murmurs and sounds associated with heart disease)
    e. Coronary arteriography (determines extent of coronary artery disease)
    f. Ventriculography (determines ventricular function)
    g. Aortography (determines the size of the aortic lumen and aorta valve)

V. Pathological States and Nursing Management
  A. *Arteriosclerosis*
   1. Arteriosclerosis is a chronic thickening and hardening of the walls of the arteries.
   2. The patient may present with:
      a. Pain
      b. Elevated B.P.
      c. Cyanosis
      d. Dyspnea
      e. Absent pulses
   3. Arteriography or angiography is the best diagnostic aid.
   4. Nursing care includes:
      a. Providing warmth
      b. Administering vasodilating drugs and antihypertensive agents
      c. Providing exercise
      d. Preventing infection
      e. Preventing emboli formation
      f. Patient education
  B. *Angina pectoris*
   1. Angina is caused by atherosclerosis, hypertension, aortic valvular disease, anemia, shock or thyrotoxicosis
      a. The decreased blood flow leads to chest pain
      b. Functional ability of the ischemic cell is not permanently lost
   2. The patient may present with:
      a. Chest pain
      b. Arrhythmias
      c. Dyspnea
   3. Diagnostic data includes history, physical and electrocardiogram
   4. Nursing care includes:
      a. Prevention of pain
      b. Prevention of complications
      c. Administration of medication
      d. Bedrest and quiet environment
      e. Patient education
  C. *Myocardial infarction*
   1. Myocardial infarction is the complete occlusion of an artery with resultant myocardial death.
      a. Infarctions are classified as subendocardial or transmural.
      b. They are referred to by location: anterior, posterior, inferior, lateral and septal.
   2. The patient may present with:
      a. Chest pain
      b. Pain radiating to jaw, arm, neck, back or epigastrium
      c. Orthopnea
      d. Vomiting
      e. Dyspnea
      f. Cyanosis
      g. Anxiety

3. Diagnostic data includes history, physical, EKG, enzyme evaluation and CBC.
4. Nursing care includes:
    a. Airway management
    b. Maintenance of circulation
    c. Arrhythmia detection
    d. Prevention of complications
    e. Hemodynamic monitoring
    f. Prevention of venous stasis
    g. Pain relief
    h. Maintaining a quiet environment
    i. Instituting advanced life support, if necessary

D. *Congestive heart failure and pulmonary edema*
  1. Heart failure is mechanical failure and may be either right- or left-sided.
      a. In left-sided failure, the myocardium fails to pump blood from the lungs into the systemic circulation.
      b. In right-sided failure, the heart fails to pump blood to the lungs, and venous return is impeded.
  2. The patient may present with:
      a. Left heart failure
          1. Dyspnea
          2. Orthopnea
          3. Paroxysmal-nocturnal dyspnea
          4. Acute pulmonary edema
          5. Fatigue
          6. Nocturia
          7. Elevated pulmonary artery diastolic pressure and pulmonary capillary wedge pressure
      b. Right heart failure
          1. Fatigue
          2. Dependent edema
          3. Liver engorgement
          4. Anorexia
          5. Jugular vein distention
  3. Diagnostic data includes history, physical, chest x-ray and liver function tests.
  4. Nursing care includes:
      a. Establishment and maintenance of airway and ventilation
      b. Reduction of venous congestion through administration of medications, and maintenance of fluid and electrolytes
      c. Observation for complications
      d. Monitoring for changes in cardiopulmonary status and development of dysrhythmias

E. *Pericarditis*
  1. Pericarditis is an inflammation of the pericardium that results in fibrotic changes and calcification.
  2. The patient may present with:
      a. Chest pain
      b. Cough
      c. Hemoptysis

      d. Fever
      e. Cyanosis or pallor
      f. Dysrhythmias
      g. Friction rub
   3. Diagnostic data includes a differential diagnosis between pericarditis and MI.
      a. EKG changes in pericarditis do not result in Q waves.
      b. Friction rub and pulsus paradoxus are heard in pericarditis.
      c. Echocardiography may reveal pericardial effusion.
      d. Leukocytes are elevated.
   4. Nursing care includes:
      a. Relief of pain
      b. Observation for signs of tamponade
      c. Observation for dysrhythmias
      d. Monitoring and assessment of hemodynamic changes
      e. Administration of antipyretic measures
F. *Hypertensive crisis*
   1. Hypertensive crisis is a significant rise in the blood pressure, producing a crisis situation.
   2. The patient may present with:
      a. Diastolic pressure above 120 mm Hg
      b. Impaired renal function
      c. Severe retinopathy and papilledema
      d. Restlessness
      e. Headache
      f. Epistaxis
      g. Nausea and vomiting
      h. Weakness
      i. Mentation changes
   3. Diagnostic data includes history and physical, 24-hour urine study, EKG and radiologic studies such as IVP and renal angiogram.
   4. Nursing care includes:
      a. Administration of medications
      b. Prevention of complications
      c. Close monitoring of VS
G. *Shock*
   1. Shock is characterizied by poor tissue perfusion.
   2. It is caused by a decrease in venous return or a decrease in the heart's ability to pump.
   3. Shock may be classified as:
      a. ***Cardiogenic***
      b. ***Hypovolemic***
      c. ***Septic***
      d. ***Neurogenic***
   4. The patient may present with:
      a. Systolic pressure below 80 mm Hg
      b. Metabolic acidosis
      c. Oliguria or anuria
      d. Decreased stroke volume and pulse pressure

5. The best diagnostic aid is laboratory data: ABG, urinalysis and serum analysis.
6. Nursing care includes:
   a. Maintenance of airway and adequate oxygenation
   b. Maintenance of fluid and electrolyte balance, as well as acid-base balance
   c. Administration of medications
   d. Advanced life support measures, as necessary

H. *Pacemakers*
  1. Pacemakers are classified as *temporary* or *permanent.*
  2. *Temporary pacemakers*
     a. Techniques for insertion include:
        1. *Transvenous endocardial*
        2. *Epicardial*
        3. *Emergency*
     b. The patient in need of temporary pacing may present with dizziness, fainting, bradycardia and arrhythmias.
     c. History, physical and EKG provide the best diagnostic data.
     d. Nursing care is aimed at support.
        1. Preoperative care includes a brief explanation, administration of sedation and establishment of I.V. lines.
        2. Postoperative care includes:
           a. Accurate documentation
           b. Immobilization of arm, catheter and pacer
           c. Electrical safety measures
           d. Monitoring of rhythm
           e. Observation for infection
           f. Life-support measures, as needed
  3. *Permanent pacemakers*
     a. Permanent pacemakers are used in long-term treatment of symptomatic chronic heart block.
     b. Permanent pacers are inserted by one of three methods:
        1. Transvenous endocardial
        2. Thoracotomy epicardial
        3. Subxiphoid, transxiphoid or transmediastinal epicardial pacing
     c. The patient presents the same as for temporary pacing.
     d. EKG, history and physical are the best diagnostic aids.
     e. Nursing care is divided into three phases:
        1. Preoperative:
           a. Monitor temporary pacemaker.
           b. Provide emotional support.
           c. Teach family and patient.
        2. Postoperative:
           a. Accurately chart.
           b. Observe pacemaker function.
           c. Observe for dysrhythmias.
           d. Limit activity following insertion of transvenous pacer.
           e. Prevent complications.

3. The rehabilitative phase includes psychological intervention and patient teaching.
4. *Types of pacemakers*
   a. Two basic types: *fixed* and *demand rate*
   b. Can stimulate atrium or ventricle
      1. *Atrial* are used to stimulate atria when AV conduction is functioning properly.
      2. *Ventricular*-stimulating mechanism delivers continuous stimuli to ventricles.
   c. *Atrial* and *ventricular* provide sequential delivery of a stimulus to the atria and ventricles.
5. *Electrical complications* include:
   a. Electrical leakage from line-powered equipment
   b. Sensitivity to electrical fields
      1. Magnetic fields
      2. Alternating currents
      3. Low conducted currents

I. *Surgical intervention*
1. Cardiac surgery (adult)
   a. Clinical symptoms differ with the anomaly; however, general symptoms include fatigue, dyspnea and pain.
   b. Nursing care includes:
      1. Airway maintenance and ventilation
      2. Arrhythmia detection
      3. Monitoring of circulatory problems
      4. Observation and intervention in coagulation problems
      5. Maintenance of acid-base balance, as well as fluid and electrolyte balance
      6. Emotional support
2. Vascular surgery
   a. Carotid occlusive disease can be diagnosed by a bruit or thrill over the carotids and angiography. Surgical procedure is endarterectomy.
   b. Occlusive disease of the terminal aorta and iliac is diagnosed by arteriography. Surgical procedure is aortoiliac thromboendarterectomy or bypass.
   c. Diseases of the femoral and popliteal arteries present with intermittent claudication in the lower leg and are diagnosed by arteriography.
   d. An aneurysm is a dilatation of the vessel wall.
      1. Types of aneurysms:
         a. *True* (abdominal thoracic)
            1. Outpocketing aneurysm
            2. Fusiform aneurysm
         b. *Traumatic*
   e. Nursing care in vascular surgery is aimed at maintaining the graft.

VI. Care Common to Cardiovascular Problems
A. Observe changes in cardiac circulation.
B. Hemodynamic monitoring may be done in the following ways:
   1. Central venous pressure (CVP)

2. Pulmonary artery wedge pressure, which reflects left ventricular function
3. Intra-ortic balloon pump (IAPB), which reduces afterload and increases coronary perfusion
    a. May be used in cardiogenic shock or postcardiac surgery
    b. Complications include clotting of femoral artery, ischemia of foot distal to insertion site, wound infection, renal failure, trauma to main vessels, thrombocytopenia, azotemia.

C. Nursing interventions in hemodynamic monitoring:
  1. Maintain head of bed below 45 degrees.
  2. Evaluate vital signs hourly.
  3. Prevent leg flexion at groin.
  4. Inspect catheter for kinking or disconnection.
  5. Reduce anxiety.
  6. Observe waveforms.

D. Maintain fluid and electrolyte balance.
E. Provide physical and emotional rest.
F. Prevent infection.
G. Maintain nutrition.
H. Begin rehabilitation.

CHAPTER SIX
RENAL SYSTEM

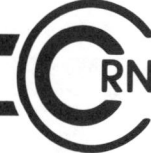

BEHAVIORAL OBJECTIVES

After reading the *Renal System,* the nurse will be able to:
- Identify the anatomical structures of the kidney
- Name the four primary functions of the kidney
- List in sequence the steps involved in urine formation, beginning with renal artery perfusion
- Identify the functions of each of the following structures:
  nephron
  proximal tubule
  Henle's loop
  distal tubule
  juxtaglomerular apparatus
- Identify three ways in which the kidneys assist in maintaining acid-base balance
- Define the following terms:
  acute cortical necrosis
  acute tubular necrosis
  oliguria
  anuria
  azotemia
  osmolarity
  diuresis
  peritoneal dialysis
  hemodialysis
  AV fistula
  AV shunt

TOPICAL OUTLINE
RENAL SYSTEM

- I. The Renal System: Overview 365
- II. Renal Anatomy 365
    - Location 365
    - Size 365
    - Renal fascia 365
    - Gross structures 366
        - Renal cortex 366
        - Renal medulla 366
        - Renal pelvis 366
    - Nephron 367
        - Glomerulus 367
        - Renal tubules 368
- III. Renal Physiology 369
    - Glomerular filtration 369
    - Constituents of glomerular filtrate 370
    - Tubular reabsorption and secretion 370
        - Proximal tubule 370
        - Henle's loops 371
        - Distal tubule 371
        - Collecting tubules 371
    - Regulation of water balance 372
    - Regulation of blood pressure 373
    - Regulation of electrolytes 375
        - Sodium 375
        - Potassium 375
        - Calcium and phosphate 375
        - Magnesium 376
        - Chloride 376
    - Excretion of waste products 377
    - The kidney and acid-base balance 377
        - Phosphates as renal buffers 378
        - Secretion of ammonia 379
        - Acidosis 379
        - Alkalosis 379
- IV. Assessment of the Renal System 380
    - Gross cerebral function 380
    - Specific cerebral function 380
    - Inspection 380
    - Palpation 380
    - Percussion 380
    - Auscultation 381
    - Renal assessment 381
        - Level of consciousness 381
        - Voiding pattern 381
        - Control of stream 381
        - Dysuria 381

        Toilet habits   381
        Evaluation of vital signs   382
    Laboratory and radiologic studies   382
V. Pathological States and Nursing Management   384
    Acute renal failure   384
        Pathophysiology: general   384
        Pathophysiology: specific   386
        Clinical presentation   386
        Diagnostic data   386
        Nursing care   386
    Chronic renal failure   387
        Pathophysiology   387
        Clinical presentation   388
        Diagnostic data   388
        Nursing care   388
    Pyelonephritis   388
        Pathophysiology   388
        Clinical presentation   389
        Diagnostic data   389
        Nursing care   389
    Glomerulonephritis   389
        Pathophysiology   389
        Clinical presentation   390
        Diagnostic data   390
        Nursing care   390
    Nephrotic syndrome   391
        Pathophysiology   391
        Clinical presentation   391
        Diagnostic data   391
        Nursing care   391
    Hypertension   392
        Pathophysiology   392
        Clinical presentation   392
    Renal insufficiency   392
        Pathophysiology   392
        Clinical presentation   393
        Diagnostic data   393
        Nursing care   393
    Dialysis   393
        Peritoneal dialysis   394
        Hemodialysis   395
        Nursing care   396
VI. Care Common to Renal Problems   397
    Maintenance of fluid balance   397
    Monitoring fluid balance   398
    Maintenance of electrolyte balance   398
    Maintenance of nutrition   399
    Maintenance of renal perfusion   399

Maintenance of acid-base balance   399
     Prevention of complications   400
Program Assessment: Science and Situation   403
Key Point Recognition Answers   411
PASS Answer Sheet   417
Survey Summary   419

THE RENAL SYSTEM: OVERVIEW

The *renal system* comprises the **kidneys, ureters, bladder** and **urethra.** The major function of the renal system is to excrete wastes from the body. This is accomplished through the regulation of fluid and electrolytes, which are excreted through urine formation and micturition. The renal system can easily adapt to variations in fluid load. The renal system, a life-maintenance system, regulates the internal environment of the body.

KEY CONCEPT: The renal system, which is essential to life, regulates the internal environment of the body.

RENAL ANATOMY

LOCATION

The kidneys are bean-shaped, retroperitoneal structures that lie on either side of the vertebral column. They extend from the 11th or 12th thoracic vertebra to the 2nd lumbar vertebra. The right kidney is lower than the left because of the right lobe of the liver lying just above it (Fig. 6-1).

The medial border of each kidney, called the **hilus,** is concave. The hilus is an entrance for the renal blood vessels and the renal pelvis.

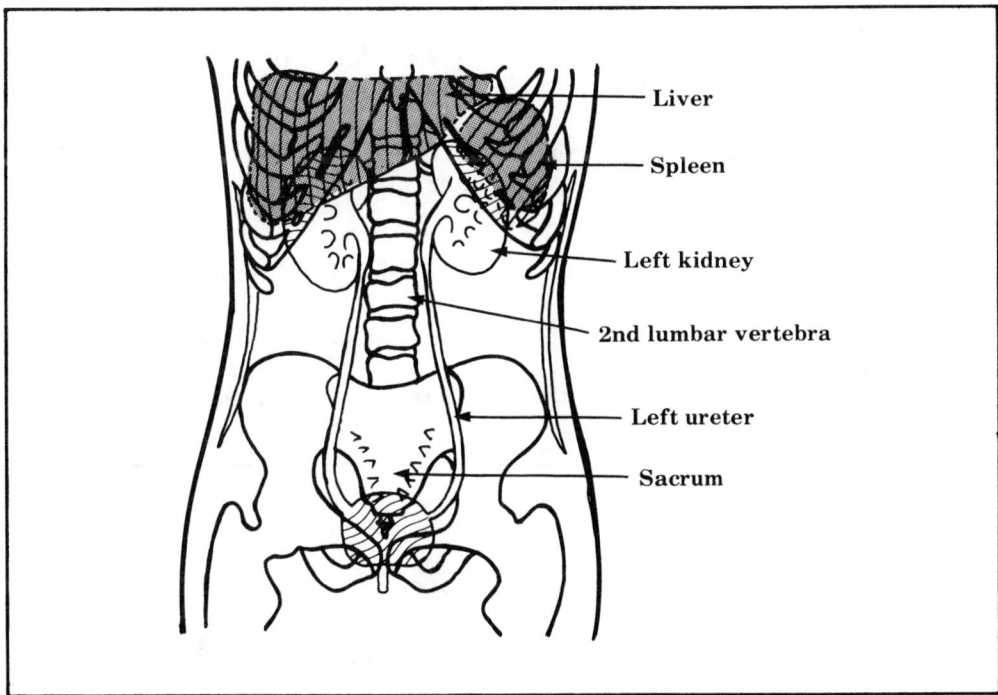

Fig. 6-1. Location of kidneys

SIZE

Each adult kidney weighs approximately 120 to 150 gm, is 10 to 12 cm long, 5 to 6 cm wide (from the hilus to the cortex), and is 3 to 4 cm thick.

RENAL FASCIA

Coverings and various structures surrounding it protect the kidney from direct trauma and limit blood loss when injury is sustained. Anteriorly, a thick cushion of intestines protects the kidneys. The ribs provide protection posteriorly.

The kidney's outermost covering is composed of a thin membranous sheet, the **renal fascia.** The renal fascia surrounds a thick mass of adipose tissue called **perirenal fat.** Loosely attached to the renal cortex is the innermost covering, the *fibrous renal capsule.* It is a smooth, thin membrane. Further protection is provided by *pararenal fat,* adipose tissue located outside the renal fascia.

KEY POINT RECOGNITION
Write true or false by each statement. Answers are at the end of this chapter.

_____ 1. The kidneys extend from the 9th thoracic vertebra to the 11th or 12th thoracic vertebra.

_____ 2. The left kidney is lower than the right kidney because of the liver which lies just above it.

_____ 3. The renal blood vessels enter the kidney through the hilus.

_____ 4. The renal fascia is the outermost covering of the kidney.

_____ 5. Perirenal fat is located outside the renal fascia for the purpose of protection.

GROSS STRUCTURES
Renal Cortex
The *renal cortex* (Fig. 6-2) is the outer layer of the kidney. It is mainly composed of glomeruli arranged on vertical arterioles and convoluted portions of the proximal and distal tubules. The cortex extends from the renal capsule to the medulla, and down between the renal pyramids of the medulla toward the renal pelvis.

Renal Medulla
The middle layer of the kidney is the *renal medulla.* It is composed of 8 to 18 triangular wedges called *pyramids.* The apices of the pyramids are directed toward the renal pelvis.

The pyramids have a striated appearance because they are composed of portions of both Henle's loop and the collecting ducts of the nephron.

Renal Pelvis
The *renal pelvis* is the inner layer of the kidney. It is the main reservoir for the renal collecting system.

The renal pelvis lies at the base of the kidney and is composed of fingerlike sacs that extend into the medulla. Each of these sacs is known as a *calyx.* As the calyces progress toward the collecting ducts that lead to the ureters, the calyces become larger.

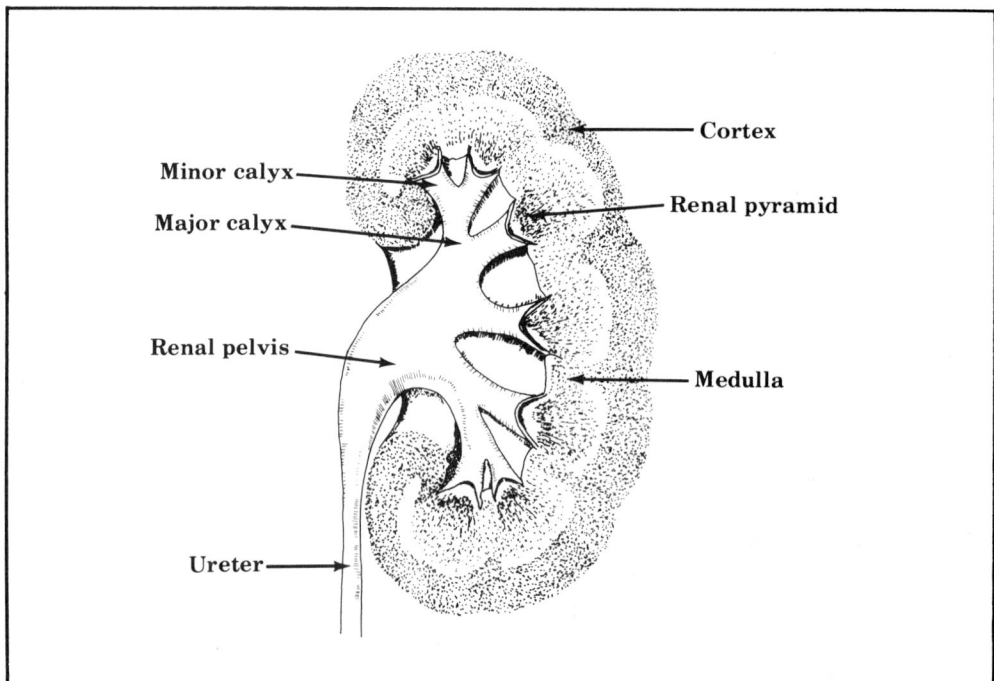

Fig. 6-2. Kidneys: gross structures

KEY CONCEPT: The three layers of the kidney are: renal cortex (outer); medulla (middle); and renal pelvis (inner).

KEY POINT RECOGNITION
Write true or false by each statement. Answers are at the end of this chapter.

_____ 1. The renal cortex is mainly composed of glomeruli and convoluted portions of the proximal and distal tubules.

_____ 2. The renal medulla is composed of pyramids.

_____ 3. The renal pelvis is the main reservoir for the renal collecting system.

NEPHRON

The *nephron* (Fig. 6-3) is the functional unit of the kidney. Each kidney contains approximately 1 million nephrons that are similar in both structure and function. Structurally, each nephron is composed of a *glomerulus, proximal tubule, Henle's loop, distal tubule* and *collecting tubule.* These structures operate as one independent functioning unit. In the presence of massive nephron destruction (70 to 75 percent), the remaining nephrons will compensate and maintain normal renal function with no ill effect to the patient.

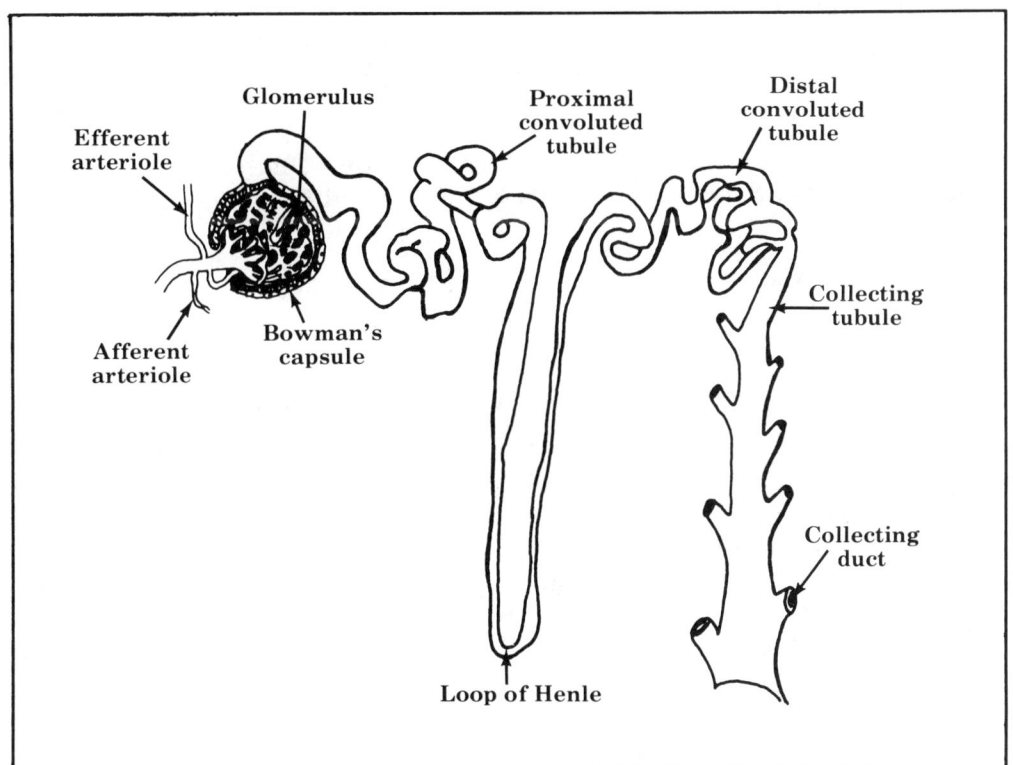

Fig. 6-3. Nephron

Glomerulus

The vascular component of the nephron is the *glomerulus.* It is composed of a spherical capillary tuft. This capillary tuft is formed by the division of the *afferent arteriole.*

An epithelial-lined membrane, called *Bowman's capsule,* envelops the small, spherical capillary mass.

The capillary tuft of the glomerulus is composed of many capillary loops. These loops are important to kidney function; they provide a large surface area for glomerular filtration. Outflow of blood is provided for as the capillary loops join to form the efferent arteriole.

Renal Tubules
Proximal Convoluted Tubule (PCT)
The PCT lies in the cortex next to the glomerulus. It is lined with cuboidal epithelial cells. The terminal portion descends into the renal medulla and emerges as the descending Henle's loop. The PCT receives the glomerular filtrate from the glomerulus.

Henle's Loop
The glomerular filtrate then passes into the next portion of the tubular system called Henle's loop. It is a sharp, hairpin loop that consists of a descending limb with a thin segment and a thick ascending limb. The length of the loop depends upon the location of its glomerulus within the cortex. As the ascending limb enters the renal cortex, the tubule once again becomes convoluted.

Distal Convoluted Tubule (DCT)
The *distal convoluted tubule* is found in the renal cortex. It empties into the collecting ducts that lead to the ureters and bladder.

The DCT contains a specialized cell group called the **macula densa.** The macula densa is composed of granular cells with closely packed nuclei. At one point, the distal tubule is positioned between the afferent and efferent arterioles. The *macula densa* and the combination of the vascular poles of the glomerulus form the *juxtaglomerular apparatus* or JG cells. It is the juxtaglomerular apparatus that controls the kidney's secretion of *renin*.

Collecting Tubule
The *collecting tubule* is the final portion of the renal tubule. It joins the collecting ducts in the medulla. At this point, urine collects and empties into the renal pelvis.

KEY CONCEPT: The nephron is the functional unit of the kidney and is composed of the glomerulus, PCT, Henle's loop, DCT and collecting tubule.

KEY POINT RECOGNITION
Write true or false by each statement. Answers are at the end of this chapter. A score below 80% indicates the need for further study.

_____ 1. Each kidney contains approximately 100,000 nephrons.

_____ 2. The nephrons have a vast capacity for compensation in the face of nephron destruction.

_____ 3. Bowman's capsule, a component of the nephron, is a spherical capillary tuft.

_____ 4. The blood flowing out of the glomerulus flows through the efferent arteriole.

_____ 5. The proximal convoluted tubule receives the glomerular filtrate.

_____ 6. Henle's loop is part of the renal tubule.

_____ 7. The macula densa is a specialized group of cells within the proximal tubule.

_____ 8. The juxtaglomerular apparatus controls the secretion of renin.

RENAL BLOOD FLOW
The *renal arteries* enter the kidney at the hilus (Fig. 6-4). Located at the level of the second lumbar vertebra, these large vessels allow high rates of blood flow.

The kidneys are perfused with 1,200 ml of blood per minute. This constitutes 20 to 25 percent of the total cardiac output.

The renal arteries divide at the hilum to form an *anterior* and *posterior* branch. Further division of these branches forms the *interlobar* arteries. The interlobar arteries direct blood to the junction of the medulla and cortex. At this point the arteries divide again to become the *afferent arterioles,* thus feeding the glomeruli.

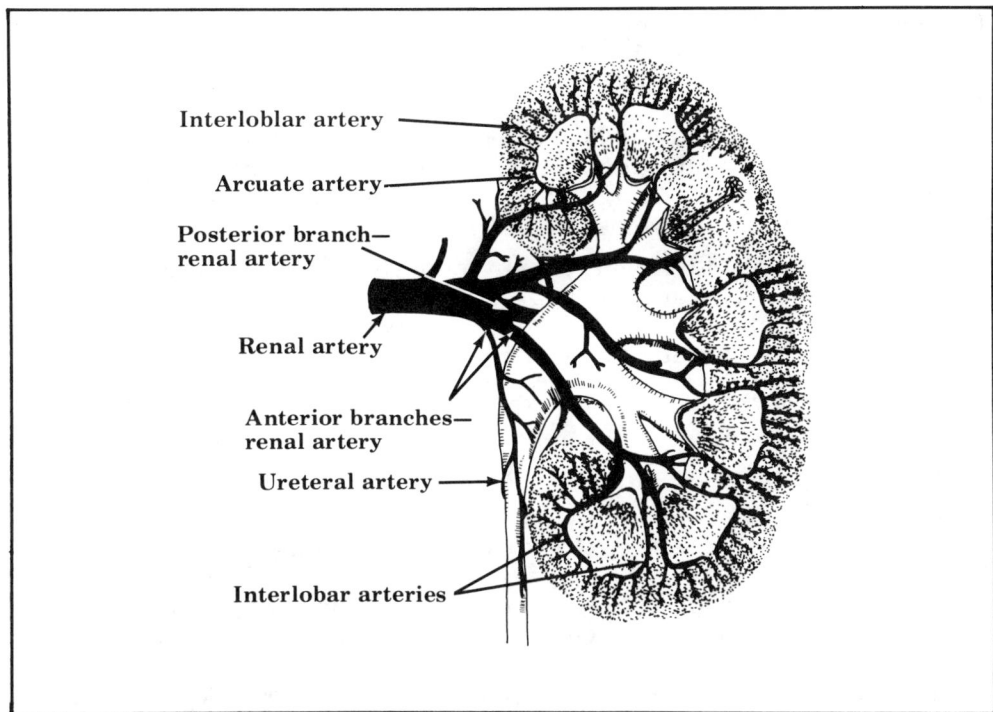

Fig. 6-4. Renal blood flow

The *renal capillaries* surround the tubules. These vessels arise from the efferent arterioles in the outer cortex. Taking a slightly different route, the *efferent arterioles* from the juxtaglomeruli continue into the medulla, follow Henle's loop, return to the cortex and, finally, empty into the veins.

The *renal veins* are large vessels that originate at the posterior and anterior sides of the sinus and terminate at the inferior vena cava.

KEY CONCEPT: The renal arteries perfuse the kidneys with 1,200 ml of blood/minute (20 to 25% of the total cardiac output).

KEY POINT RECOGNITION
Write true or false by each statement. Answers are at the end of this chapter.

_____ 1. Renal arteries allow high rates of blood flow.

_____ 2. The kidneys are perfused with 1,200 ml of blood/minute.

_____ 3. The afferent arterioles feed the glomeruli.

_____ 4. The renal capillaries arise from the efferent arterioles.

RENAL PHYSIOLOGY

The functions of the kidney include:
- Maintenance of plasma osmolarity and pH
- Maintenance of electrolyte concentrations
- Excretion of the waste products of protein metabolism

It is the continual ability of the kidney to save or excrete water, to eliminate excess hydrogen ions, to regenerate bicarbonate and to absorb or secrete electrolytes that allows for dynamic plasma homeostasis.

GLOMERULAR FILTRATION
The glomerular filtration of plasma is the beginning of urine formation and is directly related to renal blood flow. Renal blood flow equals 20 to 25 percent of the total cardiac output, or 1200 ml/minute. Therefore, if both the hematocrit and

plasma constitutents, such as glucose, amino acids, electrolytes, urea, and creatinine, are at normal levels, 125 ml of plasma pass through the glomeruli every minute. Conversely, if cardiac output falls by as little as 10 percent, renal blood flow decreases, as does the renal plasma flow. When cardiac output falls, the glomerular filtration rate should also decrease, but a built-in control or autoregulation maintains the filtration rate. This autoregulation is accomplished by a rise in the efferent arteriolar resistance and a decrease in the afferent arteriolar resistance, resulting in increased vascular resistance.

The glomerular capillaries are highly permeable to many molecules, with the exception of blood cells and proteins. The nonfilterable molecules are retained by the capillary membrane and move with the remaining plasma into the efferent arteriole. The filtered water and molecules compose the glomerular filtrate.

The rate at which glomerular filtrate is formed is called the ***glomerular filtration rate*** (GFR).

CONSTITUENTS OF GLOMERULAR FILTRATE

Three basic substances are filtered through the glomeruli: electrolytes, nonelectrolytes and water. The electrolytes include sodium (Na^+), potassium (K^+), chloride (Cl^-), calcium (Ca^{++}), magnesium (Mg^{+++}), bicarbonate (HCO_3^-) and phosphate (HPO_4^-). Nonelectrolytes are the end products of protein metabolism (urea, uric acid, ammonia and creatinine), glucose and amino acids.

KEY CONCEPT: The functions of the kidney are to maintain acid-base regulation, to maintain electrolyte concentrations and to excrete the waste products of protein metabolism. This occurs at the level of the nephron and begins with the glomerular filtration of plasma.

KEY POINT RECOGNITION

Write true or false by each statement. Answers are at the end of this chapter.

_____ 1. Renal blood flow equals 50 percent of the total cardiac output.

_____ 2. Autoregulation prevents the GFR from decreasing with the cardiac output.

_____ 3. The glomerular capillaries are permeable to proteins and blood cells.

_____ 4. The basic substances filtered through the glomeruli are electrolytes and water.

TUBULAR REABSORPTION AND SECRETION

The renal tubules reabsorb over 99 percent, or 124 to 125 ml/minute, of the glomerular filtrate, producing 1 ml of urine/minute, or 1 to 1.5 liters/day. Both active and passive transport play a role in the reabsorption and secretion of constituents in the tubules. Active transport occurs when a substance is transported against a concentration gradient and requires energy to exchange ions. Passive transport occurs when a substance is absorbed or secreted without requiring energy.

Proximal Tubule

Sixty to eighty percent of the glomerular filtrate is reabsorbed in the proximal tubule (PCT). The majority of sodium, calcium, phosphate and magnesium ions, uric acid, glucose and amino acids are reabsorbed by active transport. Urea passively diffuses from the tubule to the peritubular blood. The diffusion of urea is related to the passive diffusion of water from the proximal tubular fluid. When water is reabsorbed, the concentration of urea increases, causing the urea to diffuse from the tubule. Chloride is passively reabsorbed by following the positively charged sodium ions through the tubular lumen. This process is necessary for maintenance of electrical neutrality. Glucose and amino acids are reabsorbed in the PCT unless their serum concentration exceeds the renal threshold. Ninety percent of the bicarbonate is reabsorbed.

Reabsorption rate depends upon the length of time the filtrate is present. In a hypovolemic situation, the GFR decreases, reabsorption increases and urine output decreases. Conversely, if the body is hypervolemic, the GFR increases and tubular absorption decreases, resulting in increased urine output. Fine tuning of this regulatory act is mediated by the hormones aldosterone, antidiuretic hormone (ADH) and, possibly, natriuretic hormone.

Organic acids and drugs are secreted at the PCT. The secretion of hydrogen is important to acid-base regulation. Creatinine is actively secreted in the proximal tubule.

Henle's Loop

When the glomerular filtrate reaches Henle's loop, it is greatly reduced in volume because of the large percentage of water reabsorption in the proximal tubule. As the filtrate passes through the descending limb of Henle's loop, water diffuses into the bloodstream, and sodium enters the filtrate from the blood, resulting in a more hypertonic filtrate. At the ascending limb, chloride and sodium are actively transported into the interstitium and the renal medulla adjacent to the Henle's loop.

If the rate of flow reduces through Henle's loop because of conditions such as hypovolemia, excessive amounts of sodium and chloride are given up to the renal medulla. This results in decreased urine volume and increased concentration of solutes except sodium.

The functional relationship between Henle's loop, collecting tubules, medullary interstitial tissue and peritubular capillaries makes the countercurrent multiplier system possible. This very complex system concentrates or dilutes the urine. Concentration or dilution of urine is accomplished by the countercurrent mechanism, which maintains the hyperosmolar gradient in the renal medullary tissues.

Distal Tubule

The selective process of reabsorption and secretion is completed in the distal and collecting tubules, with the final adjustments of sodium made in the DCT. As the filtrate enters the DCT, it is hypotonic to plasma. This is due to the transport of sodium and chloride from Henle's loop into the interstitium of the medulla. Active sodium reabsorption in the DCT is enhanced by aldosterone. Chloride is transported either passively or by ion exchange.

Uric acid and potassium are secreted from the blood into the distal tubule. Approximately 6 percent of the filtered potassium load is excreted in the urine.

Collecting Tubules

Water reabsorption is one of the prime functions of the collecting tubules. The absorption of solute-free water in the collecting tubules is dependent upon the activity of ADH. ADH is discussed in the sections on water and blood pressure regulation.

Potassium and hydrogen ions, as well as ammonia, are secreted. The secretion of ammonia is a control mechanism for the excretion of hydrogen ions. This mechanism will be discussed in the acid-base section.

KEY CONCEPT: The renal tubules reabsorb over 99% of the glomerular filtrate and produce 1 ml of urine/minute by active and passive reabsorption and secretion of glomerular filtrate and its constituents.

KEY POINT RECOGNITION
Write true or false by each statement. Answers are at the end of this chapter. A score below 80% indicates the need for further study.

    _____ 1. The renal tubules reabsorb the glomerular filtrate at the rate of 125 ml/minute.

    _____ 2. Sixty to eighty percent of the glomerular filtrate is reabsorbed in the PCT.

    _____ 3. Urea is reabsorbed by the PCT.

    _____ 4. Normally, glucose and amino acids are diffused from the PCT.

_____ 5. Reabsorption rate is dependent upon the length of time the filtrate is present in the PCT.

_____ 6. If the GFR decreases, reabsorption increases in the PCT and results in a decreased urine output.

_____ 7. Creatinine is actively secreted in the PCT.

_____ 8. Entering Henle's loop, the glomerular filtrate volume is reduced because of water reabsorption in the PCT.

_____ 9. The filtrate becomes more hypertonic at the descending limb of Henle's loop.

_____10. Urine is concentrated or diluted by the countercurrent mechanism.

_____11. Reabsorption and secretion is completed in the DCT and collecting tubules.

_____12. Final adjustments of sodium are made in the collecting tubules.

_____13. Aldosterone enhances sodium reabsorption in the DCT.

_____14. Water reabsorption is a main function of the collecting tubules.

_____15. Potassium and hydrogen ions are secreted into the lumen of the collecting tubules.

REGULATION OF WATER BALANCE

The body maintains fluid balance and concentration via the thirst-neurohypophyseal-renal axis. Three mechanisms are responsible for this regulation: **Thirst** regulates the intake of fluid. **Antidiuretic hormone** (ADH) helps control the osmolality of extracellular fluid and sodium concentration. The **countercurrent mechanism** of the kidney adjusts urine osmolality.

Ninety percent of all excreted urine is water. The total solute concentration is fairly constant at 60 gm/day. The homeostatic mechanisms of the body provide for wide fluctuations in water and solute intake and output by providing the kidney with the ability to produce concentrated or diluted urine. For example, concentrations of plasma and body fluids are maintained within a narrow limit. When large volumes of ingested water cause body fluids to become diluted, the kidney responds by excreting excess water and diluting the urine. The converse is also true. In dehydration, the urine is highly concentrated with decreased water loss. This reabsorption and retention of water is the body's means for returning the body fluids to normal concentration levels.

Osmolality and osmolarity are terms used to express concentration in terms of 1,000 grams of water, in units of milliosmole (mOsm) per liter. **Osmolality** refers to the amount of water in one liter of solution and does not vary with temperature. The **osmolarity** of a solution is dependent upon the solution's temperature and the space occupied by the solids in 1,000 grams of water. The terms are often used interchangeably when referring to the concentrations of body fluids.

KEY CONCEPT: It is the responsibility of the kidneys to maintain the concentration of body fluids at 285 mOsm/L.

The ADH mechanism (Fig. 6-5) is essential in maintaining the volume and osmolarity of extracellular fluid (ECF). ADH is synthesized in the supraoptic nuclei of the hypothalamus. The formed ADH travels to the posterior pituitary for storage and is released via a blood connection between the hypothalamus and the pituitary (hypophyseal portal system). It is believed that the supraoptic area of the hypothalamus overlaps with the thirst center. This would integrate the thirst mechanism and osmolality monitoring with the release of ADH.

The mechanism is dependent upon vessel stretch or osmoreceptors for an initial response. These sensor cells, located in the hypothalamus and left atria, stimulate an increase in the release of ADH when there is a need to conserve water. This occurs when filling pressures in the heart or blood flow decrease, or when the osmolarity of the plasma increases. Water will be reabsorbed at the distal and collecting tubules, resulting in maintenance of the circulating blood volume, a decrease in body fluid osmolality and a concentrated, low-volume urine.

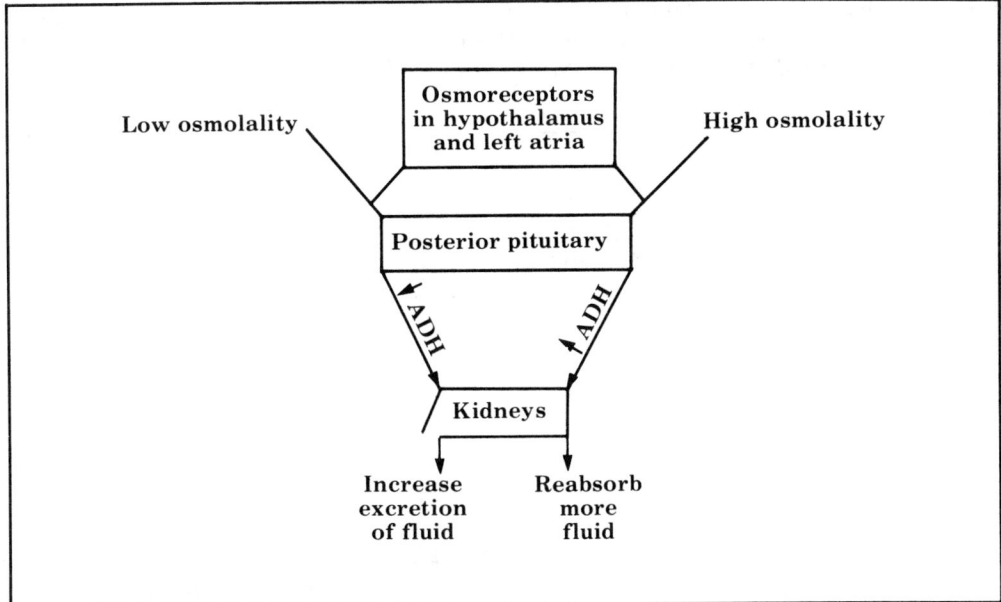

Fig. 6-5. ADH mechanism

The reverse occurs in low plasma osmolarity. ADH secretion is inhibited when volume expansion secondary to an increased water intake exists. Tubular reabsorption of water decreases and a dilute, large-volume urine is excreted.

KEY CONCEPT: Three mechanisms are responsible for the maintenance of fluid balance and concentration: thirst, ADH and the countercurrent system of the kidney.

KEY POINT RECOGNITION

Write true or false by each statement. Answers are at the end of this chapter. A score below 80% indicates the need for further study.

_____ 1. Fluid balance and concentration are maintained via the thirst-renal axis.

_____ 2. Thirst regulates the intake of fluids.

_____ 3. Ten percent of all excreted urine is water.

_____ 4. In overhydration, the body responds by concentrating the urine and excreting large amounts of water.

_____ 5. ADH is synthesized in the posterior pituitary.

_____ 6. When the body perceives a need to conserve water, the release of ADH is inhibited.

_____ 7. When ADH is released, water is reabsorbed at the distal and collecting tubules.

REGULATION OF BLOOD PRESSURE

An adequate circulating plasma volume is essential for the maintenance of a perfusion-level blood pressure. Important mechanisms within the kidney and endocrine systems respond to hypoperfusion states to conserve or increase circulating blood volume.

A vital part of the kidney-endocrine system is the *juxtaglomerular apparatus* (JGA). The JGA is a group of specialized cells in the nephrons, located in the inner cortex of the kidney adjacent to the medulla. The nephrons housing JG cells retain sodium and thus have a greater capacity for concentrating urine. The cells of the JGA monitor arterial pressures in the afferent and efferent arterioles, as well as the sodium content in the distal tubule. Granules of inactive renin are found in JG cells. It is the monitoring effect, the secretion of renin and the response of aldosterone that make up the blood pressure regulating system, or the *renin-angiotensin-aldosterone mechanism* (Fig. 6-6).

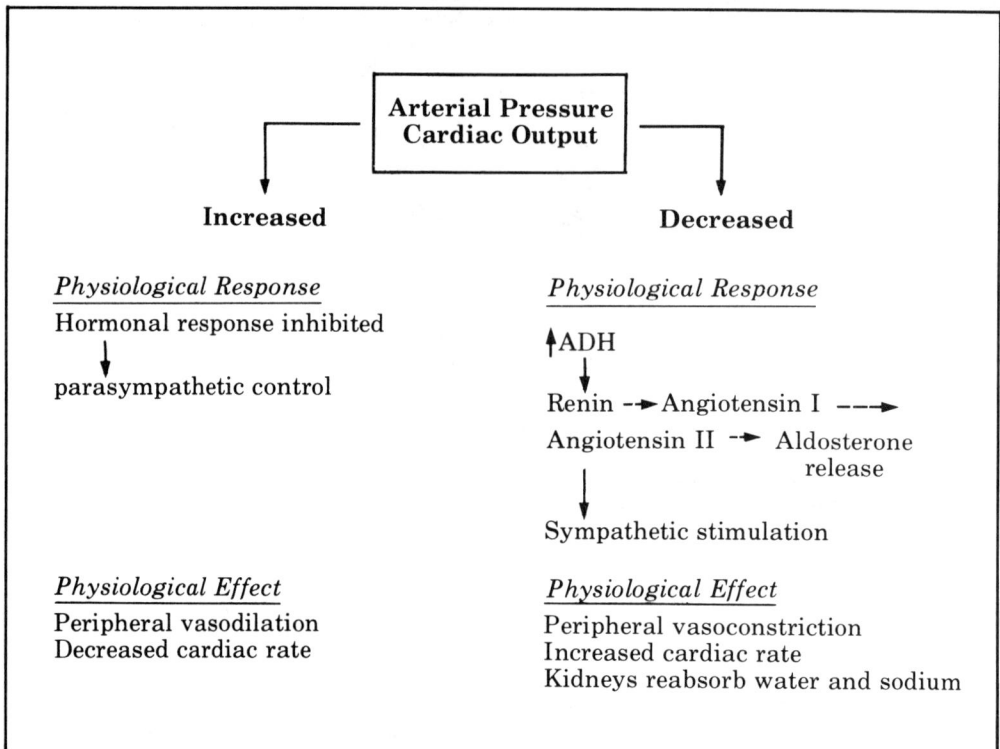

Fig. 6-6. Renin-angiotensin-aldosterone mechanism

A decrease in the GFR results in low pressure in the afferent arterioles. The sympathetic nervous system is stimulated to release catecholamines. The amount of serum sodium decreases as it passes through the JG cells. With this altered tubular fluid flowing through the JGA, a domino effect of the renin-angiotensin-aldosterone mechanism occurs. The JGA secretes renin, which causes an increased amount of angiotensin I to be released. Angiotensin I converts to angiotensin II. Circulating angiotensin II, a potent vasoconstrictor, produces an increase in arterial blood pressure. Specifically, pressure is increased by the following physiological responses: vasoconstriction of renal and peripheral arterioles; retention of water, which occurs when the adrenal cortex is stimulated and secretes aldosterone. Aldosterone causes DCT reabsorption of sodium, which retains water, resulting in increased circulating volume.

Blood pressure is also regulated by ADH's response to decreased filling pressures of the heart or increased plasma osmolarity. Release of ADH causes the reabsorption of water in the DCT and CT, thus assisting in the expansion of fluid volume in an effort to increase arterial blood pressure.

 KEY CONCEPT: The ability of the kidney to assist the body in maintaining homeostasis in hypoperfusive states is dependent on the feedback mechanisms of the renin-angiotensin-aldosterone mechanism and ADH.

KEY POINT RECOGNITION
Write true or false by each statement. Answers are at the end of this chapter. A score below 80% indicates the need for further study.

     _____ 1. The JGA is located in the adrenal cortex.

     _____ 2. JG cells monitor pressure and have granules of inactive angiotensin in them.

_____ 3. A decreased sodium level in tubular fluid will trigger the renin-angiotensin mechanism.

_____ 4. JG cells secrete renin, which changes angiotensin I to angiotensin II, causing an increase in pressure.

_____ 5. Aldosterone is secreted in response to high blood pressure and causes the excretion of sodium via the urine.

REGULATION OF ELECTROLYTES

Sodium

Sodium is the major extracellular cation. Normal serum concentration of sodium is 136 to 143 meq/L. Normal sodium content of urine is 40 to 80 meq/L. Greater than 99 percent of filtered sodium is reabsorbed in the tubules. If renal perfusion is decreased, tubular reabsorption of sodium increases, and the urine sodium content drops to 10 to 20 meq/L. Sixty-five percent of filtered sodium is reabsorbed in the proximal tubule. The final 3 to 4 percent of sodium is reabsorbed in the collecting tubule or ducts.

Sodium excretion depends on GFR and secretion of aldosterone. However, the regulation of salt excretion is primarily dependent upon the renin-angiotensin-aldosterone mechanism. A low pulse pressure in the afferent arterioles stimulates the sympathetic nervous system to secrete catecholamines. The glomerular filtrate containing catecholamines and low sodium stimulates the secretion of renin as it passes the JGA. Angiotensin I is released and converted to angiotensin II. It stimulates the secretion of aldosterone, resulting in tubular reabsorption of sodium.

Aldosterone secretion and sodium reabsorption are further regulated by hyperkalemia, the total amount of sodium in the body and the adrenocorticotropic hormone (ACTH).

Sodium reabsorption is decreased at the tubules if there is an increased GFR, inhibition of aldosterone or secretion of ADH.

Potassium (K^+)

Potassium is the major intracellular cation. Serum potassium is normally 3.5 to 5 meq/L.

Potassium is actively reabsorbed in the proximal tubule. Approximately 12 percent of the filtered potassium is actively and passively secreted in the distal tubule. Ten to fifteen percent of potassium is excreted in the urine, compared to the 1 to 2 percent of sodium that is excreted.

Several factors influence the amount of potassium excreted: hypokalemia, hyperkalemia, acidotic and alkalotic states and urine volume.

Aldosterone regulates potassium through a feedback mechanism. An elevation in serum potassium stimulates the secretion of aldosterone. At the DCT and CT, an ion exchange between sodium and potassium occurs. Sodium is reabsorbed and potassium is excreted.

In hypokalemia, the kidney tries to reabsorb potassium. However, the amount of potassium excreted is influenced by urine volume. Increased GFR and volume results in excretion of a large amount of potassium ions. If a large output is generated, the potassium excretion increases, even in the presence of severe hypokalemia.

KEY CONCEPT: When administering potent diuretics, observe serum K^+ levels. The generation of a large urine output, even in the presence of hypokalemia, causes the kidney to excrete potassium. Supplemental potassium may be necessary to avoid hypokalemic arrythmias.

Calcium (Ca^{++}) and Phosphate

Normal serum calcium is 8.5 to 10.5 mg/dl. Calcium is necessary for transmission of nerve and muscle impulses, blood coagulation, bone formation and cellular permeability.

Approximately 90 percent of filtrate calcium is reabsorbed. Primary factors influencing calcium reabsorption include parathyroid hormone (PTH), vitamin

D and the effects of corticosteroids and diuretics. The parathyroid hormone responds to a decrease in ionized serum calcium. A decrease in serum calcium stimulates the secretion of PTH, resulting in increased tubular reabsorption of calcium and phosphate excretion. PTH also mobilizes calcium in the bones. In patients with renal pathology, this may produce demineralization of the bones.

Vitamin D is necessary for the absorption of calcium from the small intestine. Administration of steroids interferes with the absorption of calcium in the intestine.

Diuretics also affect calcium regulation. Generally, an increase in urine volume results in decreased calcium excretion. This is because of the reduction in total fluid volume and the resultant decreased GFR. Specifically, thiazides increase calcium reabsorption in the DCT while Lasix (furosemide) inhibits calcium reabsorption.

The normal serum concentration of phosphate is 3.0 to 4.5 mg/dl. Phosphate ions are found in the bone and are necessary for intracellular energy-producing reactions.

Active phosphate reabsorption takes place in the PCT. Phosphate reabsorption depends upon the sodium concentration and is inversely related to the GFR. Increased GFR results in decreased reabsorption, while decreased GFR results in increased reabsorption.

Parathyroid hormone inhibits the tubular reabsorption of phosphate. Phosphates are inversely proportional to serum calcium.

KEY CONCEPT: Observe for changes in serum calcium in the presence of diuresis or when administering steroids or diuretics.

Magnesium (Mg$^+$)

Normal serum concentration of magnesium is 1.5 to 2.5 meq/L. It is the second major intracellular ion. Like calcium, magnesium is dependent on the sodium ion for reabsorption. The amount of magnesium reabsorbed by the kidney is inversely proportional to the serum sodium level. Increased serum magnesium results in decreased reabsorption. Decreased serum magnesium results in increased reabsorption.

Chloride (Cl$^-$)

Normal serum concentration of chloride is 98 to 100 mg/dl. Chloride is a negatively charged ion. It is paired with sodium, following its pathway through the nephron. Because it assists in the balancing of the bicarbonate ion, chloride's excretion is influenced by alterations in acid-base status. For example, in the presence of acidosis, the chloride ion is excreted and the bicarbonate ion is reabsorbed, preserving the electrochemical balance. In alkalosis, the chloride ion is reabsorbed and the bicarbonate ion is excreted.

KEY POINT RECOGNITION

Write true or false by each statement. Answers are at the end of this chapter. A score below 80% indicates the need for further study.

_____ 1. Sodium is the major intracellular cation.

_____ 2. More than 99 percent of sodium is reabsorbed in the tubules.

_____ 3. Three to four percent of sodium is reabsorbed in the PCT.

_____ 4. Sodium excretion is dependent on GFR and the secretion of aldosterone.

_____ 5. Aldosterone secretion is regulated by hyperkalemia, ACTH and the total amount of sodium in the body.

_____ 6. Sodium reabsorption is decreased if the GFR is decreased.

_____ 7. Sodium reabsorption is decreased if ADH is secreted.

_____ 8. Normal serum potassium is 3.5 to 5.5 meq/L.

_____ 9. Potassium is actively secreted in the PCT.

_____10. One to two percent of filtered potassium is excreted in the urine.

_____11. Increased serum potassium stimulates aldosterone secretion, resulting ultimately in potassium reabsorption and sodium excretion.

_____12. Potassium excretion is increased in the presence of a large urine output. This occurs even in a severe hypokalemic state.

_____13. About 90 percent of calcium is reabsorbed.

_____14. Decreased serum calcium stimulates PTH secretion, resulting in reabsorption of calcium in the tubules.

_____15. PTH may contribute to demineralization of the bone in patients with chronic renal failure.

_____16. Increased urine output results in decreased calcium excretion.

_____17. Increased GFR results in decreased reabsorption of phosphate.

_____18. PTH enhances reabsorption of phosphate.

_____19. Increased serum magnesium level results in decreased reabsorption of magnesium.

_____20. Magnesium is dependent on sodium for the reabsorption process.

_____21. Chloride excretion is influenced by changes in the body's acid-base status.

_____22. In the presence of acidosis, chloride is reabsorbed.

EXCRETION OF WASTE PRODUCTS

One of the primary functions of the kidney is to excrete the waste products of protein metabolism. The waste products excreted in urine number over 200. Urea and creatinine are the major excreted products capable of measurement.

Urea is a nitrogenous waste product of protein metabolism. Urea is filtered and reabsorbed throughout the nephron. Urea is measured via the blood urea nitrogen (BUN) level in the blood. Urea excretion is influenced by its presence in the filtrate flow, by secondary to clinical states of catabolism, such as trauma, burns, infection and fever, or by certain drugs or alterations in diet. In volume depletion or any cause of decreased filtrate flow, urea may be reabsorbed.

Creatinine is a waste product of muscle metabolism. It is primarily filtered out of the blood by the kidneys and is not secreted or reabsorbed to any degree. Creatinine's rate of excretion is equal to the GFR. Because it is equally produced and excreted, the serum and urine levels of this product are excellent indices of renal function.

KEY POINT RECOGNITION

Write true or false by each statement. Answers are at the end of this chapter. A score below 80% indicates the need for further study.

_____ 1. Urea is freely filtered and reabsorbed throughout the nephron.

_____ 2. Urea excretion may be influenced by fever or severe burns.

_____ 3. Urea is freely excreted in volume depletion.

_____ 4. Creatinine is freely reabsorbed by the kidneys.

_____ 5. Creatinine's rate of excretion is inversely related to the GFR.

THE KIDNEY AND ACID-BASE BALANCE

The body maintains a state of acid-base balance through the integration of body processes involving the kidneys, lungs and body buffers, such as bicarbonate, blood and plasma proteins. The kidney's role in this dynamic process is to stabilize fluid volume while also responding to the body's need to conserve or excrete hydrogen ions. Four basic mechanisms accomplish this delicate balance: direct excretion of hydrogen ions; reabsorption of bicarbonate; excretion of hydrogen ions with renal buffers; and excretion of ammonia.

A very small amount of hydrogen as a free acid is present in the urine. The amount directly excreted is less than 1 meq/day.

Ninety percent of all filtered bicarbonate (HCO_3^-) is reabsorbed in the proximal tubule by the sodium and hydrogen ion exchange (Fig. 6-7). In the tubular cell, carbon dioxide (CO_2) combines with water (H_2O) in the presence of carbonic anhydrase to form carbonic acid (H_2CO_3):

$$CO_2 + H_2O \xrightarrow{Ca} H_2CO_3$$

The carbonic acid (H_2CO_3) then dissociates to form the hydrogen ion (H^+) and bicarbonate (HCO_3^-):

$$H_2CO_3 \longrightarrow H^+ + HCO_3^-$$

Hydrogen is secreted into the lumen of the tubule in exchange for sodium, which is absorbed into the tubular cell. The bicarbonate (HCO_3^-) remains. The Na^+ unites with the HCO_3^-, and they leave the cell as sodium bicarbonate ($NaHCO_3$) and enter the tubular lumen:

$$Na^+ + HCO_3^- \longrightarrow NaHCO_3$$

The hydrogen that was secreted into the tubular lumen combines with the $NaHCO_3$ coming from the cell and forms sodium and carbonic acid (H_2CO_3):

$$H^+ + NaHCO_3 \longrightarrow Na + H_2CO_3$$

The sodium re-enters the cell and combines with more bicarbonate. The carbonic acid (H_2CO_3) remains in the lumen.

The carbonic acid dissociates into CO_2 and H_2O:

$$H_2CO_3 \longrightarrow CO_2 + H_2O$$

The carbon dioxide re-enters the cell, and the water is excreted. The CO_2 that had moved back into the cell then combines with water to form carbonic acid. And the process is repeated:

$$CO_2 + H_2O \longrightarrow H_2CO_3.$$

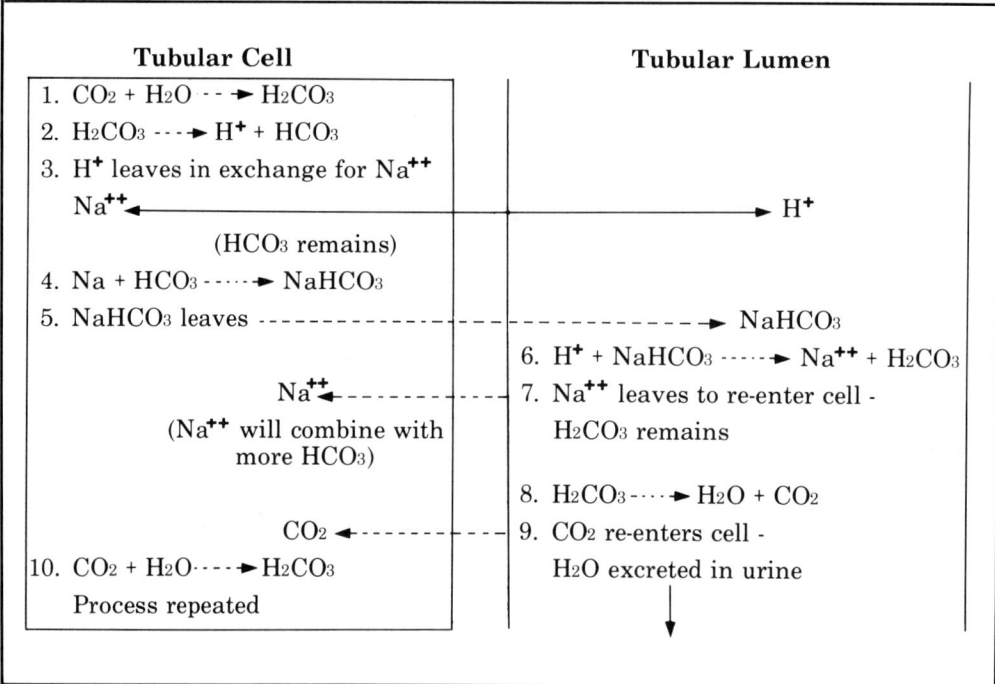

Fig. 6-7. Reabsorption of bicarbonate

Phosphates as Renal Buffers

Phosphates are filtered by the glomerulus and act as buffers for the excretion of hydrogen ions. The process is as follows:

Phosphate (HPO_4) is secreted into the tubular lumen and combines with a hydrogen ion to form hydrogen phosphate, which is excreted:

$$HPO_4^{(-2)} + H^+ \longrightarrow H_2PO_4^{-1}$$

Carbonic acid (H_2CO_3) can combine with dibasic sodium phosphate (Na_2HPO_4) in the tubule to form sodium bicarbonate ($NaHCO_3$) and monobasic sodium phosphate (NaH_2PO_4):

$$H_2CO_3 + Na_2 + HPO_4 \longrightarrow NaHCO_3 + NaH_2PO_4$$

The sodium bicarbonate is reabsorbed and the sodium phosphate is excreted. The hydrogen ion (H^+) alone can combine with dibasic sodium phosphate to produce sodium and monobasic sodium phosphate (NaH_2PO_4):

$$H^+ + Na_2 + HPO_4 \longrightarrow Na + NaH_2PO_4$$

Sodium re-enters the cell and the sodium phosphate is excreted in the urine. This is another way to rid the body of excess hydrogen ions.

Secretion of Ammonia

Ammonia (NH_3) is produced in the distal tubular cells. It diffuses into the tubular lumen and attaches to a hydrogen ion to form the ammonium ion:

$$NH_3 + H^+ \longrightarrow NH_4$$

The ammonium ion (NH_4) may then be excreted with sulfates or join with sodium chloride ($NaCl$) to produce ammonium chloride and sodium:

$$NH_4 + NaCl \longrightarrow NH_4Cl + Na$$

Ammonium chloride is excreted in the urine and the sodium re-enters the cell.

Acidosis

In response to increased secretion of hydrogen ions into the tubular lumen during cellular acidosis, all bicarbonate and sodium is reabsorbed. There is also an increase in the excretion of phosphate and an increased production of ammonia to accommodate the excretion of hydrogen ions. The hydrogen ion may also be excreted as carbonic acid (H_2CO_3). Urine pH will be less than 5.0 because of the higher than usual concentration of hydrogen ions in the urine.

Alkalosis

In an alkalotic state, there is decreased hydrogen ion secretion and an excess amount of bicarbonate ions in the tubules. The excess bicarbonate is excreted in the urine, resulting in a pH greater than 7.0.

Ammonia production is also decreased.

KEY CONCEPT: The kidneys play a dynamic role in acid-base regulation through maintaining fluid volume and the life sustaining pH range, responding to the body's need to conserve or excrete hydrogen ions.

KEY POINT RECOGNITION

Write true or false by each statement. Answers are at the end of this chapter. A score below 80% indicates the need for further study.

_____ 1. A large amount of hydrogen is present in the urine as a free acid.

_____ 2. Ninety percent of all filtered bicarbonate is reabsorbed in the PCT through sodium and hydrogen ion exchange.

_____ 3. CO_2 and H_2O form H_2CO_3 in the presence of carbonic anhydrase.

_____ 4. H_2CO_3 dissociates and forms H^+ and HCO_3^-.

_____ 5. After H^+ and HCO_3^- formation, H^+ is then secreted into the lumen of the tubule in exchange for Na^+.

_____ 6. The NCO_3^- and Na^+ combine and enter the tubular lumen as sodium bicarbonate.

_____ 7. The H^+ combines with the $NaHCO_3^-$ to form sodium and carbonic acid.

_____ 8. Ultimately, the carbonic acid dissociates into CO_2 and H_2O. The water re-enters the cell, the CO_2 is excreted and the process begins again.

_____ 9. Phosphates act as buffers for the excretion of bicarbonate ions.

_____10. Ammonia is produced in the distal tubular cells.

_____11. Ammonium chloride is excreted in the urine.

_____12. Bicarbonate and sodium are reabsorbed in response to an increase in the secretion of H^+ ions.

_____13. To accommodate the excretion of H^+ ions in acidosis, ammonia production is decreased.

_____14. In alkalosis, there is decreased hydrogen ion secretion and an excess amount of bicarbonate in the tubules.

_____15. Ammonia production is increased in alkalosis.

ASSESSMENT OF THE RENAL SYSTEM

Physical assessment of the patient experiencing renal dysfunction is basically the same as the assessment of any other patient. Significant *medical* problems, *current therapies, family history* and *review of systems* are included. Particular attention must be paid to the presenting complaint, its duration and character, and the circumstances surrounding exacerbations and remissions. The following symptoms require further investigation: infections, hypertension, pulmonary disorders, nausea, vomiting, weakness, fatigue, weight loss, edema and changes in mentation.

Specific signs of altered functioning in specific renal disorders may include:

Urinary tract disorders—dysuria, abnormal appearance of urine, such as hematuria, pyuria, biliuria, myoglobinuria, frequency or urgency of urination, nocturia, polyuria, incontinence, oliguria and pain in the flank or groin area

Uremia—nausea, vomiting, pruritus, weight loss with muscle wasting, bleeding, asterixis, peripheral neuropathy, uremic breath and uremic frost

The *physical examination* should include assessment of the following:

GROSS CEREBRAL FUNCTION

Check for consciousness, awareness, orientation, memory and judgment.

SPECIFIC CEREBRAL FUNCTION

Check conversational ability and attention span.

INSPECTION

Check skin for abnormal color.

Check skin for capillary integrity.

Check for skin turgor.

Check for presence of edema (periorbital, localized, anasarca, pulmonary).

Check respirations for air hunger.

Check urinary output for quantity and characteristics.

Check muscles for tremors, weakness, wasting and tetany due to hypocalemia.

Check for asterixis (flapping or hyperextended wrists and fingers).

Check cardiac status for dysrhythmias.

Check mucous membranes for color and hydration.

PALPATION

Palpate for size, shape and location of kidneys.

Palpate for tenderness.

Palpate area over bladder for fullness.

Palpate nailbeds for capillary refill.

PERCUSSION

Percuss for tenderness, pain, mass and ascites.

AUSCULTATION

Listen for bowel sounds (hyperactive, hypoactive, absent).

Listen for breath sounds (intensity, rales).

Listen for heart sounds (murmurs, pericardial rub).

Listen for abdominal bruits.

KEY CONCEPT: Physical assessment of the patient with a renal problem should include assessment of: gross and specific cerebral functions, in addition to inspection, palpation, percussion and auscultation of the renal system.

KEY POINT RECOGNITION

Write true or false by each statement. Answers are at the end of this chapter. A score below 80% indicates the need for further study.

_____ 1. Dysuria, polyuria, hematuria and pyuria may indicate a renal disorder.

_____ 2. Urine is checked for quantity and characteristics.

_____ 3. Periorbital edema, anasarca and pulmonary edema may indicate renal disorders.

_____ 4. Asterixis may indicate a uremic state.

_____ 5. Tetany may indicate hypercalcemia.

RENAL ASSESSMENT

Level of Consciousness

Under any condition, the *level of consciousness* (LOC) is the single most important determinant of neurological status. To assess level of consciousness, the following must be determined:

Arousability

Orientation

Ability to follow commands

Voiding Pattern

After the LOC has been determined, nursing assessment of the renal system begins with a detailed description of the voiding pattern. This includes:

Duration of the problem, its onset and description

Observation of the urinary stream

Bladder distention, abdominal fullness, bladder size and fullness

Control of Stream

Next, the control of the urinary stream is assessed:

Can the patient void on command?

Does the patient have the sensation to void?

Are there areas of irritation or breakdown?

Are there other problems associated with the inability to control urinary stream (spinal cord injury, urinary tract infection)?

Dysuria

Dysuria is a sign of urinary tract infection. Dysuria is described as burning upon urination, which is sometimes accompanied by frequency and urgency. Question the patient regarding painful urination.

Toilet Habits

Toilet habits include assessing whether the patient can perform toileting safely and independently. Will the patient need adjunctive equipment? Will an indwelling catheter be necessary?

Evaluation of Vital Signs

The blood pressure may be normal or elevated. Rarely in renal dysfunction is *hypotension* seen unless bleeding or sepsis is present. *Hypertension* may be seen in chronic renal failure, the nephrotic syndrome or hypertensive renal disease. *Tachycardia* and *pyrexia* may be present if there are infections of the urinary tract. These may be self-limiting and return to normal as the infection clears. *Respiratory* changes are uncommon. Illnesses that reduce renal function and perfusion may alter vital signs. These illnesses do not necessarily involve kidney tissue directly. The reduction in urinary output and a reduction in the clearance of materials are the indicating factors. Reduction in renal function may be secondary to hypovolemia, cardiac failure and septic shock.

Laboratory and Radiologic Studies

Laboratory studies in renal disease are varied and tailored to be presumptive diagnosis at hand (Fig. 6-8):

Test	Normal Value*	Variation with Renal Disorder**
Serum		
Na	135-148 meq/L	Va-May ↑
K	3.5-4.8 meq/L	↑
Cl	96-110 meq/L	Va-May ↑
CO_2	24-28 meq/L	↓
Osmolarity	280-295 mOsm/Kq/L	Va
Calcium	8.5-10.5 mg/100 ml	↓
Magnesium	1.6-2.2 meq/L	N-May ↑
Phosphorus	2-4.5 mg/100 ml	↑
Glucose	70-110 mg/dl	Va
Hemoglobin	12-16 gm/100 ml	↓
Hematocrit	40-50%	↓
BUN	10-20 mg/100 ml	↑ 10:1 Ratio
Creatinine	.6-2.0 mg/100 ml	↑
Urine		
Specific gravity	1.010-1.025	Va-May ↓
pH	4-7	Va
Glucose	L0.25 mg/percent	Va
Protein	L100 mg/day	Va
RBCs	0-2 HPF (high power field)	Va
WBCs	2-3 HPF	Va
Na	40-80 meq/L	Va
K	40-80 meq/L	↓
Cl	80-120 meq/L	↓
Osmolarity	600-1400 mOsm/L	↓
Creatinine clearance	80-125 ml/min	↓
Color and clarity	clear	cloudy infection
Culture and sensitivity	negative	foamy albumin
Acetone		diabetes
Casts		

*Ranges for normal values may vary for certain parameters based on laboratory methods and standards for institutions.

** ↑—Increase
↓—Decrease
Va—Variable
N—Normal

Fig. 6-8. Laboratory studies: renal function

BUN (blood urea nitrogen) is the end product of protein metabolism. Nitrogen is an endogenous waste product. An increased BUN indicates a decreased glomerular filtration rate, a high protein intake, or a catabolic state. Normal: 8 to 18 mgm/dl.

Serum creatinine reflects the balance between creatinine production and filtration by the renal glomerulus. Elevated creatinine is seen in all diseases of the kidneys in which there is nephron destruction of 50 percent or more.

Electrolytes-*Sodium* is a cation found in extracellular fluid. It helps regulate acid-base balance. Sodium protects the body from excessive fluid loss. Hypernatremia may result from excessive intravenous sodium infusion. Hyponatremia may be due to the loss of sodium from the kidneys from the use of diuretics. Decreased serum sodium is also seen in patients who are acidotic secondary to chronic renal insufficiency. Patients who continue to reabsorb water from the distal tubules and excrete concentrated urine may be suffering from antidiuretic hormone (ADH) dysfunction. Normal: 136 to 142 meq/L.

Potassium is a primary cation of intracellular fluid. It helps regulate acid-base balance, osmotic pressure and cellular membrane potential. Hyperkalemia is frequently associated with renal failure. Hypokalemia reflects total body depletion of potassium, which is seen in potassium-losing nephropathy and renal tubular acidosis. Hyperchloremia and aminoaciduria often accompany hypokalemia. Normal: 3.8 to 5.0 meq/L.

Chloride, an extracellular ion, regulates acid-base balance and osmotic pressure. Hyperchloremia is frequently associated with renal tubular acidosis, decreased CO_2 content and hypokalemia. Hypochloremia is associated with hypokalemia and alkalosis. Normal: 95 to 103 meq/L.

The CO_2 *content* is checked to determine the presence of acid-base abnormalities. Elevated CO_2 content indicates respiratory acidosis or metabolic alkalosis. Low CO_2 content is associated with metabolic acidosis, such as uremic acidosis, diabetic ketoacidosis, lactic acidosis and renal tubular acidosis or respiratory alkalosis. Normal: 24 to 30 mm/L.

Radiologic studies are distinct and are briefly discussed here:

Flat plate: The kidney, ureters and bladder (KUB) are radiographed to determine their size, shape and position.

Intravenous pyelogram: An IVP is performed by an invasive injection of dye into a vein. This is done to visualize the urinary tract for obstruction, tumors, cysts, congenital abnormalities or hypertension of the renal vasculature.

Retrograde pyelography: This study visualizes the urinary collecting system for obstruction. Uretheral catheters are passed up the ureters into the renal pelvis.

Retrograde urethrography: This is performed to determine the status of the urethra.

Renal scan: This is a noninvasive radiographic procedure used to determine renal perfusion and function.

Cystoscopy: This is an invasive procedure used to detect pathology of the urethra or bladder.

Diagnostic ultrasonography: This is a noninvasive procedure to detect masses, obstructions and malformations of structures in the urinary tract.

Computerized axial tomography: A CAT scan is a noninvasive procedure in which multiple radiographs are interpreted by a computer. The use of multiple radiographs based on density provides a three-dimensional view of abnormalities.

Voiding cystourethrography: This study is used to determine if there is reflux of urine into the ureters on voiding.

Renal arteriogram: This is accomplished by an invasive injection of dye. This study helps determine abnormalities or tumors in the renal vasculature.

Renal biopsy: This is an invasive procedure performed to determine the type and stage of renal pathology.

KEY CONCEPT: Nursing assessment of the patient with a renal dysfunction includes evaluation of history, physical, laboratory and radiologic findings.

KEY POINT RECOGNITION
Write true or false by each statement. Answers are at the end of this chapter. A score below 80% indicates the need for further study.

_____ 1. Elevated creatinine indicates nephron damage.

_____ 2. An elevated blood urea nitrogen level indicates increased glomerular filtration.

_____ 3. Blood urea nitrogen is the end product of protein metabolism.

_____ 4. Normal BUN level is 90 to 120 mgm/dl.

_____ 5. Diuretics may cause hyponatremia.

_____ 6. Hypochloremia frequently occurs in the presence of hypokalemia and alkalosis.

_____ 7. An elevated serum CO_2 content indicates serum alkalosis.

_____ 8. BUN and creatinine studies are important determinants of renal function.

_____ 9. Nursing assessment of patients with a renal problem includes checking the voiding pattern, toilet habits and control of urination.

_____ 10. Hypotension is common in patients with chronic renal failure.

PATHOLOGICAL STATES AND NURSING MANAGEMENT

ACUTE RENAL FAILURE

Pathophysiology: General

Renal failure is defined as the sudden cessation of the kidneys in excreting the waste products of cell metabolism. Renal failure is generally caused by one of three etiological factors: **prerenal, intrarenal** or **postrenal** conditions (Fig. 6-9).

	Prerenal	Intrarenal		Postrenal
Urine		cortical	medullary	
Sodium	↓ 10 meq/L	↓ 10 meq/L	↑ 20 meq/L	varies
Specific gravity	↑ 1.020	varies	1.010-1.015	varies
Protein	minimal to none	moderate to heavy	minimal to moderate	varies
Sediment	normal	RBC, WBC	epithelial cells, tubular cells, rare RBC	varies
Serum BUN	↑	↑	↑	↑
Creatinine	↑	↑	↑	↑

↑—increase
↓—decrease

Fig. 6-9. Acute renal failure: pre-renal, intrarenal, postrenal

Prerenal conditions decrease circulating blood flow through the kidneys and decrease perfusion to the affected renal tissue. Precipitating factors leading to **prerenal** conditions are hemorrhage, sepsis, burns, mismatched blood transfusion causing lysis of hemoglobin, massive crushing injuries, acute pancreatitis and dehydration. The decrease in renal perfusion leads to oliguria or anuria.

Intrarenal conditions, or intrinsic renal failure, result from injury to the kidney cells. Cortical injury causes swelling of the renal capillaries and cellular proliferation, resulting in a decreased glomerular filtration rate. A decreased glomerular filtration rate occurs as a result of glomeruli obstruction due to the edema and cellular debris. Acute cortical necrosis refers to infarction of the entire nephron, a result of prolonged renal ischemia. This is commonly seen in complications of pregnancy, such as abruptio placentae, post-partum hemorrhage, toxemia or septic abortion. Medullary injury develops as a result of long standing ischemia or nephrotoxic injury. Nephrotoxic injury may affect the epithelial layer. This layer is capable of regeneration. However, injuries involving nephrons and peritubular capillaries may cause permanent damage since this layer does not regenerate. Intrarenal conditions are often precipitated by acute post streptococcal glomerulonephritis, acute cortical necrosis, systemic lupus erythematosus, endocarditis, abruptio placentae, abortions and malignant hypertension. Acute tubular necrosis resulting from nephrotoxicity follows ingestion or inhalation of chemical substances, such as bichloride of mercury, ethylene oxide (antifreeze) and carbon tetrachloride. Drugs may also cause nephrotoxicity. Common offenders are aminoglycosides, aspirin and phenacetin.

Whatever the cause, acute renal failure usually follows a clinical course composed of three stages: oliguria, diuresis and recovery (Fig. 6-10).

	Oliguric Phase	**Diuretic**	**Recovery**
Symptoms	Na + H$_2$O Overload Weight gain Paroxysmal nocturnal dyspnea Dyspnea on exertion Anorexia Nausea Vomiting Diarrhea Mental disturbances Lethargy Uremic frost Metabolic acidosis	Urine output 400 ml/day Na+K depletion Changes in mental acuity Degree of thirst Skin turgor Tachycardia Changes in mucous membranes	Absent
Lab Studies	Urine concentrated Urine/plasma osmolarity ratio 2:1 ↑ BUN ↑ Creatinine ↑ Na, K ↑ Phosphate ↓ Hemoglobin ↓ hematocrit	↑ BUN ↓ Na ↓ K ↓ H$_2$O	Normal

Fig. 6-10. Stages of acute renal failure

Oliguria is usually the result of a surgical, medical or obstetrical problem. Oliguria is seen within 48 hours after the injury or several days after exposure to nephrotoxic chemicals. Prerenal output is less than 400 ml per day. Oliguria may result from shock, decreased plasma volume or a decrease in the renal blood flow through the kidneys. In prerenal oliguria, damage is to the parenchyma. The oliguric urine is concentrated. The urine-plasma osmolarity ratio is above 2:1. Prerenal oliguria may progress to acute tubular necrosis, changing the ratio to 1:1. The urine plasma urea concentration ratio is greater than 20:1 in prerenal oliguria and less than 10:1 in acute tubular necrosis.

Diuresis, or the diuretic stage, is defined as urine output above 400 ml/day. The output per day rarely exceeds 4,000 ml. The high urine volume is due to osmotic diuresis produced by blood urea concentration and the impaired ability of the tubules to conserve water and salt. Severe deficits of potassium, sodium and water may lead to death if they are not corrected. The diuretic stage may continue for two to three weeks.

The *recovery* stage lasts up to one year. During this stage, the concentrating ability of the kidneys improves. There may be permanent reduction in the glomerular filtration rate.

Acute tubular necrosis, acute cortical necrosis, decreased glomerular filtration and altered blood flow distribution are all pathophysiological states of acute renal failure. Acute vasomotor nephropathy is a condition of acute renal failure.

In acute vasomotor nephropathy, there is a decrease in the glomerular filtration rate and an uneven distribution of blood flow through the kidney. This leads to ischemia and toxic renal failure.

Pathophysiology: Specific
Acute Tubular Necrosis (ATN)

Renal failure with acute tubular necrosis is the result of tubular obstruction and back diffusion of tubular fluid. Two types of lesions are associated with acute tubular necrosis: necrosis of the tubular epithelium, in which the basement membrane remains intact and usually follows ingestion of nephrotoxic chemicals; and the necrosis of tubular epithelium and the basement membrane, which occurs with renal ischemia. ATN is the pathological diagnosis seen in 25 percent of acute renal failure. In contemporary nephrology, the condition is felt to be vasomotor nephropathy.

Acute Cortical Necrosis (ACN)

Acute cortical necrosis is an infarction of the entire nephron. The result is irreversible renal failure. The glomerular filtration rate decreases as a result of glomerular edema and cellular debris.

Decreased Glomerular Nephropathy

In decreased glomerular filtration, the decreased filtration rate leads to an increase in the tone of involved afferent arterioles. The decreased glomerular capillary pressure causes filtration to cease. The end result is an increase in vascular resistance and a decrease in renal blood flow.

Altered Blood Flow Distribution

In acute renal failure, the blood flows primarily through the inner cortex and medulla. In chronic renal failure, blood is diverted into the outer cortex, allowing for sufficient glomerular filtration.

Clinical Presentation

The clinical presentation is extremely variable and dependent on the specific disease process. Changes in mentation, such as confusion, lethargy and stupor, may occur. Nausea, vomiting, anorexia, constipation, diarrhea, deep or rapid respirations, pulmonary edema, tachycardia, dysrhythmias, pericarditis, dry skin and pruritis may be observed. The most common preceding symptom of acute renal failure is the sudden onset of renal dysfunction manifested by an extreme alteration in urine output and concentration.

Diagnostic Data

Patient history is an important diagnostic aid when determining the etiology of acute renal failure. Routine laboratory tests, such as CBC and urinalysis, are valuable in assessing possible renal involvement. BUN and creatinine are the most single important determinants of renal function. A triple renal scan and renal ultrasound may be ordered if an obstruction is suspected.

Nursing Care

The major nursing responsibilities are:

(1) Maintain fluid and electrolyte balance. Correct and maintain adequate

hydration. Correct electrolyte imbalance. Correct acid-base imbalance.
(2) Prevent shock. Monitor intake, output and vital signs. Assure adequate hydration.
(3) Prevent infection. Use strict aseptic technique.
(4) Maintain nutritional status.
(5) Provide meticulous skin care.
(6) Treat hypertensive states.
(7) Prevent complications.

KEY CONCEPT: Acute renal failure may present different clinical pictures according to the specific etiology. The overall nursing goals are to maintain the patient during the acute stage and to prevent further complications.

KEY POINT RECOGNITION
Write true or false by each statement. Answers are at the end of this chapter. A score below 80% indicates the need for further study.

_____ 1. Renal failure is the sudden inability of the kidneys to excrete the waste products of cell metabolism.
_____ 2. Prerenal failure is the reduction in blood flow through the kidneys.
_____ 3. Intrarenal failure results from injury to the kidney cells.
_____ 4. In intrarenal failure, the glomerular filtration rate is increased.
_____ 5. Acute tubular necrosis is an infarction of the entire nephron.
_____ 6. Medullary injury may result from renal ischemia or nephrotoxic injury.
_____ 7. Postrenal failure is due to an obstruction in the urinary collecting system.
_____ 8. The diuretic stage of acute renal failure appears within 48 hours following the initial insult.
_____ 9. Urinary output falls to less than 400 ml per day during the oliguric phase of renal failure.
_____10. Oliguric urine is dilute.
_____11. Prerenal oliguria may progress to acute tubular necrosis.
_____12. In the diuretic stage, the high urine volume is due to osmotic diuresis.
_____13. Acute tubular necrosis may occur following the ingestion of carbon tetrachloride.
_____14. Acute vasomotor nephropathy denotes an increase in glomerular filtration.
_____15. In acute renal failure, blood flows primarily into the outer cortex, bypassing the cortex and medulla.
_____16. BUN and creatinine are valuable diagnostic aids.
_____17. Nursing care is directed toward recognition of imbalances and prevention of complications.

CHRONIC RENAL FAILURE
Pathophysiology
Chronic renal failure is the slow, progressive development of renal dysfunction. The nephrons lose their ability to maintain the volume and composition of body fluids. Chronic glomerulonephritis, pyelonephritis, uncontrolled hypertension, renal diseases secondary to systemic disease, drugs, toxic agents and infections may cause chronic renal failure. There is a decrease in glomerular filtration, with a resultant rise in serum phosphate and a decrease in ionizable calcium. The products of protein metabolism accumulate in the blood. Renal osteodystrophy, uremic bone disease, develops as a result of calcium, phosphate and parathyroid changes. Sodium and water retention occurs, leading to conges-

tive heart failure, pulmonary edema and hypertension. Metabolic acidosis results from the retention of bicarbonate and the kidney's inability to excrete hydrogen ions.

Initially, BUN and creatinine are within normal limits. As the disease progresses, the BUN and creatinine rise because of destruction of the nephron.

The exact mechanism of impaired kidney function in chronic renal failure is not known. There are two theories:

(1) All the nephrons are affected in varying degrees. The nephrons responsible for specific functions are destroyed or impaired.

(2) When nephrons are diseased, they are totally destroyed and become nonfunctional. The unaffected nephrons remain intact and continue to perform normally.

According to the second hypothesis, the kidney attempts to compensate. The filtration process shifts to the remaining functioning units, causing hypertrophy. The healthy nephrons increase the glomerular filtration rate, the solute load and tubular reabsorption. This compensatory mechanism can continue until advanced uremia ensues. The filtration rate and solute load of each nephron becomes so high that a balance between filtration and tubular reabsorption cannot be maintained. The kidney's ability to concentrate or dilute urine in response to the body's needs becomes more limited.

Clinical Presentation

The clinical presentation begins with mild fatigue, headache, generalized malaise, gastrointestinal disturbances and bleeding tendencies. As the disease progresses, the patient becomes increasingly lethargic, develops Kussmaul's respirations, coma and convulsions. The appearance of a white frost, "uremic frost," on the skin is a grave sign. This white frost is urate crystals. If untreated, death will result.

Diagnostic Data

A rise in serum BUN and creatinine is an important diagnostic aid. A creatinine clearance of 5 to 10 ml/min. indicates that the glomerular filtration rate is less than 10 percent.

Nursing Care

The aim of nursing care is to maintain homeostasis:

(1) Regulate protein, fluid, sodium and calcium. Restrict potassium and phosphate. Maintain adequate caloric intake. Administer vitamin supplements.

(2) Administer aluminum hydroxide antacids, which bind phosphorus in the intestinal tract.

(3) Monitor blood pressure. Observe for hypertension and pulmonary edema.

(4) Protect from injury.

(5) Provide emotional support for the patient and family.

(6) If appropriate, provide referral or teach about dialysis.

PYELONEPHRITIS

Pathophysiology

Pyelonephritis is a bacterial infection of the renal pelvis, interstitial tissue and tubules. Pyelonephritis may be chronic or acute. Escherichia coli is the most common organism causing urinary tract infections. The organism enters via the urethra and ascends to the bladder, ureters and renal pelvis. Fluid accumulates under the renal pelvis, causing inflammation and obstruction of the urinary outflow tract. Scarring of the ureters and atrophy of the renal parenchyma may result. Precipitating factors are sex, age, pregnancy, vesicourethral reflux and phenacetin abuse.

Clinical Presentation

A sudden onset of general malaise, fever, chills, back pain and flank tenderness, elevated serum white blood cells, pyuria and a history of dysuria, frequency and urgency, is indicative of pyelonephritis. When acute pyelonephritis is complicated by obstruction, the incidence of bacteriuria increases. These patients must be treated with drug therapy until cultures are negative.

Chronic pyelonephritis usually results from untreated or recurrent pyelonephritis. It is usually diagnosed after the patient presents with symptoms of chronic renal insufficiencies or hypertension. A decrease in the concentrating ability of the kidney, polyuria, nocturia and a low specific gravity are seen early in pyelonephritis.

Diagnostic Data

The most important laboratory studies are the urine culture, urine analysis with WBC casts and serum elevation of white blood cells.

Nursing Care

The major goals of nursing care are early detection of the illness, proper therapy and the correction and treatment of underlying systemic disease.

(1) Patient education should include instructions to seek medical care if early signs of pyelonephritis reappear, such as fever, costovertebral tenderness, cloudy urine, dysuria or frequency.

(2) Proper collection of urine specimens is important to accurate studies.

(3) Administer medications, especially antibiotics.

(4) Instruct the patient in proper toilet habits to prevent further bacterial contamination.

(5) Encourage adequate fluid intake.

KEY CONCEPT: Nursing care for pyelonephritis is aimed at the reduction and control of the bacterial infection in an effort to prevent renal damage.

KEY POINT RECOGNITION

Write true or false by each statement. Answers are at the end of this chapter. A score below 80% indicates the need for further study.

_____ 1. Pyelonephritis is defined as a viral infection of the bladder.

_____ 2. The most common causative agent of urinary tract infections is the streptococcus.

_____ 3. Pyelonephritis may lead to scarring of the ureters and atrophy of the renal parenchyma.

_____ 4. Common symptoms of pyelonephritis include general malaise, fever, dysuria, frequency and flank pain.

_____ 5. Chronic pyelonephritis results from untreated or recurrent pyelonephritis.

GLOMERULONEPHRITIS

Pathophysiology

Glomerulonephritis often follows an acute inflammatory disease of the glomerulus of the kidneys. It may be due to primary renal disease or secondary to glomerular lesions as seen in systemic lupus erythematosus.

Acute glomerulonephritis is usually an immune response to group A beta-hemolytic streptococcus. If often occurs two to three weeks poststreptococcus throat infection. Formation of the antigen-antibody complex prevents filtration through the glomerular tubules. Deposits are left on the basement membrane, causing injury and inflammation of the membrane. Polymorphonuclear leukocytes, platelets, phagocytes and lysomal enzymes are attracted to the membrane. This causes proliferation of the endothelial cells and congestion of the porous glomeruli. Hematuria and proteinuria develop because of the escape of blood and protein through the porous glomerular capillary. Renal cells become ineffective and die.

Chronic glomerulonephritis is responsible for the greatest number of patients undergoing chronic dialysis or renal transplants. It is the leading cause of renal failure. Chronic glomerulonephritis is caused by the progressive destruction of glomeruli from long-standing glomerular nephritis.

In advanced chronic glomerulonephritis, the kidneys reduce to approximately one-fifth of their normal size. The surface becomes scarred and granular. Microscopic examination shows interstitial fibrosis, atrophy of the tubules and a thickening of the arterial walls.

Clinical Presentation

The course of chronic glomerulonephritis varies from 2 to 40 years, with the end stage being uremia and death. The patient with chronic glomerulonephritis generally complains of recurrent dependent edema, headache, dyspnea on exertion, blurred vision, nocturia, weakness, fatigue and weight loss. The patient with acute glomerulonephritis complains of shortness of breath, headache, weakness and anorexia. Dependent edema, hypertension and decreased urinary output may also be present.

Diagnostic Data

Early in chronic glomerulonephritis, a urinalysis reveals albumin, casts and blood. As the disease progresses and only a few intact nephrons remain, the urinalysis may be negative for protein and blood. The specific gravity of the urine becomes fixed and the blood's nonprotein nitrogen level increases.

Acute glomerulonephritis is diagnosed by an elevation in the BUN and creatinine levels and an elevated antistreptolysin O titer. A urinalysis reveals protein and red blood cells, retention of wastes and an increased specific gravity.

Nursing Care

Nursing care is aimed at teaching the individual to live a healthful lifestyle.
 (1) Maintain fluid balance.
 (2) Promote dietary changes: restrict sodium, potassium and protein intake.
 (3) Administer medication. Explain the importance of prophylactic treatment.
 (4) Prevent further complications.
 (5) Prevent further infections.
 (6) Promote follow-up.

KEY CONCEPT: Exposure to any infection may cause the reoccurrence of glomerulonephritis and must be avoided.

KEY POINT RECOGNITION

Write true or false by each statement. Answers are at the end of this chapter. A score below 80% indicates the need for further study.

_____ 1. Glomerulonephritis follows an acute inflammatory disease of the glomerulus of the kidneys.

_____ 2. Acute glomerulonephritis is an immune response to group A beta-hemolytic streptococcus.

_____ 3. The leading cause of renal failure is acute glomerulonephritis.

_____ 4. Chronic glomerulonephritis is caused by the progressive destruction of glomeruli due to long-standing glomerular nephritis.

_____ 5. In advanced chronic glomerulonephritis, the kidneys become enlarged.

_____ 6. Chronic glomerulonephritis causes the surface of the kidney to become scarred and granular.

_____ 7. The patient with chronic glomerulonephritis may present with signs of polyuria, oliguria, proteinuria and hypertension.

_____ 8. Azotemia and edema rarely occur in chronic glomerulonephritis.

_____ 9. Chronic glomerulonephritis presents with a fixed, elevated specific gravity.

_____ 10. A decreased serum antistreptolysin O titer and decreased urea nitrogen level are present in chronic glomerulonephritis.

NEPHROTIC SYNDROME

Pathophysiology

Nephrotic syndrome is a condition caused by massive proteinuria. The glomerular basement membrane becomes damaged, causing an increase in permeability. Protein crosses the membrane. The nephrotic syndrome leads to degeneration and necrosis of the renal tubules. Hypoalbuminemia may develop as a result of 5 to 15 gm of protein being lost in the urine. This lack of serum albumin decreases colloid osmotic pressure, causing a fluid shift from the intravascular space to the interstitial space. The shifting of fluid leads to generalized edema, hypovolemia, decreased renal perfusion and decreased glomerular filtration rate. The body's compensatory response to hypovolemia stimulates aldosterone and ADH release, which causes the reabsorption of sodium and water and perpetuates the problem.

Clinical Presentation

The clinical presentation is characterized by edema, anasarca, proteinuria, elevated serum lipids, hypertension, hematuria, loss of appetitie and fatigue. Women experience amenorrhea and other reproductive disorders.

Diagnostic Data

The patient presents with severe generalized edema and proteinuria. Urinalysis findings reveal proteinuria and albumin and globulin protein fractions (lipiduria), as well as hypoalbuminemia and elevated serum crystals.

Nursing Care

(1) The control of the nephrotic syndrome is based upon reducing the albuminuria and mobilizing edema.
(2) Accurately administer steroids and diuretics.
(3) Increase protein intake by dietary intervention.
(4) Restrict sodium.
(5) Observe for hypokalemia.
(6) Maintain the patient with severe edema on bedrest.
(7) Prevent complications related to immobility.
(8) Prevent infection.
(9) Provide comprehensive patient teaching.
(10) Provide meticulous skin care.

KEY CONCEPT: Reduction of albuminuria and maintenance of body processes are primary goals in the treatment of the nephrotic syndrome.

KEY POINT RECOGNITION

Write true or false by each statement. Answers are at the end of this chapter. A score below 80% indicates the need for further study.

_____ 1. The nephrotic syndrome is caused by the lack of protein in the urine.

_____ 2. In nephrotic syndrome, the glomerular basement membrane becomes less permeable.

_____ 3. Nephrotic syndrome leads to necrosis of the renal tubules.

_____ 4. Hypoalbuminemia may develop in nephrotic syndrome.

_____ 5. Hypoalbuminemia decreases colloid osmotic pressure.

_____ 6. Nephrotic syndrome is characterized by edema, anasarca, proteinuria and hypertension.

_____ 7. In nephrotic syndrome, hypokalemia may develop.

HYPERTENSION
Pathophysiology

Hypertension is the sustained elevation of blood pressure above 90 mm Hg diastolic or 140 mm Hg systolic. **Essential hypertension** is hypertension in which the etiology and pathogenesis are unknown. **Malignant hypertension** is severe hypertension with diastolic pressure above 120 to 130 mm Hg, grade IV retinopathy and renal dysfunction, such as proteinuria, hematuria or azotemia.

As a result of long-term hypertension, the lumen of the intrarenal blood vessels narrows. The small arteries and arterioles sclerose, causing destruction and atrophy of the glomeruli, tubules and nephrons.

A decrease in renal blood flow and glomerular filtration rate stimulates the renin-angiotensin-aldosterone mechanism. Angiotensin and aldosterone release and tubular reabsorption of sodium and water increase the blood pressure further.

Clinical Presentation

If *diastolic* blood pressure is above 90 mm Hg, and *systolic* blood pressure is above 140 mm Hg, signs and symptoms of chronic renal failure are present. It is possible for hypotension to be present with normal cardiac output and blood volume. However, if the mean arterial pressure falls below 40 mm Hg, renal perfusion is compromised. In malignant hypertension, a pressure less than 150/90 mm Hg results in decreased glomerular filtration rate caused by renal arteriolar constriction.

RENAL INSUFFICIENCY
Pathophysiology

Renal insufficiency is a reduction in renal function. However, this reduction is compatible with life. Precipitating factors are plasma loss, cardiac failure, renal occlusion, hypovolemia, hypotension or vasoconstriction.

Hypovolemia may result from blood loss, gastrointestinal fluid loss, third spacing phenomenon, fluid and electrolyte imbalance or shock. Excessive use of diuretics and sepsis are clinical states that lead to an inadequate circulating volume and prerenal failure. This reduced circulating volume reduces arterial pressure and decreases filtration in the afferent arterioles. The reduction in arterial pressure causes the baroreceptors in the aortic arch and carotid sinus to effect a sympathetic nervous system response. The osmoreceptors and baroreceptors stimulate the pituitary to release antidiuretic hormone. The added release of aldosterone increases tubular reabsorption of sodium and water. This is the body's attempt to conserve plasma volume and maximize urine concentration.

Sepsis is a pathological state resulting from microorganisms in the blood. Sepsis-induced hypovolemia is due to capillary leakage and third space shifting of fluid. Patient presentation can be misleading because the associated weight gain, edema and increased central venous pressure would not seem to indicate a hypovolemic state. However, renal insufficiency will result if sepsis is not treated properly.

Cardiac failure produces a physiological state similar to hypovolemia. This state is a result of pump failure and the concurrent reduction in cardiac output. As cardiac output falls, sympathetic activity increases, causing renal vasoconstriction of the afferent and efferent arterioles. Renal blood and glomerular filtration rates decrease. The filtration fraction rises. Protein concentration in the peritubular capillaries rises, which increases renal vascular resistance and lowers postglomerular capillary hydrostatic pressure. The resultant effect is an increase in proximal tubular sodium reabsorption.

Renal arterial occlusion is a bilateral mechanical obstruction of the renal arteries caused by one of two etiological factors: **thrombus** or **embolus.**

In case of thrombus or embolus, the decreased blood flow causes a cessation of urinary output, anuria and necrosis of the renal parenchyma.

Anuria is a diagnostic aid because it rarely occurs in other types of kidney failure.

Clinical Presentation

The clinical presentation is extremely variable and dependent on the cause. Shocklike symptoms may occur, but are more common in hypovolemia and cardiac failure. Weight gain, edema and an increase in the central venous pressure may be seen in sepsis. The most common symptoms are hypotension, tachycardia, diaphoresis, cyanosis and mentation changes.

Diagnostic Data

Laboratory studies revealing electrolyte imbalances and proteinuria are the best diagnostic aids. A complete history and physical are necessary to determine the cause and extent of renal insufficiency. Routine laboratory tests are valuable to determine overall patient condition.

Nursing Care

The major nursing responsibilities when caring for a patient with renal insufficiency include:

(1) Assess neurological status, including continuous monitoring for mental changes.
(2) Assess circulation, including continuous monitoring of blood pressure, cardiac status and vital signs.
(3) Assess and maintain fluid and electrolyte balance.
(4) Prevent complications.
(5) Monitor urinary output and intake.
(6) Provide emotional support to the patient and family.

KEY CONCEPT: Hypertension and renal insufficiency have varying clinical presentations. Nursing care is aimed at prevention.

KEY POINT RECOGNITION

Write true or false by each statement. Answers are at the end of this chapter. A score below 80% indicates the need for further study.

_____ 1. Hypertension is the sustained elevation of blood pressure above 120 mm Hg diastolic or above a systolic of 160 mm Hg.

_____ 2. Malignant hypertension is severe hypertension with concomitant renal dysfunction.

_____ 3. The lumen of the intrarenal blood vessels may narrow as a result of hypertension.

_____ 4. The renin-angiotensin-aldosterone mechanism may be stimulated by a decrease in renal blood flow and glomerular filtration rate.

_____ 5. Although cardiac output and blood volume are normal, hypotensive states are possible in malignant hypertension if the blood pressure falls below 150/90.

_____ 6. Renal insufficiency is a reduction in renal function that is incompatible with life.

_____ 7. Hypovolemia may precipitate renal insufficiency.

_____ 8. Pump failure may precipitate renal insufficiency.

_____ 9. Plasma loss may precipitate renal insufficiency.

_____10. Sepsis can produce hypovolemia and precipitate renal insufficiency.

_____11. Renal arterial occlusion is a mechanical obstruction of the renal arteries.

_____12. Anuria is rare in renal arterial occlusion.

DIALYSIS

Dialysis is the utilization of a semipermeable membrane to remove accumulated toxins and water from the body when the kidneys are not functioning. Water and solutes move across the semipermeable membrane by osmosis, diffusion and ultrafiltration.

Dialysis is indicated in fluid overload when there is an accumulation of waste products in the serum; and in acid-base electrolyte imbalances that cannot be controlled by nondialytic methods. Candidacy for dialysis is established by meeting the following criteria:

(1) A blood urea nitrogen (BUN) level greater than 100, associated with a proportional rise in serum creatinine of 10 or more

(2) Fluid overload that predisposes to cardiac failure and pulmonary edema

There are two major types of dialysis: peritoneal dialysis and hemodialysis. The type used will depend upon factors such as availability of hemodialysis, bleeding disorders, recent abdominal surgery or the presence of adhesions.

Peritoneal Dialysis

Peritoneal dialysis allows for the removal of toxic substances and excessive fluid by using the peritoneal lining of the abdominal wall and organs as the semipermeable membrane. It is indicated for fluid overload, electrolyte and acid-base imbalance associated with acute renal failure, and exogenous poisoning (providing the substance is dialyzable). Peritoneal dialysis is contraindicated in the presence of bleeding disorders or recent abdominal surgery.

The dialysate consists of: hypertonic glucose solution (1.5 to 4.25 gm/100 ml); electrolytes in the normal concentration of serum; and a buffer, such as acetate or lactate.

Potassium and ***heparin*** are usually not present in commercially prepared solutions; however, they may be added to the solution. Heparin prevents clotting of the catheter. Lidocaine may be added to decrease the abdominal pain or cramping associated with peritoneal dialysis. Infusion of the concentrated peritoneal solution causes a movement of molecules across the peritoneal lining from an area of greater concentration to an area of lesser concentration. This is called diffusion. The movement of fluid from an area of lesser concentration to an area of greater concentration occurs by osmosis. Both occur simultaneously.

The use of hypertonic glucose results in the osmosis of fluid and the diffusion of waste products into the bath. Urea nitrogen, potassium, chloride, sodium, creatinine, phosphates, uric acid, bicarbonate, calcium and magnesium are cleared during peritoneal dialysis.

Procedure

A percutaneous catheter is inserted into the peritoneal area via a trocar. After insertion of the percutaneous catheter, one or two liters of dialysate solution are infused into the peritoneal cavity. The fluid is allowed to remain within the cavity for 20 to 45 minutes, allowing for diffusion and osmosis. After the prescribed time, the solution is allowed to drain by gravity from the abdomen. The procedure is repeated until the correct clinical state is achieved.

Nursing Care

Prior to insertion of the catheter, the patient's weight is recorded. Careful explanation should be given to the patient regarding the procedure, risks and expected outcomes. The patient is instructed to void. If unable to void, urinary catheterization may be necessary. An empty bladder decreases the likelihood of bladder perforation during the insertion of the trocar.

After the catheter is inserted, the nurse should stabilize the external catheter against the abdominal wall and apply a sterile dressing. The dressing should be changed, using aseptic technique, every 24 hours or every time it gets wet. The area is inspected daily for signs of inflammation or infection.

During the procedure, the patient is observed for changes in sensorium, vital signs and cardiovascular or respiratory status. As the solution is released from the abdomen, documentation should be made as to the amount and characteristics of the dialysate. Any deviation from the instilled fluid should be reported. If the fluid drained from the peritoneum is amber or brownish it may indicate perforation of the bladder or bowel. Bloody drainage is common during the first few exchanges; however, persistent bleeding may indicate abdominal hemorrhage or uremic coagulopathy. Cloudy fluid associated with the abdominal pain and elevated temperature indicates infection or peritonitis. Infection is treated systemically or intraperitoneally with antibiotics. Periodic cultures of the drained fluid may be ordered to rule out infection of the peritoneal cavity.

Pain may occur during any phase of the dialysis cycle. Decreasing the flow rate or amount of dialysate during infusion may control the pain. Also, the addition of lidocaine to the solution may elevate the abdominal discomfort. Care should be taken to avoid introduction of air, which accumulates under the diaphragm, creating pressure described as a cramplinglike pain and shortness of breath.

Vital signs are monitored to detect changes in baseline blood pressure and pulse, which may indicate impending shock or overhydration.

Hyperglycemia is the result of a high concentration of glucose in the dialysate solution. Dialysis patients should be monitored for elevation in blood sugar. Special care should be taken in monitoring blood sugar in diabetic patients undergoing dialysis.

Care must be taken to prevent complications resulting from immobility during peritoneal dialysis. Good skin care, range of motion and attention to respiratory status are necessary to prevent complications.

Hemodialysis

Hemodialysis is an extracorporeal technique using a semipermeable membrane to remove toxic substances, waste products and excess fluid from the systemic circulation. The principles are essentially the same as for peritoneal dialysis. Hemodialysis adds ultrafiltration to the osmosis and diffusion principles, which allows the passage of fluid through a membrane by means of a pressure gradient. Depending on the type of machine, the fluid will either be forced out of the blood and into the dialysate when the positive pressure on the blood side of the membrane is created, or negative pressure on the dialysis side will suck waste products out of the blood into the bath solution.

Hemodialysis is used for the following situations: when peritoneal dialysis is contraindicated; in chronic renal failure when medication and diet no longer control the symptoms; or if rapid removal of toxic substances is desired. Hemodialysis is also the method of choice for acute renal failure caused by trauma or infection.

Hemodialysis is contraindicated in individuals unable to tolerate systemic heparinization or patients whose cardiovascular system will not tolerate rapid changes in extravascular fluid volume.

Procedure

To initiate hemodialysis, a vascular access to an arterial and venous vessel is necessary. Arterial pressure is required to enable the blood flow to reach the dialyzer.

The most common techniques used are the AV shunt and AV fistula (vas catheter and femoral Shaldon catheter.)

An AV shunt is composed of a silastic tube and a teflon vessel tip. The tube and tip are inserted into an artery and vein, then joined together to form an extracorporeal circulation. The external tubing is interrupted for attachment to the dialysis lines or placement on the artificial kidney.

An AV fistula is surgically produced by the anastomosing of a vein and an artery that lie in close proximity. The radial artery and cephalic vein are used most often. The connection provides adequate arterial pressure for dialysis.

Both the shunt and the fistula have advantages and disadvantages. The shunt is the method of choice in acute renal failure for immediate dialysis. It may be utilized immediately following the anastomosis. A fistula is internal, thus decreasing the risk of infection and hemorrhage. An AV shunt is external. It may clot or disconnect, resulting in massive blood loss.

A dialysate bath similar to peritoneal dialysis is used for hemodialysis. Commerical preparations vary; the majority utilize a solution without glucose.

The vascular access provides sufficient arterial pressure to bring blood to the machine, where it will come in contact with the membrane and the dialysate bath. After the cleansing phase of the bath, the solution is returned to the patient via the venous route. This completes the procedure.

The system is heparinized to prevent anticoagulation during the procedure. A loading dose, usually 2,000 units, is administered. Continuous heparinization is done by bolus or constant infusion pump at the rate of 1,000 to 3,000 units every hour while the patient remains on the machine. Dosage varies to meet the needs of the patient. Optimal clotting time on the machine is 12 to 20 minutes. Heparinization is usually discontinued one hour prior to termination of the procedure. This allows the patient's clotting time to return to normal. Protamine can be used to reverse heparinization.

Nursing Care

Vascular access. If the patient has an AV shunt, patency must be checked every two hours by auscultation or palpation. A bruit is heard and a thrill is felt. If absent, the physician is notified. Routine flushing of the shunt with heparinized saline may be done to prevent clotting.

Since shunts are external, care is taken to avoid infection. Dressings are changed every 24 hours, using strict aseptic technique. Equipment should always be kept at the bedside to clamp the shunt tubing if a disconnection occurs. The immediate application of clamps is necessary to prevent massive blood loss.

If an AV fistula is used, patency is checked by auscultation and palpation. A bruit is auscultated and a thrill is felt. The skin area should be observed for discoloration, infection or bleeding, and changes should be reported immediately.

With a shunt or a fistula in use, venipunctures, intravenous therapy, injections and blood pressure reading should *never* be performed on the affected arm.

Care during hemodialysis is aimed at monitoring the patient for changes or complications. Vital signs, vascular access function, clotting times and temperature of the patient are checked. The temperature of the dialysate bath is checked frequently.

Hypotension associated with fluid loss or a shift in electrolytes is common. If hypotension occurs, the procedure is slowed and normal saline is administered.

A sudden onset of chest pain, dizziness or ringing in the ears may indicate an air embolus. If suspected, the patient should be turned on the left side and placed in the Trendelenburg position. This should lodge the embolus in the right ventricle, facilitating entry into pulmonary circulation.

Hematoma development at the vascular access site is common. Cold is applied initially, followed by application of heat to dissolve the accumulation of blood under the skin.

KEY CONCEPT: Knowledge of the disease process, coupled with technical skills, allows the nurse to be fully accountable for the safe and competent care of the patient with renal disease.

KEY POINT RECOGNITION

Write true or false by each statement. Answers are at the end of this chapter. A score below 80% indicates the need for further study.

_____ 1. Dialysis utilizes a semipermeable membrane to remove toxins and water.

_____ 2. Patients with a blood urea nitrogen level greater than 100 are possible candidates for dialysis.

_____ 3. Peritoneal dialysis uses the peritoneal lining of the abdominal wall as the semipermeable membrane.

_____ 4. Peritoneal dialysis can be utilized on any patient needing dialysis.

_____ 5. Peritoneal dialysis solution contains hypertonic glucose.

_____ 6. Hemodialysis solution contains hypertonic glucose.

_____ 7. Heparin is added to peritoneal dialysis solution to prevent clotting.
_____ 8. Urea nitrogen, potassium, chloride, sodium, creatinine and bicarbonate are some of the particles removed during peritoneal dialysis.
_____ 9. Hyperglycemia rarely occurs during peritoneal dialysis.
_____10. The development of pain during peritoneal dialysis is a grave sign; dialysis should be stopped immediately.
_____11. Hemodialysis does not utilize a semipermeable membrane.
_____12. Hemodialysis is contraindicated in individuals unable to tolerate systemic heparinization.
_____13. Hemodialysis utilizes either an AV shunt or an AV fistula for circulatory access.
_____14. An AV shunt is the surgical anastomosing of a vein and an artery.
_____15. AV fistulas have a higher risk of infection and hemorrhage than AV shunts.
_____16. If an AV shunt disconnects, massive blood loss can occur.
_____17. **Optimal clotting during hemodialysis is 12 to 20 minutes.**
_____18. AV shunts may become infected.
_____19. With a shunt, blood for lab work may be drawn through the shunt.
_____20. A venipuncture or blood pressure reading should never be performed in the arm with a fistula.
_____21. Fluid loss from dialysis can result in hypotension.
_____22. A sudden onset of chest pain and dizziness may indicate an air embolus in the dialysis patient.
_____23. Warm soaks should be applied initially to hematomas at the vascular access site.
_____24. Normal saline is administered to correct hypotensive states due to the fluid loss of dialysis.
_____25. Patency of an AV shunt is ascertained by auscultation, palpation and inspection.

CARE COMMON TO RENAL PROBLEMS

MAINTENANCE OF FLUID BALANCE

Body weight is an important indicator of fluid balance. Changes in body weight may be an important sign of overhydration or dehydration. *Overhydration* may result in weight gain and edema. Subjective signs of overhydration include: elevated blood pressure, anasarca, ascites, neck vein distention, dyspnea and stupor due to water intoxication.

Dehydration may result in weight loss and poor skin turgor. Subjective signs of dehydration include: decreased blood pressure, stupor due to hypovolemia and flat neck veins or no neck vein distention.

The primary objective of *fluid management* is to meet the tissue hydration needs without causing fluid overload.

Assessment of the patient's fluid status includes examination of: skin turgor, mucous membranes, blood pressure and cardiac and respiratory status.

The best indicator of fluid status is the patient's weight. Therefore, the patient with a renal problem must be weighed daily. Fluids are ordered and administered according to fluid loss, taking into consideration insensible water loss, urinary output, drainage and bowel loss. Fluid replacement is calculated using a standard formula. The formula used by many clinicians to calculate fluid replacement or adjustment on an hourly basis is: output from the previous hour plus 20 to 30 ml. (Hourly Intake X Previous Hour's Output + 20 to 30 ml.)

Accurate documentation of the patient's intake and output, plus daily weight, are essential. Pulmonary edema is a common manifestation of fluid overload in acute renal failure, especially in the presence of existing cardiac pathology. The treatment for pulmonary edema secondary to acute renal failure is dialysis, oxygenation and mild sedation.

MONITORING FLUID BALANCE

Fluid balance may be monitored in the following ways:

Measure body weight to provide a guideline for fluid replacement or fluid restriction.

Record intake and output, including fluid loss from lungs, skin and bowels, which usually totals 750 to 800 ml per day. Also consider the fluid generated metabolically (from carbohydrate metabolism) which is usually 300 to 350 ml per day.

Assess renal ability through measurements of urine volume, creatinine clearance, specific gravity, osmolarity, electrolytes and protein.

Monitor fluid replacement.

MAINTENANCE OF ELECTROLYTE BALANCE

Many factors influence electrolyte balance. Conditions that can cause an imbalance include: nasogastric drainage, vomiting, diarrhea and diuretic therapy.

Damaged nephrons cannot appropriately secrete and reabsorb specific ions. This produces electrolyte imbalances, which can result in lethal complications.

Potassium. Hyperkalemia is a dangerous imbalance that results from decreased glomerular filtration. Cardiac dysrhythmias are the primary clinical manifestation of hyperkalemia. Dietary intake of potassium is restricted to 60 mg or less/day. Drugs, fluids and foods containing potassium are avoided. Hyperkalemia may be treated with Kayexalate™, intravenous calcium chloride, sodium bicarbonate or a combination of glucose and insulin.

Kayexalate is an ion-exchange resin that can be administered orally or as a retention enema. It exchanges sodium for potassium. It reduces potassium levels but can contribute to volume overload.

If serum potassium exceeds 6.5 meq/L, emergency measures are necessary. During the acute phase, the treatment of choice is intravenous calcium chloride, sodium bicarbonate or the combination of glucose and insulin. A 10 percent solution of calcium, using 0.5 ml/kg of body weight over a 10-minute period, may be used to counteract the potassium-induced irritability of the heart. The infusion is discontinued if the heart rate decreases by 20 or more beats per minute. The infusion may be resumed after the pulse returns to normal.

A 7.5 percent solution of sodium bicarbonate may be given intravenously. It is calculated at 3 ml/kg of body weight.

The combination of 50 percent glucose, using 1 ml/kg of body weight, and regular insulin infused over one hour may shift the potassium from the extracellular fluid compartment into the intracellular fluid compartment.

Hypokalemia may occur during the diuretic phase of acute renal failure. The patient may excrete as much as 3 to 4 liters of urine per day. The loss of potassium is due to the restoration of tubular absorption and the excretion of large volumes of urine. The serum potassium level is watched closely to avoid dysrhythmias due to hypokalemia.

Sodium. Hypernatremia occurs in acute renal failure as a result of minimal sodium loss associated with oliguria and the stimulation of aldosterone. Sodium intake is limited to 500 to 1,500 mg/day. An elevated serum sodium is usually treated with fluid management and dialysis.

Calcium. Hypercalcemia in acute renal failure is rare unless there is existing pathology that produces an elevated serum calcium.

Hypocalcemia, a serum level less than 8.5 mgm/100 ml, is often a result of excessive gastrointestinal loss from diarrhea or nasogastric suction. Multiple transfusions of citrated blood or the rapid reversal of acidosis may lead to a hypocalcemic state. Treatment is the administration of intravenous calcium. Patients with hypocalcemia may present with tetany and bronchospasms.

Phosphate. Phosphate elevation, hyperphosphatemia, is a serum level greater than 5.5 mg/100 ml. Hyperphosphatemia is the inability of the diseased renal tubules to excrete phosphate. The reabsorption is inversely proportional to the glomerular filtraton rate. As the glomerular filtration rate decreases, the reabsorption of phosphate is increased; therefore, less phosphate is lost in the urine. Since phosphates are poorly dialyzed, the serum level is controlled by restricting dietary intake of phosphates and administering aluminum hydroxide. The aluminum hydroxide binds the phosphates in the intestine, limiting its absorption and thereby increasing calcium levels.

Monitoring electrolyte balance is accomplished by: monitoring electrolyte reports; providing for and monitoring electrolyte replacement, which includes both medication administration and dietary replacements; encouraging adequate hydration; and observing for signs of imbalance, such as tetany, in hypocalcemia.

MAINTENANCE OF NUTRITION

Providing for adequate nutrition includes the intake of: adequate calories, essential vitamins and amino acids, and adequate protein, carbohydrates and fats.

Starvation or catabolic states. Prolonged periods of starvation or catabolic states can significantly increase the morbidity and mortality rate of patients with acute renal failure.

A diet high in carbohydrates, caloric content of 1,500 to 2,000 calories per day, essential amino acids, essential vitamins and controlled amounts of sodium, potassium and phosphorus, is the ideal method of maintaining a proper nutritional state for the patient with renal dysfunction. However, this is sometimes impossible because of azotemia. Azotemia produces a depressed sensorium and gastrointestinal disorders that make oral feedings difficult.

The use of tube feedings and parenteral infusions offers an alternative to oral feedings. However, the hyperosmolarity of the tube feeding solutions produces severe diarrhea. The diarrhea associated with tube feedings may be minimized if the feeding is diluted with water in a ratio of 1:1. The concentration may be increased over a three-day period until a full-strength solution is tolerated by the patient.

Hyperalimentation is used when total parenteral nutrition is required. The standard solution is not appropriate for patients with acute renal failure. This solution usually contains electrolyte additives and protein hydrolysate. When protein hydrolysate is used as a nitrogen source, azotemia may be accelerated. Hyperalimentation for patients with acute renal failure should contain crystalline amino acids and no additional electrolytes. Water-soluble vitamins and folic acid may be added. All of these ingredients are added to a high concentration of glucose to provide the sufficient caloric and protein content necessary to reverse the catabolic state. Hyperalimentation requires careful administration to prevent complications such as sepsis and hyperglycemia.

Monitoring of the nutritional status may be done in the following ways. Monitor the diet. Provide dietary replacements. Maintain hyperalimentation.

MAINTENANCE OF RENAL PERFUSION

Maintaining renal perfusion includes the control of: **hypertension,** by monitoring B.P., salt intake, water and drug therapy; **hypotensive states,** by administering volume expanders or vasopressors to correct low blood pressure; and **renal hypoperfusion,** by administering drugs to increase cardiac-renal flow.

MAINTENANCE OF ACID-BASE BALANCE

Baseline arterial blood gases are necessary to provide a comparison for future readings. Arterial blood gases must be assessed for acid-base imbalance.

Acidosis is often present in renal failure. In acidotic states, observe for hyperkalemia.

Alkalosis is rarely seen in renal disease. If alkalosis is present, the patient will very likely be hypokalemic too. Alkalosis is usually associated with vomiting, diuresis and hypokalemia.

Metabolic renal acidosis is secondary to the acid waste products of protein catabolism. Lactic acidosis is the result of impaired hepatic metabolism, lactate or decreased perfusion with anaerobic metabolism. This results in hyperkalemia, hyperphosphatemia and the loss of bicarbonate. An arterial blood gas with a pH of 7.3 or less and a bicarbonate of 15 meq/L or less indicates respiratory compensation. The treatment aimed at correcting the imbalance begins with the administration of intravenous sodium bicarbonate. The amount of bicarbonate given depends upon the deficit. Sodium bicarbonate may be used initially, but long-term correction for a patient with lactic acidosis secondary to acute renal failure is dialysis.

Monitoring acid-base balance is most effectively accomplished by analyzing arterial blood gases and serum bicarbonate.

PREVENTION OF COMPLICATIONS

Many factors influence the complications associated with renal dysfunction. The majority of deaths in acute renal failure are secondary to the complications listed below:

Cardiovascular—pericarditis, dysrhythmias, CHF, MI

Neurological—uremic encephalopathy, seizures, stroke, coma

Infection—respiratory, sepsis, urinary tract infection, skin infection

Hematological—bone marrow depression, hemolysis, bleeding tendencies, hypovolemia

Cardiovascular. The primary complication involving the cardiovascular system is cardiac dysrhythmias resulting from hyperkalemia. Other complications include congestive heart failure, hypertension and pulmonary edema.

Pericarditis, the accumulation of fluid around the pericardium, may develop in approximately 18 percent of patients with acute renal failure. The patient presents with pleuritic pain, which increases on deep inspiration, fever, tachycardia and a pericardial friction rub. The severity of the symptoms depends upon the rate of accumulation and the quantity of fluid. If undiagnosed, complete heart failure with tamponade may result. Diagnosis is suggested by muffled heart sounds, hypotension, paradoxical pulse and enlarged cardiac silhouette on x-ray. The treatment includes dialysis, pericardicentesis and intrapericardial steroids in intractable cases. The clinical condition of these patients may require pericardicentesis or a pericardectomy to remove the accumulated fluid.

Cardiac dysrhythmias result from hyperkalemia. The earliest EKG change is the development of tall peaked T waves. As the patient becomes more hyperkalemic, the EKG reveals ST segment depression, a prolonged P-R interval, shortening of the Q-T interval and a widening of the QRS. If untreated, cardiac standstill will occur.

Treatment includes restriction of oral potassium intake; the administration of Kayexalate; intravenous calcium chloride, sodium bicarbonate or the combination of glucose and insulin; and dialysis.

Neurological. The development of uremic encephalopathy is not completely understood. It is likely to occur with a rapid onset of azotemia. This is considered a preterminal state. Acute renal failure complicated by cerebral ischemia, hypoxemia, sepsis or severe metabolic dysfunction predisposes to neurological involvement. The patient develops apathy and altered sensorium. As the condition deteriorates, asterixis develops and progresses to convulsions and coma.

Convulsions are controlled with the intravenous administraton of diphenylhydantoin (Dilantin), valium or phenobarbital. Caution must be exercised to prevent oversedation. The early use of dialysis in renal failure has decreased the incidence of uremic encephalopathy.

Infection. Infection, secondary to dialysis, is responsible for 50 to 90 percent of the deaths in acute renal failure. The primary sources of infection include wounds, the urinary tract and the respiratory system.

Healing is slow in uremic patients. Therefore, special attention should be given to intravenous sites, peritoneal dialysis sites, external AV shunts and wounds. The development of a respiratory infection is secondary to central nervous system depression caused by the uremic state or from oversedation. Immobility increases the accumulation of bronchial secretions, contributing to the development of pulmonary infection. Strict attention to oral hygiene, pulmonary toilet and suctioning technique may prevent respiratory complications.

The use of an indwelling catheter in an oliguric patient provides a greater risk for the development of a nosocomial infection. If an indwelling catheter is used, strict aseptic technique is essential.

Hematological. Anemia in acute renal failure is the result of three factors: bone marrow depression due to decreased production of erythropoietin by the failing kidney; hemolysis from an abnormal chemical environment, which reduces the life span of red blood cells to half; and bleeding tendencies due to a qualitative deficiency in platelets and vitamin K, which result in gastrotintestinal hemorrhage.

Blood replacement is ordered in response to the patient's symptoms, rather than in laboratory values only. Transfusions consist of fresh, frozen plasma or packed red blood cells that are less than 48 hours old. The age of the cells is vital. Older cells result in the elevation of the serum potassium level.

Hypovolemia. Hypovolemia requires the replacement of plasma or blood to increase circulating blood volume and renal blood flow.

Cardiac failure is usually treated with medications to increase cardiac output, thereby increasing kidney perfusion. Inotropic agents, drugs that reduce afterload and the intra-aortic balloon pump are commonly used to treat cardiac failure.

If a mechanical obstruction is causing the renal ischemia, an attempt is made to relieve the obstruction.

In the clinical state of hypotension, the aim is to raise the arterial blood pressure and increase perfusion through the kidneys. However, the use of vasopressors in hypoperfusion states should be instituted only after volume has been replaced. Vasopressors are used in individuals who do not respond to conventional therapy.

Nephrotoxicity. When intrinsic renal failure results from nephrotoxicity, the offending drug must be discontinued. The goal is to remove the patient from the substance or chemical responsible for creating toxicity to the renal parenchyma.

Complications can be prevented in the following ways:

Watch for signs of infection.

Use strict aseptic technique.

Immediately recognize and treat complications.

Monitor laboratory studies for changes.

Monitor EKG for changes.

Watch for sensorium changes.

Uremic syndrome. The uremic syndrome is the retention of nitrogenous metabolites. Retention is a secondary effect of renal failure. The following may help deter the occurrence of the uremic syndrome:

Prevent metabolic acidosis.

Prevent electrolyte imbalance.

Prevent hypertension.

Prevent dehydration.

Prevent infection.

Reduce protein intake.

KEY CONCEPT: Continuous and thorough patient assessment is essential to the management of renal problems.

KEY POINT RECOGNITION

Write true or false by each statement. Answers are at the end of this chapter. A score below 80% indicates the need for further study.

1. Changes in fluid balance can be measured by weight loss or gain.
2. Electrolyte imbalance can be caused by massive tissue destruction.
3. Renal perfusion can be maintained by controlling hypertensive and hypotensive states.
4. Alkalosis is frequently seen in renal failure.
5. Uremic syndrome results from retention of nitrogenous metabolites.
6. **Pulmonary edema is a common manifestation of fluid overload.**
7. Kayexalate can only be administered orally.
8. The emergency treatment of hyperkalemia includes the intravenous administration of calcium gluconate combined with insulin.
9. Hyperkalemia commonly occurs during the diuretic phase of acute renal failure.
10. Hypernatremia is associated with oliguria in acute renal failure.
11. Hypocalcemia is rare in renal dysfunctions.
12. Hypocalcemia is the result of excessive gastrointestinal fluid loss.
13. Hyperphosphatemia results from the inability of the diseased renal tubules to excrete phosphate.
14. Phosphates are readily dialyzed.
15. Aluminum hydroxide binds phosphates in the kidneys.
16. Azotemia produces a depressed sensorium and gastrointestinal disorders.
17. The standard solution for hyperalimentation is appropriate for patients with renal disorders.
18. Hyperalimentation solution for patients with renal failure should contain protein hydrolysate.
19. Hyperalimentation for patients with renal failure should contain crystalline amino acids.
20. In the uremic syndrome, the retention of nitrogenous wastes is a secondary effect of renal failure.
21. If acidosis occurs in renal failure, observe for hyperkalemia.
22. Alkalosis in renal disease is usually associated with vomiting, diuresis or hypokalemia.
23. Metabolic acidosis in renal failure is often secondary to the accumulation of the acid waste products of protein catabolism.
24. Pericarditis, congestive heart failure and pulmonary edema are common complications of renal failure.
25. Renal failure complicated by cerebral ischemia, hypoxemia, sepsis or severe metabolic dysfunction predisposes the patient to neurological involvement.
26. Infection secondary to dialysis is responsible for only a small percentage of deaths in renal failure.
27. Immobility may increase the occurrence of infection.
28. Anemia in renal failure can be caused only by bone marrow depression.
29. Transfusing the patient in renal failure with fresh frozen plasma increases the serum potassium level.
30. If nephrotoxicity is suspected, the causative agent must be identified and removed.

PASS
Program Assessment: Science and Situation

1. The innermost covering of the kidney is loosely attached to the
    a. perirenal fat.
    b. renal cortex.
    c. adipose tissue.
    d. renal fascia.

2. A nephron is composed of the following:
    a. Bowman's capsule, afferent and efferent arterioles
    b. renal pyramid, calyx, glomerulus
    c. glomerulus, proximal tubule, Henle's loop, distal tubule, collecting tubule
    d. glomerulus, juxtaglomerular apparatus, Henle's loop

3. Blood enters the glomerulus via the
    a. afferent arteriole.
    b. efferent arteriole.
    c. proximal tubule.
    d. Henle's loop.

4. The kidneys are perfused with blood at the rate of
    a. 1,200 ml/minute.
    b. 1,200 ml/hour.
    c. 600 ml/minute.
    d. 600 ml/hour.

5. Glomerular filtrate is best described as
    a. identical to urine.
    b. a precursor of urine and composed of water, electrolytes and the waste products of protein metabolism.
    c. a precursor of urine and composed of protein and the waste products of protein metabolism.
    d. a precursor of urine and composed of plasma, water and blood cells.

6. The renal tubules normally reabsorb
    a. over 50% of the glomerular filtrate.
    b. over 75% of the glomerular filtrate.
    c. over 85% of the glomerular filtrate.
    d. over 99% of the glomerular filtrate.

7. The majority of the reabsorption of the glomerular filtrate takes place in the
    a. collecting duct.
    b. Henle's loop.
    c. proximal tubule.
    d. distal tubule.

8. ADH secretion is increased:
    (1) if there is a need to conserve water
    (2) if there is decreased renal blood flow and decreased atrial filling pressures

(3) in the presence of increased serum osmolarity
(4) in the presence of decreased serum osmolarity
   a. 1, 4
   b. 1, 2, 4
   c. 1, 2, 3
   d. 1, 3

9. The juxtaglomerular apparatus
   a. contains inactive granules of renin.
   b. responds to a decrease in sodium ion concentration in the glomerular filtrate.
   c. has a longer Henle's loop for greater urine concentration.
   d. all of the above

10. The substance directly responsible for peripheral vasoconstriction and increased aldosterone secretion is
    a. angiotensinogen.
    b. renin.
    c. angiotensin II.
    d. angiotensin I.

11. Sodium reabsorption is decreased at the tubules when
    a. the GFR is increased.
    b. aldosterone is inhibited.
    c. ADH is secreted.
    d. all of the above

12. The amount of potassium excreted in the urine is dependent upon the:
    (1) volume of urine excreted
    (2) availability of sodium ions
    (3) acid-base status
    (4) level of serum potassium
       a. 1, 2, 3, 4
       b. 1, 3, 4
       c. 2, 3, 4
       d. 1, 2, 4

13. The reabsorption of the chloride ion is dependent upon the:
    (1) acid-base status
    (2) amount of available sodium ions
    (3) secretion of ADH
    (4) amount of available magnesium ions
       a. 1, 2
       b. 1, 2, 4
       c. 2, 3, 4
       d. 1, 2, 3

14. Which of the following substances is freely filtered by the kidneys and has an excretion rate equal to that of the GFR?
    a. bicarbonate
    b. urea

c. calcium
d. creatinine

15. Which of the following mechanisms help the kidney maintain acid-base balance?
    (1) reabsorption of bicarbonate
    (2) renin-angiotensin-aldosterone mechanism
    (3) excretion of hydrogen ions
    (4) excretion of ammonia
    a. 1, 2, 4
    b. 1, 3, 4
    c. 3, 4
    d. 1, 4

16. Ninety percent of all filtered bicarbonate is reabsorbed in the proximal tubule through
    a. Na^{++} and K^+ ion exchange.
    b. phosphate and H^+ ion exchange.
    c. Na^{++} and H^+ ion exchange.
    d. the secretion of ammonia.

17. Which one of the following heart sounds may be auscultated on a patient with renal failure in the absence of any other known cardiac pathology?
    a. pericardial rub
    b. systolic murmur
    c. diastolic murmur
    d. atrial gallop

18. Which of the following is the most accurate index of renal function?
    a. BUN
    b. serum electrolytes
    c. urine electrolytes
    d. serum creatinine

19. The single most useful test for the measurement of glomerular filtration is
    a. urea clearance.
    b. creatinine clearance.
    c. uric acid clearance.
    d. protein clearance.

20. Renal failure is defined as
    a. urine output less than 400 cc/24 hours.
    b. the absence of urine output.
    c. the inability of the kidneys to adequately excrete products of cell metabolism.
    d. the inability of the kidneys to excrete the water necessary to accommodate the waste products of cell metabolism.

21. The most common infecting organism in the urinary tract is
    a. proteus vulgaris.
    b. group A-beta-hemolytic streptococcus.
    c. Klebsiella pneuminiae.
    d. Escherichia coli.

22. In progressive renal failure, workload shifts to the remaining functioning nephrons. When this occurs, which of the following compensatory events take place?
    (1) hypertrophy of the working nephrons
    (2) an increase in the GFR through the functioning nephrons
    (3) an increase in the solute load
    (4) an increase in tubular reabsorption
    a. 1, 3
    b. 1, 2, 3
    c. 3, 4
    d. all of the above

23. Nephrotic syndrome is chiefly characterized by
    a. proteinuria.
    b. oliguria.
    c. an elevated serum creatinine and BUN.
    d. hematuria.

24. The generalized edema associated with nephrotic syndrome is the result of
    a. fluid overload.
    b. a decreased GFR.
    c. pump failure.
    d. fluid shift secondary to hypoalbuminemia.

25. Which of the following conditions can result in prerenal failure?
    (1) obstruction of the renal artery
    (2) congestive heart failure
    (3) decreased circulating blood volume
    (4) severe burns
    a. 4 only
    b. 1, 2, 3
    c. 3, 4
    d. 2, 3, 4

26. Prerenal failure associated with cardiac failure is the direct result of
    a. obstruction of the renal vessels.
    b. decreased cardiac output and decreased renal perfusion.
    c. fluid overload leading to glomerular solute overload.
    d. an increased retention of Na^+.

27. Which symptom usually indicates a bilateral mechanical obstruction of the renal arteries?
    a. oliguria
    b. anuria
    c. proteinuria
    d. hematuria

28. Renal failure that is the result of injury or necrosis to the renal parenchyma is classified as
    a. chronic.
    b. postrenal.
    c. intrinsic.
    d. acute.

29. Which of the following is considered the primary cause of acute intrinsic renal failure?
    a. injury to the kidney cells
    b. renal insufficiency
    c. decreased perfusion to the renal tissue
    d. obstruction

30. Which of the following is *not* (usually) a cause of nephrotoxicity?
    a. barbiturates
    b. ethyline oxiell (antifreeze)
    c. carbon tetrachloride and ethyl alcohol
    d. aminoglycosides

31. The pathological change resulting in acute cortical necrosis is due to the
    a. necrosis of the glomerular basement membrane.
    b. infarction of the entire nephron.
    c. increased permeability of the basement membrane.
    d. necrosis of tubular epithelium.

32. Acute tubular necrosis secondary to which etiology has the potential for regeneration of the injured tissue?
    a. glomerular nephritis
    b. renal insufficiency
    c. nephrotoxicity
    d. CHF

33. Which of the following theories are considered responsible for acute vasomotor nephropathy?
    (1) increased glomerular filtration
    (2) decreased glomerular filtration
    (3) altered blood flow distribution
    (4) infarction of the entire nephron
    a. 1, 3
    b. 2, 3
    c. 1 only
    d. 4 only

34. Which of the following events occur as a result of decreased glomerular filtration in acute renal failure?
    (1) an increase in the tone of afferent arterioles
    (2) necrosis of tubular epithelium
    (3) reduction in glomerular capillary pressure
    (4) reduction in vascular resistance
    a. 1, 3
    b. 1, 4
    c. 2 only
    d. 1, 3, 4

35. Which of the following is a cause of postrenal failure?
    a. prostatic obstruction
    b. neurogenic bladder
    c. vasoconstriction of renal vasculature
    d. renal calculi

36. Oliguria is defined as
    a. no urine output.
    b. urine output less than 250 cc/day.
    c. urine output less than 400 cc/day.
    d. urine output greater than 1,000 cc/day.

37. Which one of the following clinical states is not considered high risk for the development of acute renal failure?
    a. major burns
    b. severe left ventricular dysfunction
    c. diabetes ketoacidosis
    d. malignant hypertension

38. Which of the following is the most common preceding sign of acute renal failure?
    a. sudden onset of renal dysfunction
    b. altered sensorium
    c. pericardial friction rub
    d. uremic frost

39. Azotemia is defined as
    a. a urine output of less than 400 cc/day.
    b. the presence of nitrogenous products in the blood.
    c. fluid overload resulting in pulmonary edema.
    d. convulsions secondary to uremic encephalopathy.

40. Which of the following is *not* a cardiac dysrhythmia or disturbance usually seen with hyperkalemia?
    a. tall peaked T-waves
    b. ST segment dysussion
    c. atrial fibrillation
    d. widened QRS

41. Which of the following is the best indication of a patient's fluid status?
    a. blood pressure
    b. weight
    c. mucous membranes
    d. skin turgor

42. In oliguric renal failure, which of the following is recommended to calculate fluid replacement?
    a. I = 0 plus 50 cc/hour
    b. I = 0
    c. I = 0 plus 20 to 30 cc/hour
    d. 10 cc per hour

43. Which of the following are indications for dialysis?
    (1) urine output less than 400 cc/24 hours
    (2) BUN greater than 100 mg
    (3) BUN greater than 100 with proportional rise in serum creatinine of 10 or more
    (4) symptomatic fluid overload compromising cardiovascular and pulmonary status

a. 3, 4
b. 1, 3
c. 2, 4
d. 1, 4

44. In peritoneal dialysis, the optimum dwell time of dialysate fluid is
    a. one hour.
    b. 20 to 45 minutes.
    c. 15 to 20 minutes.
    d. 10 minutes.

45. Which of the following is *not* true of an AV shunt?
    a. There is risk of infection.
    b. There is risk of clotting.
    c. It may disconnect and result in severe bleeding.
    d. It cannot be used for 3 to 4 weeks after creation.

46. Uncontrollable hypertension secondary to renal failure is due to:
    (1) increase in serum renin level
    (2) increase in renal blood flow
    (3) increase in the GFR
    (4) increase in tubular reabsorption of sodium
    a. 1, 2
    b. 1, 3
    c. 1, 4
    d. 1, 2, 4

47. In the diuretic phase of acute renal failure, high urine volume is due to:
    (1) the decreased blood urea concentration
    (2) osmotic diuresis secondary to an increased blood urea concentration
    (3) the impaired ability of the tubules to conserve water and salt
    (4) the uneven distribution of blood flow throughout the kidney
    a. 1, 3
    b. 2, 3
    c. 1, 3, 4
    d. 3, 4

48. In chronic renal failure, there is a(n)
    a. decrease in the GFR, decrease in ionizable calcium and a rise in serum phosphate.
    b. increase in the GFR, decrease in ionizable calcium and a decrease in serum phosphate.
    c. decrease in the GFR, ionizable calcium and serum phosphate.
    d. increase in the GFR and ionizable calcium, and a decrease in serum phosphate.

49. The hematuria and proteinuria of acute glomerulonephritis is due to
    a. deposits of the antigen-antibody complex on the endothelial cells.
    b. interstitial fibrosis.
    c. the escape of blood and protein through the porous glomerular capillary.
    d. sclerosis of the arterioles and atrophy of the glomeruli.

50. Sodium reabsorption is decreased at the tubules if there is:
    (1) an increase in the GFR
    (2) inhibition of aldosterone
    (3) secretion of aldosterone
    (4) secretion of ADH
    a. 1, 3, 4
    b. 1, 2
    c. 1, 3
    d. 1, 2, 4

KEY POINT RECOGNITION ANSWERS

Location, size and fascia
1. False—The kidneys extend from the 11th or 12th thoracic vertebra to the 2nd lumbar vertebra.
2. False—The right kidney is lower than left.
3. True
4. True
5. False—Perirenal fat is adipose tissue located outside the renal fascia. Perirenal fat is surrounded by the renal fascia. Both serve as protection for the kidney.

Gross structures
1. True
2. True
3. True

Nephron
1. False—There are 1 million in each kidney.
2. True
3. False—Bowman's capsule is a membrane that envelops the capillary tuft of the nephron.
4. True
5. True
6. True
7. False—The macula densa are found in the DCT.
8. True

Renal blood flow
1. True
2. True
3. True
4. True

Glomerular filtration
1. False—20 to 25 percent or 1200 ml/minute
2. True
3. False—They are highly permeable, but not to proteins and blood cells.
4. False—electrolytes, nonelectrolytes and water

Tubular reabsorption and secretion
1. True
2. True
3. False—Urea is passively diffused from the tubule to the peritubular blood.
4. False—They are reabsorbed.
5. True
6. True
7. True
8. True
9. True
10. True

11. True
12. False—Final adjustments of sodium are made in the DCT.
13. True
14. True
15. True

Regulation of water balance
1. False—Thirst-neurohypophyseal-renal axis
2. True
3. False—90 percent
4. False—Urine is diluted and excess water is excreted.
5. False—ADH is synthesized in the hypothalamus and is released from the pituitary.
6. False—It is stimulated.
7. True

Regulation of blood pressure
1. False—JG cells are located in the nephrons of the inner cortex adjacent to the medulla.
2. False—They have granules of inactive renin.
3. True
4. True
5. False—Aldosterone is released in response to the body's need to reabsorb sodium.

Regulation of electrolytes
1. False—It is the major extracellular cation.
2. True
3. False—65 percent
4. True
5. True
6. False—Sodium reabsorption is decreased if the GFR is increased.
7. True
8. True
9. False—It is actively reabsorbed in the PCT.
10. False—10 to 15 percent
11. False—Hyperkalemia stimulates aldosterone secretion, resulting in sodium reabsorption and potassium excretion.
12. True
13. True
14. True
15. True
16. True
17. True
18. False—PTH inhibits tubular reabsorption of phosphate.
19. True
20. True
21. True
22. False—Chloride will be excreted.

Excretion of waste products

1. True
2. True
3. False—In volume depletion, urea may be absorbed.
4. False—Creatinine is freely filtered by the kidney.
5. False—Creatinine's rate of excretion is equal to the GFR.

The kidney and acid-base balance

1. False—A small amount of free acid is present in the urine.
2. True
3. True
4. True
5. True
6. True
7. True
8. False—No! The H_2O is excreted and the CO_2 re-enters the cell to again combine with H_2O to form carbonic acid. STUDY THIS SECTION AGAIN!!
9. False—Phosphates act as buffers for the excretion of hydrogen ions.
10. True
11. True
12. True
13. False—There will be an increase in the production of ammonia.
14. True
15. False—It is decreased.

Assessment of the renal system

1. True
2. True
3. True
4. True
5. False—Tetany may be due to hypocalcemia.

Renal assessment

1. True
2. False—An elevated BUN indicates decreased glomerular filtration.
3. True
4. False—Normal BUN is 8 to 18 mgm/dl
5. True
6. True
7. True
8. True
9. True
10. False—Hypertension may be seen with chronic renal failure.

Acute renal failure

1. True
2. True
3. True
4. False—The glomerular filtration rate is decreased.

5. False—Infarction of the entire nephron is called acute cortical necrosis.
6. True
7. True
8. False—The oliguric stage is seen within 48 hours following the initial insult.
9. True
10. False—Oliguric urine is concentrated.
11. True
12. True
13. True
14. False—In acute vasomotor nephropathy, there is a decrease in glomerular filtration rate.
15. False—In acute renal failure, blood flow is primarily through the inner cortex and medulla.
16. True
17. True

Chronic renal failure: pyelonephritis
1. False—Pyelonephritis is a bacterial infection of the renal pelvis, interstitial tissue and tubules.
2. False—The most common organism causing urinary tract infections is Escherichia coli.
3. True
4. True
5. True

Glomerulonephritis
1. True
2. True
3. False—The leading cause of renal failure is chronic glomerulonephritis.
4. True
5. False—The kidneys reduce in size by nearly one-fifth.
6. True
7. True
8. False—Azotemia and edema are seen in chronic glomerulonephritis.
9. True
10. False—An elevated antistreptolysin O titer and elevated serum urea nitrogen levels are seen in chronic glomerulonephritis.

Nephrotic syndrome
1. False—Nephrotic syndrome is caused by massive proteinuria.
2. False—The glomerular basement membrane becomes thick, causing an increase in permeability.
3. True
4. True
5. True
6. True
7. True

Hypertension and renal insufficiency
1. False—Hypertension is the sustained elevation of blood pressure above a diastolic of 90 mm Hg or systolic of 140 mm Hg.
2. True

3. True
4. True
5. True
6. False—Renal insufficiency is a reduction in renal function that is compatible with life.
7. True
8. True
9. True
10. True
11. True
12. False—Anuria is a diagnostic aid in determining renal arterial occlusion.

Dialysis
1. True
2. True
3. True
4. False—Peritoneal dialysis is contraindicated in the presence of bleeding disorders or recent abdominal surgery.
5. True
6. False—Hypertonic glucose is not necessary.
7. True
8. True
9. False—Patients are monitored for hyperglycemia. This may occur during peritoneal dialysis.
10. False—Pain may occur during any phase of the dialysis cycle.
11. False—Hemodialysis is an extracorporeal technique using a semipermeable membrane.
12. True
13. True
14. False—The surgical anastomosing of a vein and an artery is called an AV fistula.
15. False—An AV fistula is internal, thus decreasing the risk of infection and hemorrhage.
16. True
17. True
18. True
19. False—Venipunctures, intravenous therapy, injections or blood pressure readings must never be done in the arm with an AV shunt.
20. True
21. True
22. True
23. False—Cold should be used initially.
24. True
25. True

Care common to renal problems
1. True
2. True
3. True
4. False—Acidosis is frequently seen in renal failure.
5. True

6. **True**
7. False—Kayexalate may be given orally or as a retention enema.
8. False—Emergency measures for the treatment of hyperkalemia include intravenous administration of calcium chloride, sodium bicarbonate or the combination of glucose and insulin.
9. False—Hypokalemia is common.
10. True
11. False—Hypercalcemia is rare.
12. True
13. True
14. False—Phosphates are poorly dialyzed.
15. False—Aluminum hydroxide binds phosphates to the intestinal wall.
16. True
17. False—The standard hyperalimentation solution is not appropriate.
18. False—Hyperalimentation solution should not contain protein hydrolysate.
19. True
20. True
21. True
22. True
23. True
24. True
25. True
26. False—Infection secondary to dialysis is responsible for 50 to 90 percent of the deaths.
27. True
28. False—Anemia may be caused by bone marrow depression and hemolysis.
29. False—Transfusions of fresh frozen plasma should not contribute to hyperkalemia.
30. True

PASS ANSWER SHEET

1. b
2. c
3. a
4. a
5. b
6. d
7. c
8. c
9. d
10. c
11. d
12. b
13. a
14. d
15. b
16. c
17. a
18. d
19. b
20. c
21. d
22. d
23. a
24. d
25. c
26. b
27. b
28. c
29. a
30. a
31. b
32. c
33. b
34. a
35. c
36. c
37. d
38. a
39. b
40. c
41. b
42. c
43. a
44. b
45. d
46. c
47. b
48. a
49. c
50. d

SURVEY SUMMARY
RENAL SYSTEM

I. The *renal system* is responsible for fluid and electrolyte regulation; it has an excretory function; and is composed of the *kidneys, ureters, bladder* and *urethra*.

II. Anatomy
   A. *Renal anatomy*
   1. The bean-shaped kidneys lie on either side of the vertebral column at the 11th or 12th thoracic vertebra and extend to the 2nd lumbar vertebra.
   2. Each kidney weighs approximately 120 to 150 gm and is 10 to 12 cm in length.
   3. Various coverings protect the kidney:
      a. *renal fascia*
      b. *perirenal fat*
      c. *fibrous renal capsule*
      d. *pararenal fat*
   4. The gross structures of the kidney include the:
      a. *renal cortex* or outer layer
      b. *renal medulla* or middle layer
      c. *renal pelvis* or inner layer
   5. The *nephron* is the functional unit of the kidney and is composed of the *glomerulus, proximal convoluted tubule, Henle's loop* and *distal convoluted tubule*.
   6. *Renal blood flow* is approximately 20 to 25 percent of total cardiac output.
      a. The *renal arteries* are large, high-flow vessels perfusing the kidney with 1,200 ml per minute.
      b. The *renal veins* are large vessels that empty into the inferior vena cava.

III. Physiology
   A. The kidney, through fluid and electrolyte control, maintains plasma homeostasis.
   B. The ultrafiltrate of plasma is glomerular filtrate.
   1. The rate at which the glomerular filtrate is formed is called the glomerular filtration rate (GFR) and is related to renal blood flow.
   2. The constituents of glomerular filtrate include electrolytes, nonelectrolytes and water.
   C. Tubular reabsorption and secretion
   1. The tubules reabsorb 99 percent of the glomerular filtrate produced.
      a. 124 to 125 ml of filtrate are reabsorbed per minute.
      b. 1 ml or 1 to 1.5 liters per day of urine are produced.
   2. 80 to 85 percent of the glomerular filtrate is reabsorbed in the proximal tubule.
      a. Reabsorption is dependent upon the GFR.
         1. If GFR is increased, tubular reabsorption is decreased, resulting in an increased urine output.
         2. If GFR is decreased, tubular reabsorption is increased, resulting in a decreased urine output.

b. Creatinine, organic salts and drugs are secreted in the proximal tubule.
3. The major function of Henle's loop is the concentration or dilution of urine. This is accomplished by the countercurrent mechanism of the kidney.
4. The selective process of reabsorption and secretion takes place in the distal tubules and collecting tubules.
   a. Final adjustments of sodium are made in the DCT.
   b. Water reabsorption is a prime function of the collecting tubule and is dependent upon the activity of ADH.
D. Regulation of water balance is maintained via the thirst, ADH and countercurrent mechanisms.
   1. Thirst regulates fluid intake.
   2. ADH controls osmolality of ECF and sodium concentration.
   3. The countercurrent mechanism of the kidney adjusts urine osmolality.
E. Blood pressure regulation by the kidney is dependent upon special feedback mechanisms.
   1. The renin-angiotensin-aldosterone mechanism
      a. JG cells secrete renin, which converts angiotensin I to angiotensin II, resulting in increased blood pressure via vasoconstriction.
      b. Aldosterone is secreted and results in tubular reabsorption of water in the DCT and CT.
F. Regulation of electrolytes
   1. Sodium is the major extracellular cation.
      a. Sodium regulation is dependent upon the GFR, aldosterone secretion, third factor and ADH secretion.
      b. The renin-angiotensin-aldosterone mechanism is primary in the regulation of sodium excretion.
   2. Potassium is the major intracellular cation.
      a. Influencing factors in potassium regulation are hypokalemia, hyperkalemia, acidotic and alkalotic states, and urine volume.
      b. Aldosterone secretion causes cations to be exchanged with Na^+ reabsorbed and K^+ excreted.
   3. 90 percent of filtered calcium is reabsorbed. Factors influencing reabsorbtion include:
      a. PTH (parathyroid hormone)
      b. Vitamin D
      c. Effects of steroids and diuretics
   4. Reabsorption of phosphate takes place in the PCT and is inversely related to the GFR.
      a. Increased GFR results in decreased reabsorption.
      b. Decreased GFR results in increased reabsorption.
   5. Magnesium is dependent on sodium for reabsorption.
   6. Chloride is important in the regulation of acid-base.
      a. It is excreted in acidosis.
      b. It is reabsorbed in alkalosis.
G. A primary function of the kidney is excretion of the waste products of protein metabolism.
   1. Urea is a nitrogenous waste product and is both filtered and reabsorbed in the nephron.

2. Creatinine is a waste product of muscle metabolism and is freely filtered by the kidneys.
H. The kidney has an important role in maintaining acid-base balance.
1. Four mechanisms help to accomplish this:
a. Direct excretion of H^+ ions
b. Reabsorption of bicarbonate:
1. $CO_2 + H_2O \xrightarrow{CA} H_2CO_3$
2. $H_2CO_3 \rightarrow H^+ + HCO_3$
3. $Na^+ + HCO_3 \rightarrow NaHCO_3$
4. $H^+ + NaHCO_3 \rightarrow Na + H_2CO_3$
5. $H_2CO_3 + CO_2 + H_2O$
6. $CO_2 + H_2O \rightarrow HCO_3$ (process begins again)
c. Excretion of hydrogen ions with renal buffers:
1. $HPO_4{}^2 + H^+ \rightarrow H_2PO_4$
2. $H_2CO_3 + Na_2 + HPO_4 \rightarrow NaHCO_3 + NaH_2PO_4$
3. $H + Na_2 + HPO_4 \rightarrow Na + NaH_2PO_4$
4. Sodium re-enters the cell and sodium phosphate is excreted in the urine.
d. Excretion of ammonia:
1. $NH_3 + H^+ \rightarrow NH_4$
2. $NH_4 + NaCl \rightarrow NH_4Cl + Na$
3. Ammonium chloride is excreted in the urine and sodium re-enters the cell.
2. In response to acidosis, bicarbonate and sodium are reabsorbed.
3. In response to alkalosis, bicarbonate is excreted in the urine.

IV. Assessment of the renal system should include:
   A. *Assessment of gross cerebral functioning*
   B. *Specific cerebral functioning*
   C. *Inspection*
      1. Skin color
      2. Body edema
      3. Urinary output
      4. Asterixis
   D. *Palpation*
      1. Size, shape and location of kidneys
      2. Tenderness
      3. Bladder fullness
   E. *Percussion*
      1. Tenderness
      2. Mass, or tumor
      3. Ascites
   F. *Auscultation*
      1. Bowel sounds
      2. Breath sounds
      3. Heart sounds
   G. *Assessment includes evaluating:*
      1. *Level of consciousness*
         a. Arousability
         b. Orientation

          c. Ability to follow commands
       2. *Voiding pattern*
          a. Duration of problem
          b. Observation of urinary stream
          c. Bladder distention for fullness
       3. *Control of stream*
          a. Void on command
          b. Sensation to void
          c. Skin irritation or breakdown
          d. Associated problems
       4. *Toilet habits* are assessed for:
          a. Safety
          b. Independence
          c. Use of equipment
          d. Use of indwelling catheter
       5. *Evaluation of vital signs*
       6. *Evaluation of laboratory and radiologic studies:*
          a. Serum
          b. Urine
          c. Radiologic studies

V. Pathological states and nursing management
   ### A. *Acute renal failure*
   1. Acute renal failure is the cessation of kidney function and is caused by prerenal, intrarenal or postrenal conditions.
   2. The three phases of acute renal failure are oliguric, diuretic and recovery.
   3. Acute renal failure includes the following pathological conditions:
      a. Acute tubular necrosis
      b. Acute cortical necrosis
      c. Acute vasomotor nephropathy
      d. Decreased glomerular filtration
      e. Altered blood flow distribution
   4. The patient may present with:
      a. Changes in mentation
      b. Lethargy
      c. Stupor
      d. Nausea, vomiting
      e. Deep or rapid respirations
      f. Pulmonary edema
      g. Tachycardia
      h. Dysrhythmias
      i. Pericarditis
      j. Dry skin
      k. Pruritis
   5. Important diagnostic data includes:
      a. History
      b. BUN
      c. Creatinine
      d. Intravenous pyelogram

6. Nursing care of the patient in acute renal failure includes:
   a. Maintenance of fluid and electrolyte balance
   b. Prevention of shock
   c. Prevention of infection
   d. Maintenance of nutritional status
   e. Meticulous skin care

B. *Chronic renal failure*
   1. Chronic renal failure is an insidious, progressive development of renal dysfunction.
   2. The patient presents with mild fatigue, headache, gastrointestinal disturbances and bleeding tendencies.
   3. Important laboratory findings are a rise in serum BUN and creatinine.
   4. Nursing care in chronic renal failure includes:
      a. Careful regulation of protein, fluid and sodium
      b. Continuous blood pressure monitoring for hypertension
      c. Maintaining a safe environment
      d. Emotional support for patient and family
      e. Patient teaching and referral, as indicated
      f. Preventing complications.

C. *Pyelonephritis*
   1. Pyelonephritis is a bacterial infection of the renal pelvis, interstitial tissue and tubules.
   2. Presenting signs include general malaise, fever, chills, back pain and flank tenderness.
   3. Definitive diagnosis is made by urine culture and the serum elevation of white blood cells.
   4. Nursing care specific to pyelonephritis includes:
      a. Patient education
      b. Proper collection of specimens
      c. Proper toilet habits
      d. Encouraging fluid intake

D. *Glomerulonephritis*
   1. Glomerulonephritis follows an acute renal inflammatory disease.
   2. There are two classifications of glomerulonephritis:
      a. Acute glomerulonephritis
      b. Chronic glomerulonephritis
   3. Clinical presentation
      a. Chronic—proteinuria, hypertension, blurred vision, weight loss
      b. Acute—hematuria, proteinuria
   4. Diagnostic data include urine specific gravity, serum protein nitrogen level and antistreptolysin 0 titer.
      a. Chronic—A high specific gravity albumin, casts, blood and protein are found in the urine.
      b. Acute—Hematuria, proteinuria, elevated antistreptolysin 0 titer, and an elevated BUN and creatinine are present.
   5. Nursing care specific to glomerulonephritis includes:
      a. Maintenance of fluid balance
      b. Proper nutrition with restriction of sodium and protein intake
      c. Administration of medication to prevent infection

  d. Prevention of further complications, including infections
  e. Encouraging follow-up care
  f. Patient education
 E. *Nephrotic syndrome*
  1. The nephrotic syndrome is a condition caused by massive proteinuria.
  2. Presenting signs include edema, anasarca, proteinuria, hematuria, anorexia and fatigue.
  3. Diagnostic data includes laboratory studies for albumin and globulin protein fractions.
  4. Nursing care specific to the nephrotic syndrome includes:
   a. Administration of steroids and diuretics
   b. Control of the nephrotic syndrome by reducing albuminuria
   c. Restriction of sodium
   d. Increasing protein intake
   e. Bedrest for severe edema
   f. Prevention of complications associated with immobility
   g. Meticulous skin care
   h. Emotional support
 F. *Hypertension*
  1. Hypertension is the sustained elevation of blood pressure above a diastolic of 90 mm Hg or systolic of 140 mm Hg.
  2. Presenting signs are blood pressure readings.
  3. The two classifications of hypertension are:
   a. Essential hypertension
   b. Malignant hypertension
 G. *Renal insufficiency*
  1. Renal insufficiency is a reduction in renal function that is compatible with life.
  2. Presenting signs include weight gain, edema, hypotension, shock-like symptoms, tachycardia, diaphoresis, cyanosis and mentation changes.
  3. Definitive diagnosis is made by laboratory studies, history and physical.
  4. Nursing care includes:
   a. Monitoring for changes in neurological states
   b. Maintaining circulation
   c. Maintaining fluid and electrolyte balance
   d. Monitoring urinary output
   e. Providing emotional support to patient and family
 H. *Dialysis*
  1. Dialysis is the utilization of a semipermeable membrane to remove toxins and water.
  2. The two types of dialysis are:
   a. Peritoneal dialysis
   b. Hemodialysis
  3. Nursing care includes:
   a. Prevention of circulatory overload
   b. Prevention of complications—infection, hemorrhage
   c. Patency of fistula or shunt
   d. Monitoring for changes during procedure

e. Emotional support and teaching for the patient and family

VI. Care common to renal problems

  A. *Maintenance of fluid balance*
   1. Body weight is an important indicator of fluid balance.
   2. Observe for overhydration and dehydration.
   3. Monitor fluid balance.
   4. Assess renal ability.
   5. Record intake and output.
   6. Monitor fluid replacement.

  B. *Maintenance of electrolyte balance*
   1. Many factors influence electrolyte balance.
   2. Potassium:
      a. Hyperkalemia can be corrected by diet and medications.
         1. Kayexalate
         2. Emergency: I.V. administration of CaCl, sodium bicarbonate or the combination of glucose and insulin
   3. Hypernatremia is treated by fluid management and dialysis.
   4. Hypocalcemia is treated with I.V. administration of calcium.
   5. Phosphate levels are controlled by diet and with the administration of aluminum hydroxide.

  C. *Maintenance of nutrition* is accomplished by:
   1. Tube feedings
   2. Hyperalimentation
   3. Monitoring of nutrition
   4. Providing adequate calories, vitamins, proteins, carbohydrates and fats

  D. *Maintenance of renal perfusion* is accomplished through the:
   1. Control of hypertension
   2. Control of hypotensive states
   3. Control of renal hypoperfusion

  E. *Maintenance of acid-base balance* is accomplished by:
   1. Obtaining baseline arterial blood gases, monitoring changes and instituting treatment
   2. Acidosis is often present in renal states.
   3. Alkalosis is rare in renal disease and is usually associated with vomiting, diuresis, and hypokalemia.

  F. *Prevention of complications* requires close observation and immediate intervention. Common complications include:
   1. Cardiovascular
      a. Dysrhythmias
      b. Pericarditis
   2. Neurological
      a. Convulsions
      b. Asterexis
      c. Coma
   3. Infection
      a. Secondary to dialysis
      b. Respiratory infections
   4. Hematologic-anemia

5. Hypovolemia
6. Nephrotoxicity
   a. Medications
   b. Chemicals
7. Uremic syndrome.

CHAPTER SEVEN
ENDOCRINE SYSTEM

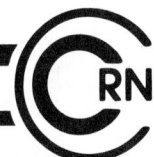

BEHAVIORAL OBJECTIVES

After reading the *Endocrine System,* the nurse will be able to:
- Identify the anatomy of the endocrine system
- Describe the function of structures related to the endocrine system
- Describe the physiology of the endocrine glands
- State the anatomical location and major functions of the following glands:
  pituitary
  thyroid
  parathyroid
  pancreas
  adrenals
- Identify the hormones associated with the adenohypophysis, neurohypophysis, thyroid gland, parathyroid gland, pancreas, adrenal glands and adrenal medulla
- Identify specific signs of altered functioning in the endocrine system
- State the components of physical assessment as they relate to the endocrine system
- State laboratory and radiologic studies as they relate to endocrine disorders
- Describe the pathophysiology of the following states:
  diabetes insipidus
  secretion of inappropriate ADH
  thyrotoxic crisis
  hypoparathyroid
  diabetic ketoacidosis
  hyperketotic hyperosmolar coma
  hypoglycemia
  adrenal crisis
- Identify clinical manifestations and diagnosis findings associated with:
  diabetes insipidus
  secretion of inappropriate ADH
  thyrotoxic crisis
  hypoparathyroidism
  diabetic ketoacidosis
  hyperketotic hyperosmolar coma
  hypoglycemia
  adrenal crisis
- Develop a nursing care plan for these conditions:
  diabetes insipidus
  secretion of inappropriate ADH
  thyrotoxic crisis
  hypoparathyroidism
  diabetic ketoacidosis
  hyperketotic hyperosmolar coma
  hypoglycemia
  adrenal crisis
- List the common problems associated with endocrine disorders

TOPICAL OUTLINE
ENDOCRINE SYSTEM

I. The Endocrine System: Overview 431
II. Anatomy and Physiology 432
    Endocrine glands 432
        Pituitary (hypophysis) 432
        Thyroid 432
        Parathyroid 432
        Pancreas 432
        Adrenals 433
    Hormones 434
        Hormones associated with the hypophysis 434
        Hormones associated with the neurohypophysis 436
        Hormones associated with the thyroid gland 437
        Hormones associated with the parathyroid gland 437
        Hormones associated with the pancreas 438
        Hormones associated with the adrenal glands 438
III. Assessment of the Endocrine System 441
    Gross cerebral functions 441
    Specific cerebral function 441
    Level of consciousness 441
    Inspection 442
    Palpation 442
    Percussion 442
    Auscultation 442
IV. Pathological States and Nursing Management 444
    Diabetes insipidus 444
        Pathophysiology 444
        Clinical presentation 444
        Diagnostic data 444
        Nursing care 444
    Secreton of inappropriate ADH (SIADH) 445
        Pathophysiology 445
        Clinical presentation 445
        Diagnostic data 445
        Nursing care 446
    Thyrotoxic crisis 446
        Pathophysiology 446
        Clinical presentation 446
        Diagnostic data 446
        Nursing care 446
    Hypoparathyroidism 447
        Pathophysiology 447
        Clinical presentation 447
        Diagnostic data 447
        Nursing care 447
    Diabetic ketoacidosis 447
        Pathophysiology 447

        Clinical presentation   448
        Diagnostic data   448
        Nursing care   448
    Hyperketotic hyperosmolar coma (HHNK)   449
        Pathophysiology   449
        Clinical presentation   449
        Diagnostic data   449
        Nursing care   449
    Hypoglycemia   449
        Pathophysiology   449
        Clinical presentation   449
        Diagnostic data   450
        Nursing care   450
    Adrenal crisis   450
        Pathophysiology   450
        Clinical presentation   450
        Diagnostic data   450
        Nursing care   450
V. Care Common to Endocrine Problems   453
    Airway and ventilation   453
    Fluid and electrolyte balance   453
    Neurological status   453
    Patient and family education   454
Program Assessment: Science and Situation   455
Key Point Recognition Answers   463
PASS Answer Sheet   469
Survey Summary   471

THE ENDOCRINE SYSTEM: OVERVIEW

The endocrine system is essential to the integration of body systems. It is through the secretion of hormones that the endocrine system interfaces with the nervous system to fine-tune or adjust physiological responses to the environment. This important homeostatic system includes the following glands:

Pituitary
Thyroid
Parathyroid
Pancreas
Adrenals

These glands (Fig. 7-1) are responsible for growth, development, fluid and electrolyte balance, metabolism, acid-base balance and reproduction.

Name	Location	Hormone
Pituitary (hypophysis) Adenohypophysis* Neurohypophysis+	Cranial cavity in sella turcica below hypothalamus	*GH, TSH, ACTH, FSH, LH, ICSH, PRL, MSH +ADH, Oxytocin
Thyroid	Neck between the second and third tracheal rings	TSH
Parathyroid	Posterior plane of thyroid	Parathormone
Pancreas	In abdomen between the spleen and duodenum	Glucagon Insulin
Adrenals Cortex* Medulla+	Apex of each kidney	*Glucocorticoid *Mineralocorticoid *Androgen +Epinephrine +Norepinephrine

Fig. 7-1 Endocrine glands

ANATOMY AND PHYSIOLOGY

ENDOCRINE GLANDS

Pituitary (Hypophysis)

Once believed to be the "master gland," the **hypophysis** (pituitary gland) is located in the **sella turcica** below the **hypothalamus.** The pituitary is almond-shaped and composed of two major segments: the anterior portion **(adenohypophysis)** and the posterior portion **(neurohypophysis).** The adenohypophysis is connected to the hypothalamus (the true master gland) by the vascular system. The hypothalamus sends **releasing factors** (chemicals keyed to cause the release of hormones from the target organ) via the arterial blood supply to the adenohypophysis. Once received by the adenohypophysis, these releasing factors stimulate the release of specific hormones from the adenohypophysis.

This same system, working in reverse, governs the inhibition of the release of these hormones. When sufficient blood hormone levels are achieved, the hypothalamus ceases to release the specific releasing factor for that hormone. This **negative feedback system** allows regulation of hormone release based on the concentration of that hormone present in the circulation.

KEY CONCEPT: Lack of a sufficient hormone concentration causes release of the releasing factor and, therefore, release of the specific hormone. Adequate hormone concentration causes inhibition of the release of releasing factor and inhibits release of the hormone.

The neurohypophysis is connected to the hypothalamus by a band of neural tissue. The hypothalamus produces both posterior pituitary hormones, **antidiuretic hormone (ADH)** and **oxytocin,** which are then stored and released by the neurohypophysis. The physiological effects of each hormone trigger its release from the neurohypophysis. These physiological effects are also the mediators of the negative feedback cycle that inhibits the release of these hormones.

Thyroid

The **thyroid** is composed of two lateral lobes connected by a fine filament of tissue called the **isthmus.** The thyroid is located between the second and third cartilaginous rings of the trachea and can be palpated in the anterior midline of the neck. It is a highly vascular organ. The high rate of blood flow is necessary to thyroid hormone synthesis.

Parathyroid

The **parathyroid glands** are composed of four flattened, oval bodies located in the posterior plane of the thyroid gland, one on the upper side of each thyroid lobe and one on the lower side of each lobe. The parathyroid hormone **parathormone** is secreted by chief cells in response to blood calcium levels. A negative feedback system stops secretion of parathormone when the calcium level is adequate. To work effectively, parathormone requires the presence of adequate amounts of **vitamin D.**

Pancreas

The **pancreas** is composed of three sections: the **head, tail** and **body.**

The pancreas is located in the posterior compartment of the abdomen between the spleen and the duodenum. The pancreas has two types of secretory cells responsible for hormone secretion: the **acinar cells,** which serve an exocrine function (external secretion); and the **islet cells,** which serve an endocrine function (internal secretion). The **acinar cells,** being exocrine glands, will not be discussed. The islet cells are of two basic types: **alpha cells** and **beta cells.**

The alpha cells secrete **glucagon,** which functions to raise the blood glucose level by stimulating glyconeogenesis and glycogenolysis. The beta cells are concerned with the secretion of **insulin,** which enhances glycogen storage, transports glucose into the cell, stimulates the metabolic rate and decreases blood glucose levels.

Adrenals

The *adrenal glands* are a pair of triangle-shaped glands. They are found in the retroperitoneal space, one at the apex of each kidney. The adrenal glands are composed of two sections: the *cortex* and the *medulla.*

The outer portion of the gland, the *cortex,* makes up about 80 percent of the volume of the adrenal gland. It consists of three distinct layers, each producing its own hormone. The hormones are: *glucocorticoids, mineralocorticoids* and *androgens.*

Glucocorticoid and androgen are stimulated and regulated by ACTH secretion. ACTH plays a small part in the regulation of mineralocorticoid, but the major regulator is the *renin-angiotensin* system, which triggers mineralocorticoid release in response to a decreased blood volume.

The inner section, the *medulla,* produces: *epinephrine* and *norepinephrine.*

These hormones (also called catecholamines) are regulated by neural stimuli from the autonomic nervous system.

KEY CONCEPT: Hormonal secretion or inhibition is a highly specialized physiological process that responds to changes in homeostasis.

KEY POINT RECOGNITION

Write true or false by each statement. Answers are at the end of this chapter. A score below 80% indicates the need for further study.

_____ 1. The hypophysis is located in the sella turcica below the hypothalamus.

_____ 2. The two major segments of the pituitary are the adenohypophysis and neurohypophysis.

_____ 3. The neurohypophysis is also called the anterior portion of the pituitary.

_____ 4. The neurohypophysis is connected to the hypothalamus by the vascular system.

_____ 5. The hypothalamus sends releasing factor to the adenohypophysis.

_____ 6. Adequate hormone concentration results in inhibition of the releasing factor.

_____ 7. The negative feedback system allows regulation of hormone, based on the concentration of the hormone in the circulation.

_____ 8. ADH and oxytocin are produced in the neurohypophysis.

_____ 9. The trigger for release of ADH is hypervolemia and hypotonicity.

_____ 10. The thyroid's two lateral lobes are connected by the isthmus.

_____ 11. The thyroid is located between the fourth and fifth tracheal rings.

_____ 12. A low blood flow to the thyroid is conducive to hormone synthesis.

_____ 13. The parathyroid glands are located in the posterior portion of the pituitary.

_____ 14. When blood calcium levels are adequate, parathormone is secreted.

_____ 15. Acinar cells serve an exocrine function.

_____ 16. Islet cells are of two types: alpha and beta.

_____ 17. Glucagon raises blood glucose by stimulating glyconeogenesis and glycogenolysis.

_____ 18. Insulin is vital in the transportation of glucose into the cell.

_____ 19. The adrenal medulla produces epinephrine and norepinephrine.

_____ 20. The major regulator of mineralocorticoid is ACTH.

_____ 21. Catecholamines are regulated by neural stimuli.

_____ 22. Glucocorticoid is stimulated by ACTH secretion.

HORMONES

Hormones Associated with the Hypophysis

The hormones associated with the *adenohypophysis* are:

Growth hormone (GH), also called **somatotropic hormone (STH)**

Thyroid stimulating hormone (TSH)

Adrenocorticotropic hormone (ACTH)

Follicle stimulating hormone (FSH)

Luteinizing hormone (LH)

Interstitial cell stimulating hormone (ICSH)

Prolactin (PRL)

Melanocyte stimulating hormone (MSH)

Growth hormone, also called *somatotropic hormone,* is the major hormone released by the adenohypophysis. This hormone is responsible for growth and development in humans and has earned the pituitary gland the reputation as the "master gland." It was believed that the pituitary was responsible for growth and development and that all aspects of GH were under the control of the pituitary. It is now known that GH release is stimulated by a hypothalamic releasing factor known as *growth hormone releasing factor* (GHRF). GH release can also be stimulated by exercise, hypoglycemia and decreased amino acid levels. The common factor in all the releasing mechanisms is the need for energy and the need for the use of fat stores to produce energy.

Growth hormone, which is responsible for initiating protein anabolism, conserving carbohydrates and mobilizing fat stores, affects *all body cells.* The effects of growth hormone are stimulation of **bone** and **cartilage growth, protein-linked activities,** such as muscle mass growth and tissue generation, **use of fat for energy** with the resultant **sparing of carbohydrates,** and the **growth of the human body.**

Under normal circumstances, the growth spurts seen in puberty result from GH. However, if excess GH is released in childhood, the result is *gigantism,* an excess and abnormal growth and development pattern. In adulthood, after the closure of the epiphyseal plates, the result of excess GH secretion is *acromegaly,* an abnormal growth pattern resulting in excessive growth of hands, feet, jaw and internal organs. Diminished amounts of GH secreted during childhood result in *dwarfism,* while decreased secretion during adulthood leads to *decreased organ weight.*

Inhibition of GH release is brought about by *growth hormone inhibiting factor* (GHIF or somatostatin), a chemical produced by the hypothalamus, or by long periods of *elevated corticosteroid levels,* which promote protein breakdown for energy production, or *hyperglycemia.*

Thyroid stimulating hormone (TSH) increases the growth and function of the thyroid cells. Excess TSH results in an increase in the size of the thyroid gland and **hyperthyroid symptoms: tachycardia, weight loss, increased appetite, diarrhea, tremors, weakness** and **heat intolerance.**

Decreased TSH release results in a decrease in the size of the thyroid gland and the typical symptoms of **hypothyroidism: lethargy, fatigue, weight gain, constipation, cold intolerance, cardiomegaly, cardiac failure** and **diminished mental acuity or altered mental status.**

TSH is released from the adenohypophysis by the presence of *thyrotropin releasing factor* (TRF), produced by the hypothalamus. TSH release is also stimulated by depressed levels of circulating thyroid hormone and by cold temperatures. TSH release is inhibited by adequate or elevated levels of thyroid hormone and by sympathetic nervous system stimulation.

Patients presenting with signs of either hypo- or hyperthyroidism must be carefully studied to determine the primary site of the problem. Elevated or decreased thyroid hormone levels, while responsible for the symptomatology, often are secondary to hypothalamic dysfunction, resulting in elevated or depressed levels of TRF. Testing for response to thyroid releasing factor is a relatively safe and easy method for determining the primary cause of the symptoms. A TRF-like drug is injected I.V., and serial blood samples are tested for concentration of thyroid hormone. The results of the study enable the clinician to determine if the problem lies in the thyroid (excess—deficient thyroid hormone production), the hypothalamus (excess—deficient TRF production) or in the inability of the adenohypophysis to react correctly to the levels of TRF present. Side effects of the test, which rarely last longer than five minutes, may be transient tachycardia, blood pressure changes, flushing and, rarely, cardiac arrhythmias.

Adrenocorticotropic hormone (ACTH) acts on the cells of the adrenal cortex. Its functions are multiple: **stimulation of growth and function of the adrenal glands, stimulation of production and release of glucocorticoids from the adrenal cortex, stimulation of production of mineralocorticoids by the adrenal cortex** and **stimulation of production of androgens by the adrenal cortex.**

ACTH is released from the adenohypophysis by the action of *corticotropin releasing factor* (CRF), produced by the hypothalamus. Decreased plasma cortisol levels, hypoglycemia and stress can also stimulate the release of CRF from the hypothalamus. Increased plasma cortisol levels inhibit the release of CRF and, therefore, inhibit the release of ACTH.

The major effect of ACTH is on the production of *glucocorticoids.* Elevation of ACTH levels results in a syndrome similar to Cushing's disease. The clinical findings are **weakness, fatigue, depression, fat deposits** in the face and trunk (moon-face and dowager's hump), with simultaneous wasting of the extremities, **elevation of blood glucose and blood pressure** and **decreased immune response.**

The effect of elevated ACTH levels on the production of mineralocorticoids and androgens is minimal and produces no clinical signs.

Decreased ACTH levels result in an Addisonian-type clinical picture featuring **hypotension, hypoglycemia, weight loss, weakness** and **increased skin pigmentation.**

In addition, the adrenals atrophy, and there is a decrease in the production of both mineralocorticoids and glucocorticoids.

Follicle stimulating hormone (FSH) stimulates the maturation of ovarian follicles or sperm by its action on the cells of the ovaries or testes. Release of FSH from the adenohypophysis is stimulated by *follicle stimulating factor* (FSF), produced by the hypothalamus. Elevated FSH levels result in the onset of early or precocious puberty. The mechanism causing inhibition of release of FSH is unknown, but the clinical picture of inhibition presents as delayed or absent puberty. Postmaturation, inhibition of FSH release, may result in amenorrhea.

Two similar hormones are produced by the adenohypophysis, dependent on the sex of the individual. *Luteinizing hormone* (LH) is produced in *females only*. Its purposes are to increase secretion of estrogen and progesterone, and to stimulate the of growth of the corpus luteum. By acting directly on the cells of the ovaries, LH prepares the ovary for release of an ovum and sets up the proper hormonal conditions for fertilization and development of the embryo. The sequelae of increased levels of LH are unknown, but it has been theorized that one effect may be the development of pseudo-pregnancy or disruption of the normal cycle by the continuous production of estrogen and progesterone. Decreased levels of LH result in immaturity of the corpus luteum and markedly decreased levels of estrogen and progesterone. *Luteinizing hormone releasing factor* (LHRF) is responsible for the release of LH, but the mechanism responsible for inhibition of LH release has not yet been identified.

Interstitial cell stimulating hormone (ICSH) is produced in *males only*. Its actions are to stimulate production of testosterone and to aid in the development of male sex characteristics. It acts directly on the cells of the testes. Closely related to LH, the release of ICSH is stimulated by LHRF. The factors that inhibit its release are unknown. Elevated ICSH levels do not appear to produce any clinical signs, except the possibility of increased testosterone levels.

Decreased ICSH levels result in decreased testosterone production and the failure to develop secondary male sexual characteristics.

Prolactin (PRL) is the only adenohypophyseal hormone known to be inhibited rather than released under normal circumstances. The site of production of *prolactin inhibiting factor* (PIF) is not clear; but it is theorized that it may be the adenohypophysis, since it is known that certain tumors of the anterior pituitary produce lactation as a side effect. Prolactin stimulates lactation, and release of prolactin is caused by the inhibition of PIF during labor and breast feeding, or in the case of an adenohypophyseal tumor. Under normal circumstances, lactation does not occur because of the inhibition of LH by the effect of prolactin inhibiting factor. It is only when this suppressive factor is removed that lactation is stimulated. The end organ of prolactin is the breast. Inappropriate or excessive lactation is the result of secretion or elevation of prolactin. Normally, failure to lactate is due to PRL inhibition. Lactation is inhibited or absent in postpartum women with decreased PRL levels.

Melanocyte stimulating hormone (MSH) is responsible for the production and deposit of skin pigmentation by direct action on skin cells. MSH is released from the adenohypophysis by the action of decreased plasma cortisol levels; CRF may play a role in the release of MSH. Increased MSH levels result in skin hyperpigmentation. Inhibition of MSH is the result of increased plasma cortisol levels and may also result from the presence of a possible inhibiting factor produced by the hypothalamus. Decreased levels of MSH result in inadequate skin pigmentation.

Hormones Associated with the Neurohypophysis

The hormones associated with the neurohypophysis are: *antidiuretic hormone* (ADH) and *oxytocin.*

Antidiuretic hormone (ADH) is also called *vasopressin.* Working on the kidneys (collecting ducts and distal tubules), ADH increases water reabsorption and inhibits diuresis. An additional effect of ADH release is constriction of the smooth muscles of the arterioles, resulting in increased arterial systolic pressure. ADH also has an effect on the G.I. tract, leading to abdominal cramping. ADH is manufactured by the hypothalamus, but stored and released by the neurohypophysis. It is released when an increase in serum osmolarity is detected by the osmoreceptors in the hypothalamus. These osmoreceptors detect serum hyperosmolarity and stimulate the neurohypophysis to release ADH. Appropriate serum osmolarity does not stimulate osmoreceptors, and no release signal is sent. Under normal circumstances, the negative feedback system is very sensitive and the proper serum concentration is maintained. However, in certain disease states (meningitis, apical lung tumors and some types of cerebral mass lesions), the amount of ADH released is excessive in relation to the serum osmolarity. This condition is known as *syndrome of inappropriate antidiuretic hormone* (SIADH). The results of SIADH are free-water intoxication (hypervolemia) and dilutional hyponatremia secondary to the lack of appropriate diuresis.

Lack of release of ADH results in a syndrome known as *diabetes insipidus* (DI). Under normal circumstances, ADH release is inhibited when the serum osmolarity is within the normal range. In the pathological states of edema, compression or destruction of the hypothalamus or neurohypophysis, or the edema occurring after pituitary surgery, ADH production is markedly decreased or totally halted (hypothalamic site), or ADH release is halted or impaired (pituitary site). The lack of ADH results in uncontrolled diuresis. Remember that ADH controls water reabsorption only, so this diuresis is all free water, and the patient rapidly develops dehydration and hypernatremia. The specific gravity of urine in DI is generally below 1.005 and little sodium is excreted in the urine. Because a free-water diuresis exists, fluid replacement must be with hypotonic solutions. If able to speak, the patient will complain of thirst; only water should be used to orally replace volume. Juices and other solutions high in sodium should be avoided because the patient is already hypernatremic.

Oxytocin is the second hormone of the neurohypophysis. Inhibition of oxytocin release is the normal state in the nonpregnant, non-nursing female. The mechanism of inhibition is not clearly understood. Oxytocin release is caused by the initiation of labor and by breast feeding. Oxytocin acts on the cells of the uterus to produce uterine contractions and the cells of the breast to induce lactation. The effects of increased oxytocin release are poorly understood, although some researchers feel it may contribute to excessive uterine contractions. Decreased oxytocin results in insufficient lactation and a failure to initiate adequate uterine contractions during labor.

Hormones Associated with the Thyroid Gland

The thyroid gland is responsible for the production of three hormones: *thyroxine* (T_4), *triiodothyronine* (T_3) and *thyrocalcitonin* (calcitonin).

Thyroxine is the major hormone secreted by the thyroid and is composed of iodine and tyrosine, and is bound to proteins in the systemic circulation.

Release of T_4 is initiated by the release of *thyrotropin releasing factor* (TRF), which stimulates the secretion of *thyroid stimulating hormone* (TSH), as does exposure to cold temperatures. T_4 inhibition is caused by inadequate amounts of TSH and can also be inhibited by elevation of serum glucocorticoid levels.

T_4 acts on all body cells to stimulate protein synthesis, speed fat and carbohydrate metabolism, accelerate bone growth and stimulate the production of cyclic AMP within the muscle cells.

Elevated T_4 levels produce the symptoms associated with *hyperthyroidism:* weight loss with increased appetite; muscle tremors and weakness; tachycardia; exophthalmos; heat intolerance; diarrhea; menstrual irregularities; and hypertrophy of the thyroid gland.

In children, sharply elevated growth patterns are seen.

Decreased levels of T_4 produce the symptoms characteristic of *hypothyroidism:* decreased metabolic activity with lethargy; fatigue and weight gain; cardiomegaly and failure; cold intolerance; dry skin and lack of perspiration; periorbital edema; mental changes, such as memory lapses and decreased concentration and attention span; atrophy of the thyroid gland; and constipation.

Triiodothyronine is also an iodine-tyrosine compound bound to plasma proteins. It is four times more potent than T_4 in its actions and effects, but in all other respects it is identical to T_4, producing the same symptoms in elevated or depressed states.

Thyrocalcitonin is manufactured and released by the C cells of the thyroid gland. It is released in response to the serum calcium-magnesium balance. Thyrocalcitonin release is caused by elevated serum calcium levels, elevated magnesium levels and elevated serum glucagon levels. Supression is caused when there is damage to the C cells of the thyroid gland. Thyrocalcitonin exerts its effects on bone and renal tissue. It achieves reduction of serum calcium levels by inhibiting bone lysis and increasing urinary excretion of calcium, phosphates, sodium, chlorides and magnesium.

Increased levels of thyrocalcitonin produce decreased serum calcium, inhibition of bone lysis and wasting of calcium, magnesium, sodium, chloride and phosphates via urinary excretion.

Decreased thyrocalcitonin levels result in increased bone lysis and elevation of serum calcium, and depression of urinary excretion of calcium and the other associated ions.

Hormones Associated with the Parathyroid Gland

Parathormone (PTH) is the only known hormone associated with the parathyroid gland. Parathormone release is stimulated by depressed serum calcium levels and elevated serum phosphate and magnesium levels. Parathormone release is inhibited by elevated serum calcium levels and by inadequate vitamin D levels. Adequate levels of vitamin D are required for parathormone to act on the target cells.

Parathormone works on the cells of the kidney, gastrointestinal tract and bone. It causes decreased reabsorption of phosphate and increased absorption of calcium. In addition, parathormone decreases bone reabsorption of calcium, increases absorption of calcium by the G.I. tract and enhances excretion of bicarbonate from the renal tubules.

Elevated parathormone levels produce increased serum calcium, leading to fatigue, lethargy, weakness, headache, excessive urination and the formation of renal calculi. Decreased PTH results in lowered calcium levels, tremor, tetany and the associated signs of hypocalcemia.

Hormones Associated with the Pancreas

The hormones associated with the pancreas are **glucagon** and **insulin**.

Glucagon is secreted by the alpha cells of the islet portion of the pancreas. Release of glucagon is stimulated by hypoglycemia, starvation, increased levels of amino acids, elevation of catecholamine levels and excessive exercise. Inhibition and its mechanism are unclear, except in cases where the islet cells are rendered nonfunctional. Glucagon raises blood glucose levels by stimulating glycogenolysis and glyconeogenesis, and inhibiting glycolysis. Working on the liver cells, glucagon elevates serum glucose levels, but it also employs fatty acid oxidation to elevate circulating glucose.

Insulin is produced by the beta cells of the islet and is needed for transport of glucose into the cell; initiation of protein synthesis; fatty acid storage; and reduction of cellular metabolism of triglycerides.

Insulin release is triggered by hyperglycemia and elevated levels of ACTH, growth hormone, gastrin and glucagon. Failure to secrete insulin (one of the primary mechanisms in diabetes mellitus) is not totally understood, but it may result from an inherited or acquired defect in the beta cells.

An immunological theory of diabetes has been suggested. Some patients may produce insulin in adequate amounts, but produce an antibody that blocks the action of insulin. Insulin's primary target organ is the liver; but it also plays a role in the metabolic processes of almost all other body cells. Elevated insulin levels result in hypoglycemia. Decreased levels result in hyperglycemia, acidosis and ketosis, which result from the by-products of "alternate pathway" production of glucose. These alternate pathways are called into play when the body cells are unable to use the available serum glucose because the lack of insulin does not permit transport into the cells. The cells, believing that insufficient glucose is present, signals the liver to produce more glucose. Thus, fat and protein are metabolized by glyconeogenesis to provide glucose.

Hormones Associated with the Adrenal Glands
The Adrenal Cortex

The hormones of the adrenal cortex include **glucocorticoids, mineralocorticoids** and **androgens.**

Glucocorticoids are the hormones released by the adrenal cortex that are responsible for decrease in inflammation, depressed protein synthesis and stimulation of glyconeogenesis.

This is often called the "steroid effect." **Cortisol** is the primary glucocorticoid produced by the adrenals. Production is stimulated by ACTH, CRF, trauma, stress and infection.

The inhibition of glucocorticoid release is due to a negative feedback mechanism resulting from adequate blood levels. The hypothalamus is signaled and ACTH levels are reduced. The glucocorticoids affect all body cells. Increased levels present a syndrome (Cushing's) consisting of weakness; fatigue; irritability; depression; thinning of the skin; fat deposits in the face and trunk with wasting of the extremities; elevation of blood pressure and blood glucose; and inhibition of the immune system.

Decreased levels result in a syndrome (Addison's) presenting as hypotension; hypoglycemia; weight loss; weakness; stimulation of melanocyte stimulating hormone (MSH); skin pigmentation; and fatigue.

Mineralocorticoids are produced by the adrenal cortex. The primary hormone is **aldosterone.** It is released by the effect of the renin-angiotensin system, hyponatremia and hyperkalemia.

Mineralocoticoids act on the distal and collecting tubules of the kidney to conserve sodium, excrete potassium and conserve fluid to increase extracellular volume.

Increased mineralocorticoids result in hypertension, hypokalemia and weakness. Decreased mineralocorticoids result in hyponatremia and dehydration because of excess fluid loss via the kidneys and sweat glands.

Androgens are the third type of hormone produced by the adrenal cortex. Their physiology is not totally understood, but in normal amounts, they have little effect on any body system except the reproductive organs. In excess, they result in precocious puberty in males and masculinization in females. Decreased levels result in feminization and lack of sexual development in the male.

The Adrenal Medulla

The hormones of the *adrenal medulla* include *epinephrine* and *norepinephrine*. Collectively, the hormones of the adrenal medulla are also known as *catecholamines*.

Epinephrine is the primary hormone of the adrenal medulla. It is released through stimulation of the sympathetic nervous system and stimulation of insulin and histamine. Inhibition is the result of adrenal dysfunction.

Epinephrine acts on the smooth muscles, the vascular system and various other body cells. Its normal effects are positive chronotropic and inotropic effects on cardiac cells; dilatation of blood vessels supplying the heart and skeletal muscles; constriction of the blood vessels supplying the abdominal viscera and skin; decreased peristalsis and secretion by the G.I. tract; elevation of blood glucose; constriction of the sphincter muscles; pupillary dilatation; increased perspiration; and dilatation of the bronchioles with increased rate and depth of respirations.

Increased epinephrine levels exaggerate the normal effects, while a decrease has minimal or no effect. However, decreased epinephrine levels do contribute to a decreased fight or flight response.

Norepinephrine is also produced by the adrenal medulla. It is identical to epinephrine in release mechanisms, effects and sequelae, except norepinephrine exhibits a greater effect on the skeletal muscles with less effect on the cardiac cells, decreased metabolic effect and increased peripheral resistance.

KEY POINT RECOGNITION

Write true or false by each statement. Answers are at the end of this chapter. A score below 80% indicates the need for further study.

_____ 1. Somatotropic hormone is released by the adenohypophysis.

_____ 2. GH is stimulated by the hypothalamic releasing factor GHRF.

_____ 3. GH is responsible for initiation of protein anabolism.

_____ 4. GH affects bone and cartilage by inhibiting growth.

_____ 5. Excess GH in childhood results in gigantism.

_____ 6. Somatostatin of GHIF inhibits the release of GH.

_____ 7. Hyperglycemia stimulates the release of GH.

_____ 8. Tachycardia, weight gain, weakness and mental slowing are symptoms of hyperthyroidism.

_____ 9. TSH may be released in the presence of cold temperatures.

_____10. Sympathetic nervous system stimulation is a stimulus for release of TSH.

_____11. Abnormal thyroid levels may be secondary to hypothalamic dysfunction.

_____12. ACTH is released from the adenohypophysis by the action of CRF.

_____13. Hypoglycemia and stress can stimulate the release of corticotropin releasing factor from the hypothalamus.

_____14. Increased plasma cortisol levels indirectly inhibit the release of ACTH.
_____15. Elevation of ACTH levels results in the following signs and symptoms: weakness, depression, dowager's hump, blood glucose elevation and decreased immune response.
_____16. FSH is released by the adenohypophysis in the presence of follicle stimulating factor.
_____17. Luteinizing hormone acts on the ovaries to set the hormonal conditions necessary for fertilization and development of the embryo.
_____18. Interstitial cell stimulating hormone stimulates lactation.
_____19. ICSH is stimulated by luteinizing hormone releasing factor.
_____20. Prolactin is stimulated by PIF.
_____21. Increased plasma cortisol levels stimulate the release of melanocyte stimulating hormone.
_____22. ADH (vasopressin) decreases water reabsorption and inhibits diuresis.
_____23. ADH release results in decreased arterial systolic pressure.
_____24. The osmoreceptors respond to hyperosmolarity by sending a message to the pituitary to release ADH.
_____25. Free-water intoxication and dilutional hyponatremia are the result of excessive ADH release in relation to serum osmolarity.
_____26. Hypothalamic edema may result in the increased production of ADH.
_____27. Diabetes insipidus is a condition in which inappropriate diuresis results in dehydration and hypernatremia.
_____28. The patient with diabetes insipidus is hypernatremic and hypovolemic.
_____29. Oxytocin is inhibited in the lactating female.
_____30. T_4 is composed of iodine and tyrosine.
_____31. TRF inhibits the secretion of TSH, which in turn causes release of thyroxine.
_____32. Thyroxine is inhibited by elevated levels of serum glucocorticoids.
_____33. T_4 stimulates protein synthesis and speeds fat and carbohydrate metabolism.
_____34. Elevation of T_4 levels results in weight loss, cardiomegaly, exophthalmos, decreased concentration and heat intolerance.
_____35. T_4 is four times more potent than T_3.
_____36. Thyrocalcitonin is released by elevated serum calcium, magnesium and glucagon levels.
_____37. **Increased levels of thyrocalcitonin produce decreased serum calcium.**
_____38. Calcitonin is produced in the hypothalamus and released by the C cells of the thyroid.
_____39. Parathormone is released when serum calcium levels are depressed.
_____40. Decreased levels of vitamin D stimulate the release of parathormone.
_____41. Parathormone causes decreased reabsorption of phosphate and increased absorption of calcium.
_____42. Release of glucagon is stimulated by hyperglycemia and excessive exercise.
_____43. Glucagon stimulates glycogenolysis and glyconeogenesis, and inhibits glycolysis, which results in the raising of blood glucose levels.
_____44. Insulin is necessary for the initiation of protein synthesis and fatty acid storage, as well as for the transport of glucose into the cell.

_____45. Elevated ACTH levels trigger the release of insulin.
_____46. Inadequate insulin levels result in the metabolism of fat and protein.
_____47. Cortisol is the primary glucocorticoid produced by the adrenal cortex.
_____48. An effect of glucocorticoid release is stimulation of glyconeogenesis.
_____49. Cortisol production may be stimulated by severe trauma.
_____50. Adequate glucocorticoid levels ultimately result in the inhibition of glucocorticoid release through the reduction of ACTH.
_____51. Signs and symptoms of increased glucocorticoid levels include hypoglycemia, hypotension, increased skin pigmentation and fatigue.
_____52. The primary mineralocorticoid is aldosterone.
_____53. Hyperkalemia and hyponatremia inhibit the release of aldosterone.
_____54. Aldosterone is important in the conservation of sodium and potassium.
_____55. Increased levels of mineralocorticoid result in hypertension and hypokalemia.
_____56. Decreased levels of androgens result in lack of sexual development in the male.
_____57. Epinephrine exerts a positive inotropic effect on heart cells.
_____58. Epinephrine is released through the stimulation of the parasympathetic nervous system.
_____59. Epinephrine release results in an increased rate of respirations.
_____60. Norepinephrine release results in increased peripheral vascular resistance.

ASSESSMENT OF THE ENDOCRINE SYSTEM

Assessment of the patient experiencing metabolic dysfunction is not very different from the assessment of any other patient. Significant medical problems, current therapies, family history and a review of systems are all included. Particular attention must be paid to the presenting complaint, its quantity, quality, location, aggravating and deviating factors, and the setting in which it occurs. The following symptoms require further investigation: headache, dizziness, visual changes, dyspnea, palpitations, fatigue, lethargy, weakness, tremors and muscle cramps.

Specific signs of altered functioning in the endocrine system may include an increase or decrease in appetite and thirst; polyuria, oliguria and nocturia; changes in skin and hair texture, skin pigmentation and hair distribution; intolerance to heat or cold; and personality changes.

The physical examination should include assessment of the following:

GROSS CEREBRAL FUNCTIONS
Level of consciousness, awareness, memory, orientation, judgment

SPECIFIC CEREBRAL FUNCTION
Speech pattern, attention span, and coordination

LEVEL OF CONSCIOUSNESS
Under any condition, the level of consciousness is the single most important determinant of neurological status. To assess level of consciousness, the following must be determined: *ease of arousal, orientation, response to verbal, visual or painful stimuli.*

After the level of consciousness has been determined, pupillary response must be checked for size, shape and consensual reaction.

Next, the muscular tone is examined for weakness, tremors, cramping, wasting and equal strength.

INSPECTION

Height and weight in relation to family history and chronological age

Distribution of subcutaneous fat

Facial expression and body movement, periorbital edema

Condition of mucous membranes and tongue

Skin turgor, pigmentation, texture, general condition (dry/oily) and presence of lesions

Motion of thyroid as the patient swallows

PALPATION

Touch the skin for temperature and hydration. Check for:

Presence of enlarged or nodular thyroid, thrill or over-thyroid arteries

Presence of abdominal or suprarenal masses

Heart rate and rhythm, blood pressure

Respiratory rate and rhythm

PERCUSSION

Percuss for:

Masses

Changes in size, contour and characteristics of the thyroid, kidney and other abdominal organs

AUSCULTATION

Check thyroid gland for bruits.

Evaluate vital signs.

The blood pressure may be hypotensive, hypertensive, or normotensive. Rarely in endocrine dysfunction is **hypotension** seen. When present, it usually indicates a pathology affecting the endocrine system. This pathology may be a lack of aldosterone, cortisol or insulin, causing fluid and electrolyte imbalances and circulatory collapse.

Hypertension may be present and is often a diagnostic finding secondary to head trauma, surgery or other intracranial pathology. This is a compensatory mechanism to ensure perfusion of an edematous brain. Also, a marked increase in systemic adrenergic activity, as seen in thyrotoxic crisis, elevates the blood pressure.

Bradycardia is common in mass lesions or edema, which create a downward pressure on the brainstem. This clinical picture may be seen as a result of tumors of the hypothalamic-neurohypophyseal system.

Hyperthermia may be seen as a result of compression of the hypothalamus. Thyrotoxic crisis or nonketotic hyperosmolar coma are situations in which hyperthermia may result. These febrile states are usually accompanied by tachycardia and tachypnea. *Hypothermia* is often present in profound injury that results in brain death.

Respiratory changes are common with metabolic diseases. *Cheyne-Stokes* respirations are rhythmic hypo- and hyperventilation, alternating with periods of apnea. The entire sequence is a crescendo-decrescendo response to alterations in pCO_2 levels that frequently occurs with bilateral corticol lesions. *Kussmaul breathing* is deep, gasping respirations associated with diabetic ketoacidosis.

LABORATORY AND RADIOLOGIC STUDIES

Laboratory studies in metabolic disease are varied and tailored to the presumptive diagnosis. Some of the laboratory studies used are:

Urinalysis to determine osmolarity, specific gravity, calcium phosphate, 17 ketosteroids, 17 hydroxycorticoids, glucose, culture and sensitivity

Serum to determine osmolarity, sodium, potassium, chloride and protein levels, WBC, hemoglobin, hematocrit, glucose, calcium, phosphate, T_4, T_3, protein-bound iodine, BUN and plasma (cortisol level, 17 hydroxycorticoids, plasma ACTH and MSH levels, culture and sensitivity free fatty acids)

Arterial blood to determine pH, pCO_2, bicarbonate level

Radiologic studies are more distinct and are briefly discussed in the following:

Skull Series: These radiographs are used to determine metastatic disease and fractures, and to determine the configuration of the sella turcica as a gross screen for pituitary abnormalities.

Chest and abdominal radiographs: These are used to detect metastatic disease or an infectious process.

Long bone series: This series is used to detect changes in bone density.

CT scan: This is a noninvasive procedure where multiple films are interpreted by computer. A three-dimensional view of the brain is provided and used to detect intracranial pathology, and tumors of the organ, bone or tissue.

Pancreatic scan: This scan detects some pathological changes within the pancreas.

Thyroid scan: This scan determines the absorption capabilities of the thyroid gland.

Adrenal arteriography: This study is used to detect any thrombosis of the adrenal arterial vasculature.

Other tests, such as electroencephalography, brain scan and electrocardiography are especially useful in detection of pituitary abnormalities and brain masses.

KEY CONCEPT: Assessment of the patient with an endocrine disorder includes evaluation of level of consciousness, findings on physical examination, vital signs, laboratory and radiologic studies, as well as noting any deviations from the norm.

KEY POINT RECOGNITION

Write true or false by each statement. Answers are at the end of this chapter. A score below 80% indicates the need for further study.

_____ 1. Intolerance to environmental changes is never indicative of endocrine disorders.

_____ 2. The skin is inspected for pigmentation changes, which may indicate an endocrine disorder.

_____ 3. Exophthalmos means protruding eyeballs.

_____ 4. The thyroid gland is auscultated for the presence of a bruit.

_____ 5. The abdomen is palpated for the presence of suprarenal masses.

_____ 6. Under any condition, assessment of the level of consciousness is the single most important factor to be assessed.

_____ 7. Hypotension is present when the aldosterone level is elevated.

_____ 8. Hypotension is often present in hypoglycemia.

_____ 9. A decrease in systemic adrenergic activity may result in hypertension.

_____10. Tumors of the hypothalamic-neurohypophyseal system may cause bradycardia.

_____11. Hyperthermia may be present in thyrotoxic crisis or nonketotic hyperosmolar coma.

_____12. Kussmaul breathing is often present in a patient suffering from diabetic ketoacidosis.

PATHOLOGICAL STATES AND NURSING MANAGEMENT

DIABETES INSIPIDUS

Pathophysiology

Diabetes insipidus is a defect in either the synthesis of ADH (in the hypothalamus) or a defect in the release of ADH (from the pituitary). It can occur, though rarely, from a primary renal defect, resulting in the inability of the renal tubules to respond to ADH therapy, causing excessive water excretion.

The most common precipitating factor of DI is trauma, either structurally or surgically, to the hypothalamic-pituitary system. Surgery in the neurohypophyseal region obviously influences the production of ADH. Surgery or trauma to the adenohypophysis affects ADH production by causing edema in the neurohypophysis. Tumors in the hypothalamic-pituitary system can also produce diabetes insipidus. Other precipitating factors are inflammation, degenerative disease (Hodgkin's, sarcoidosis, syphilis) and metastatic lesions arising from breast or lung neoplasms.

DI can be transient or permanent, depending on the etiology. Transient DI, generally after trauma or surgery to the adenohypophysis, can be treated symptomatically with fluid replacement. Permanent or transient DI that does not resolve within a few days requires ADH replacement therapy.

Clinical Presentation

The clinical presentation of DI is generally of sudden onset and includes dilute polyuria (up to 25 liters per day) and increased thirst. Thirst is subjective and will only be evident if the patient is awake enough to recognize thirst. The urine is very dilute (specific gravity below 1.005) because the effect of ADH secretion is water diuresis without concomitant electrolyte excretion.

Diagnostic Data

Diagnostic findings may include marked dehydration if the condition has persisted undetected and untreated for a period of hours to days. Laboratory studies will show a decrease in urine osmolality, an increase in serum osmolality and an elevation of the serum sodium level. These laboratory findings are secondary to inappropriate water diuresis, resulting in urine low in electrolytes and relative systemic water depletion, causing relative hypovolemic hypernatremia.

Other diagnostic aids may include visual field testing. If the lesion is in the hypothalamic area and of sufficient size, it may compress the optic chiasm, resulting in bitemporal visual field loss (bitemporal hemianopsia). Vasopressin infusion testing will result in an increase in urine osmolality by 10 percent or more after administration.

Nursing Care

Nursing management of the patient with DI includes:

(1) Accurately record intake and output.
(2) Measure specific gravity.
(3) Carefully titrate fluids:

   Possibly elect to allow the patient to "drink to thirst." Only water should be offered, since electrolyte concentration in serum is elevated. An alternate method is to replace each hour's output with a hypotonic I.V. solution equal to the previous hour's output, plus 50 cc. Calculate and include in the hourly replacement formula fluid loss due to continuous nasogastric drainage.

(4) Perform diagnostic testing.

   Water deprivation test: Maintain rigid fluid restriction. Monitor weights and vital signs. Monitor for dehydration and hypovolemic shock. Collect all blood and urine specimens ordered for testing of sodium content, osmolality and specific gravity.

The patient with DI will continue to exhibit water diuresis with fluid restriction. The urine osmolality and sodium content will remain decreased. The serum sodium and osmolality will remain elevated and continue to elevate as exogenous fluid restriction continues. Complications include fluid overload and severe hypernatremia.

Saline infusion test: Administer prescribed saline infusion at the ordered rate. Monitor for fluid overload and vital signs. Collect timed specimens of blood and urine for analysis. The patient with DI will continue to exhibit water diuresis; however, the serum sodium will rise precipitously as the urine sodium remains markedly decreased.

(5) Administer medications.

Vasopressin (ADH) replacement:

DDAVP (deamino-D-arginine vasopressin) is a nasal spray with minimal side effects and a long antidiuretic action.

Lysine vasopressin, a nasal snuff, may be erratically absorbed and is contraindicated in patients with nasal-transsphenoidal surgery for pituitary problems.

Vasopressin tannate, in an oil base, must be warmed and accurately and carefully mixed, or the injection will consist entirely of the oil base. Painful swelling may appear at the injection sites. Given at bedtime, it decreases urinary output and allows uninterrupted sleep.

For short-term replacement, aqueous pitressin may be administered intramuscularly.

Chlorpropamide stimulates the release of ADH from the pituitary and enhances its effect at the kidney. It requires an intact, functional pituitary gland and may induce hypoglycemia.

KEY CONCEPT: Clinical presentation of DI is intense thirst and polyuria. Nursing care is aimed at recording weight, intake and output; careful titration of fluids; measurement of specific gravity; and administration of medication.

SECRETION OF INAPPROPRIATE ADH (SIADH)
Pathophysiology

Secretion of inappropriate ADH (SIADH) results from either increased production or secretion of ADH. The excessive secretion of ADH does not respond to plasma osmolality (the usual stimulus to release) and results in an increase in total body fluid volume because of decreased excretion of water.

Precipitating factors leading to SIADH are head trauma, meningitis, metastasis from lung and pancreatic tumors, respiratory infections, Addison's disease, hypothyroidism, hypopituitarism and drug therapy (vasopressin, chlorpropamide, vincristine, clofibrate and the thiazides).

Clinical Presentation

Presenting signs include headache, lethargy, disorientation, weakness, decrease in deep tendon reflexes, nausea and vomiting, anorexia, diarrhea and seizures.

Diagnostic Data

Diagnostic findings reveal hyponatremia, potassium, chlorides and osmolality due to the dilutional effect of increased body water. The urine sodium, osmolality and specific gravity are increased, reflecting the normal excretion of electrolytes accompanied by decreased free-water excretion. A water loading test may be done to provide definitive confirmation of the diagnosis. A free-water challenge is given; if SIADH is present, the patient will excrete less than 50 percent of the fluid bolus given, and the urine will not become more dilute than prior to the loading.

Nursing Care
Nursing management includes:
(1) Assess general status.
(2) Assess fluid and electrolyte balances:
Restrict fluids.
Carefully record intake and output.
Hypertonic saline infusion and furosemide (Lasix) I.V. may be used for acute symptomatic episodes of hypervolemia.
Monitor for symptoms of water intoxication: confusion, disorientation, weakness, vomiting, seizures and coma.
Avoid administration of free water in any form (enema, NG flush, mixed with tube feedings).

KEY CONCEPT: Because of the increase in total body fluid volume, nursing care is aimed at assessment of fluid and electrolyte balance.

THYROTOXIC CRISIS
Pathophysiology
Thyrotoxic crisis results when excessive amounts of thyroid hormones are released, causing exaggerated adrenergic activity. Causative factors include excessive intake of thyroid hormone supplements, cessation of antithyroid medications, subtotal thyroidectomy, exacerbation of hyperthyroidism by stress, trauma or infection, manipulation of hyperthyroid gland and ketoacidosis.

Clinical Presentation
The clinical presentations may vary. The patient may complain of tremors, weakness, emotional lability, psychosis, palmar erythema and diaphoresis; and present with an elevated temperature. Nausea, vomiting and weight loss may be present. Hypertension, tachycardia, systolic murmurs and hyperkinesis may also be present. As the condition deteriorates, delirium, stupor and coma develop.

Diagnostic Data
Diagnostic findings may reveal the signs mentioned in clinical presentations, plus thyroid enlargement, presence of thyroid bruit or thrill, and elevated pulse pressure. Lab studies will show normal or elevated serum calcium and glucose, elevated white blood cell (WBC) count and hemoglobin, T_4, T_3 and PBI. Thyroid scanning will be positive if over 90 percent of the 131-I injected into the bloodstream is absorbed by the thyroid. 131-I uptake is also increased and the excretion is decreased.

Nursing Care
The goal of nursing management is to provide supportive care, as well as to prevent complications and progression of the crisis.
(1) Regulation of metabolic activity is vital.
Decrease hyperthermia, but avoid aspirin, which increases free thyroxine levels.
Maintain hydration.
Provide a quiet environment.
(2) Decrease sympathetic stimuli through monitoring cardiac rate and rhythm, and blood pressure.
Use positive inotropic agents.
Use antihypertensives and beta-adrenergic blockers.
(3) Maintain nutrition to meet increased need for carbohydrates, protein and B-complex.
(4) Use iodine agents and antithyroid medications to decrease hormone production and release.

(5) Avoid use of iodine (topical, I.V.) prior to diagnostic testing.

(6) Monitor cardiac rate and rhythm, and blood pressure.

KEY CONCEPT: Nursing must provide supportive care and prevent complications associated with thyrotoxic crisis.

HYPOPARATHYROIDISM
Pathophysiology

Hypoparathyroidism results from a defect in the release of PTH. This leads to hypocalcemia and altered neuromuscular function. Hypoparathyroidism may be caused by surgery or manipulation of the thyroid or parathyroid glands, radiation injury occurring after treatment with 131-I, or following acute pancreatitis. In some cases the cause is unknown.

Clinical Presentation

Classically, the patient presents with numbness and tingling in the distal extremities, muscle cramps in the hands and feet, and carpopedal spasm. Nausea, vomiting, abdominal pain, laryngeal stridor and dyspnea, confusion, lethargy and emotional changes may also be present. In advanced cases, patients may exhibit seizure activity.

Diagnostic Data

The patient will present with symptoms of tetany: Chevostek's sign (tremor of muscles innervated by facial nerve VII after the nerve is tapped); and Trousseau's sign (carpopedal spasm when circulation of the upper arm is disrupted).

The definitive diagnosis is made by a serum calcium less than 8.5 mg/dl with an increase in serum phosphate, low urinary calcium and phosphate, prolongation of Q-T interval on EKG, and generalized dysrhythmia.

Nursing Care

Nursing management includes:

(1) Assess and monitor airway and ventilation, especially if laryngeal spasm or stridor is noted.

(2) Maintain calcium levels:

Use a large-diameter I.V. Calcium is irritating to tissue; therefore, be extremely sensitive to signs of infiltration.

Administer it slowly. Monitor cardiac rate and rhythm.

Do not mix it with saline, which induces increased calcium excretion. Vitamin D is useful to increase absorption of orally administered calcium. Carefully monitor the patient receiving concurrent digitalis preparations.

(3) Monitor respiratory and emotional states. Hyperventilation results in alkalosis and increased ionized calcium, which is not utilizable, therefore increasing the chances of tetanic symptoms.

(4) Take seizure precautions:

Follow prophylactic safety measures.

DIABETIC KETOACIDOSIS
Pathophysiology

Diabetic ketoacidosis (DKA) is a complete lack of or marked reduction in the amount of insulin available in the systemic circulation. This hypoinsulinemia results in failure of glucose transport into the cell for utilization. The failure causes elevated serum glucose levels (hyperglycemia) with diminished intracellular glucose. The cellular deficiency and products of cellular metabolic activity stimulate glycogenolysis, and eventually gluconeogenesis from protein stores. As protein and fat stores are utilized, free fatty acids enter the hepatic circulation. The end product of this metabolism is keto-acid, acetoacetic acid and betahydroxybutyric acid.

Causes in the known diabetic can include failure to take adequate insulin or insulin resistance. Pancreatitis may be a cause of DKA in both the diabetic and nondiabetic patient. Other causes of DKA in the diabetic patient are those requiring an increase in insulin supply (i.e., stress, surgery, trauma, infection, pregnancy). Sudden onset of juvenile diabetes may present as DKA.

Clinical Presentation

The clinical presentation may vary from a mildly decreased level of consciousness to marked change in consciousness. There may be nausea; vomiting; weakness; dry, warm skin with poor skin turgor and dehydration; hypotension; hypothermia; and tachycardia. Acetone may be generally detected on the breath. Prior to the onset, the patient will probably have experienced polydipsia, polyuria and abdominal discomfort. Kussmaul respirations may be present. Weight loss may have been noted several days prior to the onset of current symptoms.

Diagnostic Data

Diagnostic findings include:

(1) Elevation of serum glucose (300 to 1,000 mg, maybe greater)

(2) Presence of acetone and glucose in the urine

(3) Decreased urine sodium and chloride, and elevated urine specific gravity (Glucose acts as an osmotic diuretic, preventing the excretion of some portion of the electrolytes and elevating the specific gravity by its presence.)

(4) Presence of ketones in the serum

(5) Acidosis, with a decrease in serum bicarbonate levels and a decrease in pCO_2

(6) Elevated serum potassium, which may fall precipitously when acidosis and hyperglycemia are corrected. EKG may be used to monitor changes associated with hyper- and hypokalemia.

Nursing Care

The goal of nursing management is supportive, as well as preventive.

Nursing management should include the following special measures:

(1) Monitor fluid and electrolyte balance.

Initially infuse isotonic saline, given at 200 to 1,000 cc/hr. to enhance excretion of glucose.

Monitor for fluid overload.

As glucose approaches 250 mg, change intravenous solution to 5 percent dextrose in ½ normal saline to prevent loss of potassium, cerebral edema and hypoglycemia.

Administer regular insulin by continuous infusion, 4 to 8 units/hr.

Other methods include bolus 10 to 25 units/hr., I.M. 5 to 10 units/hr., S.Q. 10 to 100 units/hr.

A loading dose of 20 units I.V. (or I.M.) may be used.

Hourly glucose and ketone levels in blood and urine should be monitored.

Monitor electrolytes: Replace potassium and bicarbonate as needed. Monitor EKG for changes associated with potassium fluctuations.

(2) Support ventilation and oxygenation.

(3) Monitor intake and output.

(4) Take seizure precautions.

(5) Identify any underlying cause, usually infection, and begin treatment.

(6) Assess G.I.; relieve dilatation by inserting NG tube, if necessary.

HYPERKETOTIC HYPEROSMOLAR COMA (HHNK)
Pathophysiology

Nonketotic hyperosmolar coma (hyperosmolar coma-nonketotic, HHNK) is caused by an insulin deficiency, causing hyperglycemia, diuresis, hyperosmolality and cellular dehydration. The minimal amount of insulin present is, however, enough to prevent the formation of ketone bodies. As the hyperglycemia persists, the resulting hyperosmolality causes a high osmotic gradient to occur at the blood-brain barrier, which results in dehydration of cerebral tissue and resulting CNS symptoms. Azotemia may also result secondary to a decreased glomerular filtration rate (GFR).

The causes of HHNK may be undiagnosed and untreated mild diabetes; diabetes of recent onset; use of steroids, diuretics or hypotonic fluids; or acute illness or stress.

Clinical Presentation

The patient with HHNK is usually more than 50 years old and presents with lethargy, stupor or coma. A short history of polyuria, polydipsia, nausea, vomiting and weight loss can generally be elicited. The patient will appear dehydrated with dry mucous membranes and poor skin turgor. The patient will be hypotensive, tachycardic, tachypneic and hyperpyrexic. In more severe cases, hyperreflexia, severe disorientation and focal seizures may be apparent.

Diagnostic Data

Laboratory studies, such as serum and urine analyses, are necessary for diagnosis. Diagnostic findings include: elevation of serum glucose (often greater than 1,000 mg/dl), elevation of serum osmolality and presence of glucose in the urine.

A normal or elevated serum sodium, and normal or decreased serum potassium may be present. Blood pH may be normal or slightly acidic, with a decreased bicarbonate and pCO_2. The hematocrit may be elevated due to dehydration.

Nursing Care

Monitor fluid and electrolyte balance.

Replace volume of 10 to 20 liters over 24 to 48 hours.

Hypotonic or isotonic fluids may be used; the debate over which is preferable continues to be unresolved. Provide additional insulin via loading dose and continuous infusion of 4 to 10 units/hr. Monitor electrolyte values, EKG and vital signs. Observe for signs of fluid overload. Slowly replace potassium; the patient may need as much as 200 to 400 meq within 48 hours.

HYPOGLYCEMIA
Pathophysiology

Hypoglycemia (hypoglycemic reaction) is infrequently treated in the critical care setting. The primary problem is a reduction in glucose levels due to a defect in glyconeogenesis, glycogenolysis or carbohydrate absorption. It may also occur after glucose is removed in large amounts through the adipose tissue, muscle or liver. Exogenous causes of hypoglycemia include postgastrectomy syndrome, alcohol use, intolerance to certain sugars (fructose, galactose), amino acid intolerance and use of certain drugs (insulin and the sulfonylureas). A certain percentage of cases are functional, but the causes are unknown (idiopathic).

Endogenous causes of hypoglycemia include glycogen storage disease (an enzyme deficiency), pancreatic disease, disease of the adenohypophysis, hepatic disease, severe CHF, glucagon deficiency, cortisol deficiency, exercise, pregnancy, fevers and, in newborns, erythroblastosis fetalis.

Clinical Presentation

The clinical presentation is extremely variable. Changes in level of consciousness, from personality changes to coma, may occur. Headache, weakness, tremors, nervousness, anxiety, blurred vision, tachycardia, pallor, nausea and any combination of the above may be present. The most common preceding sign is hunger, usually for something sweet.

Diagnostic Data

The best diagnostic data is a decreased serum glucose. Glucose tolerance testing may reveal an excessive decline in glucose levels; other tests may show increased insulin activity and decreased sensitivity to stimuli for insulin secretion.

Nursing Care

The major nursing responsibility is the restoration of glucose levels and patient education.

Specific nursing management includes:

(1) Restore glucose levels:

If unconscious, give 50 ml of 50 percent dextrose I.V. Epinephrine or glucagon may be used to stimulate liver glycolysis.

If conscious, give candy, orange juice, or coffee or tea and honey.

(2) Educate the patient to eat small, frequent meals.

Eliminate or restrict simple sugars.

Eliminate caffeine and nicotine.

KEY CONCEPT: Diseases related to pancreatic dysfunction may cause diabetic ketoacidosis, hyperkinetic hyperosmolar coma and hypoglycemia. The clinical presentation and diagnostic data vary and are dependent upon the cause.

ADRENAL CRISIS

Pathophysiology

Adrenal crisis (acute adrenal insufficiency) is the result of an acute exacerbation of chronic Addison's disease or presenting manifestation of adrenal insufficiency. The lack of aldosterone and cortisol causes fluid and electrolyte imbalances, disturbances in fat, carbohydrate and protein metabolism, and can lead to circulatory collapse.

Precipitating factors are those which deplete an already diminished adrenal reserve. This may include adrenalectomy, stress (surgery, infection, trauma, hemorrhage), rapid withdrawal of steroids, cancer chemotherapy and diseases of the hypothalamus, hypophysis and autoimmune response.

Clinical Presentation

The patient presents with hypotension; rapid, thready pulse; oliguria; and cool, clammy skin. Flaccid extremities, dehydration, weakness, lethargy, hyperpigmentation, changes in level of consciousness and restlessness may also be seen. The patient may complain of abdominal pain, weight loss, anorexia and confusion.

Diagnostic Data

Laboratory studies are the best diagnostic aid, along with a complete history and physical. An elevation in the potassium, BUN and creatinine levels is seen. A decrease in the sodium, cortisol, hemoglobin, glucose and 17-hydroxycorticoids (blood and urine) and 17-ketosteroids (urine) levels are seen.

Nursing Care

The major nursing responsibilities include the following:

(1) Maintain blood volume:

Administer hydrocortisone I.V.

Use plasma as a volume expander.

Use vasopressors to elevate B.P. once adequate volume replacement is achieved.

Monitor vital signs, CVP, pulmonary artery pressures, intake and output, and serial specific gravity.

Monitor cardiac rhythm.

(2) Reduce stress:

Control hyperpyrexia.

Provide bed rest, a quiet environment and treatment of underlying stressor.

(3) Educate the patient and family.

KEY CONCEPT: Any factor that depletes the body of adrenal reserve may cause an adrenal crisis.

KEY POINT RECOGNITION

Write true or false by each statement. Answers are at the end of this chapter. A score below 80% indicates the need for further study.

_____ 1. Diabetes insipidus is caused by too much insulin.

_____ 2. Surgery or trauma of the adenohypophysis may cause edema to the neurohypophysis.

_____ 3. Precipitating factors leading to diabetes insipidus may be tumors, inflammation and degenerative diseases.

_____ 4. Anasarca and increased thirst indicate diabetes insipidus.

_____ 5. Concentrated urine with a specific gravity above 1.012 is indicative of diabetes insipidus.

_____ 6. An increase in urine osmolarity and an increase in serum osmolarity with a decrease of serum sodium indicate diabetes insipidus.

_____ 7. Diabetes insipidus is always transient.

_____ 8. Treatment for diabetes insipidus includes fluid replacement and ADH replacement therapy.

_____ 9. The patient with diabetes insipidus will continue to exhibit water diuresis even with fluid restriction.

_____ 10. Following saline infusion test for diabetes insipidus, the serum sodium level will fall.

_____ 11. DDAVP (deamino-D-arginine vasopressin) is a nasal spray with long antidiuretic action.

_____ 12. Chlorpropamide stimulates the release of ADH from the pituitary.

_____ 13. A side effect of chlorpropamide is hyperglycemia.

_____ 14. Inappropriate secretion of ADH is caused by increased production or secretion of ADH.

_____ 15. Head trauma, meningitis, Addison's disease and hypothyroidism may cause an inappropriate secretion of ADH.

_____ 16. Deep tendon reflexes are increased in the presence of SIADH.

_____ 17. SIADH reveals decreased serum sodium, potassium and chloride, and osmolarity due to the dilutional effect of increased body water.

_____ 18. Nursing management of SIADH includes forcing fluids.

_____ 19. Thyrotoxic crisis is a lack of thyroid hormones.

_____ 20. A sudden ingestion of thyroid medication may produce thyrotoxic crisis.

_____ 21. Hyperkinesis, emotional lability, elevated temperature, palmar erythema and systolic murmurs are indicative of thyrotoxic crisis.

_____ 22. Diagnostic findings of thyrotoxic crisis may reveal thyroid enlargement, bruit and thrill.

_____23. The administration of aspirin decreases free thyroxine levels.
_____24. Hypoparathyroidism leads to hypocalcemia.
_____25. Numbness and tingling in the distal extremities are indicative of hyperparathyroidism.
_____26. Seizures may develop as a result of hypoparathyroidism.
_____27. A diagnosis of hypoparathyroidism can be made from a serum calcium level less than 8.5 mg/dl and an increase in serum phosphate.
_____28. Hypoparathyroidism may cause shortening of the Q-T interval on an EKG.
_____29. Intravenous calcium is irritating to tissue.
_____30. Intravenous calcium should be mixed with saline.
_____31. Vitamin D is useful to increase absorption of calcium given orally.
_____32. Hyperventilation results in alkalosis and increased ionized calcium.
_____33. Diabetic ketoacidosis is a lack of or reduction in the amount of insulin available in systemic circulation.
_____34. Hypoinsulinemia results in the failure of glucose to be transported into the cell for utilization.
_____35. Pancreatitis may be a cause of diabetic ketoacidosis in both the diabetic and nondiabetic patient.
_____36. The clinical picture of diabetic ketoacidosis includes hypertension, dehydration, bradycardia and an acetone or fruity smelling breath.
_____37. In diabetic ketoacidosis, the serum glucose is rarely above 300.
_____38. In the initial stage of diabetic ketoacidosis, nursing management includes the administration of hypertonic solution.
_____39. Nursing management of diabetic ketoacidosis includes monitoring glucose and ketone levels of blood and urine.
_____40. Nonketotic hyperosmolar coma is caused by an insulin deficiency.
_____41. Nonketotic hyperosmolar coma causes hyperglycemia, diuresis, hyperosmolarity and cellular dehydration.
_____42. Steroids, diuretics and hypotonic fluids may cause nonketotic hyperosmolar coma.
_____43. In nonketotic hyperosmolar coma, the patient is rarely more than 40 years old.
_____44. The patient with nonketotic hyperosmolar coma presents with hypotension, bradycardia, hypothermia and poor skin turgor.
_____45. Serum glucose of 1,000 or greater, elevated serum osmolarity and glucose in the urine are indicative of nonketotic hyperosmolar coma.
_____46. A normal or elevated serum sodium, and normal or decreased serum potassium may be present in nonketotic hyperosmolar coma.
_____47. Fluid replacement for nonketotic hyperosmolar coma may be 10 to 20 liters over 24 to 48 hours.
_____48. Hypoglycemia is a reduction in glucose levels due to a defect in glyconeogenesis, glycogenolysis or carbohydrate absorption.
_____50. Erythroblastosis fetalis is an exogenous cause of hypoglycemia.
_____51. Headache, blurred vision, pallor and tachycardia may be seen in hypoglycemia.
_____52. Hypoglycemia is diagnosed by a decreased serum glucose level.
_____53. If the hypoglycemic patient is unconscious, the treatment is administration of dextrose 50 percent.
_____54. In hypoglycemia, epinephrine or glycogen will depress liver glycolysis.
_____55. Adrenal crisis is the result of a rapid exacerbation of chronic Addison's disease.

_____56. The lack of aldosterone and cortisol causes electrolyte and fluid imbalances.

_____57. Adrenal crisis presents with hypotension, oliguria, hyperpigmentation, weight loss and dehydration.

_____58. A decrease in serum potassium, creatinine and BUN levels is common with adrenal crisis.

_____59. Blood volume may be maintained in adrenal crisis by administering hydrocortisone.

_____60. Volume expanders are contraindicated in adrenal crisis.

CARE COMMON TO ENDOCRINE PROBLEMS

Changes in patient status are important signs of impending problems. Early recognition and treatment may prevent complications resulting from the specific pathological disorder.

AIRWAY AND VENTILATION

Important indicators of respiratory embarrassment are changes in respiratory quality and in arterial blood gas levels.

Subjective signs of respiratory problems include: tachypnea; dyspnea; shallow, rapid respirations; hypoxemia; dysrhythmias; adventitious breath sounds; and sternal, intercostal or paraclavicular retractions.

The lungs are encased in the thoracic cavity. Gas exchange, or the movement of gases, takes place through a semipermeable membrane. Ventilation is dependent upon the process of respiratory gas exchange.

Monitoring airway patency and ventilation is necessary to ensure adequate gas exchange. This is accomplished by analyzing arterial blood gases, observing for changes in vital signs, observing for the development of cyanosis, observing chest movement and auscultating for abnormal breath sounds.

Methods to maintain airway patency and ventilation include: proper head-neck-jaw alignment, airway suctioning as needed and oxygenation according to serial arterial blood gases.

FLUID AND ELECTROLYTE BALANCE

Changes in laboratory electrolyte values and the development of a significant discrepancy in 24-hour fluid intake and output are indicative of a pathological disorder causing fluid and electrolyte imbalances. Subjective signs include: vomiting, hyperglycemic diuresis, polyuria, tetany, weakness, dehydration, weight changes and abnormal skin turgor.

Replacement of fluids associated with gastrointestinal loss, diuresis, surgery, infection or hypercatabolic states is essential in the maintenance of fluid and electrolyte balance.

Fluids and electrolytes are monitored via: intake and output records, daily weights, observing for cardiac dysrhythmias and careful administration of parenteral fluids.

Methods used to maintain adequate hydration and electrolyte balance include: assessment of laboratory data and frequent patient assessment for changes in skin, mentation, muscular tone, vital signs and cardiac function.

NEUROLOGICAL STATUS

Changes in level of consciousness are the most sensitive sign of increased intracranial pressure (ICP). Subjective signs include: increased headache, diplopia, seizures, nausea and vomiting.

The brain is enclosed in a rigid, bony vault. Room for cerebral edema is virtually nonexistent. Therefore, intracranial pathology due to skull fractures, subdural hematomas, subarachnoid hemorrhage or an increase in the secretion of ADH may cause increased cranial pressure.

To avoid serious complications, intracranial pressure must be carefully monitored. Monitoring may be accomplished by the use of the subarachnoid screw, ventricular drain or epidural catheter.

If ICP is present, methods must be employed to decrease the rise in pressure. Methods to decrease ICP include: ventricular drainage; elevation of the head of bed 30 degrees; hyperventilation to a pCO_2 of 25 to 30 mm Hg; administration of osmotic diuretics; administration of steroids; barbiturate-induced coma; and hypothermia.

PATIENT AND FAMILY EDUCATION

Education of the patient and family is an important part of the nurse's responsibility. Patient and family teaching includes emotional support; discussion of the disease process, its limitations and complications; explanation of medications; explanation of treatment; and awareness of community resources.

KEY CONCEPT: Continuous assessment of changes in fluid and electrolyte balance, neurological status and respiratory status are vital to managing endocrine problems.

KEY POINT RECOGNITION

Write true or false by each statement. Answers are at the end of this chapter. A score below 80% indicates the need for further study.

_____ 1. Abnormal changes in arterial blood gases may reveal respiratory or metabolic disturbances.

_____ 2. Movement of the chest is the most reliable indicator of adequate oxygenation.

_____ 3. A moderate discrepancy between intake and output in a 24-hour period is not significant.

_____ 4. Polyuria may cause fluid imbalance.

_____ 5. Hypercatabolic states may cause fluid and electrolyte imbalances.

_____ 6. Tetany may be a sign of electrolyte imbalance.

_____ 7. Parenteral therapy is monitored to forewarn fluid imbalance.

_____ 8. An increase in intracranial pressure will not alter the level of consciousness.

_____ 9. Hyperthermia is used to decrease intracranial pressure.

_____10. The patient does not need to be bothered with learning about the disease process and its treatment.

PASS
Program Assessment: Science and Situation

1. The pituitary gland is located
    a. above the hypothalamus, behind the sella turcica.
    b. below the optic chiasm and the sella turcica.
    c. below the hypothalamus in the sella turcica.
    d. below the hypophysis in the sella turcica.

2. The adenohypophysis and neurohypophysis are, respectively,
    a. the portions of the pituitary in the sinuses and the skull.
    b. the anterior and posterior hypothalamus.
    c. the anterior and posterior pituitary.
    d. the lateral lobes of the pituitary.

3. Which of the following is incorrect?
    a. The hypothalamus and the pituitary produce hormones.
    b. The hypothalamus produces hormones that are stored in the pituitary.
    c. The hypothalamus produces releasing factors for the hormones of the pituitary.
    d. The pituitary produces releasing factors for hormones stored in the hypothalamus.

4. The hormones of the adenohypophysis are
    a. GH, PRL, ADH and LH.
    b. ACTH, TSH, CRF and MSH.
    c. ACTH, TSH, STH and FSH.
    d. LH, STH, ADH and PTH.

5. Hormones of the neurohypophysis are
    a. ADH and oxytocin.
    b. ADH and cortisol.
    c. ADH and GRF.
    d. ADH and ACTH.

6. The hypothalamus controls the release of pituitary hormones by
    a. positive feedback—the appropriate level of hormone acts as a stimulus to release of releasing factors (RFs).
    b. negative feedback—the appropriate level of hormone shuts off the release of RFs.
    c. osmotic feedback—the appropriate level of hormone causes osmotic diffusion into the hypothalamus and shuts off RF release.
    d. antibody feedback—antibodies formed by hormones block the release of RFs.

7. Growth hormone
    a. is also called CRF.
    b. causes acromegaly in children.
    c. stimulates the growth of bone and cartilage.
    d. is released in hyperglycemic states.

8. Thyroid stimulating hormone (TSH)
    a. is also called thyroid reduction hormone (TRH).
    b. inhibits the growth of thyroid cells.
    c. causes gigantism in adults.
    d. is released upon exposure to cold temperatures.

9. ACTH is
    a. a naturally occurring carbohydrate.
    b. produced by the adrenal glands.
    c. responsible for the production of adrenal hormones.
    d. inhibited by stress.

10. FSH, LH and ICSH are
    a. responsible for sexual maturation and reproductive ability.
    b. produced only in pregnancy.
    c. the causes of aberrant sexual behavior.
    d. not produced after puberty.

11. Prolactin (PRL)
    a. is responsible for the cessation of lactation.
    b. is released by inhibition of inhibition factor.
    c. results in uterine contractions.
    d. produces feminization and acne in males.

12. MSH is
    a. responsible for skin pigmentation.
    b. a female sex hormone.
    c. produced by the parathyroid.
    d. produced by the hypothalamus.

13. ADH is
    a. produced by the pituitary and stored in the hypothalamus.
    b. responsible for water diuresis and sodium retention.
    c. responsible for water retention and sodium diuresis.
    d. produced in excess quantities in diabetes insipidus.

14. Oxytocin is
    a. produced in the hypothalamus.
    b. produced in the neurohypophysis.
    c. shut off to allow for lactation.
    d. released by inhibition of an inhibiting factor.

15. The thyroid is composed of
    a. two medial lobes connected by the chiasm.
    b. two posterior lobes connected by the infundibulum.
    c. two lateral lobes connected by the thyroid artery.
    d. two lateral lobes connected by the isthmus.

16. Thyroid hormones are
    a. thyroxine, thyronine and thyrotonin.
    b. thyroxine, triiodotonin and thyrotoxin.

c. thyroxine, triiodothyronine and thyrocalcitonin.
d. thyroxine, triiodothyroxine and thyrocalcitonin.

17. T_4 is
    a. more potent than T_3.
    b. a combination of iodine and trypsin.
    c. released by thyroxine.
    d. responsible for stimulation of protein synthesis.

18. T_3 is
    a. more potent than T_4.
    b. a combination of iodine and trypsin.
    c. released by thyroxine.
    d. responsible for water retention.

19. Thyrocalcitonin is
    a. produced by the parathyroid.
    b. responsible for bone maturation.
    c. released by elevated glucagon levels.
    d. produced by the acinar cells of the thyroid.

20. The parathyroid glands
    a. produce calcitonin.
    b. require vitamin D to be effective.
    c. decrease vitamin B levels.
    d. work on the cells of the liver to inhibit calcium reabsorption.

21. The pancreas is
    a. composed of two divisions, the cortex and the medulla.
    b. composed of two divisions, the alpha cells and acinar cells.
    c. composed of two divisions, the alpha cells and the beta cells.
    d. composed of two types of secretory cells, the acinar cells and the islet cells.

22. The alpha cells secrete
    a. glucagon.
    b. epinephrine.
    c. catecholamines.
    d. insulin.

23. The beta cells secrete
    a. glucagon.
    b. epinephrine.
    c. catecholamines.
    d. insulin.

24. The adrenal glands are
    a. located anterior to the kidneys.
    b. composed of two layers, the medulla and the pontine.
    c. responsible for the production of skin pigmentation.
    d. composed of two layers, the medulla and the cortex.

25. Cortisol is
    a. a mineralocorticoid.
    b. produced by the cortex.
    c. the least important glucocorticoid.
    d. produced by the adrenal medulla.

26. Aldosterone is
    a. the primary glucocorticoid.
    b. produced by the adrenal medulla.
    c. activated by the renin-angiotensin system.
    d. responsible for development of sexual characteristics.

27. Epinephrine is *not*
    a. produced by the adrenal medulla.
    b. activated by the sympathetic nervous system.
    c. produced by the acinar cells of the adrenal medulla.
    d. characterized by positive inotropic effects.

28. Norepinephrine is
    a. four times as potent as epinephrine.
    b. as effective as epinephrine, but has less effect on cardiac cells.
    c. as effective as epinephrine, but has less effect on muscle cells.
    d. a negative inotropic agent.

29. Diabetes insipidus is
    a. a disorder of the adenohypophysis.
    b. the result of head trauma to the brainstem.
    c. manifested by elevated blood pressure and water retention.
    d. manifested by hypovolemia, water diuresis and hypernatremia.

30. The cause of hypernatremia in DI is
    a. sodium retention in the intracellular space.
    b. excessive free water loss.
    c. potassium sparing and resultant sodium retention.
    d. failure of the carotid baroreceptors.

31. Patients with DI will exhibit
    a. elevated specific gravity (urine).
    b. polyuria and polydipsia.
    c. polyuria and polyphagia.
    d. edema due to sodium retention.

32. DI is
    a. always transient.
    b. untreatable without surgery.
    c. treatable with several medications.
    d. transient and recurrent.

33. Fluids for the patient in DI should be
    a. hypotonic.
    b. restricted.
    c. hypertonic.
    d. high in replacement electrolytes.

34. SIADH is
    a. increased production or release of ADH.
    b. decreased production or release of ADH.
    c. a state of dehydration and sodium wasting.
    d. a state of dehydration with sodium retention.

35. A patient with SIADH may present with
    a. lethargy, hyperreflexia, nausea and vomiting.
    b. nervousness, headache, hyperglycemia and nausea.
    c. lethargy, hyporeflexia, nausea and vomiting.
    d. dehydration, nausea, vomiting and diarrhea.

36. Findings in SIADH include
    a. decreased urine sodium, specific gravity and osmolality.
    b. increased urine sodium, specific gravity and osmolality.
    c. decreased serum osmolality, but increased serum sodium.
    d. increased serum osmolality and sodium.

37. Treatment for SIADH includes
    a. replacement of hourly output, plus 50 cc.
    b. hypotonic fluids.
    c. furosemide and albumin.
    d. fluid restriction.

38. Thyrotoxic crisis may
    a. be caused by an overdose of antithyroid medications.
    b. be the result of surgical manipulation of the thyroid.
    c. be manifested by hypotension, hypothermia and tachycardia.
    d. result in decreased calcium and glucose levels.

39. Patients with hypoparathyroidism exhibit
    a. a positive Chevostek sign, but negative Trousseau sign.
    b. a positive Chevostek sign, but a negative Brudzinski sign.
    c. a positive Chevostek sign and a positive Trousseau sign.
    d. a positive Chevostek sign and a positive Kernig's sign.

40. Which of the following is not true?
    a. Calcium in combination with saline enhances calcium excretion.
    b. Vitamin D decreases calcium absorption.
    c. Calcium and digitalis have similar effects.
    d. Hypocalcemia may result in prolongation of the Q-T interval.

41. DKA is
    a. hypoinsulinemia, which enhances the cellular utilization of glucose.
    b. hypoinsulinemia, which depresses protein mobilization and conversion to glucose.
    c. hypoinsulinemia, which mobilizes free fatty acids and results in ketone production.
    d. hypoinsulinemia, which increases cellular metabolism.

42. The following may be found in DKA, except
    a. elevation of blood glucose, urine specific gravity and urine sodium and chlorides.

    b. elevation of blood glucose, urine specific gravity and decreased urine sodium and chlorides.

    c. elevation of blood glucose, decreased urine specific gravity and urine sodium and chlorides.

    d. elevation of blood glucose, decreased urine specific gravity, decreased urine sodium, potassium and bicarbonate.

43. In DKA the serum potassium is
    a. low until the hyperglycemia is corrected.
    b. elevated for several hours after the glucose returns to normal.
    c. normal but becomes elevated after the hyperglycemia is corrected.
    d. elevated but falls rapidly after the hyperglycemia is corrected.

44. Treatment of the patient in DKA consists of
    a. rapid infusion of large volumes of hypertonic fluid to promote diuresis of glucose.
    b. initial use of solutions containing 5 percent dextrose to prevent rebound hypoglycemia.
    c. I.V. bolus of rapid-acting insulin at 25 to 100 units/hr. until the glucose reaches 100 mg/dl.
    d. initial infusion of large volumes of hypotonic fluids and use of continuous infusion of low-dose insulin.

45. HHNK is
    a. insulin deficiency.
    b. a total lack of insulin.
    c. overproduction of insulin.
    d. ingestion of massive amounts of glucose.

46. The symptoms of HHNK include
    a. hyperglycemia, hyperosmolality (serum) and glucosuria.
    b. hyperglycemia, serum hypo-osmolality and glucosuria.
    c. hypoglycemia, serum hyperosmolality and glucosuria.
    d. hyperglycemia, serum hyperosmolality without glucosuria.

47. Treatment of HHNK includes all of the following, *except*
    a. replacement with hypotonic or isotonic fluids.
    b. insulin by continuous infusion.
    c. fluid restriction.
    d. potassium replacement.

48. Adrenal crisis is
    a. a result of exacerbation of Addison's disease.
    b. a result of exacerbation of Cushing's disease.
    c. a result of exacerbation of pheochromocytoma.
    d. a result of chronic inflammation of the adrenal medulla.

49. Symptoms of adrenal crisis are
    a. edema, nervousness, weight gain and hyperpigmentation.
    b. hypotension, dehydration, hyperpigmentation and lethargy.
    c. hypotension, polyuria, dehydration and weight loss.
    d. hypotension, dehydration, polyuria and hypopigmentation.

50. Treatment of adrenal crisis includes all of the following, *except*
    a. administration of mineralocorticoids.
    b. administration of glucocorticoids.
    c. administration of volume expanders.
    d. administration of antipyretics.

KEY POINT RECOGNITION ANSWERS

Endocrine Glands

1. True
2. True
3. False—Neurohypophysis = posterior pituitary
   Adenohypophysis = anterior pituitary
4. False—The adenohypophysis is connected to the hypothalamus by the vascular system.
5. True
6. True
7. True
8. False—ADH and oxytocin are produced in the hypothalamus, then stored and released from the neurohypophysis.
9. False—The trigger for release of ADH is the physiological effect, which is the result of hormone action.
10. True
11. False—Second and third tracheal rings
12. False—High blood flow
13. False—Parathyroid glands are located in the posterior plane of the thyroid.
14. False—A negative feedback system stops parathormone secretion when blood calcium levels are adequate.
15. True
16. True
17. True
18. True
19. True
20. False—The major regulator of mineralocorticoid is the renin-angiotensin system.
21. True
22. True

Hormones

1. True
2. True
3. True
4. False—GH stimulates bone and cartilage growth.
5. True
6. True
7. False—Hyperglycemia inhibits the release of GH.
8. False—Symptoms of hyperthyroidism include tachycardia, weight loss, increased appetite, diarrhea, tremors, weakness and heat intolerance. Weight gain and mental slowing are symptoms of hypothyroidism.
9. True
10. False—Sympathetic stimulation inhibits TSH release.
11. True
12. True
13. True
14. True
15. True

16. True
17. True
18. False—ICSH stimulates the production of testosterone and aids in the development of male sex characteristics.
19. True
20. False—Prolactin is inhibited under normal circumstances. PIF inhibits the release of prolactin.
21. False—Decreased plasma cortisol levels stimulate the release of MSH.
22. False—Vasopressin increases water reabsorption and inhibits diuresis.
23. False—ADH release results in increased arterial systolic pressure.
24. True
25. True
26. False—Hypothalamic edema may result in the decreased production of ADH.
27. True
28. True
29. False—Oxytocin release is caused by the initiation of labor and by breast-feeding.
30. True
31. False—TRF stimulates the secretion of TSH, which in turn causes the release of thyroxine.
32. True
33. True
34. False—Elevated T_4 levels may result in weight loss, muscle tremors, tachycardia, exophthalmos, heat intolerance, diarrhea and menstrual irregularities.
35. False—T_3 (triiodothyronine) is four times more potent than T_4 (thyroxine).
36. True
37. True
38. False—It is produced and released by the C cells.
39. True
40. False—Adequate vitamin D levels are necessary for action of parathormone on target cells.
41. True
42. False—Release of glucagon is stimulated by hypoglycemia and excessive exercise.
43. True
44. True
45. True
46. True
47. True
48. True
49. True
50. True
51. False—These are signs of decreased levels of glucocorticoids.
52. True
53. False—Hyperkalemia and hyponatremia stimulate the release of aldosterone.
54. False—Aldosterone helps to conserve sodium and water. Potassium is excreted.
55. True

56. True
57. True
58. False—It is released through the stimulation of the sympathetic nervous system.
59. True
60. True

Assessment of the Endocrine System
1. False—Intolerance to environmental changes may be indicative of an endocrine dysfunction.
2. True
3. True
4. True
5. True
6. True
7. False—A lack of aldosterone causes hypotension.
8. True
9. False—An increase in systemic adrenergic activity may cause hypertension.
10. True
11. True
12. True

Pathological States and Nursing Management
1. False—Diabetes insipidus is caused by a defect in the release of ADH from the pituitary or a defect in the synthesis of ADH in the hypothalamus.
2. True
3. True
4. False—Marked dehydration, polyuria and increased thirst are indicative of diabetes insipidus.
5. False—Dilute urine with a specific gravity below 1.005 is indicative of diabetes insipidus.
6. False—A decrease in urine osmolarity and an increase in serum osmolarity with elevation of serum sodium levels are indicative of diabetes insipidus.
7. False—Diabetes insipidus may be transient or permanent.
8. True
9. True
10. False—Following saline infusion test for diabetes insipidus, the serum sodium level will rise as the urine sodium level remains decreased.
11. True
12. True
13. False—Side effect of chlorpropamide is hypoglycemia.
14. True
15. True
16. False—SIADH causes a decrease in deep tendon reflexes.
17. True
18. False—Nursing management of SIADH includes fluid restriction and monitoring for symptoms of water intoxication.
19. False—Thyrotoxic crisis results when excessive amounts of thyroid hormones are released.
20. True

21. True
22. True
23. False—Aspirin increases free thyroxin levels.
24. True
25. False—Numbness and tingling in the distal extremities are indicative of hypothyroidism.
26. True
27. True
28. False—Hypoparathyroidism may cause prolongation of the Q-T interval on an EKG.
29. True
30. False—Do not mix calcium with saline. This induces increased calcium excretion.
31. True
32. True
33. True
34. True
35. True
36. False—Hypotension, dehydration, tachycardia and an acetone breath are indicative of diabetic ketoacidosis.
37. False—The serum glucose level may be 300 to 1,000, or higher.
38. False—Isotonic or hypotonic solutions are administered initially.
39. True
40. True
41. True
42. True
43. False—The patient is usually over 50.
44. False—The patient presents with hypotension, tachycardia, hyperpyrexia and poor skin turgor.
45. True
46. True
47. True
48. True
49. True
50. False—Erythroblastosis fetalis is an endogenous cause of hypoglycemia.
51. True
52. True
53. True
54. False—Epinephrine and glucogen will stimulate liver glycolysis.
55. True
56. True
57. True
58. False—An increase in serum potassium, creatinine and BUN is seen.
59. True
60. False—Volume expanders may be used in adrenal crisis.

Care Common to Endocrine Problems
1. True
2. False—Movement of the chest may be misleading. Arterial blood gases, color, breath sounds and vital signs should also be monitored as indicators of sufficient oxygenation.

3. False—A discrepancy between intake and output may be significant.
4. True
5. True
6. True
7. True
8. False—Changes in level of consciousness are the most sensitive sign of increased intracranial pressure.
9. False—Hypothermia may be used to decrease intracranial pressure.
10. False—Knowledge of the disease process is important for the patient to know and understand.

PASS ANSWER SHEET

1. c	26. c
2. c	27. c
3. d	28. b
4. c	29. d
5. a	30. b
6. b	31. b
7. c	32. c
8. d	33. a
9. c	34. a
10. a	35. c
11. b	36. b
12. a	37. d
13. b	38. b
14. b	39. d
15. d	40. b
16. c	41. c
17. d	42. b
18. a	43. d
19. c	44. d
20. b	45. a
21. d	46. a
22. a	47. c
23. d	48. a
24. d	49. b
25. b	50. a

SURVEY SUMMARY
ENDOCRINE SYSTEM

I. **The Endocrine System: Overview**
   A. The endocrine system is important to physiologic integration of body processes.
   B. Glands include
      1. pituitary
      2. thyroid
      3. parathyroid
      4. pancreas
      5. adrenals
      6. gonads
      7. pineal
      8. thymus

II. **Anatomy and Physiology**
   A. The Endocrine Glands
      1. *Pituitary* (Hypophysis)
         a. The pituitary is located in the sella turcica below the hypothalamus.
         b. Composed of two major segments
            1. adenohypophysis (anterior portion)
            2. neurohypophysis (posterior portion)
         c. Hormonal release is controlled by *releasing factor.*
            1. Releasing factor is released when there's a lack of hormone concentration.
            2. Negative feedback system allows for regulation of hormone concentration.
      2. *Thyroid*
         a. Composed of two lobes connected by the isthmus
         b. Located in the neck at the second and third tracheal rings
         c. It is a vascular organ and requires a high blood flow for hormone synthesis.
      3. *Parathyroid gland*
         a. Composed of four flattened, oval bodies
         b. Located in the posterior plane of the thyroid
         c. *Parathormone* is secreted by chief cells in response to blood calcium levels.
      4. *Pancreas*
         a. Composed of head, tail, and body
         b. Located between the spleen and duodenum
         c. Has two types of secretory cells
            1. Acinar
               a. exocrine function
               b. endocrine function
            2. Islet
               a. alpha cells which secrete glucagon
               b. beta cells which secrete insulin

5. **Adrenal glands**
    a. The triangular shaped glands are located at the apex of each kidney.
    b. Composed of a Cortex and Medulla
    c. Hormones of the adrenals include
        1. Cortex
            a. glucocorticoid
            b. mineralocorticoid
            c. androgen
        2. Medulla
            a. epinephrine
            b. norepinephrine

B. **Hormones**
    1. Hormones associated with the *hypophysis*
        a. *Growth hormone* (GH) is the major hormone released by the anterior pituitary.
            1. Release is stimulated by
                a. growth hormone releasing factor (GHRF)
                b. exercise
                c. hypoglycemia
                d. decreased aminoacid levels
            2. Inhibition of GH release is by
                a. growth hormone inhibiting factor (GHIF)
                b. corticosteriod long standing elevated levels
                c. hyperglycemia
            3. Excess of GH
                a. childhood—gigantism
                b. adulthood—acromegaly
            4. Decreased amount of GH
                a. childhood—dwarfism
                b. adulthood—decreased organ weight
        b. *Thyroid stimulating hormone* (TSH)
            1. Acts to bring about an increase in the growth and function of the thyroid cells.
            2. Excess TSH results in hyperthyroid symptoms and increase in gland size.
            3. Decreased TSH release results in hypothyroid symptoms and decrease in gland size.
            4. *Thyrotropin releasing factor* (TRF): depressed levels of thyroid hormone and cold temperatures stimulate release of TSH.
            5. Adequate thyroid hormone levels and sympathetic nervous system stimulation inhibits release of TSH.
        c. *Adrenocorticotropic hormone* (ACTH)
            1. Acts on the adrenal cortex to stimulate
                a. growth of the adrenal glands
                b. production and release of glucocorticoids from the adrenal cortex
                c. production of mineralocorticoids by the adrenal cortex,
                d. and initiates production of androgens by the adrenal cortex

2. ACTH is released by the action of *corticotropin releasing factor.*
3. Elevated ACTH levels result in a syndrome similar to Cushing's disease.
4. Decreased ACTH levels result in an Addisonian-type clinical picture.
  d. *Follicle Stimulating Hormone* (FSH)
   1. Released in presence of *follicle stimulating factor*
   2. Simulates the maturation of ovarian follicles or sperm
  e. *Luteinizing hormone* (LH)
   1. Released in response to *luteinizing hormone release factor* (LHRF)
   2. Increases secretion of estrogen and progesterone and stimulates growth of the corpus luteum
  f. *Interstitial cell stimulating hormone* (ICSH)
   1. Released in response to LHRF
   2. Acts to stimulate production of testosterone and aid in the development of male sex characteristics
   3. Increased levels of ICSH do not produce any clinical signs, but decreased levels result in decreased testosterone levels and failure to develop secondary male sex characteristics.
  g. *Prolactin* (PRL)
   1. The only adenohypophyseal hormone that is *inhibited* under normal circumstances
   2. *Prolactin inhibiting factor* (PIF) is thought to be produced in the adenohypophysis.
   3. PRL stimulates lactation.
  h. *Melanocyte stimulating hormone* (MSH)
   1. Released by the action of decreased plasma cortisol levels
   2. Responsible for the production and deposit of skin pigmentation
   3. Increased levels result in hyperpigmentation while decreased MSH result in inadequate skin pigmentation.
2. Hormones associated with the *neurohypophysis*
  a. *Antidiuretic hormone* (ADH)
   1. Manufactured by the hypothalamus but stored and released by the neurohypopysis in response to increased serum osmolarity
   2. *Syndrome* of *inappropriate antidiuretic hormone* (SIADH) is a condition in which excess ADH is released in relation to the serum osmolarity.
   3. Lack of release of ADH results in a syndrome known as *diabetes insipidus* (DI).
  b. *Oxytocin*
   1. Inhibition of oxytocin is the normal state in the non-pregnant, non-nursing female.
   2. Acts to produce uterine contractions and to induce lactation
3. Hormones associated with the *thyroid gland*
  a. *Thyroxine* (T_4)
   1. Major hormone of the thyroid
   2. Released by the secretion of *thyroid stimulating hormone* (TSH), release of *thyrotropin releasing factor* (TRF), and exposure to cold temperatures

3. T_4 is inhibited by inadequate amounts of TSH and elevated serum glucocorticoid levels.
4. Acts to
   a. stimulate protein synthesis
   b. speed fat and carbohydrate metabolism
   c. accelerate bone growth
   d. stimulate production of cyclic AMP within muscle cells
5. Elevation of T_4 levels results in symptoms of hyperthyroidism.
6. Decreased T_4 levels produce symptoms of hypothyroidism.

b. *Triiodothyronine* (T_3)
   1. Is identical to T_4 *except* four times more potent

c. *Thyrocalcitonin* (calcitonin)
   1. Produced and released by the C cells of the thyroid
      a. Release is controlled by the calcium-magnesium balance
      b. Suppression is due to C cell damage
   2. Reduces serum calcium levels by inhibiting bone lysis and increasing urinary excretion of calcium, phosphates, sodium, chlorides, and magnesium

4. Hormones associated with the *parathyroid gland*
   a. *Parathormone* (PTH)
      1. Released directly by depressed serum calcium levels and indirectly by elevated serum phosphate and magnesium levels
      2. Inhibited by elevated serum calcium levels and inadequate vitamin D levels
      3. Requires adequate Vitamin D levels to work on its target cells
      4. Causes decreased reabsorption of phosphate and increased absorption of calcium

5. Hormones associated with the *pancreas*
   a. *Glucagon*
      1. Secreted by the *alpha* cells of the islet
      2. Release is stimulated by
         a. hypoglycemia
         b. starvation
         c. increased levels of amino acids
         d. elevation of catecholamine levels
         e. excessive exercise
      3. Raises blood glucose levels by stimulating glycogenolysis and glyconeogenesis and inhibiting glycolysis
   b. *Insulin*
      1. Secreted by the *beta* cells of the islet
      2. Release is stimulated by
         a. hyperglycemia
         b. elevation of ACTH, GH, gastrine, and glucagon
      3. Acts to
         a. transport glucose into the cell
         b. initiate protein synthesis
         c. store fatty acid
         d. reduce cellular metabolism of triglycerides

4. *Elevated* insulin levels result in *hypoglycemia* while *decreased* levels result in *hyperglycemia, acidosis,* and *ketosis.*

6. Hormones associated with the *adrenal glands*
   a. Hormones of the adrenal *cortex*
      1. *Glucocorticoids*
         a. Primary glucocorticoid is *cortisol*
         b. Production is stimulated by
            1. ACTH
            2. CRF
            3. trauma
            4. stress
            5. infection
         c. Inhibition is through a negative feedback mechanism which ultimately reduces ACTH levels.
         d. Responsible for
            1. decreasing inflammation
            2. depressing protein synthesis
            3. stimulating glycogenesis
         e. Increased levels result in Cushing's syndrome.
         f. Decreased levels result in Addison's syndrome.
      2. *Mineral corticoids*
         a. Primary mineral corticoid is *aldosterone*
         b. Production is stimulated by
            1. renin-angiotensin system
            2. hyponatremia
            3. hyperkalemia
         c. Effect is to
            1. conserve sodium
            2. excrete potassium
            3. conserve fluid
         d. Increased levels result in hypertension, hypokalemia, and weakness.
         e. Decreased levels result in hyponatremia and dehydration.
      3. *Androgens*
         a. Effect is on male reproductive system
         b. Hormones of the *adrenal medulla* (catecholamines)
            1. *Epinephrine* (adrenalin)
               a. Primary hormone of adrenal medulla
               b. Released through the stimulation of
                  1. sympathetic nervous system
                  2. insulin
                  3. histamine
               c. Inhibition is due to adrenal dysfunction
               d. Acts on smooth muscle, vascular system and various body cells
                  1. inotropic effect on cardiac cells
                  2. dilates blood vessels supplying heart and skeletal muscles

3. constricts blood vessels supplying abdominal viscera
4. decreases peristalsis and GI secretions
5. elevates blood glucose
6. constricts sphincters
7. dilates pupils
8. dilates bronchioles
9. increases perspiration
  e. Decreased epinephrine levels have minimal or no effect.
2. *Norepinephrine*
  a. Identical to epinephrine except its effect is greater on the skeletal muscles, less on the cardiac cells, and increases peripheral vascular resistance

III. Assessment of the Endocrine System should include:
  A. Specific signs of altered functioning
    1. Changes in appetite or thirst
    2. Polyuria, oliguria, nocturia
    3. Changes in skin and hair texture
    4. Changes in skin pigmentation
    5. Changes in skin and hair distribution
    6. Intolerance to heat and/or cold.
  B. Assessment of gross cerebral functioning
    1. Consciousness
    2. Orientation
  C. Specific cerebral functioning
    1. Speech pattern
    2. Coordination
    3. Attention span
    4. Arousability
    5. Orientation
    6. Ability to follow commands
  D. Inspection
    1. General appearance
    2. Height and weight
    3. Facial expression
    4. Skin turgor
    5. Condition of eyes
    6. Mucous membranes
  E. Palpation
    1. Skin temperature
    2. Thyroid enlargement or thrill
    3. Abdominal or suprarenal masses
  F. Percussion
    1. Size and contour of tumors
  G. Auscultation
    1. Thyroid gland for bruits

H. Evaluation of vital signs
   1. Hypotension
   2. Hypertension
   3. Bradycardia
   4. Hyperthermia
   5. Respiratory changes
I. Laboratory and radiologic studies
   1. Urinalysis
   2. Serum analysis
   3. Arterial blood gases
   4. Skull, chest, abdominal and longbone films
   5. CT scan
   6. Pancreatic scan
   7. Thyroid scan
   8. Adrenal arteriography

IV. **Pathological States and Nursing Management**
   A. Diabetes insipidus
      1. The defect is in the release of ADH from the pituitary or in the synthesis of ADH in the hypothalamus.
      2. The patient may present with
         a. polyuria
         b. thirst
      3. Urinalysis and serum analysis for oxmolarity, specific gravity and sodium are diagnostic aids.
      4. Nursing care includes:
         a. recording of intake and output
         b. measurement of specific gravity
         c. titration of fluids
         d. diagnostic testing
         e. administration of medications
   B. Secretion of inappropriate ADH
      1. Results from increased production or secretion of ADH
      2. The patient presents with headache, lethargy, decrease in deep tendon reflexes, seizures, nausea and vomiting.
      3. Diagnostic data includes decreased serum sodium, potassium, chlorides and osmolarity, as well as increase in urine sodium, osmolarity and specific gravity.
      4. Nursing care includes:
         a. assessment of general status
         b. assessment of fluid and electrolyte balance
   C. Thyrotoxic crisis
      1. Thyrotoxic crisis is caused by the release of an excessive amount of thyroid hormones.
      2. The patient presents with tremors, hyperpyrexia, hyperkinesis, systolic murmurs and palmar erythema.
      3. Diagnostic data includes thyroid enlargement, bruit or thrill, and a positive thyroid scan.

4. Nursing care includes:
   a. regulation of metabolic activity
   b. decrease in sympathetic stimuli
   c. adequate nutrition
   d. administration of iodine agents and antithyroid medication.

D. Hypoparathyroidism
   1. Hypoparathyroidism results from a defect in the release of PTH.
   2. The patient may present with
      a. numbness and tingling in distal extremities
      b. carpopedal spasms
      c. nausea, vomiting
      d. abdominal pain
      e. laryngeal stridor
      f. confusion
      g. lethargy
   3. Definitive diagnosis is by serum calcium level less than 8.5 mg/dl.
   4. Nursing care includes:
      a. maintenance of airway and ventilation
      b. maintenance of calcium levels
      c. monitoring of emotional states
      d. seizure precautions

E. Diabetic ketoacidosis
   1. Diabetic ketoacidosis is a lack or reduction in the amount of insulin available in systemic circulation.
   2. The patient may present with
      a. weakness
      b. hypotension
      c. tachycardia
      d. acetone breath
      e. polydipsia, polyuria
      f. Kussmaul respirations
   3. Serum glucose is the best diagnostic aid.
   4. Nursing care includes:
      a. maintenance of fluid and electrolyte balance
      b. maintenance of airway and ventilation
      c. maintaining intake and output
      d. seizure precautions
      e. prevention of complication
      f. patient education

F. Hyperketotic hyperosmolar coma
   1. Hyperketotic hyperosmolar coma is caused by an insulin deficiency causing hyperglycemia, diuresis, hyperosmolarity and cellular dehydration.
   2. The patient will present with
      a. over 50 years of age
      b. lethargy, stupor, coma
      c. polyuria, polydipsia
      d. dehydration
      e. hypotension

f. hyperpyrexia

g. facial seizures

3. Elevation in the serum glucose and osmolarity are diagnostic aids.

4. Nursing care includes:

a. maintenance of fluid and electrolyte balance

G. Hypoglycemia

1. Hypoglycemia is a reduction in glucose levels.

2. The patient will present with

a. headache

b. blurred vision

c. hunger

d. anxiety

e. personality changes

f. changes in level of consciousness

g. pallor

3. The best diagnostic aid is a serum glucose level.

4. Nursing care includes:

a. restoration of glucose levels

b. patient education

H. Adrenal crisis

1. Adrenal crisis is the result of rapid exacerbation of chronic Addison's disease.

2. The patient may present with

a. hypotension

b. oliguria

c. flaccid extremities

d. hyperpigmentation

e. changes in level of consciousness

f. abdominal pain

g. dehydration

3. Laboratory studies are the best diagnostic aid.

4. Nursing care includes:

a. maintenance of blood volume

b. reduction of stress

c. patient and family education

V. **Care Common to Endocrine Problems**

A. Observe for changes in health status

B. Airway and ventilation

1. Airway and ventilation should be monitored for

a. changes in respiration and breath sounds

b. hypoxemia

c. dysrhythmia

d. gas movement

2. Methods to maintain airway patency and ventilation include:

a. proper head alignment

b. suctioning

c. oxygenation

C. Fluid and electrolyte balance
   1. Fluid and electrolyte balance is monitored via
      a. laboratory studies
      b. intake and output
   2. Observe for vomiting, diuresis, polyuria, tetany, weakness, dehydration.
   3. Fluid replacement is used to maintain proper hydration.
D. Neurological status
   1. Observe for signs of intracranial pressure.
   2. Intracranial pressure monitoring is accomplished by
      a. subarachnoid screw
      b. ventricular drain
      c. epidural catheter
   3. Intracranial pressure may be decreased by
      a. ventricular drainage
      b. osmatic diuresis
      c. steroids
      d. hypothermia
      e. elevating head of bed 30 degrees
      f. barbituate induced coma
E. Patient education is common to all nursing care and involves teaching about
   1. disease process, its limitations and complications
   2. medications
   3. treatment
   4. community resources

CHAPTER EIGHT
GASTROINTESTINAL SYSTEM

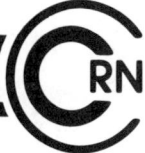

BEHAVIORAL OBJECTIVES

After reading the *Gastrointestinal System,* the nurse will be able to:

- Describe the major organs of the G.I. system and list two functions (when applicable) of each of the following: oral cavity, pharynx, esophagus, stomach, small intestine and large intestine
- Describe the accessory organs of the G.I. tract and list two functions of each of the following: gallbladder, pancreas and liver
- Explain the mechanisms of motility in the esophagus, stomach, small intestine and large intestine
- Discuss the small intestine's role in the absorption of carbohydrates, proteins and fats
- Discuss the causes of nutritional deficiencies in the patient with G.I. disturbances
- Explain the need for total parenteral nutrition for patients with certain G.I. disorders
- Explain the indications for enteral hyperalimentation and peripheral parenteral nutrition
- Discuss the importance of the history and physical for patients with G.I. disorders
- Describe the pathophysiology, clinical findings and specific nursing care for patients with the following disease states: cirrhosis, hepatic failure, bleeding esophageal varices, G.I. bleeding from peptic ulcer disease and acute pancreatitis
- State the indications for endoscopic studies and describe their current popularity as a diagnostic tool

TOPICAL OUTLINE
GASTROINTESTINAL SYSTEM

I. The Gastrointestinal System: Overview   485
II. Anatomy and Physiology   486
    Upper G.I. system   486
      Oral cavity   486
      Pharynx   487
      Esophagus   487
      Stomach   488
    Lower G.I. system   493
      Small intestine   493
      Large intestine   497
    Blood supply to the G.I. tract   501
    Nervous innervation   501
    Accessory organs of digestion   502
      Gallbladder   502
      Pancreas   504
      Liver   505
III. Physical Assessment of the Gastrointestinal System   506
    History   506
    Inspection   507
    Auscultation   508
    Percussion   509
    Palpation   509
IV. Nursing Assessment of the G.I. System   510
    Evaluation of eating   510
    Evaluation of swallowing   510
    Evaluation of digestion   510
    Evaluation of elimination   510
    Evaluation of vital signs   510
    Laboratory and radiologic studies   511
V. Pathological States and Nursing Management   512
    Cirrhosis of the liver   512
      Pathophysiology   512
      Case study   513
      Diagnostic data   514
      Nursing care   514
    Hepatic failure   515
      Pathophysiology   515
      Clinical presentation   515
      Case study   516
      Diagnostic data   516
      Nursing care   517
    Bleeding esophageal varices   517
      Pathophysiology   517
      Clinical presentation   518
      Case study   518
      Diagnostic data   519
      Nursing care   519

G.I. hemmorrhage from peptic ulcers 520
 Pathophysiology 520
 Clinical presentation 520
 Case study 521
 Diagnostic data 522
 Nursing care 522
Acute pancreatitis 522
 Pathophysiology 522
 Clinical presentation 523
 Case study 524
 Diagnostic data 525
 Nursing care 525

VI. Care Common to Gastrointestinal Problems 527
 Fluid and electrolyte problems 527
  Pathophysiology 527
  Clinical presentation 527
  Nursing care 527
 Nutritional maintenance 528
  Clinical presentation 528
  Diagnostic data 528
  Nursing care 529

Program Assessment: Science and Situation 533
Key Point Recognition Answers 543
PASS Answer Sheet 547
Survey Summary 549

THE GASTROINTESTINAL SYSTEM: Overview

The function of the gastrointestinal tract is to provide water, electrolytes and nutrients to the body and to prepare these nutrients for absorption (Fig. 8-1). The gastrointestinal system is divided into the upper G.I. system (oral cavity, pharynx, esophagus and stomach), the lower G.I. system (small intestine and large intestine) and the accessory organs of digestion (pancreas, gallbladder and liver) (Fig. 8-2).

Structure	Activity	Control	Function	Secretion
Mouth: teeth, tongue walls of cheek, palate	Chewing prepares food for swallowing and meets psychological needs.	Reflex activity- 5th cranial nerve	Breaks food into smaller portions; breaks down fibrous covering; saliva lubricates and softens; stimulates buds; bactericidal effect	Mucus; ptyalin (amylase); Hydrolyze starches by splitting off maltase
Esophagus: swallowing (deglutition)	1. Voluntary or oral occurs when the food is pressed by the tongue against the palate.	Voluntary	Movement of food	Mucus
	2. Pharyngeal begins the first-wave peristalsis, closing the epiglottis and opening the esophagus, which widens and relaxes the upper esophagus sphincter.	Involuntary glossopharyngeal nerves	Mucus lubricates; promotes passage; protects mucus	
	3. Esophageal peristaltic wave forces the bolus by contraction, momentum and gravity.	Involuntary	Neutralization of acids and bases	
Stomach	Storage, mixing and liquefaction of food into chyme; the gastric stage of digestion is stimulated by food in the stomach.	Parasympathetic nervous system vagal Hormonal stimulation-secretion of gastrin Histamine	Protein breakdown Digestion of the connecting tissue of meat Digestion of starches Digestion of fats mainly butterfats Buffering action Vitamin B_{12} absent Protein absent	Mucus; pepsin-I, II, III breakdown; proteins to polypeptides; proteoses and peptones; gastric lipase Gastrin secretion; Cholecystokinin; gastric inhibitory peptide; motilin
Small bowel	Mixing and perislaltic movement; propels chyme along the gut; aids in better digestion and absorption.	Sympathetic Parasympathetic	To complete digestion of foodstuffs; to absorb products of this digestion; activates trypsin; carbohydrate digestion; protein digestion; disaccharides to monosaccharides; neutral fats to glycerol and fatty acids	Maltase dextrinase lactose sucrase peptidases intestinal lipase Enterogastrone vasoactive intestinal peptide substance P bombesin somatosin amylase
Colon, rectum, anus	Mixing and propulsion; movements to exposure	Parasympathetic: sacral division and Tactill stomach	Absorption of H_2O and lytes in the proximal half and storage of feces in the distal half.	

Fig. 8-1 The gastrointestinal system

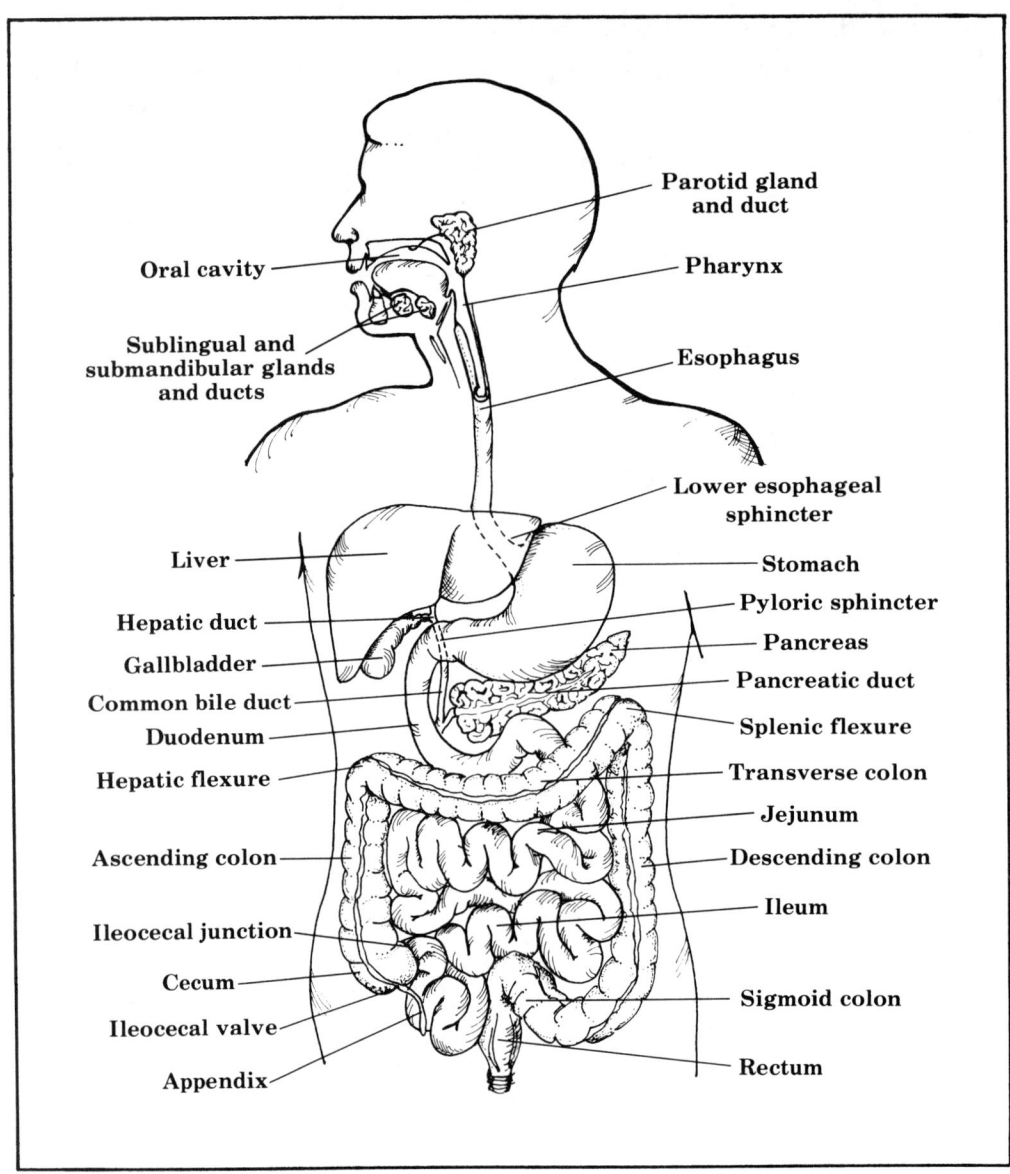

Fig. 8-2 The gastrointestinal system

ANATOMY AND PHYSIOLOGY

UPPER G.I. SYSTEM
Oral Cavity

The oral cavity begins the digestive canal and is responsible for the first step of the preparation of food for absorption. This cavity consists of the lips, cheeks, teeth, palate, gums, salivary glands and tongue. The interaction of these structures initiates the first steps of deglutition—ingestion, salivation and mastication.

The lips, cheeks, palate, gums and tongue provide the physical boundaries for the food bolus and guide the food's entry into the G.I. tract. This bolus is prevented from entering the nasal cavities by the upward movement of the palate during deglutition.

The teeth are responsible for the grinding and cutting actions of mastication. Mastication aids digestion by breaking down undigestible cellulose membranes of raw fruits and vegetables, and by greatly increasing the surface area of the food. The increased surface area allows exposure to the intestinal secretions, thereby increasing the rate of digestion.

The salivary glands secrete the watery substance saliva into the oral cavity. These glands are widely scattered within the lining of the oral cavity. Three specific glands are designated as the chief salivary glands because of their paired larger sizes. These are the **parotid, submandibular** and **sublingual glands.** These glands are categorized by the type of their secretory cells and the product they secrete, namely mucus, serous or mixed.

Saliva fulfills many functions: it begins the digestion of glycogen and starch; it retards the formation of dental caries; it activates the taste buds by dissolving the food; and it begins diluting the food toward an isotonic state.

Saliva is composed mainly of water and electrolytes. The ratio varies, depending on the rate of secretion; but saliva does remain hypotonic to body fluids. Approximately one to two liters of saliva are secreted in a 24-hour period. In addition to water, saliva contains the digestive enzyme ptyalin, an alpha-amylase that initiates starch digestion, and a glycoprotein called mucin, which provides the viscosity needed to help the food stick together.

In contrast to the other glands in the G.I. tract, salivary secretion is controlled by the autonomic nervous system. No hormones are involved. The rate of salivary secretion is increased by both sympathetic and parasympathetic stimulation.

The transportation of food from the mouth to the stomach is called deglutition (swallowing). Deglutition is a complicated process and has been divided into three stages: *voluntary, pharyngeal* and *esophageal.* The voluntary stage is the initiation of the act of deglutition and is accomplished by the tongue projecting the bolus of food from the oral cavity into the pharynx. After the voluntary stage, the rest of the deglutition process becomes automatic. The pharyngeal stage begins as the swallowing receptor areas in the pharynx are stimulated. Within one to two seconds, the trachea closes as a result of the epiglottis swinging backwards; the esophagus opens because of movement of the larynx; the hypopharyngeal sphincter relaxes; and peristalsis rapidly carries the food bolus into the upper esophagus. The deglutition process ends with the esophageal stage. Peristaltic waves propel the food bolus through the esophagus and into the stomach, as a result of the relaxation of the gastroesophageal sphincter.

Pharynx

The pharynx is divided into the **nasopharynx,** the **oropharynx** and the ***laryngeal pharynx.*** These three divisions aid in the deglutition process. The nasopharynx stretches from the nasal cavity to the soft palate. During deglutition, the soft palate is pushed upward to avoid aspiration. The oropharynx lies between the soft palates of the hyoid bone, where there is a crossing of pathways for air and food. The laryngeal pharynx continues the connection from the hyoid bone and terminates at the esophagus. The strong muscles attached to the hyoid bone pull the larynx upward and forward, which opens the esophagus. The epiglottis flings backward to prevent food from entering the trachea.

Esophagus

The most elementary segment of the alimentary canal is the esophagus, whose only function is to serve as a passageway for food from the pharynx to the stomach. This tubular structure is approximately 10 inches long, begins at the end of the laryngeal pharynx, passes through the mediastinum and diaphragm, and ends in the stomach. The esophagus is bordered anteriorly by the trachea (to which the esophagus is attached by fibroelastic membranous tissue), the pericardium and the left bronchus. The esophagus is bordered posteriorly by the thoracic vertebra and distally by the descending thoracic aorta.

The upper quarter of this collapsible tube is composed of striated muscle; the lower third is composed of smooth muscle; and the middle segment is a mixture of the two types of muscle. There are two basic layers of muscle of the esophagus: the outer longitudinal muscle layer and the inner circular muscle layer. The inner circular layer is thinner than the outer longitudinal layer in the esophagus, which is unique to this structure because the reverse is true of the remaining parts of the alimentary canal. Surrounding the lumen of the esophagus itself is the mucosa layer, consisting of a layer of stratified squamous epithelium, lamina propria and muscularis mucosa.

A narrow band of muscle fiber, called the cricopharyngeal muscle, is of great importance to ensure the functioning of the upper esophagus. This muscle, sometimes referred to as the hypopharyngeal sphincter or the upper esophageal sphincter, normally impedes air from entering the esophagus during the respiratory cycle. As the larynx moves and stretches open the esophagus during deglutition, this hypopharyngeal sphincter relaxes to allow the food bolus to enter the esophagus.

The esophagogastric junction has long been an intense area of physiological interest. Many questions have been answered by applying the data obtained from pressure-sensing catheters. There is a lower esophageal sphincter, or gastroesophageal sphincter, that normally remains tonically closed. With the initiation of deglutition, this sphincter relaxes and remains relaxed until the peristaltic wave through the esophagus is complete, thus closing the sphincter. Lack of peristalsis in the esophagus and failure of the gastroesophageal sphincter to relax following deglutition is a condition called **achalasia.** Although the specific etiology of achalasia remains unknown, there is agreement that the cause is of a neurogenic basis.

In addition to allowing the bolus of food to enter the stomach, the gastroesophageal sphincter prevents the food and gastric contents from leaving the stomach through reflux action.

Stomach

Between the esophagus and duodenum lies a large dilatation of the gastrointestinal tract called the stomach. This elongated pouch is located in the upper abdominal cavity, from the left hypochondriac region into the epigastric and umbilical regions. The shape of this organ is described as a J, but there is individual variation in its shape, according to body stature, volume of contents, phase of respiration and body posture. The stomach provides a reservoir to accept the food, secretes specific juices to enhance digestion and releases the food into the duodenum to continue the absorption process.

The anatomical landmarks of the stomach are the esophageal-cardiac juncture, the longitudinal section of the fundic stomach and the longitudinal section of the duodenum (Fig. 8-3).

The portal entrance to the stomach is known as the **cardiac sphincter.** Its relaxation is caused by the deglutition process. As gastric peristalsis strengthens, the liquified chyme leaves the stomach through the **pyloric sphincter** to enter the duodenum.

The stomach is composed of four layers: the **mucosa,** the **muscularis mucosa,** the **submucosa** and the **muscular coat.**

The mucosal layer contains a multitude of ridges called **rugae,** which are present when the stomach is empty, but disappear when the stomach is distended. The **cardiac, gastric** and **pyloric** glands are contained within the mucosal layer of the stomach. The cardiac glands are limited to the transition area between the esophagus and stomach, and are composed of mucus-producing cells. The gastric glands (oxyntic and fundic) are distributed throughout the majority of the proximal portion of the stomach. The fundic glands are composed of three types of cells that are responsible for secreting the necessary elements for the production of the gastric juice: the mucoid cells secrete mucus; the chief cells secrete pepsinogen (the precursor of pepsin) and mucus; and the parietal cells secrete hydrochloric acid. The pyloric glands, located in the distal part of the stomach, are composed of mucus-producing cells and endocrine cells that produce gastrin (the hormone responsible for the initiation of gastric secretions).

The second layer of the stomach wall, the muscularis mucosa, is a very thin layer of smooth muscle. Its function is to provide the muscular action required for the formation of the rugae. As the food enters the stomach, the rugae allow for the distension by smoothing out, consequently increasing the surface area of the stomach to enhance absorption.

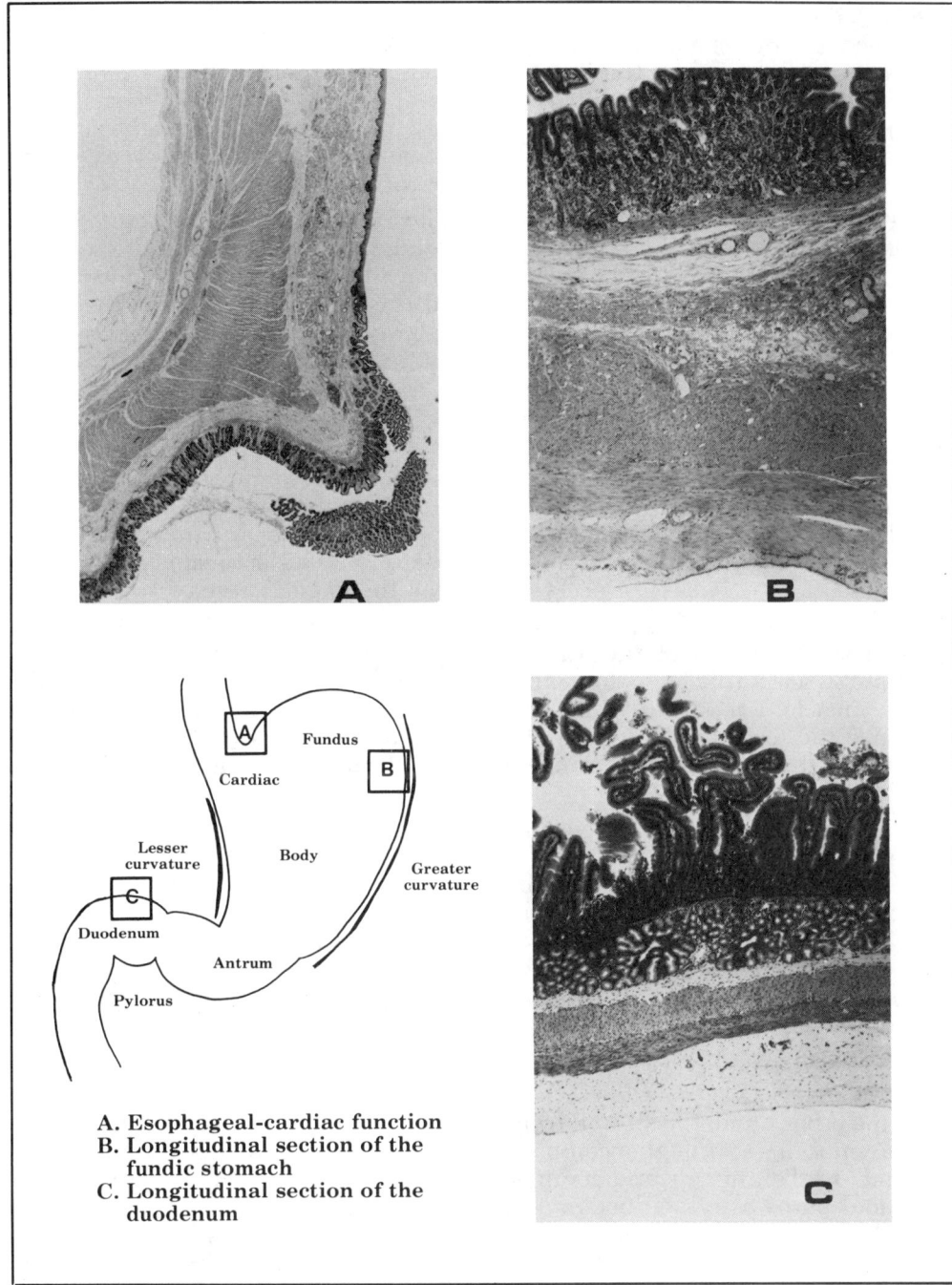

Fig. 8-3 Anatomical landmarks of the stomach

The submucosal layer of the stomach is the third layer. The larger blood vessels, nerves and lymphatics are found in this layer of loosely arranged connective tissue.

The external muscular coat completes the description of the stomach layers. This coat has three layers and is composed only of smooth muscle fibers. The longitudinal fibers are extensions of the same muscle layer of the esophagus. This external muscle encompasses the greater and lesser curvatures of the stomach. The middle circular layer is the only layer that covers the entire stomach. It also comprises the strongest layer of muscle. The inner oblique layer exhibits its strongest action in the fundus area, which diminishes as the pyloric area is approached.

Gastric Motility

As food enters the stomach, a receptive relaxation phenomenon occurs. The stomach accommodates the increased volume without increased pressure because of passive stretching. This passive stretching initiates a vagal reflex that prevents muscular activity in the body of the stomach. In addition, the relaxation spread by deglutition also permeates the fundus and body of the stomach, further enhancing accommodation of increased volume.

The digestive juices begin to break down the food as it enters the stomach and comes in contact with the stomach wall. Mixing of the food with the juices is accomplished by peristaltic waves that originate in the longitudinal muscle and spread to the circular muscle. These peristaltic contractions begin in the distal half of the stomach as weak waves. As these waves approach the antrum, both the speed and force of contractions are intensified. As these forceful contractions sweep the antrum, the pylorus narrows, allowing only a few milliliters of the liquified chyme to squirt into the duodenum. The rejected larger boluses of food are returned to the stomach for further mixing.

The primary control of the motor function of the stomach is due to ***vagal action.*** Slow electrical waves conduct approximately three times a minute in both the active and inactive stomach, originating from the intrinsic pacemaker activity of the longitudinal muscle cells. Whether peristalsis occurs is primarily determined by the release of acetylcholine by the vagus nerve.

The emptying of the stomach results from the interaction of opposing forces: The peristaltic waves of the antrum propel the chyme forward; the pylorus attempts to reject this bolus by maintaining the normal tonic contraction of the pyloric muscle. The rate at which the stomach empties depends on factors that influence the force and intensity of the antral peristalsis and the amount of pyloric constriction. These stimuli originate from either the stomach or the duodenum.

As the stomach distends from increased volume, there are more vagal discharges from stretch receptors. These vagal responses increase peristalsis, causing an accelerated rate of emptying; thus, the stomach empties at a rate proportional to its volume of material.

The release of the hormone gastrin also augments the rate of gastric emptying. Gastrin is secreted by the antral cells of the stomach. Its release promotes hydrochloric acid and pepsin production through stimulation of the parietal and chief cells. The most influential action of gastrin on gastric emptying is its resultant increase of antral motility; therefore, the stimuli from the stomach enhance the rate of emptying.

On the other hand, the stimuli from the duodenum tend to decrease the rate of gastric emptying. Through a complex series of feedback systems, the duodenum responds to the amount and composition of the chyme. Through nervous and hormonal pathways, the duodenum inhibits gastric peristalsis and constricts the pyloric sphincter in response to fat, high osmolarity and acidity; therefore, the principal action of the duodenal stimuli on gastric emptying is inhibitory.

Emotional factors also affect the rate of gastric emptying. The emptying is accelerated by aggression or anger and slowed by sadness, depression or fear.

Contents of the stomach and upper gastrointestinal tract are ejected by the act of vomiting. This complex reflux can be initiated from numerous stimuli, but the primary cause is an irritable, overdistended stomach. The control of vomiting within the central nervous system is located in the dorsolateral reticular formation of the medulla. Impulses reach this vomiting center by route of a combination of vagal and sympathetic afferents. With adequate stimulation, a concomitant wave of autonomic nervous system discharge is experienced, including tachycardia, pallor, diaphoresis, salivation and nausea. The sequence of motor events is as follows: contraction of the antrum and the stomach, with simultaneous relaxation of the rest of the stomach, sphincters and esophagus; closure of the pulmonary tree by the glottis; closure of the nasopharynx by the soft palate; and contraction of the diaphragm and abdominal muscles, resulting in a rise in intra-abdominal pressure that expels the rejected contents into the esophagus and out of the mouth.

Gastric Secretion

The digestive process begins as the ingested food is mixed with the gastric juice. The secretions of the mucous cells, the chief cells and the parietal cells combine to form the gastric juice.

Mucus and water are secreted by the mucous glands, providing a buffer system for the lining of the G.I. tract. Mucus and water form a protective barrier for the lumenal walls against self-digestion. These substances also lubricate the ingested food, enhancing tenacity, thereby promoting passage of the food particles.

Hydrochloric acid (HCl) is secreted by the parietal cells. About two liters of HCl are produced in a 24-hour period. This secretion is responsible for converting pepsinogen to pepsin. Having a pH of 1.0 to 3.5, HCl supplies the required acidity for pepsin's proteolytic action. The acid destroys many bacteria that have been ingested and negates the action of some toxins. Finally, HCl acts to denature proteins and to mollify fibrous foods, enhancing their digestion. Many hypotheses have been offered to explain the secretion of HCl. The exact mechanism is still being researched. It has been established that an active transport system is used, requiring a tremendous amount of energy to concentrate the hydrogen ions.

Intrinsic factor is also secreted by the parietal cells. The secretion of this mucoprotein is the one absolutely essential function of the stomach to preserve life. Intrinsic factor binds to vitamin B_{12} and aids absorption of this essential vitamin. Through this binding action, digestion of vitamin B_{12} is prevented. The amount of intrinsic factor produced in one hour is enough to bind with the minimum daily requirement of vitamin B_{12}.

Pepsinogen is secreted by the chief cells. This substance is the inactive precursor of pepsin. In the presence of HCl, pepsin initiates protein digestion.

The stimulation of gastric secretion occurs by the interaction of three main classes of compounds: the hormone gastrin, acetylcholine and histamine. Gastrin is released by the antral cells of the mucosa cells. Acetylcholine promotes the release of acid and increases gastric motility. Gastric distention, vagal stimulation and peptic digests stimulate the release of acetylcholine. Still under investigation, histamine has been proven to be an extremely potent acid-secretion stimulator. The gastric mucosa is not only capable of manufacturing large quantities of histamine, but also can store vast amounts. These three compounds possess similar stimulatory effects. It has been shown that all three are inhibited by atropine and by histamine (H_2) receptor blockers. It is of interest to note that cimetidine (Tagamet) belongs to the H_2 receptor antagonist classification of drugs.

Gastric secretion has been divided into stages, namely **basal, cephalic, gastric** and **intestinal.** Secretion during the basal phase (fasting state, no stimulus) has been observed to have regular fluctuations—peaks in the evening and lows in the morning. The precise cause of basal secretion remains unknown, although histamine may be involved.

During a meal, gastric secretion occurs in the remaining three stages, which are sequential with a great deal of overlap. The cephalic phase begins with the thought, taste and smell of food. Mediated by the vagus, this phase is responsible for about 10 percent of total gastric secretion.

As the food enters the stomach, the gastric phase commences. More than 70 percent of gastric acid secretion occurs in this stage. The food stimulates acid secretion by the processes of dilution and buffering of gastric acid. The result is the removal of the acid-mediated inhibition of resting gastrin and acid secretion. Vagal reflexes are stimulated by distension of the stomach and secretagogues, which are mainly protein digests. This vagal stimulation in turn serves to increase gastrin and acid release. The higher the content of protein in the ingested food, the more gastric acid is secreted. This is because proteins serve as the primary buffers in food, and with an increase of buffers in the ingested food, an increase of acid must correspond to bring the pH low enough to stop further gastrin and acid release. This feedback mechanism functions to maintain the balance necessary during the gastric phase.

Only 10 percent of the total gastric secretion occurs in the final intestinal phase. This phase begins with the chyme being propelled into the duodenum, and probably is mediated hormonally. The hormones released are enteric gastrin and possibly pancreozymin-cholecystokinin, a weak agonist of gastrin.

KEY CONCEPT: The upper G.I. system is composed of the oral cavity, pharnyx, esophagus and stomach.

KEY POINT RECOGNITION

Write true or false by each statement. Answers are at the end of this chapter. A score below 80% indicates the need for further study.

1. The oral cavity is composed of the lips, cheeks, teeth, palate, gums, salivary glands and tongue.
2. Food is prevented from entering the nasal cavities by the downward movement of the palate during deglutition.
3. Mastication increases the surface area of food.
4. The rate of digestion is increased as the surface area of the food is increased.
5. The chief salivary glands are the parotid, submandibular and secretory glands.
6. Salivation enhances the formation of dental caries.
7. Saliva is slightly hypertonic to body fluids.
8. Saliva contains water, electrolytes, ptyalin and mucin.
9. Salivary secretion is hormonally controlled.
10. The three stages of deglutition are involuntary, voluntary and esophageal.
11. The cricopharyngeal muscle impedes air from entering the esophagus during the respiratory cycle.
12. During the swallowing process, the hypopharyngeal sphincter relaxes, allowing food to enter the esophagus.
13. Achalasia is thought to be a hormonal disorder.
14. The pharynx aids in the deglutition process.
15. To avoid aspiration during swallowing, the soft palate is pushed upward.
16. The larynx is pulled upward and forward during deglutition, opening the esophagus.
17. The esophagus is approximately 6 to 8 inches long.
18. The gastroesophageal sphincter prevents food from leaving the stomach through reflux action.
19. The portal entrance to the stomach is the esophageal-cardiac juncture.
20. Liquified chyme leaves the stomach through the cardiac sphincter.
21. Rugae are present when the stomach is empty.
22. The cardiac glands are composed of mucus-producing glands.
23. The stomach is composed of five layers.
24. The fundic glands are responsible for secreting elements necessary for the production of gastric juices.
25. The parietal cells secrete pepsinogen.
26. The pyloric glands are composed of both mucus-producing cells and cells that produce gastrin.
27. The muscularis mucosa provides the muscular action necessary for the formation of the rugae.
28. Nerves and lymphatics are found in the submucosal layer of the stomach.

_____29. The external muscular coat has four layers and is composed of striated muscle.

_____30. Increased stomach volume is accommodated through vagal stimulation.

_____31. Primary control of the motor function of the stomach is through vagal action.

_____32. Acetylcholine, released by the vagus nerve, is responsible for peristaltic action.

_____33. Stomach emptying results from both the peristaltic waves of the antrum and the maintenance of the normal tonic contraction of the pyloric muscle.

_____34. Gastrin tends to decrease the rate of gastric emptying through the inhibition of pepsin production.

_____35. Nervous control of vomiting is located in the pons.

_____36. Hydrochloric acid enhances digestion by mollifying fibrous foods and denaturing proteins.

_____37. Intrinsic factor aids in the absorption of vitamin B_{12}.

_____38. Pepsinogen is the precursor of pepsin.

_____39. The interaction of gastrin, hydrochloric acid and pepsin stimulates gastric secretion.

_____40. The cephalic phase of gastric secretion begins with the thought, taste and smell of food.

_____41. More than 70 percent of gastric acid secretion occurs during the intestinal phase of secretion.

_____42. The basal phase of secretion is characterized by peaks in the evening and low secretions in the morning.

LOWER G.I. SYSTEM
Small Intestine

The largest amount of digestion and absorption takes place in the small intestine. Filling most of the abdominal cavity, the small intestine begins at the pylorus of the stomach and ends at the ileocecal valve of the large intestine. This convoluted tubule measures about 20 to 23 feet in length, with a progressively diminishing diameter. This structure is divided into three segments: the *duodenum,* the *jejunum* and the *ileum.*

The *duodenum,* measuring about 10 inches in length, is located in the epigastric and umbilical regions. This portion of the small intestine forms a C-shape, cradling the head of the pancreas in its concavity. The first inch of the duodenum is almost indistinguishable from the stomach, being covered both anteriorly and posteriorly with peritoneum. The rest is retroperitoneal.

The next 2/5 of the small intestine (about eight feet) is the *jejunum,* extending from the duodenum to the ileum.

The remaining small intestine is the *ileum,* measuring approximately 12 feet long. The jejunum and ileum gradually blend into each other.

The *ileocecal valve* connects the ileum to the cecum. The valve forms the passageway to the large intestine. The function of the ileocecal valve is similar to the gastroesophageal sphincter in controlling reflux. The ileocecal valve does not allow fecal colonic material to re-enter the ileum.

The small intestinal wall is composed of the same basic layers as the stomach: *muscular, submucosal* and *mucosal.* Although the layers are similar, many unique structural features are found within the layers of the small intestine.

The mucosal layer of the small intestine differs markedly from that in the remainder of the G.I. tract. Consisting of three layers itself, the mucous membrane contains plasma cells, numerous blood cells, blood capillaries, nerve fibers and lymphatic vessels. Composed of columnar and epithelial cells, the mucosa forms circular folds (Kerckring's folds) that project into the lumen of the intestine. These folds, which are not present in the upper part of the duodenum, reach their maximum length in the jejunum and diminish in the ileum. Their purpose is to increase the surface area for absorption.

Millions of villi project from the mucosal layer over the entire surface of the small intestine. Barely visible to the naked eye, these fingerlike projections immensely increase the surface area of the small intestine for absorptive enhancement. Visible by electron micrography, each cell of a villus has a brush border of microvilli that further multiplies the dimensions of the surface area of the small intestine. Each villus houses a vascular system surrounding a central lacteal, the lymph vessel. The villi contain at least five different kinds of cells: columnar, which absorb; goblet, which secrete mucus; undifferentiated, which proliferate and differentiate; zymogenic, which appear secretory in nature; and enteroendocrine, which produce hormones.

Between the villi are found the Lieberkuhn's crypts. The epithelial cells of these crypts produce the intestinal secretions that are reabsorbed into the villi. This exchange of fluid provides a transport for the material from the chyme to be absorbed via the villi.

Peyer's patches, or aggregated lymph nodules, are also found in the mucosal layer. These follicles form circular or oval patches and are largest and most abundant in the ileum. As with any lymph nodules, these patches synthesize antibodies and contribute to the immune response of the body.

The mucosal and submucosal layers are divided by a thin, smooth muscle called the muscularis mucosa. The submucosal layer of the small intestine is similar to that of the stomach. It consists of loosely arranged connective tissue and holds larger blood vessels and lymphatics. Nerve fibers and ganglion cells combine to form a plexus (Meissner's plexus) that connects with the myenteric plexus of the muscular layer.

The submucosal layer contains only one kind of gland, Brunner's, or duodenal, glands. Brunner's glands are found only in the duodenum and are most numerous near the pylorus. They secrete an alkaline, mucoid substance.

The muscular layer contains two easily identified smooth muscle components: an inner circular and an outer longitudinal component. The smooth muscle layers are separated by connective tissue that harbors the myenteric plexus of nerve fibers and parasympathetic ganglion cells.

Small Intestine Motility

The movement of the chyme through the small intestine is accomplished by several coinciding events. The longitudinal muscle initiates a basic electrical rhythm (BER) by means of the intrinsic pacemaker cells. These slow waves occur about 11 times a minute, although this number may vary in different parts of the small intestine. The BER does not cause the contractions, but provides the "background beat" to set the timing for the contractions.

When another stimulus is added, such as chyme distending the intestine, or irritation of the mucosal lining, this "background beat" is accentuated and, in turn, stimulates the myenteric reflex. During the upstroke of the original oscillations, a spike potential falls, which sends messages to the longitudinal muscle and then to the circular muscle, demanding their contractions. The "background beat" remains unchanged, but the intensity of the contraction is increased.

As a result of these contractions, the chyme is mixed and pushed through the small intestine. Usually, two types of movement are described: ***mixing*** or ***segmental movements,*** and ***peristaltic*** or ***propulsive movements.***

Segmentation consists of squeezing and mixing the intestinal contents by ringlike contractions of the circular muscle. A popular analogy to segmentation is the comparison of the appearance of the small intestine to a chain of link sausages. Segmentation mixes the intestinal contents with the digestive juices and brings them in contact with the mucosa so that absorption can take place.

Peristalsis is responsible for the onward and analward movement of the intestinal contents. These wavelike contractions may begin in any part of the small intestine, with a rate varying from faster in the duodenum to slower in the ileum. Distension of the intestine usually triggers peristalsis.

Small intestine functions. The most important functions of the small intestine are to **digest** and **absorb** the ingested food matter. To undersand the absorptive mechanism, several basic biochemical concepts, which will be dealt with briefly, are important.

Active transport is the process of moving a substance against a concentration gradient or against an electrical potential difference. Energy, usually in the form of ATP, is required to accomplish the movement of a substance into or out of a cell. Amino acids, Na^+, K^+, different sugars, calcium, chloride and iron ions are substances requiring active transport.

Passive diffusion is the transfer along a concentration or electrochemical gradient. No energy is required for the molecule to move from an area of high concentration to an area of low concentration. Free fatty acids and water are passively diffused.

Facilitated diffusion is movement by a carrier of a substance from a higher concentration to a lower concentration. Alone, the substance would not be able to cross the membrane; but through binding with a carrier, diffusion is possible. No energy is required.

Nonionic transport is the free movement of noncharged particles in and out of cells. Again, no energy is required for this movement. Some drugs (such as phenobarbital) and nonconjugated bile salts are mobilized through this mechanism.

It is interesting to note how different materials are absorbed. The process of absorption of a few of these important substances follows.

The absorption of water is due to passive diffusion. The small intestine has a large amount of water to deal with each day. About 1 to 2.5 liters of water are ingested, plus 8 to 10 liters of water are added as a result of the massive secretions of the G.I. tract. Most of this water is absorbed or reabsorbed, with only a fraction of it (about 150 ml) being excreted in the feces.

This voluminous water absorption is accompanied by absorption of solutes, mainly sodium and some hydrolyzed food particles. Sodium is actively absorbed in all areas of the small and large intestines. In the small intestine, sodium and water absorption is osmotic, and sodium transport takes place against a weak electrochemical gradient. In the large intestine, sodium can be absorbed against stronger electrochemical gradients at a rate sensitive to aldosterone.

Potassium absorption in the small intestine and potassium secretion in the large intestine appear to be passive. Chloride absorption is active and passive. The other major electrolytes, bicarbonate and magnesium phosphate, appear to combine properties of exchange with active and passive absorption properties.

Bodily needs dictate how much calcium the small intestine needs to absorb. A specific calcium-binding protein allows the calcium to enter the intestinal epithelial cell. The synthesis of this calcium-binding protein is stimulated by vitamin D and 1.25-dehydroxycholecalciferol, which is vitamin D after it has been processed by the liver and kidneys. Calcium can then be actively transported through the cell and into the interstitial fluid.

The absorption of iron is another bodily regulated mechanism. An adult usually ingests 15 to 20 mg of iron a day, but only 0.5 to 1.5 mg are absorbed by the small intestine by active transport. The intestinal epithelial cells absorb the iron by a specific iron-binding protein. The iron is then stored inside the cell in two forms, one that is readily absorbable and one that is slowly absorbable.

The exact mechanism of absorption of the water soluble vitamins (folic acid, vitamin B_{12}, ascorbic acid, vitamin C) remains under investigation. Among these vitamins, three mechanisms of transport—active transport, passive diffusion and carrier-mediated diffusion—appear to be represented. Absorption of vitamin B_{12} is known to be a carrier-mediated process, since its absorption in the ileum depends on its binding to the intrinsic factor synthesized by the parietal cells.

Vitamins A, D, E and K, the fat soluble vitamins, require the presence of bile salts for absorption. The mechanism of their absorption is discussed under fat absorption.

Carbohydrate Absorption

Carbohydrates supply about half of the calories ingested daily by humans. To facilitate absorption, these carbohydrates must be broken down into **polysaccharides** (starch and glycogen). This digestive breakdown is still not sufficient for absorption, since the majority of carbohydrates are absorbed in the *monosaccharide* form.

The essential pancreatic enzyme, ***amylase,*** transforms starch into the disaccharide maltose, the trisaccharide maltotriose and many oligosaccharides (short-chain polysaccharides). This part of the digestive process is completed within a few minutes after the chyme enters the duodenum.

The microvilli of the intestinal mucosal cells produce the enzymes necessary to break apart these oligosaccharides into absorbable monosaccharides: sucrase breaks sucrose into glucose and fructose; lactase breaks lactose into glucose and galactose. Glucose and galactose are then actively transported across the intestinal wall for absorption. Fructose has a carrier that facilitates its entry into the mucosal cell, utilizing facilitated diffusion for its absorption.

Protein Absorption

Proteins consist of long chains of amino acids. There are 22 common amino acids. Eight are called ***essential amino acids.*** The eight essential amino acids are ***isoleucine, methionine, leucine, phenylalanine, lysine, threonine, valine*** and ***tryptophan.*** They must be obtained from dietary ingestion since the body cannot synthesize a sufficient amount of the essential amino acids.

The digestion of proteins begins in the stomach by the acid, which denatures the protein, and by the pepsin, which initiates protein digestion by stimulating the release of gastrin and the release of pancreozymin-cholecystokinin from the duodenal mucosa. The pancreas secretes protein-splitting enzymes known as proteases, which include trypsin, chymotrypsin and carboxypolypeptidases. Each protease has a specific type of peptide linkage that it attacks. The end products are small peptides containing about four amino acids. These small peptides are further broken down into dipeptides or free amino acids by specific enzymes present in the microvilli of the intestinal mucosa. Unlike carbohydrates, some protein is best absorbed as a dipeptide and is then hydrolyzed to amino acids inside the mucosal cell. Generally, absorption of amino acids is active.

Fat Absorption

Fat in the diet is in the form of a triglyceride. Each triglyceride contains three molecules of long-chain fatty acids and glycerol. These molecules are not water-soluble, so the digestion and absorption of fats pose some unique problems.

Digestion of fats begins in the duodenum, where the pancreatic enzyme ***lipase*** comes in contact with the triglyceride. Through stages, the lipase splits the triglyceride into free fatty acid and monoglyceride.

With the completion of lipolysis, micelles must be formed. **Micelles** are very small particles composed of bile salts, fatty acids, monoglycerides, phospholipids, cholesterol and fat-soluble vitamins. These fat digestion products are enclosed in the water solution interior of the micelles. This enclosure in the micelle keeps the excess fat digestion products out of solution, but also provides transportation of these products into the jejunal mucosal cell. When the micelle comes in contact with the mucosal cell, all of the substances, except the bile salts, are readily diffused into the cell. The bile salts continue to the ileum, where they are absorbed and transported back to the liver.

As soon as the contents of the micelle are diffused into the intestinal mucosal cell, they are quickly reconstituted into triglyceride and extruded from the cell into the lymph. So why expend all the energy to break the triglyceride down if the end result is a resynthesis of a triglyceride? There appear to be two reasons: 1)

The ingested triglyceride cannot diffuse through the intestinal mucosal membrane efficiently. 2) The body is able to use endogenous fatty acids to alter the fatty acid composition of the triglyceride that is resynthesized and absorbed into the body.

Secretion in the Small Intestine

The small intestine secretions maintain a pH of about 7.0. Similar to the stomach, the small intestine has numerous mucous cells that secrete an alkaline mucus in response to chemical or mechanical irritation. The Brunner's glands in the duodenum are responsible for secreting this mucus. In addition to irritation, the stimulation of Brunner's glands include secretion and vagal stimulation. Sympathetic stimulation inhibits their secretion, so it follows that most of the stress ulcers are located in the duodenal bulb.

The epithelial cells of Lieberkuhn's crypts produce the intestinal secretions that are reabsorbed into the villi. These secretions are isotonic electrolyte fluid, similar to plasma. The epithelial cells of the intestinal mucosal contribute the digestive enzymes, including amylase, lipase, maltase, lactase, sucrase and the peptidases.

The major control for the secretion of intestinal juices is *local stimulation.* This stimulation is simply the presence of chyme in the small intestine. A second regulatory mechanism is that of *hormonal stimuli. Vasoactive intestinal peptide* (VIP) has been shown to strongly increase intestinal secretion. Its effects are quite similar to secretin.

Secretin is a hormone released from the duodenal mucosa. Its main function is to maintain the duodenal contents at a neutral pH. When the pH of the lumen of the duodenum falls below 4.5, secretin is released into the blood. This hormone is a potent stimulator of pancreatic bicarbonate, bile flow, insulin output, gastric pepsin secretion and Brunner's gland secretion. Some of the inhibitory effects of secretin include a decrease in gastric and duodenal motility, and a decrease in the gastrin-stimulated acid secretion.

Another hormone released by the duodenal mucosa is *pancreozymin-cholecystokinin* (PZ-CCK). This hormone, once thought to be two different hormones, is released into the blood in response to the presence of protein and fat digestive products in the duodenum. PZ-CCK works by securing the bile salts and pancreatic enzymes into the duodenum. The most important effects of PZ-CCK are inhibition of gastrin-stimulated acid secretion, stimulation of the pancreatic enzymes and contraction of the gallbladder.

Gastric inhibitory peptide (GIP) is released by the duodenal mucosa and acts to stimulate insulin release and inhibit gastric motility. The presence of fats and carbohydrates in the lumen signals the release of GIP.

There are many other substances in the G.I. tract that are putative hormones. Questions are still unanswered as to their importance, and their specific categorization as hormones remains under investigation.

Large Intestine

The large intestine is the final passageway for the ingested food. It is a tube that measures about 5.5 feet in length and 2.5 inches in diameter. It begins at the end of the ileum and ends at the anus. The primary functions of the large intestine are *absorption of solutes and fluid,* and *elimination of waste products.* There are three divisions of the large intestine: the *cecum,* the *colon* and the *rectum.* Beginning in the right ileac region, these divisions encase the small intestine by curving around the convolutions.

The *cecum* is described as a blind pouch 2 to 3 inches long. It hangs down at the junction of the ileum and the colon. The ileocecal valve is located at this junction between the small and large intestines and prevents feces from re-entering the ileum. The vermiform appendix arises from the medial side of the cecum. The appendix varies widely in position and size, and contains lymphoid tissue.

The *colon* is partitioned into four sections: the *ascending,* the *transverse,* the *descending* and the *sigmoid.* Beginning at the cecum, the ascending colon is situated in the right ileac region and measures about five inches long. It extends to the undersurface of the liver where it turns left, forming the hepatic flexure. This flexure forms the continuation of the colon known as the transverse section. Crossing the upper part of the abdominal cavity from the right to the left, the transverse colon is about 15 inches long. It ends at the splenic flexure where the colon turns downward, inferior to the spleen. The descending colon continues from the splenic flexure and traverses 10 inches to the brim of the pelvis in the left ileac region. The sigmoid colon, 10 to 15 inches long, extends from the pelvic brim to the rectum. This S-shaped piece of colon descends along the left pelvic wall, passes left to right across the pelvis to the right pelvic wall, where it bends, and again passes to the left to join the rectum in the midline.

The *rectum* extends from the sigmoid colon to the anal canal, descending along the hollow of the sacrum and the coccyx. Its length is approximately 5 to 6 inches. At the anorectal junction, there is a great amount of thickening of the circular muscle fibers. This thickening forms the smooth muscle ring known as the internal anal sphincter, which monitors the exit of the feces. The external anal sphincter is a cylinder of skeletal muscle that encompasses the anal canal.

The layers of the wall of the large intestine are the same as in the small intestine and stomach: **mucosal, submucosal** and **muscular.** However, some structural variations are present in the layers.

The *mucosal* layer is relatively smooth, being devoid of villi or folds. The epithelial cells are tall and columnar, and serve to absorb water and electrolytes. Goblet cells are found between the columnar cells, and their function is to produce copious amounts of mucus to lubricate the wall of the colon.

There are no major structural variations between the submucosa of the small intestine and the large intestine. This loosely arranged connective tissue holds larger blood vessels and the nerve plexus of Meissner.

The muscular layer is composed of the inner circular and the outer longitudinal layers. The inner circular layer varies in depth, being lean around the cecum and colon, but much thicker in the rectum. The longitudinal muscle fibers, although forming a continuous layer, are concentrated into three flat, strong bands called *teniae coli*. These bands are equidistant around the circumference of the bowel but are not quite as long as the large intestine. Subsequently, the large intestine is puckered into sacculations known as **haustra.**

Colonic Motility

The movement of the chyme feces is much slower in the large intestine than in the small intestine. The colon does appear to have intrinsic bioelectrical slow waves, but they remain under investigation.

Mixing movements, or ***haustrations,*** occur with the simultaneous contraction of the circular and longitudinal muscle layers. Like the segmentation in the small intestine, these haustrations slowly churn the fecal material to ensure adequate contact with the intestinal wall for absorption to take place. Secondary to the haustrations is the sauntering propulsion of the fecal material toward the anus, especially in the cecal and ascending colonic regions.

The ***propulsive*** or ***mass movements*** are responsible for the projection of the feces from the transverse colon to the sigmoid. These occur only two to three times in a 24-hour period. Distension stimulates a circular contraction, which initiates a simultaneous contraction of 8 to 10 inches or more of the distal colon, propelling the fecal material toward the anus. When the rectum is distended by the injected fecal mass, defecation is initiated.

Since the rectum is usually empty, the defecation reflex is spurred by the fecal material stretching the rectal wall. Both involuntary and voluntary responses are involved. The anal-rectal reflex, or spinal reflex, causes the internal anal sphincter to relax by receptive relaxation and the external anal sphincter to contract. The need to defecate is now a conscious process, with the individual having the capability of deciding to defecate or to suppress the urge. Now the process becomes voluntary, with the individual relaxing the external anal sphincter. A Valsalva maneuver often assists defecation with the inspiration of a deep breath, contracting the chest and abdominal muscles, which increases intraabdominal pressure. This increased pressure is transmitted to the large intestine and facilitates the passage of stool.

Pharmacological agents, diet and disease states have different effects on the motor activities of the large intestine. Inhibitory agents include a low-bulk diet and any anticholinergic drugs, such as atropine, that work by blocking parasympathetic transmission. Ganglionic blocking agents also have an inhibitory effect because of interference of the transmission of the nerve impulses. Stimulatory agents include morphine and the parasympathomimetic drugs (urecholine, neostigmine). Irritation of the colon due to increased bile salts, bacterial enterotoxins or diseased states such as ulcerative colitis, will also have stimulatory effects on the colonic motility.

Colonic Functions

The main function of the colon is absorption of water and electrolytes. The majority of this absorption occurs in the proximal half of the colon. The large intestine is presented with about 500 cc of fluid daily. It absorbs around 350 cc of this, leaving approximately 150 cc to be excreted in the feces. The large intestine is capable of absorbing up to 2 to 2.5 liters per day if the small intestinal absorption is inadequate. This voluminous water absorption is accompanied by absorption of solutes, mainly sodium and various hydrolyzed foodstuffs. Sodium is actively absorbed against larger electrochemical gradients at a rate sensitive to aldosterone. Potassium secretion appears to be passive. Chloride absorption is both active and passive. In some regions, bicarbonate appears to be secreted in exchange for luminal chloride.

The colon serves as a host for many normal flora bacteria. Their purpose is to help in the breakdown of small amounts of cellulose. The bacteria also provide a means of synthesizing important vitamins, such as K, riboflavin, nicotinic acid and folic acid. A negative action of the bacteria is their decomposition of urea to ammonia and carbon dioxide. This only poses a problem in the individual with hepatic failure.

Approximately 135 gm of feces is eliminated daily. The normal brown color of feces is due to the derivatives of bilirubin. The vast majority of the fecal material is water. Only one fourth of the daily excrement is made of solid material. Included in this solid material is sloughed epithelial cells, undigestible cellulose, dead bacteria, fat, protein and inorganic material.

KEY CONCEPT: The lower G.I. system is composed of the small and large intestines and functions to absorb nutrients and excrete body wastes.

KEY POINT RECOGNITION
Write true or false by each statement. Answers are at the end of this chapter. A score below 80% indicates the need for further study.

_____ 1. The greatest amount of digestion and absorption takes place in the large intestine.

_____ 2. The small intestine is composed of two segments: the duodenum and jejunum.

_____ 3. The ileocecal valve connects the small and large intestines.

_____ 4. The Kerckring's folds increase the surface area of the small intestine for absorption.

_____ 5. Peyer's patches synthesize antibodies.

_____ 6. Brunner's glands secrete an acetic mucoid substance.

_____ 7. An electrical rhythm is responsible for the timing of small intestinal contractions.

_____ 8. Segmental movements of the small intestine serve to mix the contents with digestive juices, as well as to bring the contents in contact with the mucosa.

_____ 9. Peristalsis is triggered by distension of the intestine.

_____10. Peristalsis occurs at a faster rate in the duodenum than in the ileum.
_____11. Energy is required for the transport of sodium and potassium into or out of a cell.
_____12. Passive diffusion is the movement along a gradient from an area of higher concentration to an area of lower concentration.
_____13. Amino acids and calcium are two examples of substances that move in and out of cells by the process of passive diffusion.
_____14. Facilitated diffusion is the movement of a substance by means of a carrier from a higher concentration to a lower concentration. Energy in the form of ATP is required.
_____15. Sodium is actively absorbed in the G.I. tract.
_____16. Potassium is passively absorbed in the small intestine, while actively secreted in the large intestine.
_____17. Calcium and iron absorption is a body-regulated mechanism.
_____18. The absorption of vitamin B_{12} is through a carrier and depends on the binding of B_{12} to the intrinsic factor synthesized by the parietal cells.
_____19. Carbohydrates must be broken down for absorption.
_____20. The majority of carbohydrates are absorbed in the polysaccharide form.
_____21. Amylase transforms starch to maltose.
_____22. Amylase is produced in the microvilli of the intestinal mucosal cells.
_____23. Sucrase breaks sucrose into glucose and galactose.
_____24. There are 22 essential amino acids.
_____25. Pepsin initiates protein digestion by stimulating the release of gastrin.
_____26. Trypsin is a protease.
_____27. Amino acids absorption is active.
_____28. Lipase splits triglycerides into free fatty acids and monoglycerides.
_____29. Micelles provide a means for fat product substances to diffuse into the mucosal cell.
_____30. Bile salts are also diffused into the cell.
_____31. The presence of chyme in the small intestine is the major control for secretion of intestinal juices.
_____32. Secretin stimulates insulin output, pepsin secretion and bile flow.
_____33. The presence of fats and carbohydrates in the duodenum signals the release of gastric inhibitory peptide.
_____34. The three divisions of the large intestine include the cecum, colon and anus.
_____35. Goblet cells of the large intestine produce large amounts of mucus.
_____36. Haustrations ensure adequate contact of the intestinal material with the intestinal wall.
_____37. Propulsive movements in the large intestine occur five to six times an hour.
_____38. Ganglionic blocking agents have an inhibitory effect on colonic motility.
_____39. Approximately 150 cc of the 500 cc of water present daily in the intestine is reabsorbed.
_____40. Normal flora bacteria of the large intestine decompose urea to ammonia and carbon dioxide.

BLOOD SUPPLY TO THE G.I. TRACT

The arterial supply of the G.I. tract stems from the *aorta*. The upper G.I. tract is supplied by the branching of the *celiac artery,* as listed below.

Celiac Branch	Supplies
Left gastric	Stomach, esophagus
Hepatic (right gastric)	Stomach
Gastroduodenal	Stomach, duodenum
Cystic	Gallbladder
Splenic	Stomach, pancreas, spleen

The middle G.I. tract is supplied by the *superior mesenteric artery*. This branch stems from the abdominal aorta and supplies the jejunum, ileum, cecum, ascending colon and part of the transverse colon.

The lower G.I. tract is supplied by the *inferior mesenteric artery*. Also from the abdominal aorta, this branch provides the transverse, descending and sigmoid colon, plus the rectum, with arterial flow.

The venous blood from the majority of the G.I. tract is emptied into the liver via the *portal venous system*. Listed below are the branches that return blood to the portal vein.

Branch	Returns blood from:
Gastric	Stomach, esophagus
Splenic	Stomach, esophagus, duodenum, pancreas, gallbladder
Superior mesenteric	Small intestine, ascending and transverse colon
Inferior mesenteric	Descending and sigmoid colon, rectum

In the liver, the portal vein gives rise to smaller branches, which drain with branches of the hepatic artery into the liver sinusoids. This drainage flows into the central vein, which forms the *hepatic vein,* which empties into the *inferior vena cava.*

KEY CONCEPT: The arterial blood supply of the G.I. tract stems from the aorta. The upper G.I. tract is supplied by the celiac artery; the middle G.I. tract by the superior mesenteric artery; and the lower G.I. tract by the inferior mesenteric artery.

Venous blood is emptied into the liver via the portal venous system, into the hepatic vein and into the inferior vena cava.

KEY POINT RECOGNITION

Write true or false by each statement. Answers are at the end of this chapter. A score below 80% indicates the need for further study.

_____ 1. The splenic branch of the celiac artery supplies the stomach, pancreas and spleen.

_____ 2. The superior mesenteric artery supplies the jejunum, ileum, cecum and part of the colon.

_____ 3. The inferior mesenteric artery supplies the colon and rectum.

_____ 4. The gastric branch of the portal venous system returns blood from the stomach and esophagus.

_____ 5. The central vein forms the hepatic vein.

NERVOUS INNERVATON

The G.I. tract contains extrinsic and intrinsic autonomic nervous system innervation. The intrinsic nerves, which are located inside the wall of the gut, are responsible for motor, secretory and sensory functions. These include the major plexuses of Meissner and Auerbach. These branch to form minor plexuses beneath the serosa, the mucosa and the circular muscle layer.

The intrinsic nerves are influenced by the extrinsic nerves of the autonomic nervous system. Parasympathetic innervation comes mainly from the vagus nerve (cranial X) and from the sacral nerves. Acetylcholine, the parasympathetic neurotransmitter, is responsible for the stimulation of all functions of the gut. Sympathetic innervation traverses via the paravertebral ganglia. These fibers innervate all organs of the gut and release norepinephrine at their end terminals.

KEY CONCEPT: The G.I. tract is innervated by extrinsic and intrinsic nerves of the autonomic nervous system.

KEY POINT RECOGNITION
Write true or false by each statement. Answers are at the end of this chapter.

_____ 1. The intrinsic nerves are responsible for motor function only.

_____ 2. Parasympathetic innervation comes mainly from the 10th cranial nerve.

_____ 3. Acetylcholine inhibits the functions of the gut.

_____ 4. The sympathetic neurotransmitter is acetylcholine.

ACCESSORY ORGANS OF DIGESTION

The anatomy and physiology of the G.I. tract are not complete without discussing the important accessory organs. These include the *gallbladder,* the *pancreas* and the *liver.*

Gallbladder

The *gallbladder* is a pear-shaped organ located in a fossa on the undersurface of the liver. This musculomembranous sac has the capacity to store about 50 cc of bile. It is anatomically divided into a fundus, which is curved and protrudes from the inferior boundary of the liver; a body; and a neck, which joins the body with the cystic duct (Fig. 8-4). The blood supply to the gallbladder arrives via the cystic artery, which is a branch of the right hepatic artery. Venous drainage is accomplished via the cystic vein. A branch of the vagus nerve provides the innervation to the gallbladder. The main function of the gallbladder is to serve as a storage tank for bile. It also has the ability to concentrate the bile.

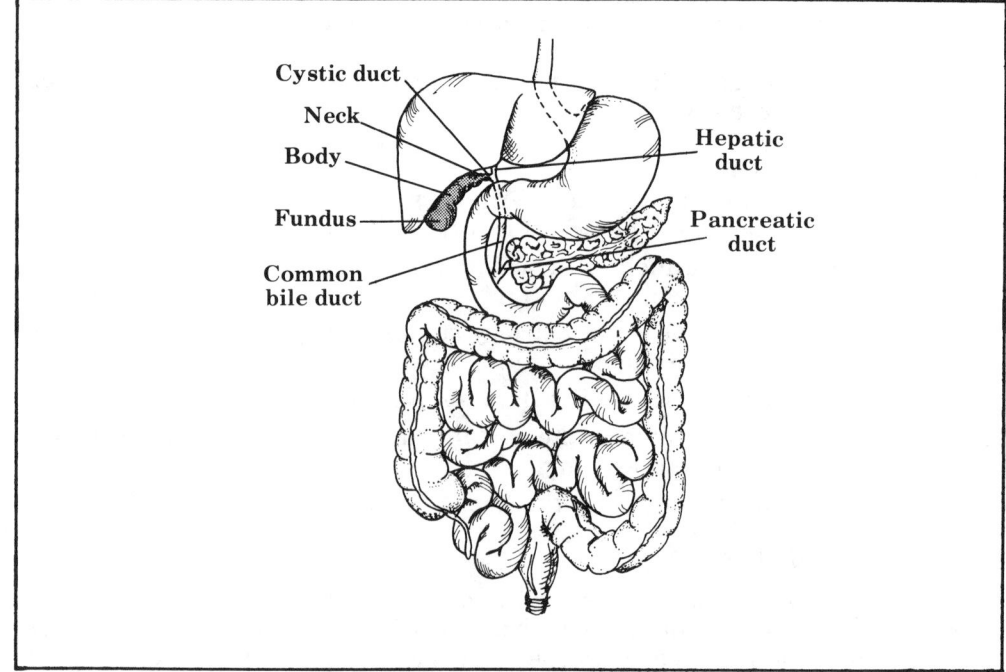

Fig. 8-4 Gallbladder

The cystic duct measures about 1.5 inches. It attaches the neck of the gallbladder to the common hepatic duct, and these two combine to form the common bile duct. At the entrance to the duodenum, the circular muscle around the terminal end of the common bile duct thickens; this area is called Oddi's sphincter. It is believed that this sphincter relaxes when the hormone cholecystokinin is released, which causes the gallbladder to contract. Cholecystokinin release is stimulated by the presence of fat or acid in the duodenum.

The liver continuously secretes bile at an average daily rate of 800 to 1,000 cc. As the bile is produced, it enters the spaces between the hepatic cells, called canaliculi. The bile flows toward the periphery of the liver lobule, where it eventually is collected into one large duct from each lobe. These two ducts combine to form the hepatic duct. Depending on the body's needs, the bile either flows into the cystic duct and to the gallbladder for storage, or continues down the hepatic duct, which becomes continuous with the common bile duct, which terminates at the duodenum.

The major constituents of bile are bile acids, water, electrolytes, bilirubin, lecithin, cholesterol and other miscellaneous metabolites. The importance of the bile salts was mentioned in the section on fat digestion and absorption. The bile salts form the micelles, which emulsify the fats and transport the fat to the mucosal wall for absorption. The bile salts are not diffused into the intestinal mucosal cells, but the majority are absorbed in the ileum and transported back to the liver for a recycling process called **enterohepatic circulation.** A small percentage of bile salts is excreted in the feces, but these are readily replaced by the continuous production occurring in the hepatic cells.

The color of bile is due to the chief bile pigment, bilirubin. The breakdown of hemoglobin causes the formation of bilirubin. The presence of bilirubin is the causative factor for the normal brown color of the feces. Any blockage in the flow of bile causes an accumulation of the bile pigments in the blood and tissues. As a result, jaundice appears.

What exactly is bilirubin? A red blood cell's life span averages 120 days. Once a red blood cell's membrane becomes fragile, it ruptures, causing a release of hemoglobin. The hemoglobin is split into globin and heme. The reticuloendothelial cells convert the heme into bilirubin and release it into the bloodstream. The bilirubin binds to albumin in the bloodstream to be transported to the liver. This form of bilirubin is fat-soluble and termed unconjugated, free or indirect bilirubin. Albumin-associated bilirubin is soluble enough for transport, but not soluble enough for efficient excretion. So the next stop for processing is the liver.

In the liver, the bilirubin is removed from the associated albumin. It undergoes a binding with glucuronic acid, a modified glucose molecule. This new formation is now water-soluble and termed conjugated or direct bilirubin. The words "direct" and "indirect" are references to laboratory tests that determine how quickly a certain reaction takes place. The conjugated bilirubin is now able to be excreted into bile.

As the bile is delivered to the intestinal tract, the intestinal microorganisms convert most of the bilirubin to urobilinogen. Some of this urobilinogen is reabsorbed and subsequently excreted in the urine, giving urine its typical amber color. The rest of the urobilinogen travels to the lower part of the intestine, where further bacterial action converts it to stercobilin. Stercobilin provides the natural brown color to the feces.

When jaundice is present, it is critical to differentiate the pathophysiology. This can be accomplished by measuring the levels of both conjugated and unconjugated bilirubin blood levels. In some institutions, the results are reported as a total bilirubin and a direct bilirubin. The indirect bilirubin can be determined by subtracting the direct bilirubin from the total bilirubin. An elevated direct bilirubin is indicative of a biliary tract obstruction, whereas an elevated indirect bilirubin is indicative of liver dysfunction.

Pancreas

The *pancreas* is located in the epigastric and left hypochondriac regions of the abdomen. It is a soft, lobulated organ that measures about four to six inches long (Fig. 8-5). The pancreas is divided into the head, which rests in the concavity of the duodenum; the body, which extends toward the spleen; and the tail, which is in contact with the spleen. The main duct of the pancreas is called Wirsung's duct, which starts in the tail and traverses the length of the organ. The Wirsung's duct joins the common bile duct, and as these two ducts pass into the wall of the duodenum, they form a short dilated area called the Vater's ampulla.

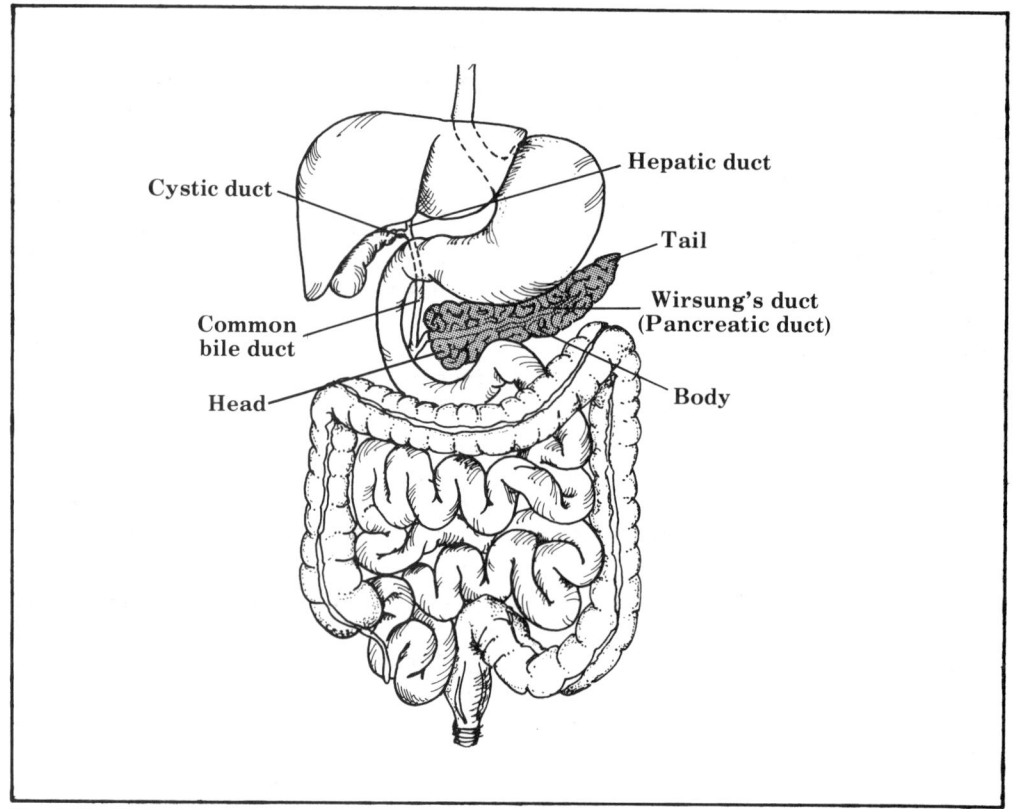

Fig. 8-5 Pancreas

The pancreas is both an *exocrine* and an *endocrine* gland. Our discussion here will be limited to the exocrine functions. Refer to the chapter on the endocrine system for coverage of the pancreas' endocrine function.

The exocrine function of the pancreas is due to the exocrine secretory units called the *acini*. The amount of pancreatic secretion adds about 1,500 cc to the total daily secretion of intestinal juices.

The acinar cells secrete a group of digestive enzymes that are capable of digesting all useful fats, proteins and carbohydrates. These pancreatic enzymes are most efficient when working in a neutral pH. The proteolytic enzymes, the major one being trypsin, are secreted in an inactive form to prevent self-digestion of the pancreas. Further catalyzing agents are required in the duodenum for the trypsin to break the amino acid bonds of the proteins. Small amounts of trypsin are secreted in an active form, but the pancreas also synthesizes a small amount of trypsin inhibitor to control the trypsin secreted. This inhibitor blocks the small amount of active trypsin until the enzyme is safely in the duodenum.

Pancreatic amylase is responsible for breaking down polysaccharides for carbohydrate absorption. Lipase breaks down triglycerides for fat absorption.

These pancreatic enzymes are transported into the duodenum in an isotonic, bicarbonate-rich electrolyte solution. This solution is another very essential production of the pancreas and is secreted by the intercalated ducts. This alkaline solution (pH around 8) has several functions: 1) it neutralizes the acid chyme in the duodenum; 2) it facilitates fat emulsification; and 3) it provides the necessary neutral working environment for the pancreatic enzymes.

Secretion of this electrolyte solution is stimulated by the hormones gastrin and secretin, and by the combination of secretin and PZ-CCK. A cholinergic vagal reflex initiated by the presence of fat and protein digests in the duodenum also stimulates pancreatic secretion.

Liver

The *liver* weighs about three pounds in an adult and qualifies as the largest organ of the body (Fig. 8-6). It is found in the upper abdominal cavity, under the dome of the diaphragm, in the epigastric and right hypochondriac regions. Four main lobes of the liver have been described. The two main lobes are the right and the left, which are divided by the falciform ligament. The right lobe is further divided into the caudate and quadrate lobes. These lobes are then divided into numerous lobules that are the functional units of the liver.

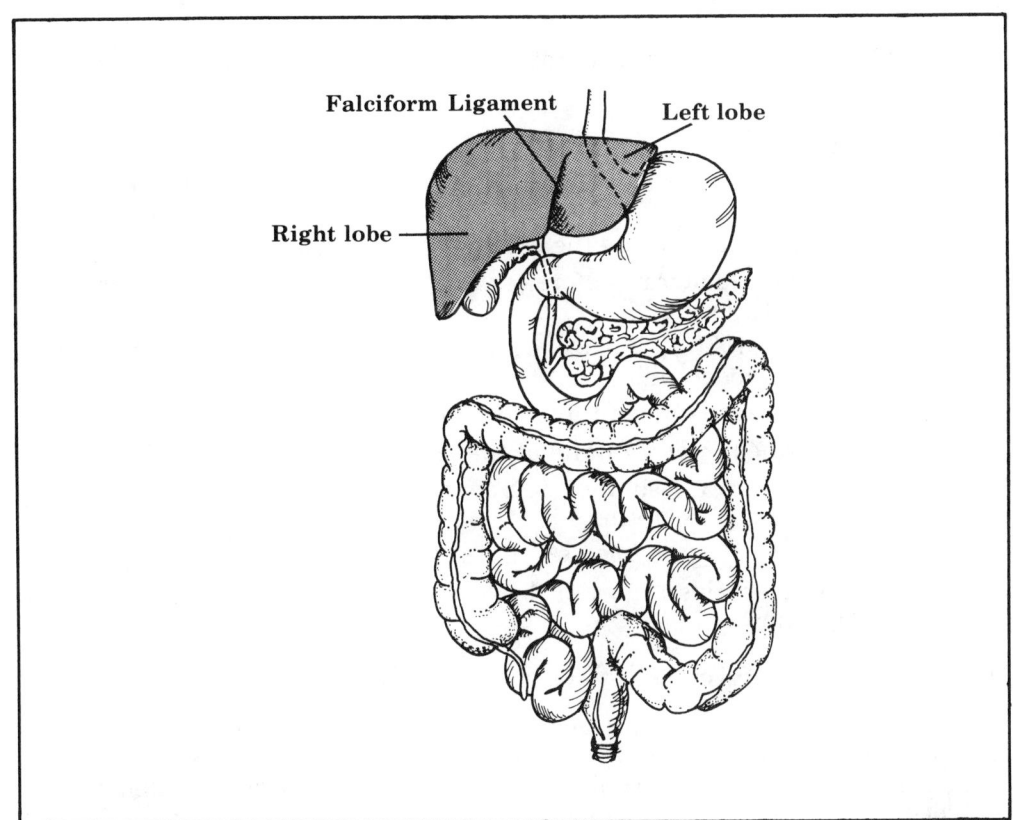

Fig. 8-6 Liver

Each lobule is constructed of thin plates of hepatic cells that branch out irregularly from the center of the lobule to its periphery. The sinusoids are found interspersed in the plates of cells. These are microscopic channels that receive blood from the hepatic artery and the portal vein. The blood then flows into the central vein of the lobule, to the hepatic vein and ultimately out the inferior vena cava. Since there are millions of sinusoids, the liver can be likened to a vast sponge. Large quantities of blood can be held in the liver at any given time, which can certainly influence the circulating blood volume.

Describing the specific functions of the liver is beyond the scope of this discussion. As it pertains to the G.I. system, the liver does not secrete digestive hormones or enzymes. Its contribution to digestion is made by its secretion of bile salts. The importance of bile salts in fat digestion has been previously covered.

Following is a list of a few of the cellular functions of the liver:
  (1) Bile secretion
  (2) Protein, carbohydrate and fat metabolism
  (3) Amino acid synthesis
  (4) Fatty acid and fat synthesis
  (5) Blood protein synthesis, including clotting factors, complement proteins and albumin
  (6) Gluconeogenesis
  (7) Glycogen storage and release
  (8) Vitamin and mineral storage
  (9) Urea formation
  (10) Drug, hormone and potential toxin processing

KEY CONCEPT: The accessory organs of the G.I. tract are the gallbladder, pancreas and liver.

The gallbladder stores bile; the pancreas secretes digestive enzymes; and the liver secretes bile salts.

KEY POINT RECOGNITION

Write true or false by each statement. Answers are at the end of this chapter. A score below 80% indicates the need for further study.

_____ 1. The gallbladder has the capacity to store 150 cc of bile.

_____ 2. The gallbladder is a storage tank for bile, but also has the ability to concentrate the bile.

_____ 3. Cholecystokinin release is stimulated by the presence of fat or acid in the duodenum.

_____ 4. The pancreas is both an exocrine and endocrine gland.

_____ 5. Exocrine secretory units of the pancreas are called acini.

_____ 6. The electrolyte solution secreted by the pancreas is stimulated by gastrin and secretin.

_____ 7. The liver does not secrete digestive enzymes.

_____ 8. The liver aids digestion by secreting bile salts, which aid in fat digestion.

PHYSICAL ASSESSMENT OF THE GASTROINTESTINAL SYSTEM

Physical assessment of the patient experiencing gastrointestinal dysfunction is not very different from the assessment of any other patient. Significant medical problems, current therapies, family history and review of systems are all included. Particular attention must be paid to the presenting complaint, its duration, character and circumstances surrounding exacerbations and remissions.

HISTORY

As with any other disease state, the history of the patient with G.I. disorders is an important part of the assessment. Naturally, the extent of the interview depends on the condition of the individual patient. Whenever possible, the following questions should be asked:

  (1) Has there been a previous hospitalization? If so, for what?
  (2) Is the patient currently taking medications? What are they?
  (3) Are there allergies to any foods or medications?
  (4) How much coffee does the patient drink?
  (4) Is there a history of G.I. bleeding? of liver disease? of anemia? of pancreatic disease?

(5) Is there a history of heart disease? high blood pressure? stroke? cancer? any chronic problems?

(6) What is the patient's present occupation?

(7) Has there been a recent exposure to someone with a contagious disease?

(8) Are alcoholic beverages drunk? How much and how often?

(9) Has there been recent weight loss or gain?

(10) Has there been any change in eating habits?

(11) Does the patient suffer from heartburn? When does it occur? What relieves it?

(12) Are there periods of nausea? When do these periods occur?

(13) Is there vomiting? When? What does the vomited material look like?

(14) Have there been any change in bowel habits? Is constipation a problem? Does the patient use laxatives? How often? Is there diarrhea? How often? What color are stools?

(15) Is there pain in the abdomen? Where is it located? Is it sharp, dull or gnawing? Does it radiate to any place? When does (did) the pain begin? Is the pain relieved by changing body position?

(16) Do the gums ever bleed spontaneously or when brushing teeth?

(17) Have there been more bruises on the skin than is usual?

(18) How many pillows are slept on at night?

While asking these questions, the astute nurse will also be making observations about the patient. The general condition of the skin gives clues to the patient's health habits and nutritional status. The level of anxiety can also be judged by the body language and responses of the patient.

It is very important to establish a good rapport with the patient during this first interview. Attempt to put the patient at ease and gain trust. Be alert for certain communication problems. If needed, engage the assistance of an interpreter. Tailor your language to the educational background of the patient. The information gained from this interview will be useless unless it is valid.

It is of paramount importance to maintain a nonjudgmental attitude when dealing with patients. This becomes difficult when the same patient is admitted routinely for alcohol-induced bleeding. The critical care nurse must realize that the physical signs of bleeding are masking a very serious psychological problem with which the patient is unable to cope. Total support and understanding must be shown to the patient.

Physical examination should include a thorough head-to-toe assessment, with emphasis placed on the *examination* of the *abdomen.* The techniques of *inspection, auscultation, percussion* and *palpation* are used when examining the abdomen. For continuity and ease of description, the abdomen is divided into sections in two ways. One way describes the abdomen in terms of quadrants formed by imaginary intersecting lines through the umbilicus. The resulting four quadrants are called the right upper, right lower, left upper and left lower quadrants (Fig. 8-7).

The second method of division sections the abdomen into nine areas for greater specificity of identifying the underlying organs. Four imaginary lines are drawn: two vertical parallel lines running from each costal margin to the inguinal ligament, and two intersecting horizontal parallel lines, one under the rib cage and one connecting the iliac crests. The resulting areas are termed the right hypochondriac, right lumbar, right inguinal, epigastric, umbilical, hypogastric, left hypochondriac, left lumbar and left inguinal (Fig. 8-8).

INSPECTION

Inspection of the abdomen is best done with the patient in a supine position, with the observer at the patient's side. The contour of the abdomen should be observed, along with a notation of symmetry. The abdominal skin should be inspected for presence of rashes, scars, vascular nevi or wounds. Dilated veins noted on the abdomen usually indicate a problem of obstruction in the inferior

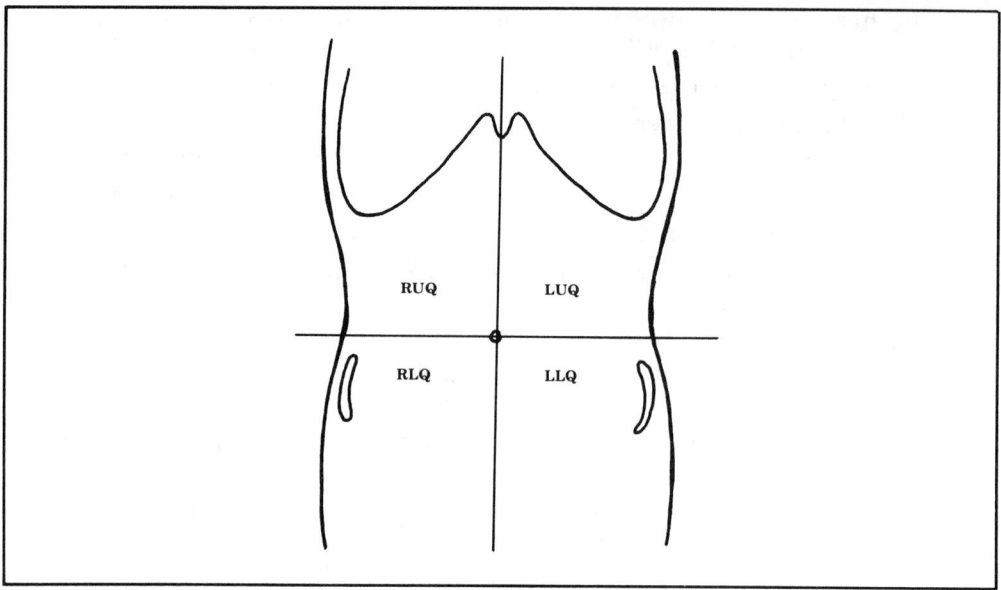

Fig. 8-7 Division of the abdomen into four quadrants

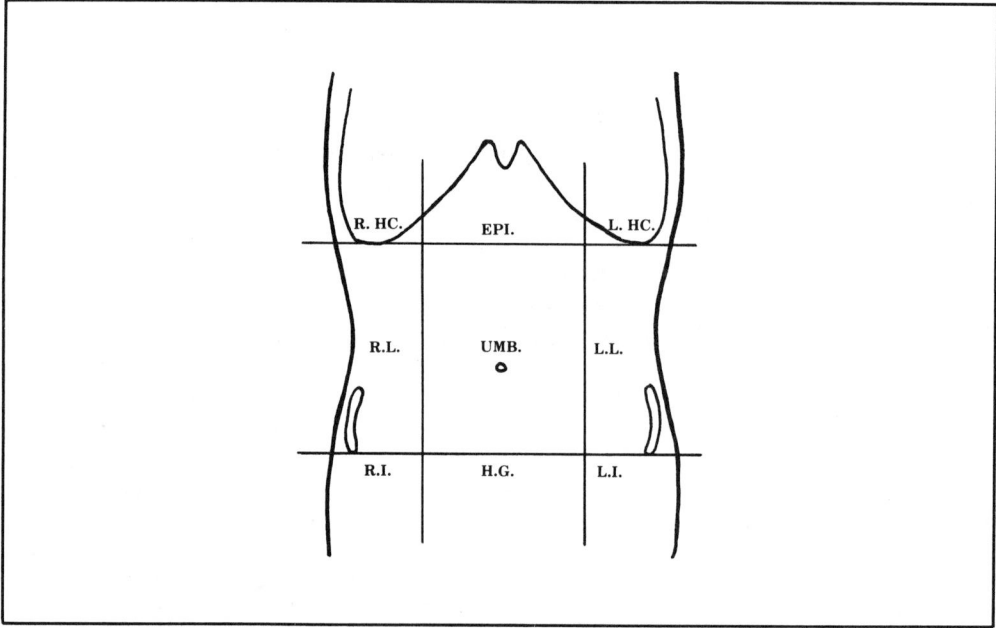

Fig. 8-8 Division of the abdomen into nine areas

vena cava. The shape and the presence of herniation of the umbilicus should be noted. If a mass is present, it may be seen if it is protuberant enough. By looking across the abdomen in the epigastric area, the normal aortic pulsation may be visualized. If the patient is quite emaciated, actual peristalsis may be viewed.

AUSCULTATION

The next step of the abdominal examination is *auscultation.* All four quadrants of the abdomen should be listened to for several minutes with the diaphragm of the stethoscope. The normal bowel sounds are caused by the movement of both air and water through the tube of the intestine. These sounds vary from barely distinguishable low reverberations to louder, high-pitched noises. With the presence of other coinciding events, certain diagnoses can be made when alterations of these normal sounds are heard. Concomitant with colicky abdominal pain, intense rushing peristalsis, termed borborygmus, is indicative of an intestinal obstruction. Other sounds that may be heard in the abdomen include a venous hum, friction rub and bruits. A venous hum is an infrequent finding, but may occur in the cirrhotic patient with a massive portal-systemic shunt from portal hypertension. It would be audible as a sustained sound in the epigastric region. Peritoneal friction rubs are also rare and are associated with irritation of the contact area between the peritoneum and the spleen. If audible over the liver, the rub may indicate a malignancy. Bruits may be heard over any of the major abdominal arteries if there is turbulent flow due to partial obstruction. It is essential to complete auscultation before proceeding to percussion and palpation, since the thumping and prodding may modify the frequency of the bowel sounds.

PERCUSSION

Percussion of the abdomen reveals the presence of air and fluid in the cavity and helps to judge the size of some abdominal organs. In the normal abdomen, the predominant finding will be the hollow tympanic sound from the air in the G.I. tract, except for the dullness found over the liver and the spleen. The area of the liver should be percussed, with an estimate of its borders made at the right midclavicular line and at the midsternal line. Different conditions interfere with the dullness of the liver, such as a pleural effusion; caution must be taken before a diagnosis of liver enlargement is made. One sign of a perforated viscus is an undistinguishable liver dullness, caused by free air under the diaphragm. The stomach, when devoid, is tympanic and can be normally percussed around the left lower rib cage. Should this area of tympany encompass a larger area and be accompanied by abdominal distension, gastric dilatation should be suspected. Splenic dullness is located posteriorly to the midaxillary line at the level of the 10th rib.

PALPATION

Palpation is the last and probably most important step in evaluating the abdomen. The patient should still be in a supine position and should have an empty bladder. Palpation is used to detect the presence and character of masses, to define the normal abdominal organs and to verify any organomegaly. To palpate the liver, place one hand under the patient at the level of the 11th rib, with pressure exerted upward. Place the other hand on the right abdominal wall below the lower margin of liver dullness, with the fingertips pushed in and up toward the right costal margin. The liver edge may be felt as the patient takes a deep breath. Normally, this edge presents as a sharp, firm object with a smooth surface. If the liver is enlarged, hard, firm and very irregular, a malignancy should be suspected. The liver in the cirrhotic patient is usually enlarged, smooth and not tender. If the edge is tender, hepatitis should be suspected. The spleen must increase its surface area several times before it becomes palpable.

Palpation is also useful in differentiating pain. Since the organs have minimal pain receptors, visceral pain is described as a generalized and dull pain. There is usually no associated muscular rigidity. An intestinal obstruction elicits visceral pain. When the peritoneum is inflamed, the associated pain is localized and sharp. This kind of pain is referred to as somatic and is elicited in conditions such as appendicitis or cholecystitis. Rebound tenderness is the excruciating pain provoked when the palpating hand is suddenly lifted off the abdomen. This pain is indicative of peritoneal inflammation. Another sign of peritoneal inflammation is the presence of involuntary rigidity of the abdominal muscles.

KEY CONCEPT: Physical assessment of the patient with a gastrointestinal disorder should include both history and physical examination. The physical examination is performed using the techniques of inspection, auscultation, percussion and palpation.

KEY POINT RECOGNITION

Write true or false by each statement. Answers are at the end of this chapter. A score below 80% indicates the need for further study.

    _____ 1. A detailed history from the patient or a reliable source is an important part of the assessment.

    _____ 2. The skin gives clues as to the health habits and nutritional status of the patient.

    _____ 3. In patients experiencing a gastrointestinal disorder, emphasis is placed on examination of the abdomen.

    _____ 4. Dilated veins noted on the abdomen usually indicate an obstruction in the inferior vena cava.

    _____ 5. A pulsation in the epigastric area is indicative of an abnormality of the aorta.

    _____ 6. With peritonitis, ileus or gangrene, bowel sounds may be hyperactive.

    _____ 7. Borborygmus is indicative of intestinal obstruction.

    _____ 8. A venous hum occurs in the absence of portal hypertension.

    _____ 9. Percussion of the stomach produces a tympanic sound.

    _____10. A cirrhotic liver is usually enlarged, nodular and tender.

NURSING ASSESSMENT OF THE G.I. SYSTEM

Nursing assessment of the gastrointestinal system helps in the preparation of a nursing care plan, contributes to the medical plan and provides for nursing intervention. Included in the assessment are: *eating, swallowing reflex, digestion, elimination* and *evaluation of vital signs.*

By chewing and mastication, the mouth, teeth, tongue, walls of the cheeks and palate prepare the food for swallowing. They break food fibers into smaller portions and stimulate taste buds. The major function of saliva is to lubricate and moisten the particles to facilitate swallowing.

EVALUATION OF EATING

To evaluate *eating,* the following must be determined:

Condition of teeth—Ill patients do not eat or salivate normally. Merely swabbing the mouth and teeth with glycerine and lemon is inadequate. Mechanical cleaning is the most effective treatment. Observe the teeth and gums for signs of infection and periodontal disease, such as pyorrhea or gingivitis. Dentures require careful cleaning with mechanical action.

Condition of the mouth—Observe for cold sores, fever blisters, canker, gingivitis, bleeding, moniliasis, thrush and lesions. Nursing care is directed toward controlling and treating the problem, reducing odorous breath, providing comfort and maintaining good nutrition.

EVALUATION OF SWALLOWING

Does the food or fluid cause any discomfort, difficulty, belching, flatulence, distention, fullness, abnormal taste or pain? Does the patient aspirate?

EVALUATION OF DIGESTION

Is any reflux of food related to eating? Is there pain, nausea, vomiting, odor to vomitus or vomitus containing digested particles?

EVALUATION OF ELIMINATION

Evaluate bowel habits, diarrhea, constipation, color of stool, odor, frequency, flatulence or pain.

EVALUATION OF VITAL SIGNS

The blood pressure may be normal or elevated. Rarely in a gastrointestinal disorder is **hypotension** seen unless bleeding occurs or hypovolemia occurs because of large fluid losses. Hypertension may be seen in **portal hypertension.**

Changes in the pulse or respiration are directly related to the pathology involved.

LABORATORY AND RADIOLOGIC STUDIES

Laboratory studies in gastrointestinal disorders are varied and tailored to the presumptive diagnosis at hand. A detailed discussion of possible studies is covered in the case studies. *Radiologic studies* are briefly discussed here.

The **upper G.I. series** may help diagnose disorders of the stomach, such as visualization of a crater in ulcerative disease. It is also useful in tracking the motility of the G.I. tract by use of fluoroscopy several hours after barium ingestion. Barium enemas may establish the presence of disorders of the colon.

Endoscopy has become the test of choice for the critically ill patient. The endoscopic examination is indicated when abnormal, but undifferentiated, G.I. radiographs have been obtained in the presence of upper G.I. bleeding. Endoscopy is also indicated to remove foreign bodies and to evaluate peptic ulcer disease. The contraindications of endoscopy include coagulation disorders, perforation and an uncooperative patient.

One of the newest endoscopic techniques is endoscopic retrograde cholangiopancreatography (ERCP). This procedure consists of placing a catheter into the Vater's ampulla to collect secretions. The pancreatic and biliary ductal systems are also visualized by the retrograde injection of contrast material. The ERCP is used for the patient with jaundice to exclude extrahepatic obstructions and to diagnose pancreatic disease.

Cholangiograms are used to evaluate the biliary ductal system. Different techniques (operative, intravenous, percutaneous transhepatic) are available for testing, but all include the injection of dye followed by fluoroscopic visualization.

Radionuclide scans have helped decrease the mortality in disease states that were formerly difficult to diagnose. Subphrenic and subhepatic abscesses become readily apparent after injection of the radioisotopes and scanning. The progression of liver disease can also be judged by this examination.

Computerized tomography is successful at locating problem areas in patients that present with the symptom of abdominal pain. Pancreatic pseudocysts, abscesses and tumors are readily diagnosed by CT scans.

Gastric analysis, to a great extent, is being replaced by more recent advances in endoscopy. It cannot establish the diagnosis of peptic ulcer disease. Gastric analysis may still be used to diagnose the Zollinger-Ellison syndrome (a tumor of the pancreas or duodenum that markedly increases gastric secretion). This test may determine the adequacy of a vagotomy or evaluate certain drug effects.

KEY CONCEPT: Nursing assessment of the patient with a gastrointestinal disorder includes the evaluation of eating, swallowing, digestion, elimination and vital signs.

Computerized tomography is successful at locating problem areas in patients that present with the symptom of abdominal pain. Pancreatic pseudocysts, abscesses, and tumors are readily diagnosed by CT scans.

KEY POINT RECOGNITION

Write true or false by each statement. Answers are at the end of this chapter. A score below 80% indicates the need for further study.

_____ 1. Laboratory data are the most important determinant of a gastrointestinal disorder.

_____ 2. An upper G.I. series is used to diagnose disorders of the stomach.

_____ 3. Endoscopic retrograde cholangiopancreatography is used for patients with jaundice to exclude extrahepatic obstructions and to diagnose pancreatic disease.

_____ 4. Gastric analysis establishes the diagnosis of peptic ulcer disease.
_____ 5. Endoscopy is contraindicated in the presence of coagulation disorders and perforation.
_____ 6. Swabbing the teeth with lemon and glycerine is adequate oral care.
_____ 7. The condition of the mouth, ability to swallow and bowel habits are important assessments of the G.I. system.

PATHOLOGICAL STATES AND NURSING MANAGEMENT

CIRRHOSIS OF THE LIVER

Pathophysiology

The general pathophysiological process of cirrhosis begins as the liver cells are destroyed. The destroyed cells are replaced by fibrous, connective tissue which is not part of the normal tissue of the liver. As this fibrotic tissue grows, it has a tendency toward overgrowth. The regenerative overgrowth completely changes the normal structure of the lobule, resulting in irregular shapes. The irregular shapes, in turn, cause a displacement or even absence of an identifiable central vein. The resultant congestion and impedance to portal blood flow lead to the often fatal sequelae of cirrhosis (Fig. 8-9).

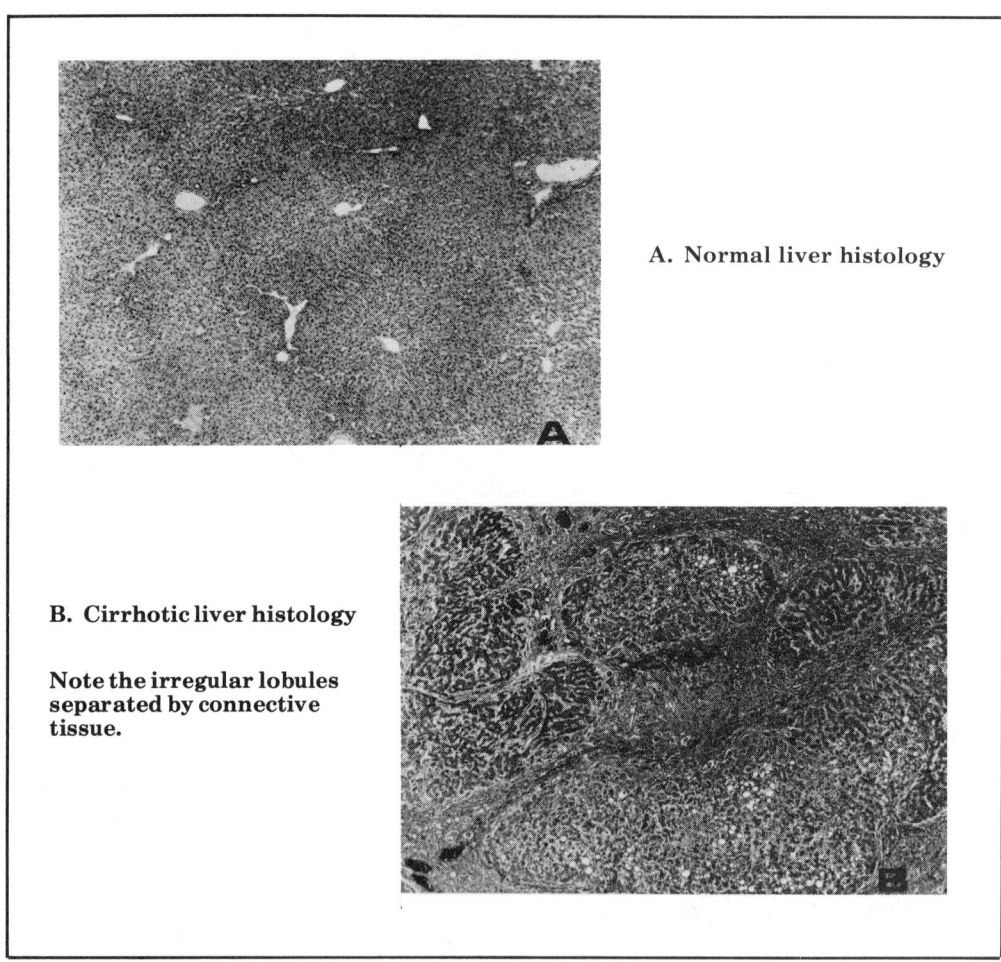

A. Normal liver histology

B. Cirrhotic liver histology

Note the irregular lobules separated by connective tissue.

Fig. 8-9 Liver histology

Three specific pathological types of cirrhosis have been described: 1) Laennec's (alcoholic, fatty), 2) postnecrotic (posthepatic), and 3) biliary (obstructive, cholangitic). The results of these specific pathological types are the same. Their differences can only be seen morphologically, obtained by liver biopsy or by postmortem examination.

Laennec's or alcoholic cirrhosis is the most common form of cirrhosis. The pathology consists of fibrosis; small, orderly nodular formations; fatty degeneration; accumulation of Mallory's alcoholic hyalin; and hepatocytic death. The Mallory's alcoholic hyalin is seen morphologically as dark, irregular figures within the liver cells. Their etiology and function remain obscure.

The major etiologic factor of Laennec's cirrhosis is alcohol. Alcohol and its metabolites have been shown to be hepatotoxins. Since alcohol is not stored in the tissues, and only a minute amount is eliminated through the lungs, skin, and kidneys, the liver is responsible for the excretion of alcohol. With massive consumption over a prolonged period of time, it is easy to see how the multifunctions of the liver can be adversely affected by this toxin. The malnutritional state that accompanies chronic alcoholism further potentiates the pathological cycle of cirrhosis.

Postnecrotic cirrhosis is the regeneration of the hepatocytes after massive destruction. The causative agents of this mass destruction are viral infection, such as chronic active hepatitis, or exposure or ingestion of toxic substances, such as some anesthetic agents or isoniazid. The regeneration typically produces wide areas of scarring, and the nodules vary in size and distribution. Hepatomegaly is not associated with postnecrotic cirrhosis, but rather the size of the liver may actually shrink because of the contraction of the scar tissue.

Biliary cirrhosis stems from scarring around each lobule. The scarring is a result of an obstruction of the bile flow from outside the liver, or of a chronic biliary infection. The injury around the bile duct causes duplication and proliferation of the bile ducts.

By understanding some of the pathophysiology of cirrhosis, it is not surprising to realize that portal hypertension is a usual consequence of this disease. The portal circulation is normally a low-pressure system. Think of portal hypertension in terms of a traffic jam on any highway. The traffic has no method of escape, and the lines become increasingly congested. Some commuters begin taking alternative routes, and eventually the alternates become just as congested. This is the demise of the blood flow in the portal circulation. The compression and displacement of the central vein by the scars and nodules do not permit normal drainage of the blood from the liver, resulting in higher pressure. The portal-systemic anastomotic channels are analagous to the alternate routes. Esophageal varix formation and hepatic coma may occur (a discussion of these entities will follow). Ascites and hydrothorax are also complications of portal hypertension from cirrhosis. Ascites is a collection of fluid within the peritoneal cavity. The fluid is a watery liquid that contains a small amount of protein. The formation of ascitic fluid is complex and controversial; but simplified, the elevated pressure within the portal system causes the fluid to seep from the liver. Because the fluid contains protein (high colloid osmotic pressure), it is accompanied by other intestinal fluids as it enters the peritoneal cavity. A hydrothorax results from the transfer of the ascitic fluid through the lymphatics into the pleural cavity.

Case Study

This hypothetical case study illustrates the diagnostic findings in a cirrhotic patient.

A 54-year-old white male was admitted to the hospital because of increasing jaundice, dark urine, ascites and light stool. He admitted to being a heavy drinker for the past 18 years, averaging a quart of whiskey a day. Six months before admission, he noted easy bruising, epistaxis and dull, intermittent abdominal discomfort. Three weeks before admission, he felt "washed out," and experienced nausea and vomiting. He denied previous transfusions, hepatitis or exposure to other chemicals or medication.

On physical examination, the patient was mentally alert and oriented. His color was jaundiced with icteric sclera. Otherwise, the head, ears, eyes, nose and throat were unremarkable. His neck and chest revealed numerous vascular or spider nevi. Pectoral alopecia and gynecomastia were evident. The heart and lungs were normal. The abdomen was large, with ascites present. The liver was enlarged with a firm, nontender, palpable edge. Splenomegaly was absent. Testicular atrophy was apparent. Scattered bruises were present on the upper and lower extremities. Palmar erythema was quite apparent. The lower extremities showed 3+ pitting edema to the knees. The neurological examination was normal. Asterixis (flapping tremor) was absent.

Admission laboratory work revealed the following: clotting times were prolonged; serum cholesterol, albumin and hematocrit were decreased; serum bilirubin, alkaline phosphotase, LDH, SGOT, SGPT and globulin were all increased. Electrolytes, BUN, and creatinine were normal. The urine was positive for bilirubin, and the stool was positive for bile, but negative for occult blood.

Diagnostic tests on this patient included an upper G.I. series that verified the presence of esophageal varices without bleeding. A Bromsulphalein (BSP) dye excretion test was positive for retention. (This test uses a dye that is normally excreted by the liver. A certain amount of dye is injected intravenously, and a sample of blood is drawn about one minute later to obtain a control level of BSP. After an additional half hour, another blood sample is drawn, and the amount of BSP is tested. Normally, a small amount should be left in the serum at this time, but with liver injury, the level will be elevated. This test must be used judiciously, though, since patients with histologically proven cirrhosis may still maintain the ability to excrete BSP.)

The extent of portal hypertension was measured on this patient via splenoportal venography. This radiologic examination allows the portal circulatory system to be seen under fluoroscopy after the injection of a dye. A liver scan also provided evidence of the hepatomegaly. A liver biopsy was not done initially because of prolonged prothrombin time; but this test *is* necessary to histologically confirm the diagnosis of cirrhosis.

The patient was placed on a 2 gm sodium, 50 gm protein, 3,000 calorie diet. Initially, multivitamins were administered intravenously to ensure intestinal transport, since this may be disrupted in the cirrhotic patient. Vitamin K was administered parenterally, and its effectiveness was monitored by daily prothrombin times. After two days of bedrest and I.V. therapy, general improvement was noted in his condition. The patient's appetite improved, his I.V. was discontinued, and he began oral vitamin therapy. Along with his wife, the patient was enrolled in a teaching program to reinforce his therapy of drugs, diet and absolute abstinence from further alcohol intake. It was stressed to the patient that even a small amount of alcohol intake might severely worsen his liver function. The patient was discharged on his sixth hospital day.

Diagnostic Data

The patient presents with a history of alcohol abuse, jaundice, malaise and ascites. Asterixis may or may not be present. G.I. series should be done unless the patient is bleeding. Bromsulphalein tests will be positive.

Radiologic studies include a routine chest x-ray, abdominal x-ray, barium enema and cholangiogram.

Special procedures to detect cirrhosis includes: **endoscopy, biopsy** and *radionuclide scan.*

Nursing Care

The major nursing responsibilities are listed below:

(1) Administer a high-caloric diet.
(2) Maintain fluid-electrolyte balances.
(3) Prevent complications.
(4) Observe for bleeding and neurological changes.
(5) Provide emotional support to the patient and family.
(6) Provide patient education.

Cirrhosis has yet to be given a universally accepted definition. Several characteristics of the disease are generally accepted: it is a severe, irreversible form of hepatic injury; it is a chronic and diffuse process involving the entire liver; and it is a process that destroys the normal architectural structure of the nodules.

HEPATIC FAILURE
Pathophysiology

As with cirrhosis, there has yet to be an accepted, precise definition of hepatic failure. Hepatic failure is a syndrome that is a consequence of massive deterioration of liver functions. This becomes an ill-defined and complex syndrome because of the various causative factors of liver failure. The causative factors can be divided into three categories: 1) conditions that cause diffuse necrosis, such as seen following exposure to hepatotoxins or in acute viral hepatitis; 2) conditions that are chronic, such as cirrhosis or chronic active hepatitis; and 3) conditions that show functional failure without necrosis of the hepatocyte.

Patients with hepatic failure may also have evidence of renal dysfunction, such as in the fatty liver of pregnancy. The pathophysiological processes of hepatic failure can be directly linked with the fact that the liver is unable to sufficiently perform its more than 100 functions.

Clinical Presentation

The clinical presentation is dependent on which functions are primarily affected and to what extent they are affected. These may range from mild jaundice to fulminant failure.

The patient may present with some form of encephalopathy or hepatic coma. The exact cause of hepatic encephalopathy has yet to be discovered. Much work has been done with the theory that an elevated serum ammonia level is a by-product of amino acid digestion and is a product of bacterial digestion of urea in the large bowel. The vast majority of ammonia is transformed to urea in the normal liver in preparation for excretion via the kidneys. But with severely compromised liver function, the ammonia is not detoxified and remains in the circulating blood. The elevated circulating ammonia may also be due to the fact that the blood bypasses the liver. (Remember those alternate routes taken by the blood when it encounters portal hypertension.) This is termed portal-systemic shunting in response to the portal hypertension or as a result of a surgical portosystemic shunt. Other agents labeled toxins also remain under investigation as potential causative agents of hepatic encephalopathy, but definitive data is not yet available.

Different stages of the encephalopathy can be observed. The development of lethargy can be a heralding sign accompanied by detectable changes in personality. The patient may oscillate between periods of flat affect to bouts of abusive behavior. Increased lethargy and flapping tremors may signal the progression of the encephalopathy. Incontinence, disconcertive behavior and even violent behavior may be exhibited. The final stage is marked by unconsciousness from which the patient cannot be aroused. Convulsions may occur, or the comatose state can lead to flaccidity.

Patients with hepatic failure may also have evidence of renal failure. The term hepatorenal syndrome may be seen in reference to this complication. The etiology of the renal failure remains a mystery, but the patient shows azotemia and oliguria. It appears to be a progressive functional failure, since no evidence of morphological changes in the kidneys themselves are apparent on tissue examination.

One of the many functions of the liver is to manufacture clotting factors. A patient with hepatic failure will have a significant deficiency of these clotting factors and will naturally have a bleeding tendency. Complications resulting from this bleeding tendency include disseminated intravascular coagulation and intracranial hemorrhage.

Any one of a number of factors can precipitate hepatic failure in an individual with marginal hepatic reserve. The most common is G.I. bleeding, since this provides a high protein load, the perfect source for increased ammonia. But even a simple acute infection can induce hepatic failure because of the liver's inability to metabolize these potentially toxic substances. In a patient with known chronic liver disease, any failure to follow the prescribed protocol of therapy could evoke hepatic failure, such as alcohol abuse or consuming a high-protein diet. Viral or toxic hepatitis and any other condition that causes acute liver damage can progress to hepatic failure. Even the procedure of a simple paracentesis may give rise to shock and hepatic failure because of a rapid loss of sodium and potassium, in conjuction with a rapid outpouring of fluid from the abdominal blood vessels in an attempt to replace the drained fluid.

A very common clinical manifestation in patients with hepatic failure is jaundice. But this does not mean that every patient with jaundice will progress to hepatic failure. Therefore, it is essential to determine the cause of the jaundice, since the therapeutic regimen depends upon the cause.

Jaundice can be caused by an increased destruction of erythrocytes. The liver is not impaired at all; it just cannot excrete the bilirubin rapidly enough to keep up with the hemolysis. This type of jaundice is known as hemolytic jaundice, and its diagnosis can be made by evaluation of laboratory data. The patient's enzymes are only minimally elevated, urobilinogen is quite elevated, hematocrit may be low and reticulocyte count is elevated.

Obstruction of the extrahepatic bile ducts may be the cause of jaundice, termed obstructive jaundice. The bilirubin is formed normally, but its passageway is blocked by something that could possibly be removed surgically (for example, stones). Laboratory data would show very little, if any, urobilinogen in the urine, but bile would be present. Elevated serum levels of SGOT, LDH and alkaline phosphatase would be seen.

The last cause of jaundice is liver cell dysfunction, known as hepatocellular jaundice. This is the kind of jaundice that will be evident in the patient with hepatic failure. The bilirubin cannot be excreted because of the damaged condition of the hepatocyte. In this case, the urine will probably be positive for bile and urobilinogen. Serum levels of fibrinogen will be low, accompanied by abnormally prolonged prothrombin times. Extreme elevation of the LDH and SGOT will be seen in conjunction with a mild elevation of the alkaline phosphatase.

Case Study

The following hypothetical case study illustrates the clinical presentation, diagnostic findings and therapy. Not unexpectedly, our patient with hepatic failure is the cirrhotic patient that was discharged from the first case study.

A 54-year-old male was admitted to the hospital in a comatose state. His wife served as the historian. He had been discharged from the hospital three weeks ago with a diagnosis of cirrhosis (refer to the cirrhotic case study for details of past history). His wife states that he attempted to adhere to his recommended diet, vitamins and abstinence from alcohol; but the past week she had noticed alcohol on his breath. She had found him unconscious in the bathroom. She denied the patient had taken any drugs, had had a recent infection or had any history of bleeding. There was no evidence of hepatitis, transfusions or exposure to chemicals.

On physical examination, the patient was unresponsive to verbal stimuli. His color was deeply jaundiced. Fetor hepaticus (characteristic musty odor) was noted during exhalation. His neck and chest had numerous vascular nevi. Bleeding was noted from his gums. Pectoral alopecia and gynecomastia were observed. Apical pulse was 110 and an S_3 gallop was audible. Respiratory rate was 36, and rales were audible bilaterally in the bases. The abdomen was large and ascitic. Both the liver and spleen were palpable. Testicular atrophy and scrotal edema were observed. Bruises were present on the upper and lower extremities. Palmar erythema was noted. Pitting edema (3 to 4+) was noticed of the lower extremities to the knees. Neurologically, the patient did not respond to verbal stimuli. Asterixis was present. Positive Babinski sign was present bilaterally. A corneal reflex was not elicited.

Diagnostic Data

Admission laboratory work revealed the following: prothrombin time was extremely prolonged; fibrinogen level was low; liver enzymes were extremely elevated; and alkaline phosphatase was minimally elevated. A urine specimen was positive for urobilinogen and bile. Electrolytes, BUN and creatinine were normal.

The patient was admitted to the critical care unit. Because of deterioration of arterial blood gases, he was electively intubated and placed on a ventilator. A Swan-Ganz catheter was inserted to monitor his fluid status. The initial readings were 42/12, with a wedge of 11. A nasogastric tube was inserted with no evidence of bleeding. The NG was attached to intermittent suction to keep the stomach empty, thereby preventing absorption of protein materials already ingested. Citrate of magnesium was instilled down to the NG tube in order to decrease cleansing of the colon to decrease the amount of nitrogenous products. One gram of neomycin was instilled down the NG tube every six hours. This poorly absorbed antibiotic decreases the intestinal flora and consequently lowers the amount of ammonia produced by these bacteria. Daily BUN and creatinine levels were monitored, since neomycin can be nephrotoxic.

Vitamin K was not given to this patient. Although his prothrombin time was prolonged, it reflected inadequate synthesis of clotting factors and adequate vitamin K. Administration of vitamin K preparations have the potential to increase the hypoprothrombinemia.

A subclavian catheter was inserted to be used for total parenteral nutrition. The solution ordered contained protein only, in the form of the essential amino acids, to reduce the protein intake. The essential calories were provided in the form of glucose.

An EEG was performed on this patient. Diffuse slowing was shown. A lumbar puncture was performed, and the fluid report showed an elevated glutamine level. The exact significance of this finding is not well defined, but it may be associated with the elevated serum ammonia levels.

The next morning, the patient was comatose, but was not flaccid. His rales had grossly increased, and his urinary output averaged 10 cc per hour. Pulmonary artery pressures were 52/20 with a wedge of 20. Furosemide was administered judiciously in an attempt to prevent hypokalemia, alkalosis and further encephalopathy. His response to the diuretic was poor. That evening, the patient had a severe hypotensive episode. Vasopressors were started, but his condition deteriorated to a cardiopulmonary arrest. Resuscitative maneuvers were to no avail.

Nursing Care

The nursing care of the hepatic failure patient is a demanding task.

(1) Protect the patient from nosocomial infections, since this complication may only increase the activity of the viscous cycle of the failure.
(2) Prevent bleeding tendency.
(3) Give special attention to the patient's skin and mucous membranes.
(4) Provide emotional support to the patient and family. Several coping mechanisms may be observed in the family's behavior. It is essential that the critical care nurse establish a rapport with the family and be able to offer support during this crisis.
(5) Maintain a safe environment; pad siderails.

KEY CONCEPT: Hepatic failure is a syndrome that is a consequence of massive deterioration of liver function. The nurse should protect the patient from infection and prevent bleeding.

BLEEDING ESOPHAGEAL VARICES
Pathophysiology

To understand the development of esophageal varices, one must understand the normal venous drainage of the G.I. tract. The portal venous blood circulates through the liver and drains out the hepatic veins to enter the systemic venous circulation of the inferior vena cava. There are areas of anastomosis that exist between the portal and systemic systems. These anastomoses exist as alternate routes of communication should there be a problem with the normal flow of blood.

One of these portal-systemic anastomoses is found in the lower third of the esophagus. Here, the portal system (esophageal branches of the left gastric vein) comes in contact with the systemic system (esophageal veins draining into the azygous veins). These two systems connect by the very small veins of the esophageal submucosal plexus. With the presence of portal hypertension, the pressure in the portal system is transmitted through this alternate route, causing dilatation of the esophageal veins. The result of this dilatation is the formation of varices.

Being veins, these vessels are used to a low-pressure system and have few compensatory methods for adapting to the high pressures. These varices are located directly beneath the mucosal layer, and at times, even protrude into the lumen. This location leaves these frail vessels susceptible to erosion from acid pepsin. Any trauma or surge of extremely elevated venous pressure could cause bleeding. Once bleeding begins, these vessels have very little ability to contract in an attempt to decrease the blood loss.

Clinical Presentation

The patient with bleeding esophageal varices presents to the emergency room with copious hematemesis that began abruptly. These patients typically do not experience abdominal pain. Because of the inability of these frail vessels to control bleeding, shock may develop quickly. All of the problems associated with shock may be seen as complications in the patient with bleeding esophageal varices. The decreased circulating blood volume may cause ischemia to the coronary arteries, resulting in a myocardial infarction. The same occurrence to the renal arteries may induce renal failure. The blood that is stagnate in the G.I. tract provides more nitrogen to be absorbed. Since this patient usually has some form of liver disease, these circumstances provide the precipitating factors needed for hepatic coma and hepatorenal syndrome.

Case Study

A 36-year-old male came to the emergency room with profuse hematemesis. He had a history of heavy drinking, but denied alcohol intake during the past three months. He had last been admitted to the hospital one year ago for bleeding esophageal varices. A diagnosis of Laennec's cirrhosis was also made at that time. He stated that for the past two weeks he had had no appetite, and he had lost five pounds during this time. He was nauseated upon arising this morning and, as he began to vomit, he noticed blood.

On physical examination, the patient was awake and alert, but obviously anxious. His skin was cool, slightly diaphoretic, and he was jaundiced. His sclera were icteric, but the head, ears and nose were unremarkable. His neck and chest revealed scattered vascular nevi. The heart rate was 130, with a blood pressure faintly audible at 80/60. Respiratory rate was 30. His abdomen was large and nontender with ascites, and splenomegaly was present. Hematemesis continued. Stool in the rectum was positive for guaiac.

Laboratory data included the following: hemoglobin and hematocrit were very low; prothrombin time was prolonged; BUN, LDH, SGOT, SGPT and alkaline phosphatase were elevated. Arterial blood gases showed slight hypoxemia and acidosis.

The patient was typed and crossmatched for four units of fresh blood. Two units were to be infused as soon as possible. A central subclavian line was established to replace lost volume. The patient's blood pressure rose to 90/60, and he was then admitted to the critical care unit.

A peripheral intravenous infusion of vasopressin was started upon arrival in the CCU. (The action of vasopressin is to decrease portal venous pressure by constricting the splanchnic vein. This allows the bleeding to be controlled.) The concentration of the drip was 100 units of vasopressin in 250 cc of D_5W, yielding 0.4 units of vasopressin/cc. The infusion of vasopressin was started at 0.3 units per minute, and the amount of bleeding was observed after 30 minutes. The patient was closely observed for any side effects, since vasopressin also causes constriction of the coronary arteries and peripheral arteries. The patency of the intravenous catheter was ensured, since infiltration of the drug has been shown to result in ischemic changes and gangrene.

Bleeding was still evident after the first 30 minutes, so the dose was increased to 0.4 units per minute for another 30-minute interval. (This titration schedule could continue until bleeding is controlled, but not exceeding the infusion of more than 0.8 to 0.9 units per minute. If peripheral infusion of vasopressin controls the bleeding, it will do so within the first 4 to 6 hours of infusion. Once the bleeding is controlled, the vasopressin is discontinued slowly by titrating down the dosage. If peripheral vasopressin is not effective, it is not unusual to see the drug infused intra-arterially, via a catheter in the superior mesenteric artery.)

Citrates of magnesium and neomycin were administered to this patient (see hepatic failure for rationale). No further bleeding was noted with the vasopressin infusing at 0.4 units per minute. His blood pressure stabilized at 110/70, with a heart rate of 96. Over the next 48 hours, the vasopressin was titrated off, and the patient was observed for an additional 24 hours in CCU. Since no further bleeding developed and his hemoglobin and hematocrit had stabilized, the patient was transferred to a medical floor for continued therapy.

Diagnostic Data

Laboratory data are an important diagnostic aid, along with a complete history and physical, to determine the extent of bleeding. Hemoglobin, hematocrit, BUN, LDH, SGOT, SGPT, alkaline phosphatase, prothrombin time and arterial blood gases should be evaluated.

Nursing Care

The initial treatment for patients with bleeding esophageal varices differs with the physician and the institution. Some physicians prefer peripheral vasopressin first, while others insert a Linton or a Sengstaken-Blakemore tube (SB) first. The SB tube is designed with two balloons, a gastric and an esophageal, that can be inflated to directly apply pressure to the bleeding esophageal varices. The gastric balloon is inflated to keep the esophageal balloon in place. A prescribed amount of traction must be maintained to the tube to prevent the gastric balloon from descending into the stomach. Special precautions must be taken to avoid necrosis to the visible nares and to the invisible esophageal and gastric walls. Suction must be readily available to prevent aspiration of pooled saliva if the patient is comatose. There is also a third port that allows for aspiration of the gastric contents.

If all available medical therapy fails to stop the bleeding, ligation of the varices may be the only choice left. These patients are very poor surgical candidates. The trauma of surgery submits these patients, who have pre-existing liver disease, to the possible complication of fulminant hepatic failure.

The goal of nursing care is to provide supportive care, as well as to prevent complications and further deterioration.

(1) Maintain the patient's airway and breathing. Prevent aspiration and pneumonia.
(2) Administer appropriate treatment as prescribed by the physician.
(3) Monitor fluid balance, hydration and electrolyte balance: electrolytes, hemoglobin, hematocrit and enzymes; measure intake and output.
(4) Monitor vital signs, especially for shock.
(5) Monitor arterial blood gases for changes and hypoxia.

KEY CONCEPT: Patients with bleeding esophageal varices present with copious hematemesis and absent abdominal pain. Shock occurs rapidly, renal failure may be evidenced and eventually hepatic coma occurs. Nursing care is aimed at maintaining the airway, instituting treatments to stop bleeding and providing emotional support.

G.I. HEMORRHAGE FROM PEPTIC ULCERS

Pathophysiology

The pathogenesis of benign peptic ulcer disease remains specifically undefined. It has been documented that neither duodenal nor gastric ulcers occur without the presence of acid. This fact has guided research to search for the mechanisms that control the parietal cell function (remember, the parietal cells of the stomach secrete HCl). Gastric and duodenal ulcerations are identical in appearance, but the debate continues as to whether they are different disease processes or the same disease process in different locations.

Increased secretion of acid and pepsin is typically found in the patient with a duodenal ulcer. The cause of this increased acid in some cases seems to be due to an increase in the amount of parietal cells present in the gastric mucosa. In other cases, the parietal cells simply secrete more acid, or these cells demand little stimulation to secrete.

On the other hand, patients with gastric ulcers usually have a normal level of acid-pepsin secretion. The defect in this situation appears to be in the defensive barrier of the mucosa. A single cause of the breakdown of the mucosal barrier has yet to be documented. Perhaps several agents are to blame, but their action is exerted on specific individuals. A few of the substances currently under investigation include aspirin, bile, ethanol, pancreatic enzymes and bile salts.

Another factor in ulcer formation is an increased autonomic stimulation. Physical or emotional stress elevates acid secretion and inhibits the Brunner's glands. This leads to a decrease of duodenal mucus, leaving the wall of the duodenum unprotected.

Endogenous or exogenous cortisones and ACTH can affect the production of mucus by either decreasing the amount or changing the type. Glucocorticoids can increase the production of pepsin and HCl.

The average life span of a gastric mucosal cell is three days, and there is constant replacement. But certain drugs, such as phenylbutazone and corticosteroids, may alter this cycle, resulting in detrimental changes in the normal homeostatic environment in the stomach and duodenum. Heavy cigarette smokers have been shown to have a higher incidence of ulcer disease, but caffeine and reserpine have yet to be proven to be ulcerogenic agents. None of these substances have been proven to be the cause of peptic ulcers, but they produce changes in the normal protective mechanism of the mucosal layer that might lead to ulceration.

Clinical Presentation

Working in a critical care unit, the nurse becomes very familiar with the patient who suddenly begins G.I. bleeding from an acute stress ulcer. The original problem may have been neurosurgical, multiple trauma, burns, major surgery or sepsis. This ulcer formation seems to differ from the chronic peptic ulcer formation in that the causative process is thought to be ischemia. These ulcerations may occur in the stomach or the duodenum, and usually are superficial; that is, they only involve the mucosal layer. Quite often, there are no warning symptoms of pain with acute stress ulcers, but the presenting sign is that of upper G.I. bleeding.

The major sites of peptic ulcers are the stomach and the duodenal bulb. Many patients with peptic ulcer disease have a typical history and symptoms, the most significant being episodic abdominal pain. Other patients may present with upper G.I. bleeding from an ulcer without antecedent symptoms. If bleeding is massive, it is usually the result of the erosion of a major artery around or within the ulcer. Duodenal ulcers are more common than gastric ulcers and are seen in patients around the ages of 40 to 50. Duodenal ulcers have not been shown to transform into malignancies. However, a small percentage of gastric ulcers have exhibited malignant transformation. Gastric ulcers tend to occur in slightly older people.

Shock is naturally the major complication for the patient with G.I. bleeding. If the bleeding is massive, vigorous resuscitation is needed to combat the sequelae of any shock state, including myocardial infarction. If the patient requires multiple blood transfusions, care must be taken to avoid any transfusion reactions.

Perforation of the ulcer leading to peritonitis is not a frequent complication, but carries an extremely high mortality rate when it does occur. Most perforations involve duodenal ulcers, with the usual site being the anterior duodenal wall. Very typically, these patients have sudden, generalized and constant abdominal pain. Within minutes, as peritonitis ensues, the abdomen of this patient shows rebound tenderness, guarding, boardlike rigidity and few, if any, bowel sounds. Immediate surgery is indicated.

Duodenal ulcers can also cause pyloric obstruction. The obstruction can be due to the inflammation of the ulcer area during the acute phase or scarring of the tissue after several episodes. The obstruction is treated with decompression of the stomach via NG suction, and fluid and electrolyte replacement. Rarely is surgical intervention needed.

Case Study

A 64-year-old male came to the emergency room with hematemesis. The patient stated that intermittently during the past six months he had been having "gnawing stomach cramps" that occurred a few hours after meals. He would obtain relief with antacids. Weeks would pass before he would again experience these symptoms. During the past two weeks, these episodes of pain had become more frequent and more severe. He had felt "sick to his stomach" intermittently and had lost eight pounds. He had been vomiting "dark brown" liquid for the past two days, but this morning the emesis had been "bloody" for the first time, and he stated that he felt "very weak." He had vomited three times before calling for an ambulance. He denied previous episodes of bleeding, liver disease or excessive alcohol intake. He denied a recent emotional upset. The only medication he took was aspirin for arthritic pain. His average intake of aspirin was 20 grains daily for the past two years. He denied cardiac or pulmonary disease.

On physical examination, the patient was awake, alert and anxious. His color was pale. His skin was cool and moist. Pallor was noticed of his sclera and mucous membranes. He complained of thirst. The head, ears and nose were normal. The chest was normal with clear breath sounds. Respiratory rate was 34. No evidence of vascular nevi was observed. The heart rate was 120, with a blood pressure of 82/50. Heart sounds were normal. Extremities were cool with no evidence of edema. His abdomen was nondistended and tender. The patient complained of pain localized in the right epigastric region. No masses were palpable. A rectal examination was performed, and the stool present was positive for guaiac.

Arterial blood gases showed the patient to be slightly acidotic and hypoxemic. Oxygen therapy was administered. The only other relevant laboratory values were an increased BUN and a markedly decreased hemoglobin and hematocrit. An ECG showed sinus tachycardia without any changes.

Two intravenous lines were established, using large bore needles. Lactated Ringer's solution was infused to replace the lost volume. The patient was typed and crossmatched for six units of whole blood and was ordered to receive three units stat. A salem sump tube was inserted and bright, red bleeding was noticed. Iced saline lavage was begun in an attempt to stop the bleeding through vasoconstriction. The patient was then admitted to the critical care unit.

Upon arrival in CCU, the patient continued to have bright red drainage from the salem sump. Constant iced saline lavage was maintained. Care was taken to express the blood clots to maintain the patency of the gastric tube. Accurate measurement of the drainage was maintained. Cimetidine 300 mg I.V. six hours was ordered.

After receiving the three units of whole blood and the I.V. fluids, the patient seemed to stabilize hemodynamically. His blood pressure was 100/60, and his heart rate was 100. His skin remained cool, but was now dry. Following two hours of lavaging, the salem sump drainage was now a coffee-ground color. Lavage was continued to empty the stomach of blood and clots in preparation for endoscopy. Visualization was enhanced with the removal of the blood.

Endoscopy was performed at the bedside. The duodenal bulb was found to be deformed and a large duodenal ulcer was visualized. No active bleeding was seen with endoscopy.

The patient's vital signs remained stable. His hematocrit after the third unit of blood was up to 30 percent. No further bleeding was noted from the salem sump, and it was discontinued the next morning. Oral antacids were administered every two hours. Three melenic stools were noted over the next 24 hours, but these were expected since blood has a cathartic action.

Over the next 24 hours, the patient remained quite stable and showed no other signs of active bleeding. He was transferred to a medical floor for continued therapy.

Diagnostic Data

Because of recent developmental advances, endoscopy has become the most valuable diagnostic aid for finding sources of bleeding. It has been shown to be superior to radiographic studies in detecting lesions. Endoscopic examinations can be documented by photography and can provide specimens for biopsy if a malignancy is suspected. One contraindication to endoscopy is the possibility of perforation. The insufflation of air into the stomach and duodenum during the procedure could cause an increase of peritoneal contamination if a perforation exists.

If endoscopy fails to locate the source of bleeding, the next diagnostic test is an angiogram. Of course, the sequence of the diagnostic tests is at the discretion of the physician and depends upon the condition of the patient. Selective angiography is usually successful at localizing the site of bleeding. The added advantage with this study is that once the catheter is in place, intra-arterial vasopressin may be administered (refer to bleeding esophageal varices for details on vasopressin therapy). The site of bleeding gastric ulcers is most often the left gastric artery, with the superior pancreaticoduodenal artery being the primary site of bleeding in duodenal ulcers.

Surgery is indicated in patients who do not respond to medical therapy. Any patient who remains hemodynamically unstable and continues to bleed after numerous transfusions usually requires surgical intervention.

Nursing Care

The goal of nursing care is to prevent *shock.*

(1) Observe for signs of G.I. bleeding.
(2) Observe for signs of shock.
(3) Maintain patient airway and breathing. Prevent aspiration and pneumonia.
(4) Monitor fluid balance, hydration and electrolyte balance. Monitor for changes. Maintain intake and output.
(5) Monitor arterial blood gases, watch for acidosis.
(6) Monitor for dysrhythmia.

KEY CONCEPT: The first line of treatment for the patient with G.I. bleeding is prevention or treatment of shock. Adequate fluid and blood replacement is essential. The next step is to find the source of bleeding so that specific therapy can be determined.

ACUTE PANCREATITIS
Pathophysiology

The pancreas is located in close proximity to other important structures in the abdomen. As might be expected, disease states of the other abdominal structures may affect the pancreas, and disease states of the pancreas may affect these other structures. Such is the case with acute pancreatitis. A wide spectrum of disease processes may be seen, ranging from slight edema of the organ to gross necrotizing and hemorrhagic changes.

A blockage of the flow of the pancreatic enzymes causes these enzymes to back up and stagnate in the ducts and acini of the pancreas. The accumulation of trypsinogen becomes so great that it negates the action of trypsin inhibitor and trypsin becomes activated. Once a small amount is activated, the activation spreads rapidly, and includes most of the proteolytic enzymes. The activated enzymes begin digesting the pancreas itself, including the fat in and around the organ.

Kallikrein, elastase, phospholipase A, and chymotrypsin are some of the enzymes that become active. Kallikrein causes vasodilatation and increased vascular permeability. Phospholipase A activates substances that are toxic to red blood cells. Elastase and chymotrypsin have been shown to cause damage to the blood vessels. Local vessels may rupture, leading to hemorrhage within the pancreas, which may be minimal or quite severe.

The precise etiology of acute pancreatitis is unknown. A multitude of conditions and processes are labeled as precipitating factors. Alcohol consumption and biliary disease remain the most frequently associated findings in acute pancreatitis. Even though the exact mechanism by which alcohol causes the changes in the pancreas is not clear, it must be considered to play an important role as an etiologic factor, since it is such a common denominator in this acute disease. Some theories label alcohol as a direct toxin to the pancreatic gland. Alcohol has been shown to increase the production of pancreatic secretions. The Oddi's sphincter has been shown to be in a state of spasm after alcohol consumption, thereby increasing the amount of compression on the already engorged ducts.

Biliary tract disease is the next most common finding in an acute attack of pancreatitis. Again, the exact mechanism remains unknown, but many theories have been proposed. Since gallstones are found in the majority of patients with acute pancreatitis, the common-channel hypothesis is one such theory. This theory claims that the cause of acute pancreatitis is a blockage of the common channel of the common bile duct and the main pancreatic duct. This blockage causes a reflux of bile into the pancreatic duct. The bile is then capable of activating the enzymes within the pancreas.

Duodenal reflux is another proposed theory. This theory concludes that there has been some damage done to the outflow tract of the pancreatic duct or to the common bile duct. This damage could be from the consumption of alcohol or from the passage of stones through these outflow tracts. Because of incompetency, bile and duodenal juices may be splashing into the pancreatic duct. One of the elements of the duodenal juice is enterokinase, an enzyme that can liberate the pancreatic enzymes.

A number of drugs have been implicated, although not well differentiated, in the etiology of pancreatitis. These include steroids, thiazide diuretics, salicylazosulfapyridine and isoniazid. Surgical, blunt or penetrating trauma may cause pancreatitis. Other etiologic considerations include familial tendencies, hyperlipidemia, infectious processes (viruses, including mumps, Coxsackie virus and infectious hepatitis, and bacteria, such as hemolytic streptococci) and hyperparathyroidism.

Clinical Presentation

As in hepatic failure, there is a wide range of signs, symptoms and complications that the patient with acute pancreatitis may exhibit. The presentation depends on the degree of damage to the ducts and acini of the pancreas.

The pain of acute pancreatitis is severe over the entire abdomen and may radiate to the back and flanks. The pain is caused by the edema and congestion of the ductules, and the release of the digested fats and proteins. Nausea and vomiting occur because of stretching and irritation of the pancreas. Abdominal distension follows, and a paralytic ileus ensues since gastric motility ceases. During the early stage, a fever is present because of the inflammatory reaction and necrosis, not from infection.

One of the complications of acute pancreatitis is hypovolemic shock. The shock state may result from the vast amount of plasma released into the peritoneum, or from the loss of blood due to hemorrhaging. Third-spacing of fluid in the atonic bowel further complicates the shock state by decreasing the circulating volume. Other complications associated with shock are acute tubular necrosis and myocardial infarction.

During an acute attack, patients may show signs of severe hypocalcemia, including tetany, neuromuscular irritability, stupor or convulsions. Part of this decreased calcium is due to the digestion of fats, which releases free fatty acids. These fatty acids quickly combine with ionized calcium. This combination does not appear to be sufficient to cause such a drastic reduction in serum calcium, but the exact mechanism remains unknown.

The necrosis of acute pancreatitis may result in the formation of an abscess. These may perforate into any surrounding organs or into the peritoneal cavity and result in peritonitis and sepsis. An abscess should be suspected with fever, a palpable mass, abdominal tenderness, an increased WBC count, nausea and vomiting. A chest radiograph may show an elevation of the diaphragm and basal atelectasis. Surgical intervention is required.

Pseudocyst formation is a common complication following a bout of acute pancreatitis. After the necrosis of tissue, cavities are left in the pancreas that are not lined with epithelial cells, but contain exudate, plasma, blood and pancreatic products. Surrounding these cavities are bits of acini that are still functioning, and these acini secrete more pancreatic juices. Since the duct is obstructed, the juices have no place to go except into the cavities, and these pseudocysts continue to grow. If the cysts become large enough to compress surrounding organs, further complications may arise and surgical intervention may be indicated.

Case Study

Following is a hypothetical case study to show the clinical presentation, diagnostic tests and treatment of acute pancreatitis.

A 66-year-old female came to the ER complaining of severe generalized abdominal pain of six hours' duration. She gave a history of gallbladder disease for the past four years, which had been treated medically. She had attended a wedding reception last evening and had indulged in a large amount of fried foods and alcoholic beverages. She normally adheres religiously to her low-fat diet, without coffee or alcohol. She began vomiting in the middle of the night, and then the pain began. She initially thought it was her gallbladder acting up, but the pain increased in intensity. When she became very sweaty, cold and was feeling extremely weak, she had her husband bring her to the ER. She denied previous cardiac or pulmonary problems. She also denied routinely taking any medication.

On physical examination, the patient was awake, alert, very restless and anxious. Her skin was cool and diaphoretic, and her color was slightly jaundiced and pale. Her head, neck, ears, eyes, nose and throat were normal. Her chest was normal with clear breath sounds. Respiratory rate was increased, at 40 per minute. Her heart rate was 136, blood pressure 86/48, and temperature 101° F. Her extremities were cool, diaphoretic and appeared slightly mottled. Her abdomen was distended, extremely tender, without bowel sounds. No ascites was observed. It was difficult to palpate the abdomen for masses because of the severity of the pain the patient was experiencing. Areas of ecchymosis were noted surrounding the umbilicus (Cullen's sign) and the groin (Grey Turner's sign). Tapping the area over the mandibular joint produced a twitching of the corner of the mouth (Chevostek's sign) and a tourniquet applied to the upper arm produced a carpal spasm (Trousseau's sign). These two signs were manifestations of a low-serum calcium.

Laboratory findings included the following: leukocytosis with increased polymorphonuclear leukocytes, elevated serum amylase, lipase, blood sugar, triglycerides, alkaline phosphotase and direct bilirubin; decreased hematocrit, serum albumin, calcium, total protein and potassium. A urine evaluation showed low calcium and high amylase. An ECG showed sinus tachycardia without ischemic changes.

Two intravenous lines were established with large bore needles and fluid resuscitation was begun. Ringer's lactate was hung in one line, with low molecular dextran in the other. The patient was typed and crossmatched for four units of whole blood to be on hold, if needed. A salem sump tube was inserted and connected to suction for control of nausea and vomiting, and to keep the pancreas at rest by decreasing pancreatic secretory activity. Demerol 75 mg I.M. was given to the patient in an attempt to alleviate the pain. Her blood pressure came up to 90/60, and the patient was transferred to the critical care unit.

In CCU, the patient continued to exhibit symptoms of shock, despite adequate fluid replacement. An abdominal radiograph verified the presence of an ileus. Since she had known biliary tract disease, the decision for immediate surgical intervention was made. Within the hour, the patient was in the operating room where a cholecystectomy was performed. The patient returned from the recovery room with a Swan-Ganz catheter in place for proper fluid management. A subclavian catheter had also been inserted for the administration of TPN, since TPN reduces pancreatic secretion of protein and fluid, and maintains nutrition. The patient was left intubated overnight and on a respirator, with frequent monitoring of arterial blood gases.

The patient was extubated in the morning. She was hemodynamically stable and no signs of complications were noted. She continued to improve, and within three days, good bowel sounds were audible. Her salem sump was discontinued, and she was started on antacids for neutralization of the gastric secretions. These were tolerated and she was advanced to small feedings of a low-fat, high-protein and high-carbohydrate diet without coffee. Improvement continued, and she was transferred to a postoperative floor for further care.

Diagnostic Data

Laboratory studies, such as complete blood count, amylase, lipase, blood sugar, triglycerides, alkaline phosphatase, electrolytes, bilirubin, urinalysis and EKG are adjuncts to establishing a diagnosis.

Nursing Care

Fluid replacement cannot be emphasized enough. These patients have tremendous volume deficiencies due to the vomiting, the loss of fluids into the peritoneal space and the third-spacing of fluids in the intestines due to its atonic condition. Colloid and crystalloid replacement solutions are indicated.

(1) Provide nasogastric suction. The pancreas is kept at rest by nasogastric suction. This keeps the stomach empty so that gastric secretions cannot stimulate pancreatic secretions. The use of anticholinergic drugs (atropine, propantheline) is controversial. Although historically these drugs have been used for the treatment of acute pancreatitis to decrease pancreatic metabolism and secretion, there is no study that has clearly given evidence of these effects.

(2) Alleviate pain. Both demerol and morphine can cause spasm of the Oddi's sphincter and significantly elevate serum amylase and lipase levels. It is important to obtain blood samples for these tests before administering any analgesics. Demerol is usually the preferred agent. Anticholinergics may be used to minimize sphincter spasm. The patient should be kept sedated with barbiturates for maximal rest, providing there is no contraindication.

(3) Prevent pulmonary complications. These may vary from ARDS, pulmonary edema and pneumonia to pleural effusion. A left pleural effusion is a common finding and can be seen on the chest radiograph. This effusion is due to diaphragmatic irritation from the inflamed pancreas. The fluid transudates from the peritoneal cavity into the pleural space.

(4) Protect from infections. The use of prophylactic antibiotics is discouraged. If a source of sepsis is identified, prompt, appropriate antibiotics should be administered.

(5) Surgery is indicated when there is known biliary disease and when there is an abdominal or pancreatic complication such as abscesses. Controversy remains concerning the use of diagnostic laparotomy and surgical resection of the pancreas.

KEY CONCEPT: Most patients do not have a smooth recovery from an acute hemorrhagic pancreatitis attack. Pancreatitis is an obscure disease, and its treatment is controversial and empirical. The major goals of therapy are to maintain an adequate circulating blood volume, to keep the pancreas at rest and to alleviate the pain.

KEY POINT RECOGNITION
Write true or false by each statement. Answers are at the end of this chapter. A score below 80% indicates the need for further study.

_____ 1. As cells of the liver are destroyed, they are replaced by fibrous, connective tissue.

_____ 2. A cirrhotic liver has a regular shape.

_____ 3. Laennec's cirrhosis is a rare form of cirrhosis.

_____ 4. Postnecrotic cirrhosis is the regeneration, after massive destruction, of the hepatocytes.

_____ 5. Hepatomegaly is associated with postnecrotic cirrhosis.

_____ 6. Biliary cirrhosis results from scarring around each lobule.

_____ 7. The portal system is a high-pressure system.

_____ 8. Ascites and hydrothorax are complications of portal hypertension due to cirrhosis.

_____ 9. Ascites is a collection of fluid within the peritoneal cavity.

_____ 10. Ascites is caused by fluid seeping from the liver.

_____ 11. The patient with hepatic failure may present with some form of encephalopathy or hepatic coma.

_____ 12. A heralding sign of encephalopathy is the development of lethargy.

_____ 13. The patient in hepatic failure may also evidence renal failure.

_____ 14. Jaundice is always a precursor of liver failure.

_____ 15. The patient in liver failure must be protected from infection.

_____ 16. Hematemesis without abdominal pain is indicative of lower G.I. bleeding.

_____ 17. Vasopressin, used to control hematemesis due to esophageal varices, is infused at a concentration of 100 units of vasopressin in 250 cc of D_5W, which yields 0.4 units vasopressin per cc.

_____ 18. If peripheral vasopressin controls the bleeding, it will do so within six to eight hours of infusion.

_____ 19. Ulcers occur in the presence of acid.

_____ 20. An increase in the secretion of acid and pepsin is indicative of a duodenal ulcer.

_____ 21. Patients with gastric ulcers have a normal level of acid-pepsin secretion.

_____ 22. Physical or emotional stress will elevate acid secretion and inhibit the Brunner's glands.

_____ 23. Glucocorticoids decrease the secretion of pepsin and HCl.

_____ 24. Acute pancreatitis is caused by activated enzymes digesting the pancreas.

_____ 25. Alcohol consumption and biliary disease are the most frequently associated findings in acute pancreatitis.

_____ 26. Alcohol decreases the production of pancreatic secretions.

_____ 27. The pain of acute pancreatitis seldom radiates.

_____ 28. In acute pancreatitis, a fever is due to infection.

_____ 29. A common complication of acute pancreatitis is hypovolemic shock.

_____ 30. The necrosis of acute pancreatitis may result in abscess formation.

_____ 31. The presence of an abscess in acute pancreatitis may result in pseudocyst formation.

_____32. During an acute attack of pancreatitis, the patient may have tetany and neuromuscular irritability.

_____33. The nurse should check for Cullen's sign by observing the area around the umbilicus for ecchymotic areas.

_____34. Colloid and crystalloid replacement solutions are contraindicated in acute pancreatitis.

_____35. Serum amylase and lipase levels can be raised by the use of morphine sulfate in patients with pancreatitis.

CARE COMMON TO GASTROINTESTINAL PROBLEMS

FLUID AND ELECTROLYTE PROBLEMS

The patient with a G.I. disorder frequently has disorders of fluid, electrolyte and acid-base balance. If not adequately monitored, these complications may become quite severe.

Pathophysiology

Whenever absorption or motility in the G.I. tract is changed by a disease state, water and electrolyte metabolisms are altered. Fluids are lost internally through third-spacing, as in an ileus; or externally through vomiting and/or diarrhea, or fistulas. This fluid is isotonic, and the loss of water, sodium and chloride depicts a loss of the main constituents of the extracellular fluid. The plasma volume decreases because of this loss of isotonic fluid and may progress to a state of hypovolemic shock if no treatment is obtained.

Clinical Presentation

Vomiting causes a loss of gastric HCl and water, which can lead to dehydration, alkalosis, hypokalemia and hyponatremia. Prolonged nasogastric suction may produce these same effects. Because of their prompt absorption, administration of soluble antacids may provoke alkalosis.

Wounds and fistulas can drain voluminous amounts of fluid (isotonic with high sodium content) per day. Hyponatremia, hypocalcemia and dehydration are common consequences.

Pancreatitis, peritonitis and paralytic ileus due to third-spacing lead to hyponatremia, metabolic alkalosis and hypovolemia. Hypocalcemia is noted in acute attacks of pancreatitis and peritonitis. Although rare, hypocalcemia can also occur if the patient receives a large amount of citrated blood over a short interval.

Diarrhea may cause hyponatremic or hypernatremic states. In the latter, the water loss exceeds the sodium loss and produces hypernatremia. Hypokalemia and metabolic acidosis are associated with severe diarrhea.

If a patient is in a state of severe, catabolic nutritional imbalance or is septic, metabolic acidosis will be present.

Although necessary treatment for some G.I. patients, certain diuretics may only further decrease serum sodium and potassium levels.

Nursing Care

In an attempt to keep the fluid and electrolyte problems under control, it is essential:

(1) That an accurate record is kept of intake and output
(2) That output includes any drainage from fistulas, tubes, bleeding, emesis or diarrhea
(3) That nasogastric tubes not be irrigated with tap water, since this may further decrease sodium
(4) To prevent the administration of tap water enema, which may decrease sodium
(5) To monitor current electrolyte status of the patient and communicate these values to the physician so that proper therapy is continued
(6) To monitor vital signs and weight

NUTRITIONAL MAINTENANCE

Patients with G.I. disorders are especially susceptible to deficiencies of nutritional requirements. Since the main function of the G.I. tract is to digest and absorb the essential carbohydrates, proteins and fats, any disease state that interferes with this process will render the patient malnourished.

Clinical Presentation

An assessment of the patient should determine nutritional state. This assessment includes a nutritional history and physical assessment. During the history interview, an evaluation of the patient's normal dietary intake is made. Often, this interview is best conducted by the dietician, with a report given to the physician. The physical assessment focuses on areas frequently affected by vitamin and nutritional deficiencies, such as nails, teeth, eyes, hair and skin. Anthropometric measurements are then taken. Included in these measurements are height, weight (with comparison to ideal body weight), mid-arm circumference (with comparison to established normal values), and triceps skinfold, which offers an estimation of the body's fat reserves.

Diagnostic Data

The depletion of protein in the patient may be measured by laboratory values obtained from serum albumin and transferrin levels. Depression of cellular immunity is an additional finding in patients with protein-calorie malnutrition and is demonstrated by a decreased lymphocyte count and a delayed hypersensitivity reaction to antigens. The skin test antigens used most often are mumps, PPD and streptokinase/streptodornase (SK/SD).

After a nutritional deficiency has been established, the causative agent of the nutritional impairment should be identified. The factors may be exposed by answering the following questions:

(1) Is the deficiency due to impairment of intake? Is the patient nauseated and vomiting? Does the patient have abdominal pain? Are medications interfering with appetite? Is the patient an alcoholic? Is depression a factor? Is a disease state (obstruction, cancer, ulcers) interfering with intake?

(2) Is the problem one of deficient absorptive mechanisms? Is the patient receiving drugs that interfere with absorption? Is there a lack of alteration of the digestive secretions and bile salts? Is the patient a diabetic? Is there evidence of increased motility?

(3) Is the patient in a state that requires more nutritional elements? Does the patient have burns? Is the patient septic? Does the patient have peritonitis? Is the patient febrile? Are there major fractures of long bones? Has the patient had major surgery?
All of these states require an additional caloric intake, anywhere from 5 to 100 percent above the average daily intake.

(4) Is the patient unable to use or store the nutrients? Is the diagnosis hepatitis? pancreatitis? cirrhosis? malignancy?

(5) Is the impairment due to excess loss or excretion from the G.I. tract?

Does the patient have a fistula or draining wound? Is the patient bleeding? Does the patient have an NG tube with voluminous amounts of drainage? Is the patient thirdspacing? Does the patient have ascites? Does the patient have a malignancy? Does the patient have a postoperative gastric resection? Malabsorption syndrome? Small gut syndrome?

(6) Is the situation one of tissue destruction? Does the patient have ulcerative disease?

One further assessment of the patient's nutritional status should be determined—nitrogen balance. Amino acids from protein in the diet serve as the source of nitrogen. A state of nitrogen balance is obtained when the amount of nitrogen consumed equals the amount of nitrogen excreted in the urine, sweat and feces. A positive nitrogen balance occurs when the amount of nitrogen consumed is greater than the amount excreted. This positive state is seen in stages of growth. A negative nitrogen balance occurs when the amount of nitrogen consumed is less than the amount excreted. This negative state can be seen in malnutrition, burns, trauma, surgery and a variety of illnesses. Corticosteroids, due to their catabolic state, may lead to negative nitrogen states. Formulas based on the amount of urea nitrogen excreted in a 24-hour period determine an estimation of the nitrogen balance of the patient.

Nursing Care

Having established that a nutritional deficiency exists, and having identified certain factors that are causing the impairment, it is essential to supply the proper nutritional requirements. This may be a relatively easy task, if the patient has a functioning G.I. tract.

(1) Provide an environment conducive to nutritional maintenance. Adequate patient teaching about a therapeutic diet may solve the problem. If possible, alterations in prescribed diets should be made for cultural and religious patterns. Providing an environment that is free from malodorous dressings may be the only stimulus needed to improve the appetite.

(2) Administer enteral hyperalimentation.

If the patient has a functioning G.I. tract, but is unable to consume nutrients for a variety of reasons, *enteral hyperalimentation* may be indicated. Patients in this category include those who are debilitated, unable to swallow (of esophageal motility problems, neurological problems or a tumor), or anorexic. By using the enteral route, one can avoid the complications of catheter insertion and sepsis that are encountered in total parenteral nutrition. Several commercially prepared formulas are available such as Compleat B, Sustacal, Ensure, Isocal, Precision, Flexical, and Vivonex. These formulas vary in protein source, calories, lactose content, and osmolality. The expertise of a clinical dietician is of value when deciding on the appropriate fluid diet for the individual patient. With the design of the soft silicone rubber feeding tubes, many of the problems with irritation from the larger NG tubes have been eliminated.

After verification of proper tube placement via x-ray, the feeding may begin. The formula is placed in plastic containers and infused with intravenous tubing, preferably by a volumetric infusion pump. To alleviate the problem of severe diarrhea caused by hyperosmolar solutions delivered into the small intestine, the enteral feeding is diluted to half strength at the onset of feeding. The concentration is increased according to the patient's tolerance. Initially, the feeding should infuse slowly and, by increasing the infusion rate daily, advance to the tolerated level. The infusion rate is reduced, or the concentration of the formula is decreased, if there is nausea, vomiting, diarrhea or abdominal cramping. Aspiration of greater than 100 cc of fluid prior to the next scheduled feeding is indicative of poor absorption and requires re-evaluation. The patient receiving enteral hyperalimentation must be monitored closely, including daily *weight, intake* and *output, electrolytes, BUN, liver function tests, glucose* and *records of aspiration.*

(3) Administer total parenteral nutrition (TPN).

If the patient has a poorly functioning G.I. tract with an anticipated long recovery phase, or if the patient has an extremely high caloric requirement, total parenteral nutrition (TPN) should be initiated. TPN is an intravenous solution containing amino acids, hypertonic glucose, vitamins, minerals, electrolytes and trace elements. Both central and peripheral administration of TPN is acceptable, with certain restrictions on the peripheral route due to the hypertonicity of the solution with resultant sclerosis of veins.

The first step in central TPN infusion is the insertion of the catheter. This procedure is *never* an emergency and must be performed with strict surgical aseptic technique. Either a subclavian or internal jugular vein is cannulated, with the former being preferred because of patient comfort and ease of care. Once proper placement is verified by x-ray, infusion of the TPN solution may begin at the prescribed rate. It must be emphasized that this catheter is *strictly* for the infusion of the TPN solution and is *not* to be used for drawing blood samples or infusing any other fluids. If infusion of additional fluids or blood is needed, a peripheral line must be established. Care of the catheter after insertion should follow hospital policy, with emphasis on the need for total aseptic technique to avoid the potential complication of sepsis.

The physician orders the formula for the TPN solution, and in most institutions, the pharmacist is responsible for preparing the solution, using the aseptic environment provided by the laminar flow hood. Various solutions are available, containing different percentages of amino acids so that therapy can be individualized. FreAmine II and Aminosyn are two common amino acid mixtures. Added to the amino acid mixture is the hypertonic glucose solution of $D_{50}W$, which provides the calories. An ideal calorie-to-nitrogen ratio should be maintained (about 150 cal/gm nitrogen) to achieve a maximal protein sparing effect. Sodium, potassium, chloride, magnesium, calcium, phosphate, vitamins and trace elements are then added to the solution. The amount of electrolytes needed varies in different patients, but more potassium is required because of its association with the intracellular movement of glucose and amino acids. Vitamins, which are necessary additives, provide substrates for metabolic processes. Vitamin B_{12} and folic acid have a tendency to change when added to TPN solution; to avoid this, they are usually administered separately. An alternative to the separate administration of folic acid and vitamin B_{12} has been the establishment of a routine vitamin protocol. Folic acid and vitamin B_{12} are added to the first liter of TPN two days a week as the only vitamin additive. The multivitamins are added to the second liter on these days. This protocol has shown satisfactory blood levels, and no change in the stability of these additives has been noted. Lipids are given twice weekly to prevent deficiencies.

The starting infusion rate usually provides from 1,200 to 2,400 cal./day. Depending on patient tolerance, the rate may be increased daily until the desired caloric intake is reached. The nurse must ensure a continuous and constant infusion rate to avoid the metabolic complications of TPN.

The use of a volumetric infusion pump is essential.

The patient receiving TPN must be monitored closely. Laboratory tests on this patient should include CBC, electrolytes, calcium, platelet count, BUN, magnesium, glucose, creatinine, total protein, albumin, phosphorus and globin. In addition, SGOT, SGPT, prothrombin time, total bilirubin and uric acid should be measured periodically. Urine glucose tests should be done every six hours. The patient must be weighed daily. An estimate of nitrogen balance should be done weekly to note the effectiveness of therapy.

The complications of TPN are due to the catheter, sepsis or metabolic disorders. Numerous problems may arise with the insertion of the subclavian catheter, including hemothorax, pneumothorax, inadvertent arterial puncture, brachial plexus irritation, air embolism and catheter embolism. The cannulation is done by an experienced physician. A postinsertion chest radiograph is essential to verify proper position and to check for potential complications.

Sepsis may be due to lack of asepsis during catheter insertion, superficial infection around the catheter after prolonged placement that is introduced into the catheter, and solution contamination. Maintenance of aseptic technique throughout all stages of administration of TPN cannot be overemphasized. The procedure varies among institutions, but when a significant temperature elevation is observed, it is recommended the TPN infusion be discontinued. To avoid hypoglycemia, $D_{10}W$ should be infused through the catheter. Cultures should be obtained from the solution and from the patient's blood, urine and sputum to identify the source. If the patient remains febrile and the source of fever cannot be identified, the catheter should be removed and sent for culture.

Hyperglycemia is one of the metabolic complications of TPN administration. This state is controlled by starting the infusion slowly, since initial hyperglycemia is expected because of stimulation of the pancreas. As the pancreas adjusts to the glucose load, a state of hyperinsulinemia occurs and the blood sugar returns to normal. After several days of TPN therapy with continued hyperglycemia and glycosuria, regular insulin should be added to the TPN, and the infusion rate should be decreased. If hyperosmolar nonketotic coma occurs, the TPN must be stopped immediately and therapy initiated, combining hydration and insulin administration.

Hypoglycemia is usually a result of abrupt cessation of the infusion of the TPN solution because of inadvertent dislodgement of the catheter or lack of solution. Reinstituting the infusion is the simplest solution, but if none is available, the infusion of $D_{10}W$ will prevent symptomatic hypoglycemia. To prevent hypoglycemia when TPN therapy is being discontinued, it is recommended that the infusion rate be tapered over several days.

Serum levels of phosphate and magnesium must be monitored to prevent deficiencies of these substances. Magnesium is necessary for cellular synthesis, and often the level drops after the initiation of TPN. The intracellular manufacture of proteins, DNA and ATP depends on phosphate. Extra phosphate may be needed to prevent the lethargy, paresthesias and possible coma of hypophosphatemia.

(4) Administer peripheral parenteral nutrition (PPN).

PPN utilizes an amino acid-dextrose solution ($D_{10}W$-$D_{20}W$), alone or in conjunction with a fat emulsion, which provides nutritional support to qualifying candidates. The tonicity of the solution is limited when infused peripherally, thus restricting the calories that dextrose supplies. The calories are supplied by Intralipid, a fat emulsion that is not irritating to peripheral veins. PPN usually provides fewer calories than TPN, making indications slightly different. PPN is indicated for patients who require total nutritional support, but in whom it is not possible to utilize a central vein cannulation; for patients who had been receiving TPN, but the central line was discontinued because of sepsis; and for patients with marginal nutritional status in whom short-term nutrition is required.

KEY CONCEPT: The patient with G.I. disorders provides the critical care nurse with numerous challenges. The major goals of therapy are to:
1. **Assess and maintain an adequate circulating volume.**
2. **Preserve fluid and electrolyte balance.**
3. **Provide adequate nutrition.**
4. **Prevent infections.**
5. **Promote return to daily activities.**
6. **Offer psychological support.**

As the patient improves from the critical period, it is imperative that the nurse begin the desperately needed patient teaching, in hopes of preventing another acute episode of the disease. Including the family in these teaching sessions may give the patient the additional support needed to deal constructively with the disease state.

KEY POINT RECOGNITION

Write true or false by each statement. Answers are at the end of this chapter. A score below 80% indicates the need for further study.

_____ 1. Vomiting causes a loss of gastric hydrochloric acid and water.

_____ 2. Diarrhea may cause a hypernatremic state.

_____ 3. Hypokalemia and metabolic acidosis may be associated with severe diarrhea.

_____ 4. Any disease state that interferes with the main function of the G.I. tract renders the patient malnourished.

_____ 5. Depression of cellular immunity is a finding in patients with protein caloric malnutrition.

_____ 6. Advantages of using the enteral hyperalimentation route are avoidance of infection and sepsis.

_____ 7. Enteral hyperalimentation may be used in patients who are unable to swallow or who are anorexic.

_____ 8. The patient receiving enteral hyperalimentation must be monitored for weight changes, intake and output, electrolytes, BUN, glucose and liver function tests.

_____ 9. Total parenteral nutrition (TPN) can be used only in patients with a functioning G.I. tract.

_____10. TPN may be used for patients requiring extremely high caloric nutrition.

_____11. FreAmine II and Aminosyn are common amino acid mixtures used in TPN.

_____12. The nurse is responsible for ensuring a continuous and constant infusion rate for TPN.

_____13. Urine glucose tests should be done every 24 hours while a patient is on TPN.

_____14. Hyperglycemia is one of the metabolic complications of TPN administration.

_____15. Hyperglycemia is usually a result of abrupt cessation of the TPN solution infusion.

_____16. The ideal calorie-to-nitrogen ratio in TPN preparation is 150 cal./gm nitrogen. This achieves a maximal protein sparing effect.

_____17. The starting infusion rate for TPN usually provides 1,200 to 2,400 calories per day.

PASS
Program Assessment: Science and Situation

1. The oral cavity consists of the
    a. lips, cheeks, teeth, palate, gums, salivary glands and tongue.
    b. teeth, gums and tongue.
    c. mouth, salivary glands and tongue.
    d. mouth, salivary glands, tongue and upper esophagus.

2. The three stages of deglutition are
    a. voluntary, esophageal and involuntary.
    b. primary, intermediate and secondary.
    c. voluntary, pharyngeal and esophageal.
    d. primary, secondary and involuntary.

3. The gastroesophageal sphincter
    a. is located at the proximal end of the esophagus.
    b. allows the food bolus to enter the stomach and prevents reflux back into the esophagus.
    c. is totally under hormonal control.
    d. normally remains open.

4. Which of the following glands located within the mucosal layer of the stomach does not secrete mucus?
    a. cardiac
    b. fundic
    c. pyloric
    d. none of the above

5. The primary control of gastric motility is
    a. hormonal action.
    b. vagal action.
    c. both a and b
    d. none of the above

6. All of the following are true about gastrin, *except* that it
    a. is secreted by the antral cells of the stomach.
    b. promotes HCl and pepsin production.
    c. increases antral motility.
    d. promotes absorption of lipids.

7. Gastric secretion is stimulated by
    a. pepsinogen, HCl and intrinsic factor.
    b. pepsin, H_2 receptor blockers and pepsinogen.
    c. histamine, HCl and mucus.
    d. gastrin, acetylcholine and histamine.

8. All of the following are true about intrinsic factor, *except* that it
    a. is secreted by the parietal cells.
    b. is a mucoprotein.
    c. binds to vitamin B_{12}.
    d. aids digestion of vitamin B_{12}.

9. The ileocecal valve
    a. connects the jejunum to the ileum and allows passage of the feces into the ileum.
    b. forms the passageway to the large intestine and controls reflux into the ileum.
    c. remains open to facilitate the passage of feces.
    d. is absent in 80 percent of adults.

10. The mucosal layer of the small intestine contains
    a. folds of Kerckring.
    b. villi and microvilli.
    c. Lieberkuhn's crypts.
    d. all of the above

11. Brunner's glands are
    a. found in the mucosal layer of the ileum and secrete an alkaline mucoid substance.
    b. found in the submucosal layer of the duodenum and secrete an alkaline mucoid substance.
    c. found in the submucosal layer throughout the small intestine and secrete a neutral mucoid substance.
    d. found in the mucosal layer of the jejunum and secrete pepsinogen.

12. Small intestinal motility is accomplished by these coinciding events:
    a. basic electrical rhythm, segmentation, peristalsis
    b. active transport, passive diffusion
    c. facilitated diffusion, segmentation
    d. mixing, propulsion, nonionic transport

13. Which of the following is true?
    a. The absorption of water is totally due to passive diffusion.
    b. When about 10 liters of water are absorbed, all but around 150 cc are reabsorbed.
    c. both a and b
    d. none of the above

14. Concerning carbohydrate absorption,
    a. carbohydrates must be broken down into polysaccharides, and most are further broken down into monosaccharides before being absorbed.
    b. pancreatic amylase is essential for breakdown.
    c. the microvilli of the intestinal mucosal cells produce the enzymes sucrase and lactase for breakdown.
    d. all of the above

15. Concerning protein absorption,
    a. some protein can be absorbed as a dipeptide.
    b. acid in the stomach, pepsin and pancreatic proteases are required.
    c. protein must be in the form of amino acid before absorption can occur.
    d. both a and b

16. Micelles
    a. are secreted by the Peyer's patches to enhance fat absorption.
    b. are very small particles composed of bile salts, fatty acids, monoglycerides, phospholipids, cholesterol and fat-soluble vitamins.

c. function to coagulate the fat digestion products.
d. allow the diffusion of all contents into the intestinal cell.

17. The purpose of the micelle formation is to
    a. transport the dipeptide to the jejunal mucosal cell.
    b. contain the bile salts in liquid to prevent their diffusion into the jejunal mucosal cell.
    c. keep the excess fat digestion products out of solution and transport them into the jejunal mucosal cell.
    d. transport the bile salts to the ileum for diffusion.

18. The epithelial cells of the intestinal mucosa contribute the digestive enzymes, including
    a. amylase and lipase.
    b. maltase and lactase.
    c. sucrase and peptidases.
    d. all of the above

19. The control for the secretion of intestinal juices is
    a. local stimulation.
    b. hormonal stimulation.
    c. both a and b
    d. none of the above

20. The primary functions of the large intestine are
    a. digestion of solutes and fluid absorption.
    b. digestion of solutes and elimination of waste products.
    c. elimination of waste products and absorption of solutes and fluid.
    d. absorption of fluid and solutes.

21. The motor activities of the large intestine are inhibited by
    a. morphine and urecholine.
    b. neostigmine and bile salts.
    c. atropine and ganglionic blocking agents.
    d. low bulk diet and bacterial enterotoxins.

22. The normal flora bacteria in the colon
    a. provide a means of synthesizing vitamin K, riboflavin, nicotinic acid and folic acid.
    b. decompose urea to ammonia and carbon dioxide.
    c. breakdown small amounts of cellulose.
    d. all of the above

23. Choose the correct venous flow of blood in the liver.
    a. portal vein, liver sinusoids, central vein, hepatic vein, inferior vena cava
    b. portal vein, hepatic vein, liver sinusoids, inferior mesenteric, inferior vena cava
    c. hepatic vein, liver sinusoids, inferior vena cava
    d. hepatic vein, liver sinusoids, central vein, inferior vena cava

24. The function(s) of the gallbladder is (are)
    a. to connect the common hepatic duct with the pancreatic duct.
    b. to store and concentrate bile.

c. to store and concentrate triglycerides and amino acids.

d. to connect the common bile duct with the pancreatic duct.

25. The major constituents of bile are
    a. bile salts, water and electrolytes.
    b. bile acids, water, electrolytes, bilirubin, cholesterol and lecithin.
    c. bile salts, miscellaneous metabolites, bilirubin, water and electrolytes.
    d. bile acids, water, electrolytes and bilirubin.

26. Indirect bilirubin is
    a. albumin-associated and not soluble enough for efficient excretion.
    b. unconjugated and fat soluble.
    c. both a and b
    d. none of the above

27. Direct bilirubin is
    a. water soluble, conjugated and excreted into bile.
    b. unconjugated and fat soluble.
    c. albumin-associated and unconjugated.
    d. fat soluble and conjugated

28. An elevated direct bilirubin is indicative of
    a. liver dysfunction.
    b. biliary tract obstruction.
    c. both a and b
    d. none of the above

29. The exocrine function of the pancreas is due to the secretory units called the
    a. islets.
    b. beta cells.
    c. acini.
    d. alpha cells.

30. The pancreas secretes a group of digestive enzymes
    a. that works most efficiently in a neutral pH.
    b. that is capable of digesting all useful fats, carbohydrates and proteins.
    c. that includes proteolytic enzymes, lipase and amylase.
    d. all of the above

31. The pancreas also produces an isotonic, bicarbonate-rich electrolyte solution that
    a. neutralizes the acid chyme in the duodenum and facilitates fat emulsification.
    b. bathes the pancreas to maintain a neutral environment.
    c. maintains a pH of 10.
    d. serves as a protection for the pancreatic enzymes.

32. The contribution from the liver to digestion includes
    a. secretion of proteolytic enzymes.
    b. secretion of bile salts.
    c. gluconeogenesis.
    d. all of the above

33. Other functions of the liver include
    a. vitamin and mineral storage.
    b. metabolism of protein, carbohydrate and fat.
    c. a and b
    d. none of the above

34. When the liver becomes cirrhotic,
    a. the hepatic vein is eroded.
    b. liver cells are destroyed and replaced by connective tissue.
    c. the sinusoids become regular in shape.
    d. all of the above

35. The difference between the pathological types of cirrhosis (Laennec's, postnecrotic and biliary) can be detected by
    a. liver scan.
    b. palpation.
    c. symptoms.
    d. liver biopsy.

36. The pathology of Laennec's cirrhosis includes
    a. fibrosis, nodular formation, fatty degeneration, Mallory's alcoholic membrane and hepatocyte death.
    b. destruction of hepatocytes, regeneration, scarring, and nodular formation.
    c. obstruction of bile flow, scarring, proliferation of bile ducts
    d. portal-systemic shunt, portal hypertension and hepatocyte death

37. Possible etiological factors in cirrhosis include
    a. alcohol and its metabolites.
    b. toxic substances.
    c. viral infections and obstruction to bile flow.
    d. all of the above

38. Potential complications of cirrhosis are
    a. portal hypertension and jaundice.
    b. portal hypertension, ascites and hydrothorax.
    c. jaundice and urobilinogen.
    d. ascites, pneumonia and CHF.

39. Medical treatment for the cirrhotic patient includes
    a. high caloric diet, exercise, and a limit of one alcoholic drink per day.
    b. rest, vitamins, restricted protein diet, and abstinence from alcohol.
    c. I.V. vitamins, exercise and abstinence from alcohol.
    d. limited alcohol, vitamins and exercise.

40. The syndrome of hepatic failure is complex and ill-defined. Causative factors include
    a. conditions that show functional failure.
    b. conditions that are chronic.
    c. conditions that cause diffuse necrosis.
    d. all of the above

41. The presenting symptom(s) of hepatic failure is (are)
    a. jaundice.
    b. encephalopathy.
    c. a range of signs from jaundice to fulminant failure.
    d. flapping tremors.

42. The elevated serum ammonia level seen in patients with hepatic failure may be due to
    a. malnutrition and excessive alcohol consumption.
    b. lack of detoxification by the liver.
    c. portal-systemic shunting.
    d. b and c

43. In a patient with marginal hepatic reserve, hepatic failure may be precipitated by
    a. G.I. bleeding.
    b. alcohol abuse and a high protein diet.
    c. hepatitis and paracentesis.
    d. all of the above

44. Hemolytic jaundice occurs when
    a. extrahepatic bile ducts are obstructed.
    b. bilirubin cannot be excreted because of liver cell dysfunction.
    c. there is an increased destruction of erythrocytes.
    d. there is gallbladder disease.

45. Laboratory findings indicative of hepatocellular jaundice are
    a. prolonged prothrombin time, elevated SGOT, LDH, urine positive for bile and urobilinogen.
    b. urine positive for bile, but little or no urobilinogen, elevated SGOT and LDH.
    c. elevated urobilinogen and elevated reticulocyte count.
    d. low hematocrit, minimally elevated SGOT and LDH.

46. The purpose of instilling neomycin down the NG in the patient with hepatic faiure is to
    a. increase the intestinal flora to lower the production of ammonia.
    b. decrease the intestinal flora to decrease the production of ammonia.
    c. increase the intestinal flora to increase the production of ammonia.
    d. decrease the intestinal flora to increase the production of ammonia.

47. The administration of furosemide to patients in hepatic failure
    a. should be restricted to decrease the congestive failure.
    b. is contraindicated.
    c. should be judicious to prevent hypokalemia, alkalosis and prevent further encephalopathy.
    d. is usually a routine bid order.

48. Esophageal varices are formed by
    a. dilatation of the small veins in the esophageal submucosal plexus at the portal-systemic anastamotic site in the lower third of the esophagus.
    b. dilatation of the esophageal branch of the left gastric artery because of portal hypertension.

c. dilatation of the azygous veins because of hypertension.

d. dilatation of the esophageal vein because of portal hypertension.

49. Bleeding of these varices may be precipitated by
    a. erosion from acid-pepsin.
    b. trauma.
    c. a surge of extremely elevated venous pressure.
    d. all of the above

50. Typically, the patient with bleeding esophageal varices will present to the ER with
    a. copious hematemesis without abdominal pain.
    b. copious hematemesis with excrutiating, diffuse abdominal pain.
    c. copious melena without abdominal pain.
    d. copious melena with excruciating diffuse abdominal pain.

51. The action of vasopressin is to
    a. increase portal venous pressure by constricting the splanchnic vein.
    b. decrease portal venous pressure by constricting the splanchnic vein.
    c. increase portal venous pressure by dilating the splanchnic vein.
    d. decrease portal venous pressure by dilating the splanchnic vein.

52. The recommended procedure for the infusion of a vasopressin drip is to
    a. start the infusion at 0.6 units/minute and titrate the dosage to stop the bleeding.
    b. start the infusion at 0.3 units/minute and observe for 30 minutes; if bleeding continues, titrate the dose to a maximum of 0.8 units/minute every 30 minutes.
    c. start the infusion at 0.8 units/minute for two hours; if bleeding continues, notify the physician.
    d. start infusion at 0.1 unit/minute, observe for two hours; if bleeding continues, notify the physician.

53. Nursing care for the patient with a Sengstaken-Blakemore tube includes
    a. continuous NG suction.
    b. intermittent inflation and deflation of the gastric balloon.
    c. maintenance of correct inflation pressures in the gastric and esophageal balloons, with traction applied to the tube to prevent descent into the stomach.
    d. continuous iced saline lavage.

54. The patient with a duodenal ulcer typically has an increased secretion of acid and pepsin caused by an
    a. increase in the amount of parietal cells in the gastric mucosa.
    b. increase in the amount of acid secreted by the parietal cells.
    c. decreased amount of stimulation needed by the parietal cells to secrete acid.
    d. all of the above

55. The pathology of gastric ulcers seems to be
    a. an increased acid-pepsin secretion.
    b. a breakdown in the defense barrier of the mucosa.
    c. an increased amount of fundic cells.
    d. a decreased amount of Brunner's glands.

56. All of the following may be factors in ulcer formation *except*:
    a. increased autonomic stimulation
    b. endogenous and/or exogenous cortisones
    c. glucocorticoids
    d. an increased number of Brunner's glands

57. The formation of an acute stress ulcer
    a. has the same pathology as peptic ulcers.
    b. involves the deep musculature of the stomach.
    c. is thought to be caused by ischemia.
    d. occurs most often in neurosurgical patients.

58. The most significant symptom of peptic ulcer disease is
    a. G.I. bleeding.
    b. abdominal cramping.
    c. episodic abdominal pain.
    d. nausea and vomiting.

59. Potential complications of peptic ulcer disease are
    a. perforation, bleeding and pyloric obstruction.
    b. peritonitis, ileus and bleeding.
    c. ileus, liver failure and intestinal obstruction.
    d. sepsis, ascites and ileus.

60. The first line of treatment for the patient with G.I. bleeding is
    a. to find the source of the bleeding
    b. to correct electrolyte imbalance.
    c. to prevent and treat shock.
    d. to perform selective angiography.

61. The pathology of acute pancreatitis includes
    a. blockage of the flow of the pancreatic enzymes, stagnation in the ducts and acini, activation of the enzymes and digestion of the pancreas.
    b. free flow of pancreatic enzymes, overabundance of trypsinogen, activation of enzymes and digestion of the pancreas.
    c. blockage of the pancreatic flow, overabundance of trypsin inhibitor and complete inactivation of the enzymes.
    d. blockage of the pancreatic flow, overabundance of bile salts and complete inactivation of the enzymes.

62. The most frequently associated findings in acute pancreatitis are
    a. steroids and biliary tract disease.
    b. trauma and steroids.
    c. alcohol and biliary tract disease.
    d. alcohol and dyazide diuretics.

63. Associated symptoms of acute pancreatitis include all of the following, *except*
    a. severe pain over the entire abdomen, with radiation to the back and flanks.
    b. nausea and vomiting.
    c. abdominal distension.
    d. febrile above 102°F.

64. The patient with acute pancreatitis will usually have all of the following laboratory data, *except*
    a. elevated serum amylase.
    b. elevated direct bilirubin.
    c. elevated calcium.
    d. decreased serum albumin.

65. Therapy for the patient with acute pancreatitis includes
    a. keeping the pancreas at rest.
    b. maintaining adequate circulating blood volume.
    c. alleviating pain.
    d. all of the above

66. When obtaining a history from the patient with a G.I. disorder, which of the following should *not* be elicited?
    a. previous G.I. problems
    b. presence of abdominal pain
    c. presence of urinary incontinence
    d. presence of heartburn

67. Bowel sounds will be absent in the following disease states, with the exception of
    a. peritonitis.
    b. ileus.
    c. gangrene.
    d. cirrhosis.

68. Colicky abdominal pain associated with borborygmus is indicative of
    a. peritonitis.
    b. intestinal obstruction.
    c. appendicitis.
    d. cholecystitis.

69. Palpation of the abdomen is useful in evaluating all the following *except:*
    a. differentiation of pain
    b. detection of presence and character of masses
    c. verifying organomegaly
    d. presence of dilated veins

70. Indications for endoscopic evaluation include
    a. upper G.I. bleeding.
    b. evaluation of peptic ulcer disease.
    c. detection of perforations.
    d. a and b

71. Vomiting may cause the following electrolyte disturbances, *except*
    a. alkalosis.
    b. hypokalemia.
    c. hyponatremia.
    d. hypercalcemia.

72. Negative nitrogen balance occurs when
    a. the amount of nitrogen consumed is equivalent to the amount excreted.
    b. the amount of nitrogen consumed is greater than the amount excreted.
    c. the amount of nitrogen consumed is less than the amount excreted.
    d. none of the above

73. Enteral hyperalimentation is indicated when
    a. the patient has a functioning G.I. tract.
    b. the patient is unable to swallow.
    c. the patient is debilitated.
    d. all of the above

74. TPN should be initiated when
    a. the patient has a poorly functioning G.I. tract.
    b. the patient has an extremely high caloric requirement.
    c. the patient is anorectic.
    d. a and b

75. Complications of TPN infusion include
    a. sepsis.
    b. catheter insertion problems.
    c. metabolic disorders.
    d. all of the above

KEY POINT RECOGNITION ANSWERS
Upper G.I. system
1. True
2. False—Upward movement of the palate
3. True
4. True
5. False—Parotid, submandibular and sublingual
6. False—It retards the formation of dental caries.
7. False—Hypertonic
8. True
9. False—It is controlled by the autonomic nervous system.
10. False—Voluntary, pharyngeal and esophageal
11. True
12. True
13. False—It is thought to be of a neurogenic basis.
14. True
15. True
16. True
17. False—10 inches
18. True
19. False—Cardiac sphincter
20. False—Pyloric sphincter
21. True
22. True
23. False—Four layers
24. True
25. False—Chief cells secrete pepsinogen. Parietal cells secrete hydrochloric acid.
26. True
27. True
28. True
29. False—It has three layers and is composed of smooth muscle.
30. False—It is accommodated by passive stretching.
31. True
32. True
33. True
34. False—Gastrin enhances the rate of gastric emptying through the promotion of increased production of hydrochloric acid and pepsin.
35. False—Dorsolateral reticular formation of the medulla
36. True
37. True
38. True
39. False—Gastric secretion is stimulated by the interaction of gastrin, acteylcholine and histamine.
40. True
41. False—Gastric phase
42. True

Lower G.I. system
1. False—Small intestine
2. False—Three segments: duodenum, jejunum and ileum
3. True
4. True
5. True
6. False—Brunner's glands secrete an alkaline mucoid substance.
7. True
8. True
9. True
10. True
11. True
12. True
13. False—Amino acids + calcium = active transport; water = passive diffusion
14. False—No energy is required.
15. True
16. False—Potassium is passively absorbed in the small intestine and passively secreted in the large intestine.
17. True
18. True
19. True
20. False—Monosaccharide
21. True
22. False—Amylase is produced in the pancreas.
23. False—Sucrase = sucrose into glucose and fructose; Lactase = lactose into glucose and galactose
24. False—Eight
25. True
26. True
27. True
28. True
29. True
30. False—Bile salts are absorbed in the ileum and transported to the liver.
31. True
32. True
33. True
34. False—Cecum, colon, rectum
35. True
36. True
37. False—They occur two to three times in a 24-hour period.
38. True
39. False—350 cc are absorbed. 150 cc are excreted in feces.
40. True

Blood supply to the G.I. tract
1. True
2. True
3. True
4. True
5. True

Nervous innervation
1. False—Motor, secretory and sensory functions
2. True
3. False—Acetylcholine is responsible for the stimulation of all functions of the gut.
4. False—Norepinephrine

The accessory organs of digestion
1. False—50 cc
2. True
3. True
4. True
5. True
6. True
7. True
8. True

Physical assessment of the gastrointestinal system
1. True
2. True
3. True
4. True
5. False—Inspection of the abdomen across the epigastric area may reveal a normal aortic pulsation.
6. False—Frequently in peritonitis, ileus or gangrene, bowel sounds are absent.
7. True
8. False—A venous hum is found in the cirrhotic patient with a massive portal-systemic shunt due to portal hypertension.
9. True
10. False—A cirrhotic liver is usually enlarged, smooth and nontender.

Nursing assessment of the G.I. system
1. False—A good history and physical are probably the most important determinants of a gastrointestinal disorder.
2. True
3. True
4. False—Gastric analysis may be used to diagnose Zollinger-Ellison syndrome.
5. True
6. False—Mechanical cleaning is most effective.
7. True

Pathological states and nursing management
1. True
2. False—The cirrhotic liver has an irregular shape.
3. False—Laennec's cirrhosis is a common form of cirrhosis.
4. True
5. False—Hepatomegaly is not associated with postnecrotic cirrhosis.
6. True
7. False—The portal system is normally a low-pressure system.
8. True

9. True
10. True
11. True
12. True
13. True
14. False—Jaundice is not always indicative of liver failure.
15. True
16. False—Hematemesis without abdominal pain is indicative of bleeding esophageal varices.
17. True
18. False—If peripheral vasopressin controls the bleeding, it will do so within four to six hours of infusion.
19. True
20. True
21. True
22. True
23. False—Glucocorticoids increase the secretion of pepsin and HCl.
24. True
25. True
26. False—Alcohol increases the production of pancreatic secretions.
27. False—The pain of acute pancreatitis may radiate to the back and flanks.
28. False—Fever is due to inflammatory reaction and necrosis.
29. True
30. True
31. False—The pseudocyst formation is due to necrotic tissue.
32. True
33. True
34. False—Colloid and crystalloid replacement solutions *are* indicated.
35. True

Care common to gastrointestinal problems
1. True
2. True
3. True
4. True
5. True
6. True
7. True
8. True
9. False—TPN may be used in patients with a non-functioning GI tract.
10. True
11. True
12. True
13. False—Urine glucose tests should be done every 6 hours.
14. True
15. False—Hypoglycemia is usually a result of abrupt cessation of TPN.
16. True
17. True

PASS ANSWER SHEET

1. a	26. c	51. b
2. c	27. a	52. b
3. b	28. b	53. c
4. d	29. c	54. d
5. b	30. d	55. b
6. d	31. a	56. d
7. d	32. b	57. c
8. d	33. c	58. c
9. b	34. b	59. a
10. d	35. d	60. c
11. b	36. a	61. a
12. a	37. d	62. c
13. c	38. b	63. d
14. d	39. b	64. c
15. d	40. d	65. d
16. b	41. c	66. c
17. c	42. d	67. d
18. d	43. d	68. b
19. c	44. c	69. d
20. c	45. a	70. d
21. c	46. b	71. d
22. d	47. c	72. c
23. a	48. a	73. d
24. b	49. d	74. d
25. b	50. a	75. d

SURVEY SUMMARY
GASTROINTESTINAL SYSTEM

I. **The Gastrointestinal System: Overview**

   A. The function of the G.I. system is to provide water, electrolytes and nutrients to the body and to prepare the nutrients for absorption.

   B. The G.I. system is divided into the:
   1. Upper G.I. system
   2. Lower G.I. system
   3. Accessory organs of digestion

II. **Anatomy and physiology**

   A. The *upper G.I. system* comprises the oral cavity, pharynx, esophagus and stomach.
   1. The *oral cavity* is responsible for the preparation of food for absorption and consists of the lips, cheeks, teeth, palate, gums, salivary glands and tongue.
   2. The *pharynx* is divided into the nasopharynx, oropharynx and laryngeal pharynx, and aids in the deglutition process.
   3. The *esophagus* is a passageway for food from the pharynx to the stomach.
   4. The *stomach* lies between the esophagus and duodenum.
      a. It acts as a reservoir to accept food, secretes digestive juices and releases food into the duodenum.
      b. The landmarks are the:
         1. Esophageal-cardiac juncture
         2. Longitudinal section of the fundic stomach
         3. Longitudinal section of the duodenum
      c. The *cardiac sphincter* is the portal of entry to the stomach, and the exit is through the *pyloric sphincter.*
      d. The four layers of the stomach include the mucosal, muscularis mucosa, submucosal and muscular coat. The cardiac, gastric and pyloric glands are within the mucosal layer.
      e. Increased stomach volume is accommodated by passive stretching, which initiates a vagal reflex, preventing muscular activity in the body of the stomach. The release of acetylcholine determines the occurrence of peristalsis.
      f. Gastric emptying is due to both peristalsis and the pylorus' attempt to reject the food bolus by maintaining normal pyloric constriction.
         1. The stomach empties at a rate proportional to its volume of material.
         2. *Gastrin* enhances the rate of gastric emptying.
         3. Duodenal stimuli on gastric emptying are inhibitory.
      g. Vomiting also empties the stomach.
         1. Nervous control is located in the dorsolateral reticular formation of the medulla.
         2. Impulses reach the vomiting center via vagal and sympathetic afferents.
      h. Gastric juice promotes digestion.
         1. *Hydrochloric acid* is secreted by the parietal cells.
            a. It converts pepsinogen to pepsin.

b. It destroys bacteria.

c. It denatures protein.

2. **Intrinsic factor** binds to vitamin B_{12} to prevent its digestion and enhance its absorption.

3. **Pepsinogen** is the inactive precursor of pepsin.

4. Gastric secretion is stimulated by the interaction of:

   a. Gastrin

   b. Acetylcholine

   c. Histamine

5. The stages of gastric secretion are:

   a. Basal

   b. Cephalic

   c. Gastric

   d. Intestinal

B. The *lower G.I. system* is composed of the small intestine and large intestine.

1. Most digestion and absorption takes place in the small intestine.

2. The small intestine begins at the pylorus of the stomach, ends at the ileocecal valve of the large intestine and measures 20 to 30 feet in length.

3. The small intestine is divided into the:

   a. Duodenum

   b. Jejunum

   c. Ileum

4. The small intestinal wall is composed of three layers:

   a. *Muscular*

      1. This layer has two smooth muscle components: inner circular and outer longitudinal.

      2. The myenteric plexus of nerve fibers and parasympathetic ganglion cells are situated in the connective tissue of the two layers.

   b. *Submucosal.* This layer contains Meissner's plexus and Brunner's glands.

   c. *Mucosal*

5. The *motility* of the small intestine is accomplished by the relationship between the following:

   a. Basic electrical rhythm

   b. Contractions

6. There are two types of small intestinal movements:

   a. *Mixing,* or sequential

   b. *Peristaltic,* or propulsive

7. The functions of the small intestine are **digestion** and **absorption.**

   a. Absorption may take place through the following mechanisms:

      1. Active transport

      2. Passive diffusion

      3. Facilitated diffusion

      4. Nonionic transport

8. Carbohydrates supply half of the daily ingested calories.

9. To facilitate absorption, carbohydrates must be broken down into *polysaccharides* and finally *monosaccharides.*
    a. *Amylase* transforms starch to maltose, maltotriose and oligosaccharides.
    b. The microvilli of the intestinal mucosal cells produce the enzymes to break the oligosaccharides into monosaccharides.
        1. *Sucrase* breaks sucrose into fructose and glucose.
        2. *Lactase* breaks lactose into glucose and galactose.
10. Protein absorption is active and accomplished by the breakdown of amino acids.
    a. There are *22 amino acids,* eight of which are essential.
    b. Protein digestion is initiated by *pepsin, gastrin* and *pancreozymin-cholecystokinin.*
    c. Protein-splitting enzymes secreted by the pancreas are:
        1. Trysin
        2. Chymotrypsin
        3. Carboxypolypeptidases
    d. Further breakdown is by enzymes in the microvilli of the intestinal mucosa.
11. Fat absorption is the process of breaking down triglycerides and resynthesizing them into triglyceride for use.
    a. *Lipase* splits the triglyceride into free fatty acid and monoglyceride.
    b. *Micelles* provide a vehicle for the fat digestion products to be diffused into the intestinal mucosal cells.
    c. Triglycerides are formed and extruded from the cells into the lymph.
12. Secretions in the small intestine are in response to chemical or mechanical irritation.
    a. Brunner's glands secrete mucus.
    b. Other areas secrete enzymes.
    c. The major control for secretion is local stimulation.
    d. Hormones also regulate secretion.
        1. Vasoactive intestinal peptide *increases* secretion.
        2. *Secretin* maintains the pH of the duodenum.
        3. *Pancreozymin-cholecystokinin* inhibits acid secretion, stimulates pancreatic enzymes and stimulates contraction of the gallbladder.
        4. *Gastric inhibitory peptide* stimulates insulin release and inhibits gastric motility.
13. The *large intestine* is 5.5 feet in length, begins at the end of the ileum and ends at the anus, and is the final passageway for food.
14. The functions of the large intestine include *absorption* of solutes and fluid, and *elimination* of wastes.
15. The three divisions of the large intestine include the:
    a. *Cecum,* which is two to three inches long.
    b. *Colon,* which has four sections: ascending, transverse, descending and sigmoid.
    c. *Rectum*
16. The layers of the large intestine include the:
    a. Mucosal
    b. Submucosal

c. Muscular
17. Colonic motility is much slower than small intestine motility.
    a. There are *mixing movements* and *propulsive movements.*
    b. Pharmacological agents, diets and disease effect colonic motility.
18. The colon serves as a host for many flora bacteria.
    a. They break down cellulose.
    b. They help synthesize vitamin K, riboflavin, nicotinic acid and folic acid.

C. Blood supply to the G.I. tract is as follows:
   1. *Arterial arises from the aorta.*
      a. The upper G.I. tract is supplied by the *ceciac artery.*
      b. The middle G.I. tract is supplied by the *superior mesenteric artery.*
      c. The lower G.I. tract is supplied by the *inferior mesenteric artery.*
   2. *Venous* blood is emptied into the liver via the *portal venous system;* into the *hepatic vein;* and into the *inferior vena cava.*

D. The G.I. tract contains extrinsic and intrinsic autonomic nervous system innervation.

E. The *accessory organs of digestion* include the gallbladder, pancreas and liver.
   1. The *gallbladder* is a pear-shaped organ that serves as a storage tank for bile.
      a. Bile secreted by the liver flows to the *hepatic duct.*
      b. It flows either into the *cystic duct* to the gallbladder or down the *common bile duct* to the duodenum.
   2. The *pancreas* is located in the epigastric region of the abdomen and aids digestion through its exocrine function.
      a. *Acinar* cells secrete digestive enzymes for digesting fats, proteins and carbohydrates.
      b. The enzymes are transported into the duodenum via an isotonic, bicarbonate-rich electrolyte solution secreted by the intercalated discs of the pancreas.
   3. The *liver* is located in the right hypochondriac region under the dome of the diaphragm.
      a. The liver has four main lobes.
      b. The liver helps digestion through the secretion of bile salts.

III. Physical assessment of the gastrointestinal system should include:

A. History
   1. Previous hospitalizations
   2. Medications
   3. Allergies
   4. Medical history
   5. Present and past occupations
   6. Exposure to contagious diseases
   7. Alcohol intake
   8. Weight changes
   9. Eating habits
   10. Bowel habits

11. Pain
12. Bleeding
B. Physical examination of the G.I. system includes:
   1. Inspection of the abdomen
   2. Auscultations of all four quadrants of the abdomen
      a. Check for normal bowel sounds.
      b. Check for a venous hum, friction rub and bruits.
   3. Percussion of the abdomen
   4. Palpation of the abdomen
      a. Check for masses, organomegaly.
      b. Check for pain.

IV. **The gastrointestinal nursing assessment includes evaluation of:**
   A. The level of consciousness
   B. Eating habits
   C. The swallow reflex
   D. Digestion
   E. Defecation and bowel habits
   F. Vital signs
   G. Laboratory and radiologic studies
      1. G.I. series
      2. Endoscopy
      3. Barium enemas
      4. Cholangiograms
      5. Radionuclide scan
      6. Gastric analysis

V. **Pathological states and nursing management**
   A. *Cirrhosis* of the liver
      1. Cirrhosis of the liver is caused by destruction of liver cells.
      2. The patient may present with:
         a. Jaundice
         b. Dark urine
         c. Ascites
         d. Light stool
         e. Enlarged liver
         f. Hypertension
      3. Diagnostic data
         a. Clotting
         b. Albumin
         c. Hematocrit
         d. G.I. series
         e. Bromsulphalein test
      4. Nursing care includes:
         a. Administer a high caloric diet.
         b. Maintain fluid and electrolyte balance.
         c. Prevent complications.
         d. Observe for bleeding and neurological changes.
         e. Provide emotional support.
         f. Provide patient education.

B. Hepatic failure
   1. Hepatic failure is caused by massive deterioration of the liver.
   2. The patient may present with:
      a. Jaundice
      b. Coma
      c. Personality changes
      d. Tremors
   3. History of cirrhosis of the liver is the best diagnostic aid.
      a. Elevated alkaline phosphatase, CDH, SGOT
      b. Decreased hemoglobin and hematocrit
      c. Urobilinogen present
      d. Decreased fibrinogen
      e. Prolonged prothrombin time
   4. Nursing care
      a. Protect from infection.
      b. Prevent bleeding.
      c. Provide emotional support.
      d. Prevent injury.
      e. Provide good skin care.
C. Bleeding esophageal varices
   1. Esophageal varices are caused by an increase of pressure in the portal system, causing dilatation of esophageal veins.
   2. The patient may present with:
      a. Copious hematemesis
      b. Shock
      c. Renal failure
      d. Myocardial infarction
   3. Laboratory studies are the best diagnostic aid.
      a. Decreased hemoglobin, hematocrit, red blood cells, white blood cells
      b. Prolonged prothrombin time
      c. Increased BUN, LDH, SGOT, SGPT
      d. Thrombocytopenia
   4. Nursing care includes:
      a. Maintain airway and breathing.
      b. Maintain fluid and electrolyte balance.
      c. Prevent further complications.
      d. Monitor vital signs.
      e. Nausea, vomiting
      f. Monitor arterial blood gases.
D. G.I. hemorrhage from peptic ulcers
   1. Peptic ulcers occur as a result of excessive secretion of gastric juices. The juices erode the mucosal lining and cause bleeding.
   2. The patient may present with:
      a. Hematemesis
      b. Shock
      c. Melina
   3. Diagnostic studies include:
      a. Decreased hemoglobin, hematocrit
      b. Increased BUN

c. Prolonged prothrombin time
4. Nursing care includes:
   a. Observe for bleeding.
   b. Observe for shock.
   c. Maintain airway.
   d. Prevent complications.
   e. Maintain fluid and electrolyte balance.
   f. Watch for acidosis.

E. Acute pancreatitis
   1. The precise urology is unknown.
   2. The patient may present with:
      a. Epigastric pain
      b. Shock
      c. Jaundice
      d. Fever
      e. Nausea, vomiting
   3. Diagnostic studies include:
      a. Leukocytosis
      b. Decreased serum and urine calcium
      c. Increased serum amylase, lipase, direct bilirubin, triglycerides
   4. Nursing care includes:
      a. Maintain airway.
      b. Maintain fluid and electrolyte balance.
      c. Maintain nasogastric suction.
      d. Alleviate pain.
      e. Prevent complications, including pulmonary.
      f. Protect from infection.
      g. Prepare for surgical intervention.

VI. Care common to gastrointestinal problems

A. *Fluid* and *electrolyte* problems
   1. Pathophysiology
      a. Fluid and electrolytes are altered in G.I. disorders.
      b. Isotonic fluid is lost internally.
      c. Plasma volume decreases because of fluid loss, resulting in hypovolemia.
   2. *Clinical presentation* is specific to the disorder involved, such as vomiting or draining fistulas.
   3. *Nursing care* includes:
      a. Accurately maintain intake and output records.
      b. Prevent irrigation of nasogastric tubes with tap water.
      c. Prevent the administration of tap water enemas.
      d. Monitor fluid and electrolyte status.
      e. Monitor vital signs.

B. Nutritional maintenance
   1. *Clinical presentation* is specific to the problem and is often elucidated during assessment.

2. ***Diagnostic data*** includes obtaining information regarding:
   a. The depletion of protein
   b. The depression of cellular immunity
   c. The causative agent of the nutritional impairment
   d. Nitrogen balance
3. Nursing care
   a. Provide an environment conducive to nutritional maintenance.
   b. Administer enteral hyperalimentation and monitor weight, intake and output, and laboratory tests.
   c. Administer total parenteral nutrition and monitor closely for complications due to the catheter, sepsis or metabolic disorders.
   d. Administer peripheral parenteral nutrition and monitor the patient.

CHAPTER NINE
HEMATOPOIETIC SYSTEM

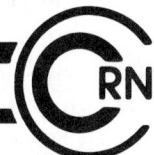

BEHAVIORAL OBJECTIVES

After reading the *Hematopoietic System,* the nurse will be able to:
- Identify the anatomy of the hematopoietic system
- Describe the function of blood and plasma
- Describe volume and volume-control related to the hematopoietic system
- Describe the blood-forming organs
- Describe normal red blood cell production, functioning and destruction
- Describe normal white blood cell production and functioning
- Identify the characteristics of the inflammatory process
- Identify the difference between cellular and humoral immunity
- Identify alterations in immunologic response
- Identify blood groups
- Identify the mechanisms related to hemostasis
- State the components of physical assessment as they relate to the hematologic system
- Identify the components of nursing assessment as they relate to the hematologic system
- Identify findings characterized by changes in erythrocytes
- Describe the pathology and clinical manifestations associated with:
  anemia
  leukemia
  lymphomas
  Hodgkin's disease
  non-Hodgkin's lymphoma
  polycythemia
  anaphylaxis
  disseminated intravascular coagulation
  hemophilia
  sickle cell disease
  multiple myeloma

TOPICAL OUTLINE
HEMATOPOIETIC SYSTEM

I. Hematopoietic System: Overview 563
II. Anatomy and Physiology 563
    Blood 563
        Components 563
        Odor, color, specific gravity, pH 563
        Function 563
        Volume and volume control 563
    Plasma 565
        Components 565
        Color 565
        Function 565
        Volume control 565
    Blood-forming organs 566
        Bone marrow 566
        Liver 566
        Spleen 566
        White pulp 567
        Marginal zone 567
        Red pulp 567
        Functions of the spleen 567
    Normal red blood cell production, function and destruction 568
        Erythrocytes 568
        Hemoglobin 569
        Producton stimulus 569
        Destruction 569
    Normal white blood cell production and function 570
    The inflammatory process 572
    Immunity 573
        Cellular immunity 573
        Humoral immunity 574
        Alterations in immunologic response 574
    Blood groups 576
    Hemostasis 577
III. Assessment of the Hematopoietic System 578
    History and general signs and symptoms 578
    Specific signs and symptoms 579
    Inspection 579
    Palpation 579
    Percussion 579
    Auscultation 579
    Evaluation of vital signs 579
    Laboratory and radiologic studies 580
IV. Pathological States and Nursing Management 582
    Anemia 582
        Pathophysiology 582
        Clinical presentation 582

Diagnostic data 582
Nursing care 583
Leukemia 585
Pathophysiology 585
Clinical presentation 585
Diagnostic data 586
Nursing care 586
Lymphomas 587
Pathophysiology 587
Hodgkin's disease 587
Non-Hodgkin's lymphoma 589
Polycythemia 589
Pathophysiology 589
Clinical presentation 589
Diagnostic data 589
Nursing care 589
Anaphylaxis 590
Pathophysiology 590
Clinical presentation 590
Diagnostic data 590
Nursing care 590
Disseminated intravascular coagulation (DIC) 591
Pathophysiology 591
Clinical presentation 591
Diagnostic data 591
Nursing care 591
Hemophilia 592
Pathophysiology 592
Clinical presentation 592
Diagnostic data 592
Nursing care 592
Sickle cell disease 592
Pathophysiology 592
Clinical presentation 593
Diagnostic data 593
Nursing care 593
Multiple myeloma 594
Pathophysiology 594
Clinical presentation 594
Diagnostic data 594
Nursing care 594
V. Care Common to Hematopoietic Problems 596
Reduced erythrocytes 596
Nursing care 596
Reduced white blood cells 596
Nursing care 596
Decreased platelet functions 596
Nursing care 596

Administration of blood   597
    Types of blood   597
    Complications related to transfusion   597
    Nursing care   597
Program Assessment: Science and Situation   599
Key Point Recognition Answers   609
PASS Answer Sheet   615
Survey Summary   617

HEMATOPOIETIC SYSTEM: OVERVIEW

Hemato is a prefix meaning blood. *Blood* is the thick, sticky substance that circulates through the heart and vessels, carrying nutrition and taking away wastes.

Blood and its production are vital to life itself. Blood carries nutrients and oxygen to the cells, helps maintain electrolyte balance by transporting electrolytes, provides heat regulation and is a defense against infection. Rarely considered a system unto itself, the blood-forming and blood-circulating organs are an organized group of related structures that function together to perform specific tasks. The organs that work as a team to help maintain *homeostasis* of the total organism are called the *hematopoietic system.*

The hematopoietic system is composed of *blood-forming organs:* bone marrow, liver, spleen, lymph nodes and thymus; and *blood-circulating organs:* heart and blood vessels.

ANATOMY AND PHYSIOLOGY

BLOOD

Components

Blood is composed of solid and liquid substances. The fluid component *plasma* is a pale yellow in color. It makes up 55 percent of the total blood volume (TBV).

The solid components are suspended within the plasma and consist of *red blood cells* (RBCs and erythrocytes), *white blood cells* (WBCs and leukocytes) and *platelets.* Forty-five percent of the TBV is made up of these solid components. Another way to describe the solid component is by percent of cells of the total blood volume, or *hematocrit.* Hematocrit is the percent of the TBV that consists of erythrocytes. Normally, hematocrit is about 42 to 45 percent, with a range of 40 to 54 percent in males and 37 to 47 percent in females.

Odor, Color, Specific Gravity, pH

Blood has a distinctive odor. Its color is various shades of red, depending on the degree of oxygenation. Venous blood is crimson. Arterial blood is bright red. The bright red color is directly related to the level of hemoglobin-oxygen saturation: the higher the oxygen level, the brighter the color. Conversely, decreased oxygen saturation will result in a darker, almost purple, color.

Blood contains clotting mechanisms. Fibrinogen, produced by the liver, is an important component of the clotting process. It is found in the plasma.

Blood is a thick, sticky substance. Blood becomes more viscous when the fluid volume or plasma is decreased, or the cells increase. Therefore, it is important to maintain the specific gravity of the blood between .048 and 1.066.

An important part of the body's ability to maintain homeostasis is through acid-base balancing mechanisms. The blood buffer system, principally composed of carbonic acid, carbonates, bicarbonates, phosphates and proteins, is one such mechanism. Therefore, maintaining normal blood pH (hydrogen ion concentration) is especially important to critically ill persons. Normal blood pH is slightly alkaline and ranges from 7.35 to 7.45.

Function

Blood transports oxygen and nutrition to the cells. Since blood is an extracellular fluid, cellular exchange of food and wastes takes place at the capillary level. It carries waste products from the cells to the organs of excretion.

In addition, blood helps maintain fluid and electrolyte balance, aids in temperature regulation and presents a defense against infection.

Volume and Volume Control

Normal blood volume is five to six liters. In the absence of pathology, the body maintains a fairly constant volume. This volume is distributed throughout the blood-circulating organs. Forty percent of the blood volume is in the venous system. The veins act as reservoirs for the circulatory system. In this capacity, they can accept large amounts of blood without significant changes in intravascular venous pressure.

Blood volume is hormonally controlled. Stretch receptors housed in the right and left atria respond to volume changes by shrinking or swelling (Fig. 9-1). If the circulating fluid is **hypervolemic,** the receptors swell and a message is sent to the posterior pituitary to halt secretion of **anti-diuretic hormone** (ADH). The kidneys respond by increasing the urinary output. Conversely, a **hypovolemic** state results in secretion of ADH and retention of water. These compensatory mechanisms are inhibited once the body begins to adapt.

Concentration	Fluid	Receptor Response	Endocrine Response	Hormone Activity	Physiological Result
Low osmolality	Increased fluids	Osmoreceptors expand	Stimulation of posterior pituitary	Decreased secretion of ADH	Diuresis
High osmolality	Decreased fluids	Osmoreceptors shrink	Stimulation of posterior pituitary	Increased secretion of ADH	Reabsorption of water

Fig. 9-1. Volume control

KEY CONCEPT: Blood is composed of plasma, red blood cells and white blood cells. It is vital to the body's ability to thrive and maintain a balanced state.

KEY POINT RECOGNITION

Write true or false by each statement. Answers are at the end of this chapter. A score below 80% indicates the need for further study.

　　　　1. The prefix meaning blood is hemato.
　　　　2. Blood carries only oxygen to the cells.
　　　　3. Blood transports electrolytes to help maintain electrolyte balance.
　　　　4. The hematopoietic system is composed of blood-forming organs.
　　　　5. The liver is a blood-forming organ.
　　　　6. The heart and blood vessels compose the blood-circulating organs.
　　　　7. The fluid components of blood are called erythrocytes.
　　　　8. White blood cells are called platelets.
　　　　9. Solid components found in blood are erythrocytes, leukocytes and platelets.
　　　10. The percentage of the total blood volume that consists of erythrocytes is called hematocrit.
　　　11. Normal hematocrit ranges from 54 to 65 percent.
　　　12. Blood varies in color due to oxygenation.
　　　13. Arterial blood is dark in color.
　　　14. The color of arterial blood is related to the oxygen saturation found in hemoglobin.
　　　15. The lower the oxygen saturation level of blood, the brighter the color.
　　　16. Fibrinogen, a component of plasma, is an important element necessary for clotting.
　　　17. The normal specific gravity of blood ranges between 1.038 and 1.076.
　　　18. The blood buffer system is composed of carbonic acid, carbonates, bicarbonates, phosphate and proteins.
　　　19. Normal blood pH is slightly acidotic.
　　　20. Normal blood pH is from 7.35 to 7.45.

_____21. Blood is an intracellular fluid.

_____22. Cellular exchange takes place at the capillary level.

_____23. Normally, there are approximately 6,000 to 10,000 ml of blood volume.

_____24. Stretch receptors found in the right and left atria are responsible for signaling changes necessary to accommodate changes in volume.

_____25. If circulating fluid is hypovolemic, receptors swell and the posterior pituitary secretes ADH.

PLASMA

Components

Plasma is the liquid part of the blood and lymphatic fluid. It is composed of serum and plasma proteins. More specifically, 92 percent is water and 6 to 7 percent is plasma protein. The specific *plasma proteins* are: **albumin, serum globulins, fibrinogen, plasminogen** and **prothrombin.**

Human blood plasma is composed of water and dissolved substances, such as electrolytes, glucose, proteins, fats, bile pigment and gases.

Color

Normally, plasma is colorless or yellowish. The yellow cast is due to the bile pigments in plasma.

Function

Plasma is the vehicle for blood cells. In this function, it carries food, antibodies, hormones, vitamins and minerals to the cells, and removes wastes from the cells. Fluid balance and pressure are regulated by osmotic pressure.

Volume Control

A dynamic relationship between the interstitial and intravascular compartments is established and maintained by the osmotic pressure gradients along a capillary bed (Fig. 9-2). This is because more plasma proteins are found intravascularly than in the interstitial space. An **osmotic pressure** is established, which draws fluid into the vessel. Each end of the capillary bed has a different pressure gradient.

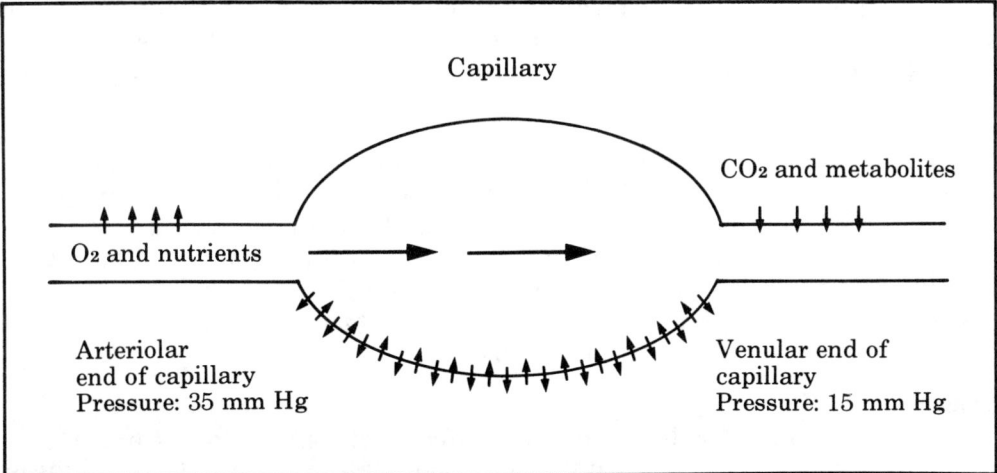

Fig. 9-2. Osmotic pressure gradient capillary bed

At the **arteriolar** end, the osmotic pressure is overridden by the blood pressure, resulting in fluid movement out of the vessels. At the *venous* end, the blood pressure is lower than the osmotic pressure, resulting in a pulling of fluid into the vessels.

Disruption in the osmotic pressure gradients due to hyperalbuminemia can cause circulatory overload, while hypoalbuminemia can result in interstitial edema. Maintaining the delicate state is necessary for fluid balance.

KEY CONCEPT: Plasma is composed of serum and plasma proteins. The osmotic pressure of the plasma protein plays an important role in maintaining fluid balance and pressure changes between the interstitial and intravascular compartments.

KEY POINT RECOGNITION

Write true or false by each statement. Answers are at the end of this chapter. A score below 80% indicates the need for further study.

_____ 1. Plasma is composed of hemoglobin.

_____ 2. The plasma proteins are albumin, globulins, fibrinogen, plasminogen and prothrombin.

_____ 3. Bile pigments found in plasma give it a characteristic yellow appearance.

_____ 4. The osmotic pressure within a vessel helps regulate fluid balance and pressure.

_____ 5. The osmotic pressure within a vessel helps maintain the dynamic relationship between the interstitial and intravascular compartments.

_____ 6. More plasma proteins are found in the interstitial fluid compartment than in the intravascular compartment.

_____ 7. The pressure gradient remains identical at both ends of the capillary bed.

_____ 8. Hyperalbuminemia can cause circulatory overload.

_____ 9. Hypoalbuminemia can result in interstitial edema.

_____ 10. The venous end of the capillary bed exerts blood pressure that is higher than the osmotic pressure.

BLOOD-FORMING ORGANS

Bone Marrow

Bone marrow is the soft tissue in the medullary cavities of long bones and in spaces between the trabeculae of cancellous bone. Marrow may be red or yellow. Yellow marrow, found in the long bones, is composed predominantly of fat cells and has little to do with blood formation. However, *red marrow* is concerned with *hematopoiesis*. Hematopoiesis is the process by which blood is produced. It is the hematopoietic function that maintains the body's blood cell level.

Liver

The *liver,* the largest organ in the body, has among its functions hematologic processes. In the fetal stage of life, erythropoiesis can take place in the liver.

Synthesis of blood constituents essential for clotting is another hematologic function of the liver. These constituents include fibrinogen and prothrombin. Antithrombins also are synthesized in the liver.

Kupffer's cells filter and destroy bacteria. As red blood cells are destroyed, the liver excretes the bile pigments and bilirubin.

Spleen

The spleen is a reddish-brown organ located in the left side of the abdominal cavity, serving as a line filter in the portal circulation. Its bloodless weight is about 80 gm; but, distended with red blood, it weighs more than 300 gm.

Blood flows through the spleen at the rate of 300 ml per minute, approximately 5 percent of the cardiac output. A little less than half of the spleen's 140 billion cells are phagocytic; however, the spleen can enlarge to meet increased phagocytic needs by multiplying the cell count up to eight times normal.

An external fibrous capsule projects trabeculae into the parenchyma, providing the framework for the arteries and veins.

The parenchyma consists of white pulp, marginal (transition) zone and red pulp. Each has three parts: vessels, reticular cells and free cells. The free cells are contained within the reticular cells.

White Pulp

A periarterial lymphatic sheath surrounds the central artery. Fibers of the periarterial lymphatic sheath catch and hold lymphocytes.

Within the sheath is the mantle, a covering of small lymphocytes surrounding the germinal centers. The vessels are branches of the central artery, which turn at a 90-degree angle for plasma skimming. Plasma is skimmed to reduce the number of red cells released in the white pulp and to concentrate the red cells to be dumped into the red pulp. Plasma is then returned to the circulation in the lymphatic system. The structural framework is a dense matrix of reticular cells supporting the germinal centers. Free cells are mostly lymphocytes.

Marginal Zone

This is a transitional zone with many end arterioles and a dense reticular network. It is well differentiated at the white pulp border, but blends with the red pulp. Free cells are blood cells from the terminal arterioles, macrophages and medium-sized lymphocytes.

Red Pulp

Vessels within the red pulp compose the majority of the terminal arterioles that dump the concentrated red cells into the cords of Bilroth. Loose connections between the endothelial cells allow movement of red cells into the venous sinuses. At the venous sinuses, blood flows into larger veins for re-entry into the portal circulation. The reticulum forms a mantle around the sinuses. Free cells are erythrocytes, granulocytes, lymphocytes and macrophages.

Functions of the Spleen

Immunity. Circulating antigens are trapped within the spleen where they interact with the concentrated immunologically active cell. The primary antibody response moves the tagged antigens, concentrated in the red pulp macrophages, to the marginal zone and then to the germinal center. This process takes four hours. The secondary antibody response follows the same sequence, but at a faster rate. The spleen is also the main producer of IgM.

Filtration. White pulp appears to be composed almost totally of plasma; therefore, antigens are engulfed in a concentration of lymphocytes. Two processes, culling and pitting, remove damaged, deformed and worn-out red blood cells from circulation. **Culling** is the selective recognition and removal of the worn-out and damaged cells. **Pitting** is the removal of rigid particles from the red cell, while preserving the cell. Red cells must deform to move through the venous sinusoids. Inclusion bodies are detached and phagocytized.

Iron is removed from degraded hemoglobin by the red pulp reticular cells. It is moved to the plasma for transport to the bone marrow for resynthesis. Excess iron is stored in the liver.

Reservoir and volume regulation. Both red pulp and venous sinuses store red blood cells. Storage of the red blood cell results in splenic enlargement. Splenic contractions restore red blood cells to the circulation. This restoration can raise the systemic hematocrit 3 to 4 percent. The mechanics of contraction are poorly understood.

Hematopoiesis. During the first five months of fetal development, the spleen produces blood cells. After this time it produces some lymphocytes and plasma cells. The germinal centers proliferate lymphocytes, but hematopoiesis, in general, is not carried out by the spleen.

KEY CONCEPT: The main blood-forming organs of the body are the bone marrow, liver and spleen.

KEY POINT RECOGNITION

Write true or false by each statement. Answers are at the end of this chapter. A score below 80% indicates the need for further study.

_____ 1. Red marrow is concerned with hematopoiesis.

_____ 2. During fetal development, erythropoiesis takes place in the liver and spleen.

_____ 3. Fibrinogen and prothrombin are synthesized in the liver.

_____ 4. Kupffer's cells are responsible for the excretion of bile pigments.

_____ 5. The white pulp of the spleen consists of lymphatic tissue.

_____ 6. When ejected into the circulating volume, the stored blood in the spleen has the capacity to raise the hematocrit 3 to 4 percent.

NORMAL RED BLOOD CELL PRODUCTION, FUNCTION AND DESTRUCTION

The hematopoietic system is responsible for producing **erythrocytes, neutrophils, lymphocytes, monocytes, eosinophils, basophils, platelets** and **cells in plasma.**

Erythrocytes

Erythrocytes, mature red blood cells, are formed by the process of ***erythropoiesis*** in the bone marrow. Mature cell production equals mature cell loss and is maintained at a steady rate of approximately 5 million per cubic milliliter. Cellular structure includes an **outer membrane** primarily composed of lipoprotein in which blood group antigens are found. The membrane is permeable to water, chloride, hydrogen and bicarbonate ions, but it is only semipermeable to sodium and potassium. Intracellular stability is maintained by active transport. The inner component, or ***stroma,*** is made up of proteins and lipids. ***Hematopoiesis*** takes place in the bone marrow of long bones until 20 years of age, and then in the vertebrae, skull, sternum and ribs.

Cell development begins with primordial stem cells, which are produced in the bone marrow. The maturation of RBCs progresses through a series of stages. Cell division is an occurrence in all of the maturational stages (Fig. 9-3).

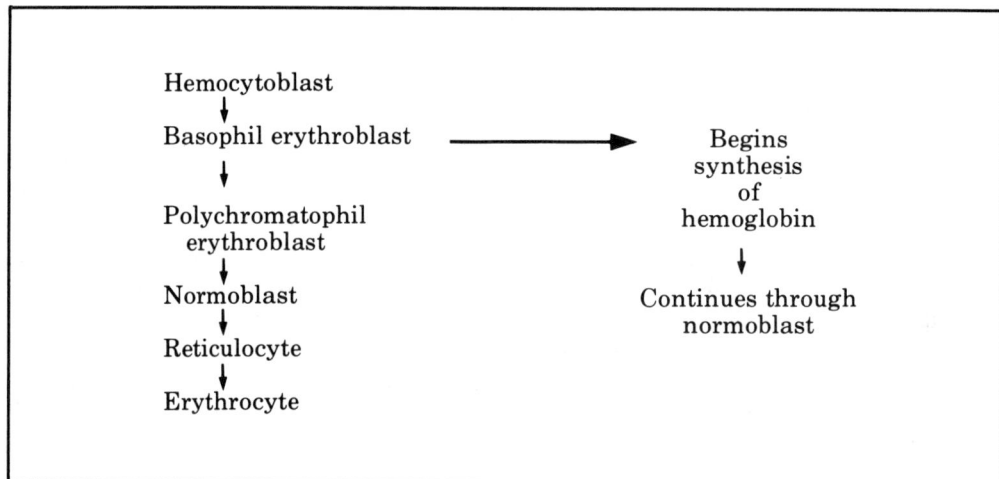

Fig. 9-3. Red blood cell maturation

Stem cells form **hemocytoblasts.** From the hemocytoblast, the first cell formed is the **basophil erythroblast.** At this level of maturation, synthesis of **hemoglobin** is begun. Throughout the maturation process, the nucleus shrinks as the hemoglobin concentration rises. Since the bone marrow does not have a large storage capacity, the mature cell, the **erythrocyte,** transudes through the capillary membrane into the capillary. This process is called **diapedesis.** In short, it is the passage of blood cells through the unruptured wall of a capillary.

Vitamin B₁₂ (cyanocobalamin), which is stored in the liver and released slowly, is required for RBC maturation. If B₁₂ is not absorbed from the G.I. tract, as in pernicious anemia, cell division and maturation are compromised, thus inhibiting RBC production.

Hemoglobin

The functional unit of erythrocytes is **hemoglobin.** Its function is to transport oxygen to the tissues.

Hemoglobin is a protein consisting of **heme,** an iron-containing pigment, and **globin.** Synthesis of hemoglobin takes place in the bone marrow. Its production occurs when iron combines with a porphyrin to form the heme molecule. Four heme molecules combine with globin to form hemoglobin. There are many types of hemoglobin. To produce the normal hemoglobins, five types of globin are used.

The amount of hemoglobin in the blood is 12 to 16 gm/100 ml of blood in the female and 14 to 18 gm/100 ml of blood in the male. The amount of hemoglobin is important in determining the amount of oxygen available to the tissues. One gram of hemoglobin can combine with 1.34 ml of oxygen. This process of oxygenation takes place in the lungs. Oxygen diffuses through the erythrocytic membrane to combine with the hemoglobin attached to the stroma. The compound formed is called **oxyhemoglobin.**

Oxyhemoglobin is an unstable compound. Therefore, when oxygen tension in the tissues is low and carbon dioxide tension is high, oxyhemoglobin releases its oxygen for the excess carbon dioxide. However, this is not a one-for-one exchange.

Production Stimulus

A lowered oxygen tension stimulates release of erythropoietin. Circulating erythropoietin acts on the bone marrow, initiating differentiation of the stem cells and hematocytoblasts. Production can reach 8 to 10 times the normal within five days.

Destruction

Destruction of RBCs is called **hemolysis.** The normal life span of RBCs is approximately 120 days. Aging increases fragility, resulting in rupture as the cells pass through constricted areas, such as the red pulp of the spleen. Hemoglobin and the cell stroma are released, ingested by reticuloendothelial cells and returned by the circulation for reuse. Bilirubin is the end product of conversion of the heme molecule. Splenectomy results in increased circulation of abnormal and old cells.

Red cells can be destroyed other than physiologically. They can be destroyed by chemical action. For example, infusion of large amounts of a hypotonic solution causes the cells to swell and hemolyze. Red cells can be traumatized mechanically by passing through machinery, or even by simple venipuncture. Increased destruction of RBCs results in increased bilirubin. When the release of bilirubin exceeds the excretion capacity of the liver, jaundice occurs.

KEY CONCEPT: Red bone marrow is concerned with hemopoiesis. An erythrocyte is a mature red blood cell. Hemoglobin is the functional unit of an erythrocyte. Hemolysis is the destruction of RBCs.

KEY POINT RECOGNITION

Write true or false by each statement. Answers are at the end of this chapter. A score below 80% indicates the need for further study.

_____ 1. Bone marrow is a hard, sticky substance.

_____ 2. Bone marrow is found in only the long bones of the body.

_____ 3. Bone marrow is red and yellow.

_____ 4. Yellow bone marrow is concerned with platelet formation.

_____ 5. Hematopoiesis is the process by which blood is produced.

____ 6. Neutrophils, lymphocytes and eosinophils are produced by the hematopoietic system.
____ 7. Erythrocytes are immature red blood cells.
____ 8. The outer membrane covering of an erythrocyte is composed of lipoprotein.
____ 9. Blood group antigens are found on the outer membrane covering of an erythrocyte.
____ 10. The outer membrane covering of an erythrocyte is semipermeable to chloride, sodium and bicarbonate.
____ 11. Stroma is made of protein and lipid particles.
____ 12. Primordial stem cells are the first stage of RBC development.
____ 13. Primordial stem cells are produced in the bone marrow.
____ 14. Cellular division only occurs in the first stage of the maturational process.
____ 15. Stem cells form basophils.
____ 16. The nucleus of an erythrocyte shrinks as hemoglobin concentration rises.
____ 17. Diapedesis is movement of a blood cell through the capillary membrane into the capillary.
____ 18. Vitamin B_{12} is required for RBC maturation.
____ 19. Vitamin B_{12} is stored in long bones and in the spleen.
____ 20. Pernicious anemia is caused by faulty absorption of vitamin B_{12}.
____ 21. The functional unit of an erythrocyte is hemoglobin.
____ 22. Hemoglobin is a protein consisting of an iron pigment and globin.
____ 23. Nine heme molecules combine with globin to form hemoglobin.
____ 24. The normal range for hemoglobin in the female is 16 to 21 gm/100 ml of blood.
____ 25. Oxygen diffuses through the erythrocytic membrane to combine with the hemoglobin attached to the stroma.
____ 26. The reticuloendothelial system removes destroyed red blood cells.
____ 27. Excess iron is stored in the spleen.

NORMAL WHITE BLOOD CELL PRODUCTION AND FUNCTION

Stem cells self-replicate and differentiate into five major types of leukocytes: **neutrophils** (62 percent), **eosinophils** (2.3 percent), **basophils** (.4 percent), **monocytes** (5.3 percent) and **lymphocytes** (30 percent).

Neutrophils, eosinophils and basophils are known as **granulocytes,** or polymorphonuclear leukocytes. They are formed in the bone marrow.

Lymphocytes and **monocytes** are produced in the lymphoid tissues of the spleen, thymus and lymph nodes.

Each type plays a specific role in protecting the body from foreign invasion. This is accomplished by one of two processes: **phagocytosis** or **immune body formation.**

Phagocytosis is the ingestion of bacteria or foreign substance. **Granulocytes** and **monocytes** are phagocytic cells. Phagocytosis is a selective process of identifying rough surface, electropositive foreign substances. Opsonins (protein antibodies) promote the adherence of phagocytes.

Neutrophils in the mature form, PMNs, are phagocytic. Immature or juvenile neutrophils are referred to as bands, because of the uniform diameters of the single lobe nuclei, which give a bandlike appearance. The bands are nonsecretory and nonproliferative. Mature neutrophils have two to five lobes connected by filaments.

Clinically, the release of immature cells is in response to inflammation or an acute infection. This is referred to as a shift to the left. The name is derived from a differential counting system. An extreme left shift is seen in myelogenous leukemia with a proliferation of myeloblasts. A shift to the right shows an increased ratio of multilobulated PMNs, indicative of vitamin B_{12}, folic acid deficiency or renal disease.

Eosinophils have weak phagocytic action. Their primary function is to promote chemotaxis, the movement of neutrophils toward the invading substance. Tissue damage is thought to release leukotoxins, which also attract neutrophils. Eosinophils have a stronger response to foreign protein, allergic reaction, and parasitic infections than other leukocytes. They may also be active in removing toxins.

Basophils respond to allergic reactions, stress and chronic inflammation. They may also release heparin, which prevents intravascular clotting.

Monocytes become fixed in tissue and enlarge to become *macrophages.* Inflammation produces rapid multiplication. They can then engulf or wall-off foreign particles.

Macrophages, which line lymph sinuses and alveolar passages, perform the same function as monocytes. Specific macrophages, *histocytes,* are found in the Kupffer's cells of the liver sinuses. They act as a filtration system for bacteria.

Lymphocytes are derived from multipotential cells that are similar to stem cells. They originate in the lymphoid structures of the bone marrow and thymus. Lymphocytes are then distributed to secondary lymphoid tissues of the spleen, lymph nodes, tonsils, pharynx and gastrointestinal tract.

Upon maturation, lymphocytes differentiate into *T* cells and *B* cells. *T* lymphocyte means thymus-dependent. *B* lymphocyte means bursa-dependent. *B* lymphocytes are named for bursa of Fabricius, the preprocessing area in birds. In humans, *B* lymphocytes are thought to be preprocessed in lymphoid tissues of the fetal liver. The *T* cells migrate and are processed through the thymus. They provide tissue and cellular immunity. The processing center for *B* cells is unknown. *B* cells are responsible for humoral immunity by mediation of immunoglobins. Processing takes place prenatally. The cells are distributed to lymphoid tissue and become enmeshed in the reticular network.

Plasma cells are differentiated successors of lymphocytes. They produce specific antibodies.

The normal lymphocyte count in the adult is 1,500 to 4,000 per mm. Infectious processes with marked lymphocytosis are pertussis, infectious mononucleosis and infectious lymphocytosis, all of which are most frequently seen in children or young adults. The cells of infectious lymphocytosis in childhood are seen in chronic lymphocytic leukemia in the adult.

KEY CONCEPT: The five major types of leukocytes are neutrophils, eosinophils, basophils, monocytes and lymphocytes. They protect the body from foreign invasion by either phagocytosis or immune body formation.

KEY POINT RECOGNITION
Write true or false by each statement. Answers are at the end of this chapter. A score below 80% indicates the need for further study.

_____ 1. Lymphocytes and monocytes are known as granulocytes.
_____ 2. Neutrophils are formed in the lymphoid tissues of the spleen, thymus and lymph nodes.
_____ 3. Neutrophils are phagocytic.
_____ 4. Basophils release heparin.
_____ 5. Monocytes enlarge to become macrophages.
_____ 6. Neutrophils differentiate into *B* and *T* cells.
_____ 7. *B* cells are responsible for tissue immunity.
_____ 8. Plasma cells are responsible for humoral immunity.

THE INFLAMMATORY PROCESS

The first line of defense is the epithelial surfaces of the body; but, if the integrity of the epithelium is broken, another defense is needed. The inflammatory process is a secondary line of defense against infection.

Inflammation is a tissue reaction to injury. It is a process in which the body begins to repair itself. It should not be mistaken for infection.

The specific signs and symptoms of inflammation include *pain, heat, erythema, swelling* and *loss of function.*

Inflammation is a process that begins almost immediately after cellular injury (Fig. 9-4). It is a local response. Histamine, serotonin and bradykinin are released by the injured tissue.

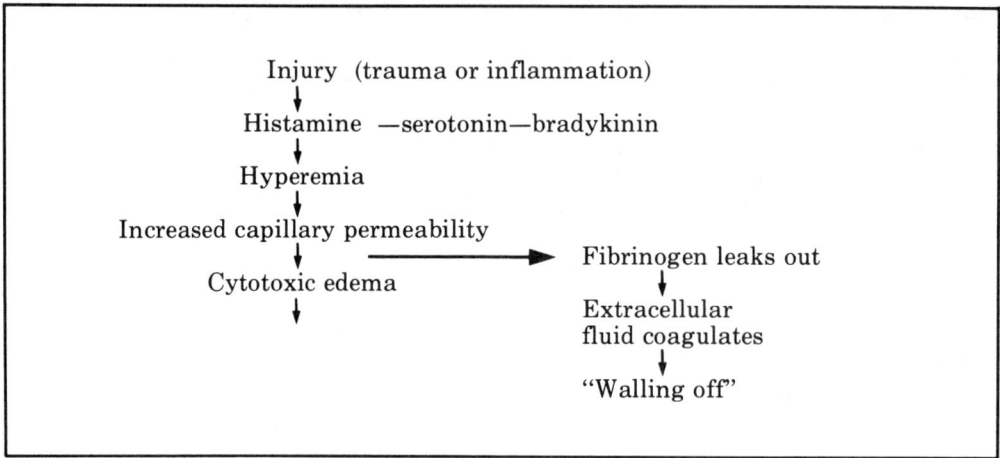

Fig. 9-4. Inflammatory process

Vascular dilatation and increased blood flow follow. There is increased capillary permeability with exudation of fluid from the intravascular space into the interstitial space. Leukocytes in the tissues increase. Fibrinogen leaks into the extracellular fluid and becomes gelatin-like. This results in a "walling off" or isolation of the injured area.

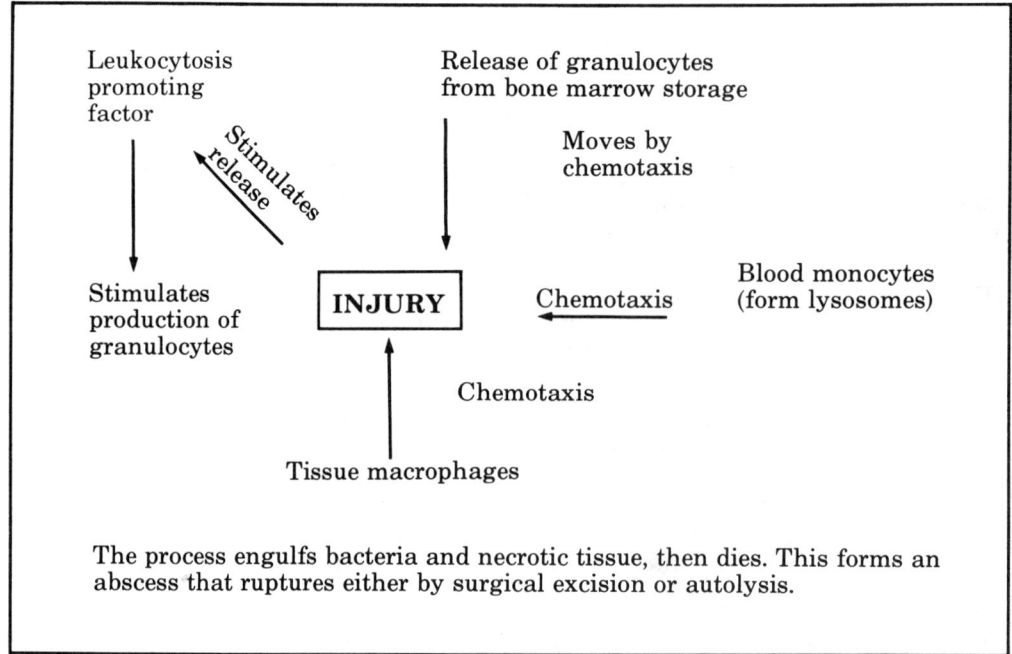

Fig. 9-5. Phagocytosis

The body's response to infection is *phagocytic* (Fig. 9-5). By phagocytosis, bacteria and necrotic tissue are engulfed. An abscess forms and is ruptured either surgically or by autolysis.

This response is initiated at the time of injury by an increased production of granulocytes; leukocytosis occurs. The leukocytes, primarily neutrophils and macrophages, are moved by chemotaxis to the injured area. Bacteria are engulfed, killed and then digested by lysosomal enzymes within the leukocytes.

Once the process and response are complete, blood vessels return to normal size, edema disappears, fibrin is digested and the leukocytes re-enter the intravascular space.

KEY CONCEPT: Inflammation is a cellular reaction to injury. Through the inflammatory process and response, the body is defended against infection or foreign invasion of injurious agents.

KEY POINT RECOGNITION

Write true or false by each statement. Answers are at the end of this chapter. A score below 80% indicates the need for further study.

_____ 1. Signs and symptoms of inflammation include pain, redness, swelling and fever.

_____ 2. The inflammatory process is initiated by the release of histamine.

_____ 3. Leukocytosis is a sign of infection, not inflammation.

_____ 4. Leukocytes are moved to the injured area by chemotaxis.

_____ 5. Bacteria are engulfed and digested by lysosomal enzymes.

IMMUNITY

Immunity is the ability of the body to defend itself against foreign organisms or toxins, most of which are proteins. *Acquired immunity* is the production of specific agents in response to invasion or sensitization. Two related, but separate, types of immunity compose the immune system: *cellular* and *humoral.*

Cellular Immunity

The basis of *cellular immunity* is the recognition of self from nonself. It involves thymic-controlled lymphocytes, or *T* cells. Cellular immunity is important in foreign tissue grafts, autoimmune processes, cancer and some allergies.

Sensitized *T* cells migrate to the antigen, swell and release lysosomal enzymes for direct destruction. Indirect confrontation by *T* cells is accomplished by the release of transfer factor, which promotes changes in small lymphocytes to specific sensitized lymphocytes. This increases their number and effect. Also released is a macrophage chemotaxic factor that attracts macrophages to the area. At this point, the process is limited by the release of migration-inhibiting factor.

The *complement system* potentiates the phagocytic action. The complement system, normally inactive, consists of nine enzyme precursors: C1 to C9. An antigen-antibody combination activates first a stage enzyme precursor. This sets in motion a sequential cascade of the C1-C9 complement. It acts by promoting phagocytosis and chemotaxis, lysing antigen cell membranes and causing antigens to agglutinate. In addition, the complement system can neutralize the molecular structure or localize the effect through an inflammatory response. Their most important function is invading the cell membrane of the antigen, since other components of the immune system cannot damage or alter the cell membrane. Lysis of cell membranes by proteolytic enzymes and opsonization of the bacterial surface by complement increase susceptibility of the tissue macrophages to phagocytic action.

Humoral Immunity

Humoral immunity is the result of circulating gamma globulins or antibodies. Invasion of an antigen stimulates release of the *B* lymphocyte specific to the invader. Following differentiation, *B* cells become mature plasma cells, which synthesize specific antibodies. Immunoglobulins (Igs) can be considered a family. Because of their specific antigen response, five classes have been identified (Fig. 9-6).

IgG—gamma

IgA—alpha

IgD—delta

IgM—mu

IgE—epsilon

Immunoglobins are antibody surface antigen receptors, which can initiate three types of antibody action: (1) direct attachment by agglutination, precipitation, neutralization or lysis; (2) activation of the complement system that attacks antigens by lysis of cell membrane, opsonization, chemotaxis, agglutination, neutralization of the inflammatory effects of hyperemia and coagulation of fibrinogen clots; and (3) activation of the anaphylactic system of antibodies. IgE immunoglobins are attached to tissue cells and blood cells, especially mast cells and basophils. An antigen reaction causes immediate swelling and rupture of the cells, thus releasing *histamine,* a slow-reacting substance of *anaphylaxis, chemotactic factor,* which attracts neutrophils, macrophages and eosinophils, and *lysosomal enzymes.* These substances establish a local inflammatory reaction.

Immunoglobulin	Function	Found
IgG	Predominant antibody Active antibacterial response Secondary response is antiviral and antitoxic	Serum and intercellular fluids
IgA	Protects body surface by preventing attachment of organisms	Serum
IgD	Protects fetus against infection	
IgM	Most active against bacteria First antibody to respond to antigen	Serum
IgE	Involved with histamine release and allergies	Serum and intercellular fluids

Fig. 9-6. Immunoglobulins

Alterations in Immunologic Response

Allergy

Allergic reactions involve IgE immunoglobins present in great numbers. An allergen is an antigen that reacts specifically with a specific IgE antibody. The allergen-reagin reaction causes an allergic response, damaging cells by swelling and rupture.

Hypersensitivity

Hypersensitivity can be induced by a genetic predisposition coupled with an external factor or *y*-prior sensitization. An immediate hypersensitive reaction is anaphylaxis. This reaction is due to chemicals acting at secondary sites. IgE reagins are attached to the tissue cells, mast cells and basophils throughout the body. Therefore, an allergen introduced systemically produces a severe, generalized response called anaphylactic shock. This is an immediate life-threatening emergency.

Intracellular reactions cause mast cell degranulation, which releases the cellular stores of histamine and eosinophil chemotactic factor of anaphylaxis (ECF-A). Eosinophils release SRS-A. Bradykinin release is related to the antigen-antibody interaction with coagulation factor XII. These three components are powerful bronchoconstrictors and increase capillary permeability. Histamine and bradykinin are vasodilators. The beta-adrenergic stimulator, epinephinre, blocks the autonomically controlled mediators.

The net effects of the mediator are generalized vasodilation and relative or absolute hypovolemia from third-spacing fluids into the interstitial spaces, secondary to increased capillary permeability, which results in shock and edema.

Another immediate hypersensitivity reaction is the *cytolytic immune response*. There is damage to the target cell as a result of a complement-fixing antibody being directed against a cell surface antigen. IgG coating of cells makes them susceptible to phagocytosis. Through a series of changes, red blood cells are destroyed. Examples of reactions resulting in hemolysis include: erythroblastosis fetalis, transfusion reaction and thrombocytopenia.

Arthus's phenomenon is a localized inflammatory response to repeated insult with central cellular necrosis. It is the result of intravascular complement fixation, causing phagocytosis of the antigen-antibody complex by granulocytes. Proteolytic enzymes are released, and platelet aggregation promotes clotting, creating a hemorrhagic necrosis. Similar reactions can occur systemically. The kidney is a common target organ, as seen with glomerular injury. Horse serum can produce a systemic anaphylactic response.

Other common sites are the skin, bone marrow, respiratory tract and G.I. tract.

In delayed reactions, the antibody is bound to the cell and cannot be transferred into the serum. Examples include tuberculin testing, contact dermatitis, tuberculosis, poison ivy and some drug allergies.

Autoimmune Diseases

Autoimmunity is the body's inability to recognize its own tissues. Antibodies are formed as if the body's own tissue is an antigen. Common autoimmune processes are rheumatic fever, lupus erythematosus, multiple sclerosis and myasthenia gravis. The process in rheumatic fever appears to be a common antigen between the streptococcus and the myocardium. Therefore, as the body produces antibodies to combat the streptococcal infection, myocardial tissue is also injured. Subsequent damage is due to the release of histamine and serotonin.

Criteria for determining the presence of an autoimmune process include: *decreased complement levels, abnormal antibodies in the serum* and affected organs having deposits of *immune complexes and complements.*

KEY CONCEPT: Immunity is the ability of the body to defend itself against foreign organisms or toxins. The two types of immunity are cellular and humoral. Potentiating the phagocytic action of the immunity process is the complement system. The immune response may be detrimentally altered by hypersensitivity or autoimmunity.

KEY POINT RECOGNITION
Write true or false by each statement. Answers are at the end of this chapter. A score below 80% indicates the need for further study.

_____ 1. B cells are the basis of cellular immunity.

_____ 2. Transfer factor causes lymphocytes to become specific and sensitized.

_____ 3. Macrophage chemotaxin factor limits the migration of macrophages.

_____ 4. The complement system aids by invading the cell membrane of the antibody.

_____ 5. Invasion of the cell membrane is necessary for macrophages to enter the cell.

_____ 6. B cells differentiate and become mature plasma cells.

_____ 7. IgG is usually the first antibody to respond.
_____ 8. IgE is involved with histamine release.
_____ 9. IgD protects the fetus against infection.
_____10. Anaphylactic shock is an immediate hypersensitive reaction.
_____11. Anaphylaxis is due to damage of the target cell as a result of a complement-fixing antibody being directed against a cell surface antigen.
_____12. Arthus's phenomenon is a local inflammatory response.
_____13. In a delayed hypersensitive reaction, the antibody is bound to the cell.
_____14. Decreased complement levels, abnormal serum antibodies, a history of streptococcal infections and myocardial damage are indicative of an autoimmune process.

BLOOD GROUPS

The blood groups can be divided into two systems: **ABO system** and **Rh system**.

Blood groups of the ABO system are O (universal donor), A, B and AB (universal recipient) (Fig. 9-7). The blood groups of the ABO system are based on the antigens and antibodies present or absent in the blood. **Agglutinogen** is the term for antigenic polysaccharides in red blood cells. **Agglutinins** are the specific plasma antibodies. Blood incompatibility is an immune reaction caused by antigen-antibody response. **Agglutination** is one mechanism of the immune reaction. The antibody acts as glue in antigen aggregation. Agglutination is a means for cross-matching blood. Incompatibility results when donor cells are agglutinated by recipient serum. Because of dilution in the recipient, donor serum does not agglutinate cells of the patient. Therefore, blood typing must be based on the agglutination of donor cells by plasma antibodies of the recipient.

Blood Group	Agglutinin	Agglutinogen
Percentage of population	Plasma antibodies	Red blood cells antigen
(universal donor) O 47%	Anti A and Anti B	---
A 41%	Anti B	A
B 9%	Anti A	B
(universal recipient) AB 3%	---	A and B

Fig. 9-7. ABO system

The **Rh system** is also based on antigen-antibody response. The Rh antigen is the strongest. The Rh factor can be positive or negative, which indicates the presence or absence of the Rh-D antigen. If an Rh negative recipient receives Rh positive blood, antibodies are formed in response to the antigen. This can occur following transfusion or delivery of a baby from an Rh negative mother and Rh positive father. Subsequent transfusions cause cells to agglutinate. Subsequent pregnancies with an Rh positive fetus and cross-placental circulation results in hemolysis of RBCs in the newborn. This condition is known as erythroblastosis fetalis. Treatment to prevent erythroblastosis fetalis involves injection of Rh positive antibodies into the mother soon after the first delivery. This blocks the initial reaction and antibody formation.

The **Coombs' test** is used to evaluate whether an Rh negative person is harboring Rh positive hemolyzing antibodies. The **direct** Coombs' test determines the presence of (IgG) antibodies fixed to RBCs. The *indirect* Coombs' test determines the presence of antibodies (IgG) in the serum.

KEY CONCEPT: The blood groups are composed of the ABO and Rh systems. Blood incompatibility is an immune reaction caused by antigen-antibody response.

KEY POINT RECOGNITION
Write true or false by each statement. Answers are at the end of this chapter. A score below 80% indicates the need for further study.

_____ 1. AB is the universal donor.
_____ 2. Agglutinogens are antigenic polysaccharides in RBCs.
_____ 3. Agglutinins are plasma antibodies.
_____ 4. The blood group B has anti-A plasma antibodies.
_____ 5. The blood group AB has both anti-A and anti-B plasma antibodies.
_____ 6. Rh positive means the presence of the Rh-D antigen.
_____ 7. Rh positive blood transfused into an Rh negative patient will initiate production of antibodies.
_____ 8. Subsequent transfusion of Rh positive blood to an Rh negative patient can result in hemolysis of the patient's RBCs.
_____ 9. The presence of IgG antibodies in the serum can be demonstrated by the indirect Coombs' test.

HEMOSTASIS

Hemostasis involves the mechanisms of *vasoconstriction, coagulation* and *clot retraction* as a means to stop bleeding.

The hemostatic *vascular components* include the constriction of arterioles and capillaries, aided by the release of serotonin at the site of injury. Platelet aggregation seals small areas. The platelets swell into irregular shapes and adhere to the collagen on the vascular wall. The plug formed is unstable.

The *coagulation mechanism* can be initiated by either of two pathways *(intrinsic* and *extrinsic)* that converge into a common sequence (Fig. 9-8). The *intrinsic pathway* (within the vessels), which includes clotting factors XII, XI and VII, is stimulated by the activation of factor XII at the surface of an injured vessel. The *extrinsic pathway* (outside the vessels) is activated by tissue damage and involves factor VII. Both pathways share factors X, V, II (prothrombin) and I (fibrinogen).

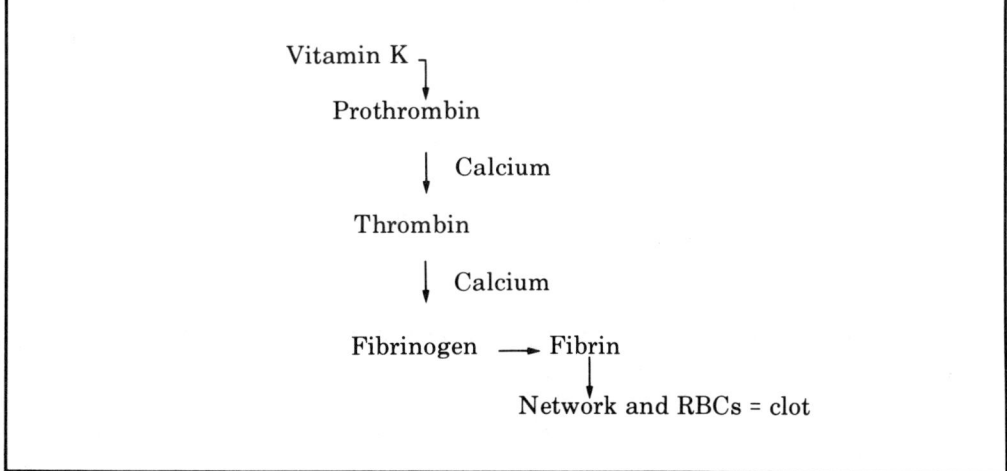

Fig. 9-8. Hemostasis: clotting

The basic mechanism of the clotting systems involves the conversion of *prothrombin* to *thrombin* by the catalytic action of prothrombin activator and calcium. Prothrombin activator is formed in a response to a ruptured blood vessel. *Thrombin* then acts as an enzyme to convert *fibrinogen* to *fibrin.* Fibrin threads make a network of red blood cells and plasma. Prothrombin and fibrinogen are both plasma proteins formed continuously in the liver. *Vitamin K* is necessary for the formation of prothrombin. In the absence of calcium, neither pathway will work.

The clot is the meshwork of fibrin threads, red blood cells and plasma. Soon after the clot is formed, it begins to retract, expressing serum. Bonding involves many platelets. The retraction also pulls together the edges of the vessel, aiding in stabilizing and hemostasis. The clot will continue to extend if it is not stopped. This is probably controlled by the absorption of most of the thrombin to the fibrin threads. The other factor is the presence of *antithrombin III,* an alpha globulin that removes thrombin from the blood. Antithrombin III blocks the effect on fibrinogen.

Heparin circulates freely and is especially abundant in the areas of the lungs and liver. It is continually being secreted by basophilic mast cells. Clotting is prevented by the action of heparin in at least four steps in the coagulation. Anticoagulant mechanisms, such as factor III, are also vital to maintain the blood's normal state.

Thrombocytes (platelets) are part of the hematopoietic bone marrow system. Megakaryocytes, the precursor cells, are very large cells that fragment into platelets within the bone marrow and are then released into the blood. Normal concentration is 200,000 to 400,000 per c. mm. Their function is to form a platelet plug to seal and repair small ruptures in blood vessels. Platelets are a crucial link in the hemostatic chain of events.

KEY CONCEPT: Hemostasis is accomplished through vasoconstriction, coagulation and clot retraction. Vitamin K and calcium are necessary to clot formation.

KEY POINT RECOGNITION

Write true or false by each statement. Answers are at the end of this chapter. A score below 80% indicates the need for further study.

_____ 1. Vasoconstriction as a hemostatic mechanism is aided by the release of serotonin at the injury site.

_____ 2. The intrinsic clotting pathway is stimulated by factor XII at the surface of an injured vessel.

_____ 3. Tissue damage initiates the extrinsic pathway.

_____ 4. Prothrombin is converted to thrombin by prothrombin activator and vitamin K.

_____ 5. Prothrombin converts fibrinogen to fibrin.

_____ 6. Vitamin K is necessary for the formation of thrombin.

_____ 7. In the absence of vitamin K, neither pathway works.

_____ 8. Antithrombin III removes thrombin from the blood.

_____ 9. Heparin aids in clotting and is constantly secreted by basophilic mast cells.

_____10. Thrombocytes form a plug to seal ruptures in blood vessels.

ASSESSMENT OF THE HEMATOPOIETIC SYSTEM

HISTORY AND GENERAL SIGNS AND SYMPTOMS

Physical assessment of the patient experiencing hematopoietic problems is not very different from the assessment of any other patient. Significant medical problems, current therapies, family history and review of systems are all included. Particular attention must be paid to the presenting complaint, its duration, character and circumstances surrounding exacerbations and remissions. The following symptoms require further investigation: fatigue, weakness, chills, fever, weight loss, diaphoresis, lethargy, tiredness and general malaise.

SPECIFIC SIGNS AND SYMPTOMS

Specific signs of altered functioning in specific hematopoietic problems may include:

Skin: prolonged bleeding, bruising, itching, pallor, jaundice

Eye: visual disturbances

Gastrointestinal: epistaxis, bleeding gums, infection of the gums, ulceration of mucous membranes, hoarseness, melena, liver disease, pain

Skeletal: pain in joints, back or bone; nuchal rigidity

Cardiorespiratory: pulmonary emboli, dyspnea, angina, hemoptysis

Genitourinary: hematuria, menorrhagia, amenorrhagia, infections

Physical examination. The physical assessment should include the following methods:

INSPECTION

Check for paleness or cyanosis of the skin, nailbeds and conjunctiva.

Check for jaundice of skin or sclera.

Check for bleeding in the form of petechiae, ecchymotic areas, epistaxis and retinal hemorrhage.

Check for ulceration of the skin.

Check for lymphatic swelling.

PALPATION

Feel for node involvement.

Feel for sternal tenderness.

Feel for bone and joint tenderness.

Feel for alterations in sensation.

PERCUSSION

Percuss for respiratory and diaphragmatic movement.

Percuss for hepatomegaly.

Percuss for splenomegaly.

AUSCULTATION

Listen for changes in heart sounds.

Listen for changes in bowel sounds.

Listen for changes in breath sounds.

EVALUATION OF VITAL SIGNS

The blood pressure may be normal or hypotensive. Rarely in hematologic disorders are alterations in the blood pressure seen. Hypotension, if observed, is a compensatory mechanism to ensure perfusion of the vital organs: kidney, brain and heart. **Tachycardia** may be present when there are changes in the circulating blood volume or hemoglobin concentration. Other compensatory cardiac mechanisms include: flow **murmurs** (usually systolic), **angina** due to an increase in oxygen demands and **tachypnea** due to an attempt to increase oxygenation.

Elevation of body **temperature** is usually indicative of an infection. This infection is often found on the skin, in the throat or in the respiratory or urinary tracts.

Level of consciousness. The level of consciousness is one of the first steps in patient assessment. To assess LOC, the following are determined: **arousability, orientation, ability to follow commands** and **pupillary response.** After the LOC has been determined, the following must be determined:

Subjective findings: vertigo, fatigue, tinnitus, syncopal episodes, urinary problems (burning, frequency), constipation, diarrhea, pain (location, type, characteristic, onset), palpitations

Objective findings: lethargy, confusion, ecchymosis, jaundice, pallor, cyanosis, ulcerations, lymphadenopathy, nuchal rigidity, tachycardia, murmurs, tenderness, splenomegaly, hepatomegaly

LABORATORY AND RADIOLOGIC STUDIES

Laboratory studies in hematopoietic disorders are the most important determinants. Laboratory tests are varied and tailored to presumptive diagnosis. Normal studies are discussed in the following:

Determinations	Reference Range	Significance
Hemoglobin	female: 12 to 14 gm per 100 ml	*Decreased* in anemia, hemorrhage or excessive fluid intake
	male: 13 to 16 gm per 100 ml	*Increased* in polycythemia, chronic obstructive pulmonary disease, and congestive heart failure
Hematocrit	female: 40 to 48%	*Decreased* in anemia and hemorrhage
	male: 42 to 50%	*Increased* in erythrocytosis, dehydration and hemoconcentration due to shock
Erythrocyte indices Mean corpuscular Vol. (MCV)	80 to 94 cubic microns	*Decreased* in microcytic anemia *Increased* in macrocytic anemia
Mean corpuscular hemoglobin (MCH)	27 to 32 micromicrogram per cell	*Decreased* in microcytic anemia *Increased* in macrocytic anemia
Mean corpuscular hemoglobin concentration (MCHC)	33 to 38%	*Decreased* in hypochromic anemia
Reticulocytes	0.5 to 1.5% of red cells	*Decreased* in conditions supressing bone marrow production: acute leukemia, late stages of severe anemias
		Increased in conditions stimulating bone marrow production: infection, blood loss, iron therapy in iron deficiency anemia, polycythemia vera
Platelet count	200,000 to 350,000 per cubic millimeter	*Decreased* thrombocytopenic purpura, acute leukemia, aplastic anemia, chemotherapy
		Increased in chronic granulocytic leukemia, hemoconcentration
Erythrocyte sedimentation rate	female: 0 to 20 mm/hr. male: 0 to 9 mm/hr.	*Increased* in tissue destruction, during menstruation, pregnancy, acute febrile diseases
Erythrocyte count	female: 4,200,000 to 5,400,000/c.mm	*Decreased* in anemias, leukemia, hemorrhage, after blood volume restoration
	male: 4,600,000 to 6,200,000/c.mm	*Increased* in diarrhea, dehydration, polycythemia, acute poisoning, pulmonary fibrosis
Prothrombin time	60 to 100% of control	*Increased* in factor X deficiency, hemorrhagic diseases, cirrhosis, hepatitis, acute toxic necrosis of the liver
Partial thromboplastin time	20 to 45 seconds	*Increased* in factors VIII, IX, X
Leukocyte alkaline phosphatase	Score of 40 to 100	*Decreased* in chronic myelocytic leukemia, chronic lymphocyte leukemia
		Increased in non-leukemic leukocytosis, myeloproliferative disease
Leukocyte count	Total: 5,000 to 10,000/c.mm	*Decreased* in aplastic anemia, agranulocytosis, chemotherapy
neutrophils eosinophils basophils lymphocytes monocytes	60 to 70% 1 to 4% 0 to 0.5% 20 to 30% 2 to 6%	*Increased* in acute infectious processes *Eosinophils* increased in collagen disease, allergy, intestinal parasitosis

Bilirubin	Total: 0.1 to 1.2 mgm/100 ml	*Increased* in liver dysfunction, hemolysis, jaundice
Direct	up to 0.3 mgm/100 ml	
Indirect	0.1 to 1.0 mgm/100 ml	

Radiologic studies are limited. They include:

Routine chest x-rays to determine abnormalities of the ribs and lung fields

Spinal radiographs to detect bony abnormalities

Flat abdomen radiographs to detect abnormalities and air in the abdomen

Lymphangiography, an invasive injection of dye into the lympathic tissue, to detect abnormalities, infection, tumors or disease process

Radionuclide scan to obtain radiographs of soft tissue, such as thyroid, brain, liver, spleen, lungs, kidneys, bone marrow and hematologic determinations.

In addition, bone marrow studies are used to detect the site of blood production and an assessment of iron stores. A bone marrow examination is diagnostic for leukemias, anemias and multiple myeloma.

KEY CONCEPT: Physical assessment of the hematologic system should include assessment of family history, medical history and medication. Performing an overall assessment includes inspection, palpation, percussion and auscultation.

KEY POINT RECOGNITION

Write true or false by each statement. Answers are at the end of this chapter. A score below 80% indicates the need for further study.

_____ 1. Prolonged bleeding and bruising of the skin may be indicative of a hematopoietic problem.

_____ 2. Epistaxis, hoarseness and ulcerations of the mucous membranes may be indicative of a gastrointestinal disorder related to the hematologic system.

_____ 3. Paleness, cyanosis and jaundice are evaluated by inspection.

_____ 4. Hepatomegaly is checked by auscultation of the liver.

_____ 5. Sternal tenderness is not an indicator of a hematopoietic problem.

_____ 6. Blood analysis is an important determinant of a hematologic disorder.

_____ 7. Changes in vital signs are important indicators of hematopoietic disorders.

_____ 8. In hematopoietic disorders, compensatory cardiac activity may include angina and systolic murmurs.

_____ 9. In hematopoietic disorders, an increase in the respiratory rate may be an attempt by the body to increase oxygenation.

_____ 10. In hematopoietic disorders, tachycardia may be due to fever or low blood volume.

_____ 11. Infection due to a hematopoietic disorder is usually not found in the respiratory or urinary tract.

_____ 12. The normal laboratory value for hemoglobin in a female is 12 to 14 gm/100 ml.

_____ 13. Hematocrit is increased in erthyrocytosis.

_____ 14. Anemia and hemorrhage cause an increase in the hematocrit level.

_____ 15. Erythrocyte indices, especially an increase in mean corpuscular hemoglobin concentration, indicates microcytic anemia.

_____ 16. Increased bone marrow production results in an increase in the reticulocyte count.

_____ 17. An increase in the platelet count may indicate hemodilution.

_____ 18. Febrile disease may increase the erythrocyte sedimentation rate.

____19. The normal erythrocyte count for males is 4,600,000 to 6,200,000 per cubic millimeter.

____20. The normal partial thromboplastin time is two to three minutes.

PATHOLOGICAL STATES AND NURSING MANAGEMENT

ANEMIA

Anemia is a reduction below the normal levels of hemoglobin or erythrocytes. Anemia is a symptom of an underlying disease process. Tissue hypoxia is the result of decreased oxygen-carrying capacity of the blood.

Pathophysiology

Anemias are caused by one of three etiologic factors: **blood loss, decreased production of erythrocytes,** or **increased destruction of erythrocytes.**

In anemias due to blood loss, the loss may be acute or chronic. When an intracorpuscular defect exists, an increase in the destruction of erythrocytes occurs. This destruction may be hereditary or acquired. Hereditary anemias include: **spherocytosis, thalassemia, stomacytosis** and **hemoglobinopathies.** Acquired anemias include: **thermal injury** and **B_{12}-iron-folic deficiencies.** In the case of decreased production of erythrocytes, the decrease of erythrocytes causes decreased hemoglobin synthesis, resulting in iron deficiency, decreased globin synthesis and decreased porphyrin.

Aplastic anemia is failure of the blood cell production involving erythrocytes, thrombocytes and granulocytes. Congenital pure red cell aplastic anemia is the exception; it is the congenital absence of erythrocyte precursors. Chemical toxins or radiation account for half of the causes of aplastic anemia. The remaining half have an unknown etiology. Fever, infection and bleeding may be seen in aplastic anemia.

Hemolytic anemia is a shortening of the life span of a red blood cell. There are congenital and acquired hemolytic anemias. Examples of hereditary hemolytic anemias are sickle cell, thalassemia, spherocytosis and glucose-6-phosphate dehydrogenase deficiency. Examples of acquired hemolytic anemias include immune and sprue cell (Fig. 9-9).

Clinical Presentation

The clinical presentation is extremely variable and dependent on the type of anemia: aplastic or hemolytic. Clinical presentation includes: pallor, cyanosis, blurred vision, tachypnea, tachycardia, anorexia, nausea, melena, hematuria, vertigo, headache, confusion and tenderness.

Clinical signs and symptoms specifically associated with:

Aplastic: fatigue, lethargy, dyspnea, cutaneous bleeding, bleeding from mucous membranes

Pancytopenia: hypoxia, infections, bleeding

Hemolysis: elevated bilirubin, jaundice, splenomegaly, hepatomegaly, pruritis

Diagnostic Data

Bone marrow biopsy is the best diagnostic aid to determine impaired cell production. Other tests to document the etiology or type include blood analysis. Blood analysis is valuable in determining the extent of reduction in erthrocytes, leukocytes and platelets. Also, the reticulocyte count is abnormal.

Hereditary	Causes	Laboratory/Clinical
Sickle cell	Blacks, some Mediterraneans Defective hemoglobin molecule Produces S Hgl Cells sickle in presence of low O_2 tension Rigid cells obstruct vessels causing ischemia and infarction	Hemoglobin electrophoresis Sickle prep Hgl: 7-10 gm Jaundice Bone marrow expansion (prominent forehead and cheek bones) Tachycardia Low flow murmurs Cardiomegaly Severe pain Infection predisposes crisis
Thalassemia	Reduction in hemoglobin formation	
Spherocytosis	Hereditary Abnormal red cell membrane leading to destruction in spleen	Small, sphere shaped red cells Splenomegaly

Glucose-6-phosphate Dehydrogenase deficiency	Abnormal G6PD-red cell enzyme
	Cell membrane unstable
	Hemolysis under stress of infection or drugs
	  antimalarial
	  sulfonamides
	  aspirin
	  thiazide diuretics
	  oral hypoglycemics
		Normal until exposure
		Elevated reticulocyte count
		Pallor
		Jaundice
		Hemoglobinuria
		Heinz bodies
		(degraded hemoglobin)

Acquired	Causes	Laboratory/Clinical
Immune	Drug-induced Antibodies react with RBC Transfusion Erythroblastosis fetalis Cell destruction or return as spherocytes	Positive Coombs' Elevated reticulocyte count Hgl: 6-9 gm

Idiopathic	Autoimmune
	  SLE
	  Lymphatic leukemia
	Drugs: methyldopa
	       penicillin	

Spur cell	Liver disease Portal hypertension	Spur-shaped RBC

Other causes:
  heart valve
  angiopathic
  infections
	RBC damaged by valve
	RBC damaged by hypertension
	Malaria
	Septic abortion
		Fragmented RBC
		
		Hemoglobinuria

Fig. 9-9. Hemolytic anemias

Nursing Care

The major nursing responsibilities for patients with anemias (Fig. 9-10 and 9-11) include:

(1) Review laboratory data relating to etiology.
(2) Watch for infection by obtaining cultures. Strict aseptic technique should be practiced to prevent cross-contamination.
(3) Maintain fluid and electrolyte balance.
(4) Observe for bleeding.
(5) Provide good skin and mouth care.

(6) Reverse isolation for severe granulocytopenia.

(7) Administer steroids and antibiotics.

(8) Provide postoperative care for the splenectomy patient.

(9) Provide care for patient following bone marrow transplants.

(10) Keep the patient warm.

(11) Conserve energy.

Signs and Symptoms	Nursing Interventions

Weakness, fatigue
  drooping posture
  slowed ambulation
  pallor of extremeties
  perspiring
  coldness
  vertigo, faintness
  joint pain
  pruritis
	Conserve strength
	  set priorities
	
	rest periods
	
	avoid stress
	
	stop before fatigued
	avoid soap, use emollients

Compensatory cardiovascular
  increased heart rate
  increased cardiac output
  shortness of breath
  decreased peripheral vascular resistance
  decreased viscosity
	Decrease workload

Pathology
  Cardiovascular:
    Angina
      secondary to ischemia
    Congestive heart failure
    High output failure
    Fainting—syncope
  Neurological:
    Cerebral vascular insufficiency
    Tinnitus
    Numbness
    Tingling
    Pounding headache
    Spots before eyes
    Drowsiness
    Irritability
    Inability to concentrate
    Poor healing
	Avoid temperature extremes
	
	Avoid bending over
	Avoid quick movements
	
	Get out of bed slowly
	
	Sit before standing
	
	Avoid infections
	Protect from trauma
	Maintain good hygiene

Fig. 9-10. Nursing intervention: anemia

Signs and Symptoms	Nursing Intervention

Thalessemia
    dark urine
    jaundice
	Rest

hepatomegaly splenomegaly	Avoid cold

pruritis
    If large hemolysis:
        fever
        headache
        pain in abdomen, back, extremities
        shock
	Prevent URI

Complications: leg ulcers, cholelithiasis	Correct acidosis

Sickle Cell
    As above, plus:
        cardiomegaly
        growth suppression
        chronic UTT
	Transfuse
	Narcotics
	Antibiotics
	O_2

Crisis:
        shock
        infarction of tissue and/or organs
        bone necrosis
        intravascular occlusion
	Partial exchange transfusion

Fig. 9-11. Nursing intervention: hemolytic anemia

KEY CONCEPT: Anemias may be caused by blood loss, decreased production of erythrocytes or increased destruction of erythrocytes.

LEUKEMIA

Pathophysiology

Leukemia is a neoplastic disease that involves the body's blood-forming organs and is characterized by a proliferation of white blood cells. There are four main types of leukemia: ***acute lymphocytic leukemia, acute myelogenous leukemia, chronic lymphocytic leukemia*** and ***chronic myelogenous leukemia.*** Etiology is unknown; however, certain conditions predispose a person to the development of leukemia: ***radiation exposure, viral infections, chemicals, immune defects*** and ***chromosomal changes.***

Progression of the disease involves the kidneys, nervous system, bone and skin. Acute leukemia refers to the presence of immature cells, whereas chronic leukemia denotes mature cells and well-differentiated white blood cells. Classification of leukemia is by cellular involvement: ***lymphocytic*** or ***myelocytic*** (Fig. 9-12). Lymphocytic leukemia is a tremendous increase in lymphocytes. The spleen and lymph nodes are enlarged. Myelocytic leukemia involves the hematopoietic bone marrow. There is a great number of myelocytes squeezing out the red cells and a marked leukocytosis with reduced red blood cells.

Clinical Presentation

The leukemia patient generally complains of fatigue, bone pain and sweating, and presents with an elevated temperature. Hepatomegaly and splenomegaly may be present. Sternal tenderness, heat intolerance, abdominal fullness, bleeding tendencies and anemia may also be present. If a fulminating infection is evident, the patient may be in ***terminal state*** or ***blastic crisis.*** Blastic crisis refers to a change in CML to a disease state of greater malignancy. It is an accelerated phase seen as a change from CML to AML.

	Acute Lymphoblastic Leukemia (ALL)	Chronic Lymphocytic Leukemia (CLL)	Acute Myelogenous Leukemia (AML)	Chronic Myelogenous Leukemia (CML)
Pathology	Proliferation of immature, functionless lymphocytes initiated in bone marrow	Proliferation of normal-appearing B cell lymphocytes	Absence of normal hematopoietic cells, proliferation of myeloblasts.	Proliferation of mature neutrophils and immature granulocytes with thrombocytosis; presence of Philadelphia chromosome (Ph) 80%
Age	Any age, peaks 4-7, abrupt onset	Uncommon before 40, gradual onset	22-24	25-60
Clinical features	Arthralgia Bone pain G.I. complaints Hepatomegaly Sternal tenderness	Asymptomatic lymphadenopathy	Arthralgia Bone pain Bleeding uncontrollable Infection uncontrollable Fever Fatigue	Heat intolerance Excessive sweating Abdominal fullness LUQ pain 2 Splenic enlargement Lymphadenopathy unusual
Chemotherapy	Multi-agent vincristine, prednisone, adriamycin, Introthecal methotrexate	Chlorambucil (most widely used) Cyclophosphamide Glucocorticoids for autoimmune hemolytic anemias	Antimetabolites cytosial arabinoside Antibiotics Methotrexate	Bisulfan Allopurinal to minimize risk of hyperuricemia
Radiation	Cranial to subdue CNS involvement	Total body radiation is alternative	Local or total prior to bone marrow transplant	Previously spleen radiated, chemo more successful
Prognosis	Maintenance therapy, 6 mercaptopurine and methotrexate Long-term survival Best response 3-7 years old	Median 6 years	Untreated 2 months Median 12 months	Median 3-5 years Blastic crisis Converts process to AML-therapy palliative

Fig. 9-12. Classification of leukemias

Diagnostic Data

A history and physical may reveal a recent viral infection, exposure to chemicals, or radiation exposure to known immune defects. However, this cannot always be elucidated by history. The patient will probably present with an elevated temperature and evidence of proliferation of white blood cells. The definitive diagnosis is made by blood and bone analysis. Because of the impaired production of cell type, anemia and thrombocytopenia occur and are often initial symptoms of a leukemia. In addition to WBC elevation, anemia, platelet reduction and abnormal phosphatase level, an elevated BUN and decreased clotting factor may also be present.

Nursing Care

The goal of nursing is to provide supportive care, as well as to prevent complications.

(1) Provide patient education by informing the patient of the basic disease process and the importance of medical follow-up.

(2) Administer appropriate drug therapy and anticipate side effects.

(3) Observe for bleeding: petechiae, ecchymosis, bleeding gums.

(4) Control pain. Severe episode may indicate blastic crisis (Fig. 9-13).

Signs and Symptoms	Nursing Intervention
Bleeding tendencies	Prevent trauma, use small needles Report and control any bleeding Avoid ASA
Infection-prone	Meticulous aseptic care Antimicrobial soaps Avoid rectal thermometers
Fatigue, weakness	Conserve strength
Mucosal ulcerations	Meticulous oral care Xylocaine solution
Chemotherapy	Know drugs and side effects
Nausea and vomiting nutrition impaired	Antiemetics Diet planning and control
Increased metabolic needs, hypercalcemia-hyperuricemia	Hydrate Allopurinol
Constipation	Mild laxatives

Fig. 9-13. Nursing intervention: leukemia

KEY CONCEPT: Nursing care is designed to provide supportive care, prevent complications and provide patient education.

LYMPHOMAS
Pathophysiology

The lymphoma is a hyperplasia of the lymphoreticular system. There are two major classifications: ***Hodgkins's disease*** and ***non-Hodgkin's lymphoma.*** Lymphomas are neoplasms arising from lymphatic tissue. They generally behave in a malignant manner.

Hodgkin's Disease
Pathophysiology

Hodgkin's disease is a histiocytic lymphoma beginning with painless enlargement of the lymph nodes. The cervical nodes are usually involved first. Hodgkin's disease composes approximately 50 percent of all lymphomas. The cause of Hodgkin's disease is unknown.

Clinical Presentation

History and physical examination may reveal systemic symptoms of fever, night sweats, generalized pruritus, anorexia and weight loss. The patient will experience an increase of pain in the lymph nodes after ingestion of alcohol. Physical examination reveals enlarged lymph nodes, spleen and liver.

Diagnostic Data

The definitive diagnosis is made by histologic evaluation of an excised node and the presence of ***Sternberg-Reed cells.*** Exploratory surgery, coupled with systemic symptoms, provides information for diagnosis and staging of Hodgkin's disease. Blood studies may indicate a reduction in the red blood cells, white blood cells and platelets. The patient with decreased blood cells may also have bone marrow and splenic involvement. A chest radiograph may show a mediastinal mass. Therapy is deferred until the disease is staged. The Ann Arbor Staging Classification is the most common classification for Hodgkin's disease (Fig. 9-14).

Stage	Definition	Treatment
I	Involvement of a single lymph node region (I) or of a single extra-lymphatic organ or site (I$_E$)	Radiation to lymph nodes and adjacent to lymphatic sites
II	Involvement of two or more lymph node regions on the same side of the diaphragm (II) or localized involvement of an extralymphatic organ or site and of one or more lymph node regions on the same side of the diaphragm (II$_E$)	
III	Involvement of lymph node regions on both sides of the diaphragm (III), which may also be accompanied by involvement of the spleen (IIIs) or by localized involvement of an extra-lymphatic organ or site (III$_E$) or both (III$_{SE}$)	A. Total Nodal Irradiation B. Chemotherapy
IV	Diffuse or disseminated involvement of one or more extralymphatic organs or tissues, with or without associated lymph node involvement	A. Chemotherapy B. Chemotherapy

The presence or absence of fever, night sweats, or unexplained loss of 10% or more body weight in the six months preceding admission are denoted by the suffix letters B and A, respectively. Biopsy-documented involvement of stage IV sites is also denoted by letter suffixes: M, marrow; L, lung; H, liver; P, pleura; O, bone; D, skin and subcutaneous tissue.

Fig. 9-14. Classification of Hodgkin's disease using Ann Arbor staging

Nursing Care

The treatment modalities are chemotherapy and radiotherapy. The exact treatment is based on the stage of the disease. The goal of nursing is to help the patient develop a realistic approach to the illness (Fig. 9-15).

Signs and Symptoms	Nursing Interventions
Nausea and vomiting	Antiemetics
Malaise	Maintain hydration Nutrition
Anorexia	High protein Low CHO
Mucosal irritation	Meticulous, frequent, gentle oral hygiene Surface anesthetics
Weakness, fatigue	Rest periods
Dry, tender, irritated skin	Avoid soap and water Emollients frequently Gentle cleansing Avoid scrubbing Use cornstarch vs. talcum Avoid adhesive Keep skin folds and contact areas dry

Fig. 9-15. Nursing intervention: radiation therapy

(1) Provide patient education regarding the disease, medication and medical follow-up.
(2) Provide emotional support to the patient and family.
(3) Prevent complications and immobility.
(4) Develop a meticulous skin regimen.
(5) Provide radiotherapy follow-up with proper skin care of markings.
(6) Observe for radiotherapy and chemotherapy effects.

Non-Hodgkin's Lymphoma

Pathophysiology

Non-Hodgkin's lymphoma is classified by histologic findings. The general node structure is classified as nodular or diffuse, and the major cell type as ***well-differentiated lymphocyte, poorly differentiated lymphocyte*** or ***undifferentiated histiocyte.***

Clinical Presentation

The disease radiates to the liver, spleen, bone marrow and other tissues in the same manner as Hodgkin's disease. Pressure and obstruction of organs and tissues cause symptoms of pain and abdominal fullness.

Diagnostic Data

Non-Hodgkin's disease is staged and treated the same as Hodgkin's disease. Treatment by radiation and chemotherapy is not as effective as in Hodgkin's disease.

Nursing Care

Nursing care needs are the same as for Hodgkin's disease.

KEY CONCEPT: Nursing personnel must provide supportive care and patient education.

POLYCYTHEMIA

Pathophysiology

Polycythemia is an overabundant production of red blood cells, white blood cells and platelets. The most common change is an increase in hemoglobin, causing an appearance of a red-purple complexion accompanied by red hands and feet.

Clinical Presentation

The patient with polycythemia generally complains of headache, weakness, dyspnea, pruritis and tearing. Bleeding from the skin and mucous membranes may also be present. Polycythemia is a relatively rare disorder, most common in persons over 50 years of age. Polycythemia may lead to thrombosis.

Diagnostic Data

The red blood count is 7 to 12 million. The skin is generally red-purple. Hemoglobin usually ranges from 18 to 24 grams and has been reported as high as 40 grams. Specific gravity ranges from 1.075 to 1.080; the normal is 1.055 to 1.065.

Nursing Care

The goal is to provide supportive care, as well as to prevent hemorrhage (Fig. 9-16).
(1) Observe the patient after phlebotomy.
(2) Administer drugs to control disease: chlorambucil, melphalan, busulfan.
(3) Offer foods low in iron.
(4) Prevent infection.
(5) Provide emotional support to the patient and family.

Signs and Symptoms	Nursing Intervention
Headache Fatigue Vertigo Angina	Symptomatic for comfort
Pedal edema Hepatomegaly Splenomegaly Paresthesia	Keep ambulatory
Claudication Pruritis Ruddy cyanosis	Reduce activities that increase venous return
Elevated systolic B.P. Dyspnea	Avoid Valsalva maneuver
Increased viscosity promotes thrombosis	Avoid temperature extremes
Excess volume, vascular engorgement	Phlebotomy
Bleeds excessively	Radioactive phosphorus (suppresses hematopoietic activity)

Fig. 9-16. Nursing intervention: polycthemia

KEY CONCEPT: Nursing must provide supportive care and prevent hemorrhage. Medications and foods containing iron should be avoided.

ANAPHYLAXIS

Pathophysiology

The most severe form of hypersensitivity is anaphylaxis. This inappropriate response to an antigen is usually manifested as a tissue-damaging overreaction to the antigen.

Clinical Presentation

The patient presents with increased irritability, dyspnea, cyanosis, convulsions, unconsciousness and death. It is common to find death due to spasms of the smooth muscles of the bronchioles. Other signs are fever, redness of the skin, pruritis and urticaria.

Diagnostic Data

In mild cases, symptoms are self-limiting. In severe cases, death may occur. Emergency treatment includes basic and advanced life support with vasopressors, corticosteroids and airway management.

Nursing Care

The goal of nursing is to prevent death (Fig. 9-17).

(1) Establish adequate airway and breathing. Because of the high incidence of respiratory impairment, most patients spend some period of time on mechanical ventilators.
(2) Administer medications.
(3) Observe for changes in vital signs.
(4) Maintain fluid and electrolyte balance.
(5) Maintain nutritional status.
(6) Prevent complications, especially bronchospasms and hypovolemia.
(7) Provide emotional and psychological support to the patient and family.

Signs and Symptoms	Nursing Intervention
Respiratory distress	Airway maintenance
Bronchospasm	Ventilation—(mechanical if necessary) may need tracheostomy
Airway obstruction	Epinephrine
Hypovolemia (third-spaced fluids)	Fluids, usually Ringer's lactate
Edema	May correct acidosis
Hives	Cardiotonic meds if indicated
Nausea, vomiting	Steroids

Fig. 9-17. Nursing intervention: anaphylaxis

KEY CONCEPT: Anaphylaxis is a true emergency necessitating immediate recognition and treatment.

DISSEMINATED INTRAVASCULAR COAGULATION (DIC)
Pathophysiology

Disseminated intravascular coagulation (DIC) is not a primary disorder, but a complication of severe injury, trauma or disease. DIC is an acute bleeding disorder resulting from defibrination. It may be initiated by the release of endotoxins or foreign material entering the bloodstream due to hypotensive states, trauma or neoplasms. The first phase of DIC is characterized by free thrombin in the blood, fibrin deposits and the aggregation of platelets. Minute thrombi are formed and obstruct circulation. These fibrin deposits destroy red blood cells.

The second phase of DIC is hemorrhage caused by depletion of clotting factors II, V, VII, IX, X and platelets. The thrombin that accelerates coagulation and converts plasminogen to plasmin eventually breaks the fibrin and fibrinogen into fibrin degradation products. This process leads to anticoagulation and bleeding.

Clinical Presentation

The first sign of DIC is purpura of the chest and abdomen. Other signs may include bleeding and shock.

Diagnostic Data

History and physical may reveal recent trauma, injury or disease process. The patient will present with purpura of the chest and abdomen. The definitive diagnosis is made by laboratory studies. The presence of thrombocytopenia, low levels of fibrinogen, and prolonged prothrombin and partial thromboplastin times indicate DIC. Other tests show low levels of factors VIII, V and abnormal red blood cells on a peripheral smear.

Nursing Care

Nursing care is aimed at treating the primary disease. The goal is to control bleeding and restore normal levels of clotting factors.

(1) Administer heparin to inhibit thrombin and allow fibrinogen and platelet levels to increase.
(2) Administer blood products to replace depleted factors.
(3) Treat sequelae including hemodialysis for renal failure.
(4) Maintain an adequate airway and breathing.
(5) Maintain fluid and electrolyte balance.
(6) Prevent complications.

(7) Observe for changes in vital signs, urinary output and cardiac function.

(8) Monitor amount and nature of drainage from tubes and incision.

(9) Provide emotional and psychological support for the patient and family.

KEY CONCEPT: DIC is an acute bleeding disorder resulting from defibrination. Immediate recognition and monitoring are important for survival.

HEMOPHILIA
Pathophysiology

Hemophilia is a hereditary coagulation disorder. The female transmits to the male both hemophilia A and B. In true hemophilia A, factor VIII is nearly absent. Hemophilia B is characterized by a deficiency of factor IX. The ability to produce thrombin and fibrin by the intrinsic mechanism is severely impaired by the absence of these important factors (Fig. 9-18).

Intrinsic	Extrinsic
Abnormal:	Normal:
Partial thromboplastin time	Prothrombin time
Platelets	Thromboplastic
Factor VIII	Factor VII
Factor IX	
Prothrombin ⟶ Thrombin	Prothrombin ⟶ Thrombin

Fig. 9-18. Hemophilia deficiencies

Clinical Presentation

The male with hemophilia has repeated episodes of bleeding. Bleeding may occur in organs, body orifices, knees, wrists and elbows. Hematuria, epistaxis, hemoptysis, hematemesis and melena may also be present.

Diagnostic Data

The definitive diagnosis is made by specific serum assay for factors VIII and IX. The partial thromboplastin time is prolonged, but prothrombin time and platelet count are normal.

Nursing Care

The goal of nursing care is to prevent bleeding and to provide patient education.

(1) Control bleeding by administering appropriate treatment: ice bags, pressure dressing, immobilization, elevation and topical coagulants.

(2) Administer fresh or fresh-frozen plasma or blood containing factor VIII.

(3) Infuse cryoprecipitate: antihemophilic factor (factor VIII).

(4) Provide emotional support to the patient and family.

(5) Observe for changes in vital signs.

(6) Observe for complications: infection and deformities.

(7) Provide patient education.

KEY CONCEPT: Hemophilia is a hereditary disorder characterized by episodes of bleeding.

SICKLE CELL DISEASE
Pathophysiology

Sickle cell disease is a congenital hemolytic anemia. The incidence of sickle cell anemia is highest in Blacks, Puerto Ricans and persons of Spanish, French, Italian, Greek and Turkish origin. Sickle cell disease is a chemical defect lying within the hemoglobin of red blood cells. The cell takes the shape of a sickle or crescent. The abnormality is in the globin fraction of the hemoglobin, where an amino acid is substituted for another in the polypeptide chain. This substitution alters the properties of the hemoglobin. The change occurs in the electrical charge, making it more soluble, therefore causing precipitation. This crystallization within the red blood cell increases the viscosity of the blood. These changes lead to hypoxia and serum acidosis.

Clinical Presentation

Sudden onset of sickling develops into a condition called *crisis.* The crisis is divided into three groups: *painful* or *thrombotic, aplastic* and *hemolytic.*

Painful crisis is due to the abnormal cell causing occlusion of small arterioles and venules. In *aplastic crisis,* the mechanism responsible for erythroblast division or maturation is depressed. This depression ultimately leads to anemia.

The patient with sickle cell generally complains of increased weakness, aching joint pain, chest pain and sudden, severe abdominal pain. Bony deformities, EKG changes resembling mitral stenosis or mitral regurgitation, icteric sclera and retardation of secondary sex characteristics may be present.

Children under the age of two with sickle cell disorder generally complain of abdominal distention, nausea, vomiting, recurrent infection, fever, failure to thrive and swelling of hands and feet. For children over two years of age, the most common complaints include joint, back and abdominal pain. Physical findings indicate pallor, lymphadenopathy, cardiomegaly, ascites, nocturia, splenomegaly and joint swelling. The definitive diagnosis of aplastic anemia is by bone marrow studies.

Hemolytic crisis involves a rapid reduction in the hematocrit level.

Diagnostic Data

History and physical examination may reveal the sickle cell disorder. However, this can not always be elucidated by history. The patient will present with abnormal crescent-shaped cells. The definitive diagnosis is made by laboratory studies. In both the trait and the disease, *sickle cell prep* and *sickledex* will be *positive. Peripheral smear* will be *normal* with the *trait,* and *positive* for sickle cells with the disease. The reticulocyte count and platelet will be increased. In addition, a urinalysis will reveal impaired concentrating ability of the kidneys.

An intravenous pyelogram reveals an increase in renal medullary blood flow and dilation of medullary blood vessels. Bone radiographs show density.

Nursing Care

Much about the therapy is supportive. In acute crisis, the treatment is to maintain **adequate hydration, fluid** and **electrolyte balance** and **pH.**

(1) Oxygen therapy may be given, but it does not reduce the pain.
(2) Administer narcotics, with care to prevent addiction.
(3) Administer intravenous fluids of dextrose 5%, which may relieve pain.
(4) Administer antibiotics.
(5) Administer blood and blood products for aplastic crisis or shock.
(6) Administer vasodilating drugs, alkaloids and, occassionally, anticoagulants.
(7) Provide emotional and psychological support for the patient and family.
(8) Provide resources for genetic counseling.

KEY CONCEPT: Sickle cell disease is a hereditary hemolytic anemia associated with defective S in the erythrocyte. This defect produces a crescent-shaped or sickle appearance to the cell.

MULTIPLE MYELOMA

Pathophysiology

Multiple myeloma is a plasma cell dyscrasia, characterized by neoplastic cells that infiltrate the bone marrow. This generally produces an ***immunoglobulin***, called ***myeloma*** or M-proteins. The bone marrow contains approximately 15 percent plasma cells, with a predominant portion being immature and multinucleated. Eventually, the plasma cells become malignant. This malignancy causes the cell to lose its ability to regulate division, leading to tumor formation within the bone. The plasma cells produce ***cryoglobulin***, an abnormal globulin. This abnormal globulin is seen in Raynaud's phenomenon. Also, renal damage, increased blood viscosity, congestive heart failure and bleeding disorders develop.

Clinical Presentation

There are a variety of symptoms, ranging from mild to severe. They include weakness, infections, skeletal pain, hemorrhage, renal failure, neurologic changes and amyloidosis. Often, lethargy and loss of weight are also present. The bones become brittle, and pathologic fractures of the hips, arms and ribs occur.

Diagnostic Data

A history and physical, plus diagnostic studies, are necessary to confirm diagnosis. Laboratory studies are useful to detect increased ESR, pancytopenia, hypercalcemia, elevation in protein electrophoresis and elevated creatinine. Urine is tested for Bence Jones protein and protein electrophoresis.

Nursing Care

The treatments for multiple myeloma are chemotherapeutic agents and radiation therapy. Radiation therapy relieves bone pain and promotes healing of pathologic fractures. The goal of nursing care is long-term management.

(1) Administer drugs: cyclophosphamide, prednisone, melphalan.

(2) Observe for side effects of bone marrow depression.

(3) Observe for signs of infection, bleeding and anemia.

(4) Maintain fluid and electrolyte balance: watch for hypercalcemia.

(5) Maintain hydration to prevent renal and neurologic damage.

(6) Control pain.

(7) Maintain mobilization.

(8) Provide emotional and psychological support to the patient and family.

(9) Provide patient education for understanding of the disease, treatment and long-term needs.

KEY CONCEPT: Nursing care is aimed at maintaining an optimal level of activity. Realistic acceptance of the disease and treatment must be initiated as soon as the diagnosis has been established.

KEY POINT RECOGNITION

Write true or false by each statement. Answers are at the end of this chapter. A score below 80% indicates the need for further study.

_____ 1. Hypoxia can occur in anemia.

_____ 2. Hypoxemia increases the production of erythrocytes.

_____ 3. Anemia due to blood loss may be indicative of a lack of available iron.

_____ 4. Spherocytosis is a hereditary extracorpuscle defect.

_____ 5. Hemoglobinopathy is an acquired extracorpuscle defect.

_____ 6. Hemolytic anemia causes premature destruction of red blood cells.

_____ 7. Aplastic anemia is always due to exposure to a chemical toxin.

_____ 8. All anemias have the same clinical presentation and laboratory abnormalities.
_____ 9. Bone marrow biopsy is important for diagnostic purposes in the suspected anemic patient.
_____10. Nursing care of the anemic patient is aimed at assessment, prevention of infection and control of bleeding.
_____11. Leukemia is a neoplastic disease.
_____12. Leukemia involves only blood-forming organs.
_____13. Acute leukemia refers to the presence of immature cells.
_____14. Chronic leukemia refers to mature cells.
_____15. Fatigue, bone pain and elevated temperature may indicate leukemia.
_____16. Severe bone pain in a diagnosed leukemia patient may indicate blastic crisis.
_____17. Patient education is one of the nursing goals for the patient with leukemia.
_____18. Elevated BUN and prolonged clotting factors may be indicative of leukemia.
_____19. Leukemia may cause a reduction in the platelet count.
_____20. Chronic lymphocytic leukemia occurs in childhood.
_____21. Hodgkin's disease is a histiocytic lymphoma.
_____22. Hodgkin's disease involves the cervical nodes only.
_____23. Systemic symptoms of Hodgkin's disease may include fever, night sweats, generalized pruritus and weight loss.
_____24. In Hodgkin's disease, enlarged nodes may diminish in size after alcohol ingestion.
_____25. The presence of Sternberg-Reed cells is indicative of Hodgkin's disease.
_____26. Non-Hodgkin's lymphoma is staged and treated the same as Hodgkin's disease.
_____27. Polycythemia is an overabundance of red blood cells.
_____28. Polycythemia causes a red-purple appearance to the skin.
_____29. A red blood count of 7 to 12 million may indicate polycythemia.
_____30. Anaphylaxis may be a true emergency.
_____31. Uncorrected anaphylaxis may result in death.
_____32. DIC results from defibrination.
_____33. Endotoxins enter the bloodstream following trauma or hypotensive states that initiate DIC.
_____34. DIC is bound thrombin and hemolysis of red blood cells.
_____35. DIC's second phase is indicated by hemorrhage.
_____36. Purpura is a latent sign of DIC.
_____37. The partial thromboplastin time (PTT) is abnormal in hemophilia.
_____38. The prothrombin time is abnormal in hemophilia.
_____39. Hemophilia is transmitted from a female to a male.
_____40. Hemophilia bleeding tendencies occur in early childhood.
_____41. Bleeding due to hemophilia is treated by transfusing with factor VIII, derived from normal plasma.
_____42. Sickle cell disease has a higher incidence among Blacks than among Whites.
_____43. Sickle cell disease indicates an abnormally shaped cell.
_____44. Sickle cell disease may cause the blood's pH to be alkalotic.
_____45. Crisis refers to a sudden event of sickling.

_____46. Painful crisis is caused by abnormal occlusion of small blood vessels.
_____47. Sickle cell disease rarely starts before 10 years of age.
_____48. Hemolytic crisis is a rapid rise in the hematocrit level.
_____49. Multiple myeloma is a plasma cell disorder.
_____50. The plasma cells produce an abnormal globulin known as cryoglobulin in multiple myeloma.
_____51. Multiple myeloma may lead to brittle bones.

CARE COMMON TO HEMATOPOIETIC PROBLEMS

REDUCED ERYTHROCYTES

Changes in the number of erythrocytes may indicate a hematopoietic problem. Findings include: **fatigue, weakness** and **orthostatic hypotension.**

Methods of treatment to increase erythrocytes include administering red blood cells.

Nursing Care

(1) Monitor cardiopulmonary status for changes.
(2) Maintain acid-base balance.
(3) Check vital signs for changes.

REDUCED WHITE BLOOD CELLS

A reduction in white blood cells can result in infection. Findings include: **elevated temperature;** formation of **pus, redness and heat; pulmonary infiltrates;** and **chest pain.**

Nursing Care

(1) Closely monitor temperature.
(2) Administer antipyretics after diagnosis is confirmed.
(3) Prevent hypothermia.
(4) Obtain culture and sensitivity studies.
(5) Use strict aseptic technique in handwashing.
(6) Administer antibiotics.
(7) Provide meticulous oral and body hygiene.
(8) Prevent cross-contamination.
(9) Administer granulocyte transfusions.

DECREASED PLATELET FUNCTIONS

Hemorrhage is a major concern with a reduction in platelets or **thrombocytopenia.** Findings include: **hematuria, G.I. hemorrhage, epistaxis, ulceration or bleeding of mucous membranes** and **cerebral vascular accident.**

Methods of treatment to increase platelet functioning include platelet transfusions.

Nursing Care

(1) Provide meticulous oral hygiene. Use a soft toothbrush and mild mouthwash.
(2) Maintain prolonged pressure at venipuncture sites and lacerations.
(3) Administer medications I.V. (not I.M. or S.Q.).
(4) Watch for mucosal irritation with nasogastric and endotracheal tubes.
(5) Prevent straining for bowel movements.
(6) Do not administer aspirin.
(7) Closely monitor mentation and vital signs for changes.

ADMINISTRATION OF BLOOD

Blood therapy is used to increase RBCs carrying oxygen, to increase blood volume and to provide proteins, coagulation factors and platelets.

Types of Blood
(1) Citrate-phosphate-dextrose whole blood provides platelets and coagulation factors.
(2) Packed red blood cells increase hemoglobin and hematocrit.
(3) Fresh frozen plasma provides clotting factors, except platelets.
(4) Cryoprecipitate provides factors VIII, XIII and fibrinogen.
(5) Platelet concentration provides platelets.
(6) Volume expanders, such as albumin and plasma protein fraction, and salt-poor albumin provide plasma-volume expansion.
(7) Granulocytes increase phagocytosis.

Complications Related to Transfusion
(1) Hives
(2) Fever
(3) Chills
(4) Pain
(5) Mentation changes
(6) Shortness of breath
(7) Shock
(8) Headache

Nursing Care
(1) Closely monitor for transfusion reaction.
(2) Maintain patient intravenous line.
(3) Monitor blood pressure, temperature and urinary output.

KEY CONCEPT: Care common to hematopoietic problems depends on the general type of disorder. The types include reduction in erythrocytes, reduction in white blood cells and reduction in platelet function. Nursing care includes closely monitoring for changes in cardiopulmonary status, vital signs and evaluation of laboratory data.

KEY POINT RECOGNITION
Write true or false by each statement. Answers are at the end of this chapter. A score below 80% indicates the need for further study.

_____ 1. Changes in erythrocyte production may be manifested by fatigue, weakness and orthostatic hypotension.

_____ 2. Platelets are administered to increase erythrocytes.

_____ 3. Infection may be due to a reduction in white blood cells.

_____ 4. A reduction in platelets may lead to hemorrhage.

_____ 5. In providing nursing care for a patient with decreased platelets, medications should be administered by deep, intramuscular injection.

_____ 6. Fresh-frozen plasma contains all clotting factors, including platelets.

_____ 7. Salt-poor albumin is a volume expander.

_____ 8. Fever, chills and hives are complications of blood transfusions.

PASS
Program Assessment: Science and Situation

1. Plasma proteins are formed in the
   a. liver.
   b. spleen.
   c. intestines.
   d. kidneys.

2. Plasma proteins consist of
   a. hemocytoblasts, serotonin and mast cells.
   b. albumin, globulin and fibrinogen.
   c. platelets, lymph and hemoglobin.
   d. neutrophils, basophils and erythrocytes.

3. Regulation of fluid balance and intravascular volume is maintained by
   a. osmotic pressure.
   b. baroreceptors.
   c. filtration.
   d. diffusion.

4. Hematocrit represents the percentage of blood that is
   a. lymph.
   b. plasma.
   c. cells.
   d. b and c

5. Bone marrow production of red blood cells is called
   a. erythroblastosis.
   b. synthesis.
   c. erythropoiesis.
   d. mitosis.

6. The inner component of the erythrocyte is the
   a. stroma.
   b. marrow.
   c. cell body.
   d. glia.

7. Hemocytoblasts are formed by
   a. reticulocytes.
   b. normoblasts.
   c. basophil erythroblasts.
   d. stem cells.

8. Movement of the mature blood cell through the capillary membrane is termed
   a. osmosis.
   b. diapedesis.
   c. diffusion.
   d. hematopoiesis.

9. Maturation of RBCs requires
   a. vitamin B₁₂.
   b. vitamin K.
   c. vitamin C.
   d. hemoglobin.

10. Synthesis of hemoglobin is begun by the
    a. reticulocyte.
    b. normoblast.
    c. mast cells.
    d. basophil erythroblast.

11. The functional unit of the erythrocyte is
    a. cyanocobalamin.
    b. the stoma.
    c. hemoglobin.
    d. protein.

12. Excess iron is stored in the
    a. intestines.
    b. liver.
    c. spleen.
    d. bone marrow.

13. Defective absorption of iron from the intestines is called
    a. sprue.
    b. anemia.
    c. cold agglutination disease.
    d. thalassemia.

14. Erythropoiesis is stimulated by
    a. diapedesis.
    b. decreased hemoglobin.
    c. lowered oxygen tension.
    d. reticulocytosis.

15. Erythropoietin is a glycoprotein that acts on the bone marrow to stimulate
    a. erythroblastosis.
    b. diapedesis.
    c. phagocytosis.
    d. differentiation of stem cells and hemocytoblasts.

16. Sympathetic stimulation of the splenic smooth muscle
    a. releases stored blood.
    b. can raise HCT 3 to 4 percent.
    c. increases circulating volume.
    d. all of the above

17. Destruction of RBCs
    a. is called hemolysis.
    b. releases the cell stroma and hemoglobin.

    c. occurs with passage of fragile cells through the red pulp.
    d. all of the above

18. Hemoglobin and the cell stoma are ingested and returned to circulation for resynthesis by
    a. diapedesis.
    b. phagocytosis.
    c. reticuloendothelial cells.
    d. erythropoiesis.

19. The end product of hemolysis is
    a. thrombin.
    b. bilirubin.
    c. creatinine.
    d. hemoglobin.

20. Excessive bilirubin produces
    a. polycythemia.
    b. anemia.
    c. jaundice.
    d. hemolysis.

21. Granulocytes are formed in the
    a. lymph nodes.
    b. thymus.
    c. spleen.
    d. bone marrow.

22. Monocytes and lymphocytes are formed in the
    a. liver.
    b. bone marrow.
    c. spleen, thymus and lymph nodes.
    d. all of the above

23. Ingestion of bacteria or foreign substances is called
    a. phagocytosis.
    b. leukocytosis.
    c. hemolysis.
    d. erythropoiesis.

24. The movement of neutrophils toward a foreign substance is known as
    a. apsinigation.
    b. chemotaxis.
    c. phagocytosis.
    d. neutrophilia.

25. Chemotaxis is the attraction of phagocytes to the injured area through a chemotactic
    a. antibody.
    b. enzyme.
    c. erythrocyte.
    d. chemical.

26. Heparin is released by
    a. basophils.
    b. eosinophils.
    c. neutrophils.
    d. monocytes.

27. Bands seen in response to infection represent
    a. stem cells.
    b. mast cells.
    c. immature or juvenile neutrophils.
    d. reticulocytes.

28. Specific histocytes found in the liver sinuses that filter bacteria from the G.I. tract are
    a. Kupffer's cells.
    b. mast cells.
    c. neutrophils.
    d. opsins.

29. Lymphocytes
    a. originate in the bone marrow in the embryo.
    b. are preprocessed in the prenatal phase.
    c. migrate to lymphoid tissue.
    d. all of the above

30. *T* cells are
    a. lymphocytes.
    b. preprocessed in the thymus.
    c. involved in cellular immunity.
    d. all of the above

31. Successor cells of lymphocytes that produce specific antibodies are
    a. mast cells.
    b. plasma cells.
    c. stem cells.
    d. *T* cells.

32. Mediation of immunoglobins for humoral immunity is the function of
    a. *B* cells.
    b. *T* cells.
    c. stem cells.
    d. mast cells.

33. Antigen-antibody reaction promotes phagocytosis by enzymatic action of
    a. humoral immunity.
    b. *T* cells.
    c. the complement system.
    d. cellular immunity.

34. The primary function of the complement system is
    a. preprocessing of *T* cells.
    b. coagulation.

c. hemolysis.
d. alteration of the cell membrane.

35. Circulating gamma globulins (antibodies) produce
    a. cellular immunity.
    b. humoral immunity.
    c. complement system.
    d. hemolysis.

36. Synthesis of specific antibodies is accomplished by
    a. plasma cells.
    b. *B* lymphocytes.
    c. *T* lymphocytes.
    d. antigens.

37. The most predominant immunoglobin is
    a. IgM.
    b. IgG.
    c. IgE.
    d. IgD.

38. An allergy is due to a deficit of
    a. immunoglobins.
    b. antigens.
    c. *B* cells.
    d. *T* cells.

39. The chemical(s) released in a hypersensitive response is (are)
    a. histamine.
    b. serotonin.
    c. bradykinin.
    d. all of the above

40. Severe generalized vasodilation with hypotension and third-spacing fluids is
    a. autoimmunity.
    b. immune reaction.
    c. anaphylactic shock.
    d. Arthus's phenomenon.

41. An example of a localized phagocytosis with hemorrhagic necrosis is
    a. Arthus's phenomenon.
    b. an allergy.
    c. anaphylaxis.
    d. cytotropic reaction.

42. The body's inability to recognize self from nonself is the definition of
    a. Arthus's phenomenon.
    b. allergy.
    c. autoimmune disease.
    d. anaphylaxis

43. Blood grouping is based on
    a. agglutination of recipient cells by donor cells.
    b. agglutination of donor cells by recipient serum.
    c. agglutination of donor cells by recipient cells.
    d. agglutination of recipient cells by donor serum.

44. Erythroblastosis fetalis
    a. results from a sensitized antigen-antibody reaction.
    b. does not occur with the first pregnancy.
    c. causes hemolysis of red blood cells.
    d. all of the above

45. The basic mechanism of coagulation is the conversion of
    a. thrombin to fibrinogen.
    b. prothrombin to thrombin.
    c. thromboplastin to fibrinogen.
    d. fibrin to fibrinogen.

46. Vitamin K is required for the formation of
    a. thromboplastin.
    b. fibrin.
    c. prothrombin.
    d. thrombin.

47. Platelets are fragments of the precursor
    a. reticulocytes.
    b. hemocytoblasts.
    c. megakaryocytes.
    d. mast cells.

48. Heparin is continuously circulated by
    a. stem cells.
    b. factor VIII.
    c. megakaryocytes.
    d. basophilic mast cells.

49. Hereditary hemolytic anemias with unstable red cell membranes leading to destruction are
    a. thalassemia and sickle cell.
    b. spherocytosis and glucose-6-phosphate dehydrogenase.
    c. aplastic and thalassemia.
    d. sprue and aplastic.

50. Hereditary anemia with a defective hemoglobin molecule found predominantly in Blacks is
    a. sprue.
    b. thalassemia.
    c. spherocytosis.
    d. sickle cell.

51. Pernicious anemia results in
    a. demyelination of dorsal and lateral columns and peripheral nerves.

b. cardiomegaly.
   c. angina.
   d. jaundice.

52. Bone marrow dysfunction can be caused by
    a. isoniazid (INH).
    b. gentamycin.
    c. chloramphenicol.
    d. all of the above

53. Blast cells are commonly seen in
    a. polycythemia.
    b. aplastic anemia.
    c. thalassemia.
    d. leukemia.

54. Reticulocytosis is seen in
    a. agranulocytosis.
    b. polycythemia.
    c. sickle cell anemia.
    d. spherocytosis.

55. Disorderly proliferation of white blood cells is
    a. leukemia.
    b. anemia.
    c. thalassemia.
    d. agranulocytosis.

56. Acute and chronic leukemia are differentiated by
    a. rate of growth.
    b. number of cells present.
    c. predominance of immature or mature cells.
    d. response to treatment.

57. Blastic crisis converts
    a. chronic myelogenous leukemia to acute myelogenous leukemia.
    c. chronic lymphocytic leukemia to acute lymphocytic leukemia.
    c. acute myelogenous leukemia to myelogenous leukemia.
    d. a and b

58. Cranial radiation may be used for the following to reduce CNS involvement:
    a. acute myelogenous leukemia (AML)
    b. chronic lymphoblastic leukemia (CLL)
    c. acute lymphoblastic leukemia (ALL)
    d. chronic myelogenous leukemia (CML)

59. The most common leukemia to attack children is
    a. CLL.
    b. ALL.
    c. AML.
    d. CML.

60. The Philadelphia chromosome is present in 80 percent of
    a. ALL.
    b. AML.
    c. CML.
    d. CLL.

61. Total body radiation for leukemia may be used
    a. prior to bone marrow transplant.
    b. as an alternative to chemotherapy CLL.
    c. to treat CML.
    d. a and b

62. Lymphoma involving both sides of the diaphragm, but excluding the spleen, is classified as
    a. stage III.
    b. stage I.
    c. stage II.
    d. stage IV.

63. The most effective chemotherapeutic agent for lymphocytic lymphoma is
    a. vincristine.
    b. methotrexate.
    c. busulfan.
    d. cytosine arabinoside.

64. Coombs' test is used to determine
    a. number of mast cells.
    b. the effectiveness of RhoGAM.
    c. sensitivity.
    d. presence of IgG antibodies in an Rh negative person.

65. The immunoglobulin that responds first to an invasion of a foreign substance is
    a. IgA.
    b. IgG.
    c. IgM.
    d. IgE.

66. The immunoglobulin responsible for anaphylactic reaction is
    a. IgD.
    b. IgE.
    c. IgA.
    d. IgM.

67. The primary treatment of D/C is
    a. Amicar.
    b. heparin.
    c. transfusion.
    d. antibiotics.

68. Hypovolemia in anaphylactic shock is the result of
    a. third spacing of fluids.

    b. hemorrhage.
    c. inappropriate ADH.
    d. diuresis.

69. Replacement of platelets and fibrin in D/C would usually be by infusion of
    a. whole blood.
    b. packed cells.
    c. cryoprecipitate.
    d. albumin.

70. The greatest danger in immunosuppressed diseases is
    a. hemorrhage.
    b. infection.
    c. allergic reaction.
    d. none of the above

KEY POINT RECOGNITION ANSWERS

Blood
1. True
2. False—Blood carries oxygen and nutrients to cells.
3. True
4. False—The hematopoietic system is composed of blood-forming and blood-circulating organs.
5. True
6. True
7. False—The fluid component of blood is called plasma.
8. False—White blood cells are called leukocytes.
9. True
10. True
11. False—The normal hematocrit range in females is 37 to 47 percent, and in males, 40 to 54 percent.
12. True
13. False—Arterial blood is bright red in color.
14. True
15. False—The higher the oxygen saturation level found in hemoglobin, the brighter the color.
16. True
17. False—The normal specific gravity of blood is 1.048 to 1.066.
18. True
19. False—Normal pH is slightly alkaline
20. True
21. False—Blood is an extracellular fluid.
22. True
23. False—Normal blood volume is 5000 ml to 6000 ml, or 5 to 6 liters.
24. True
25. False—If circulating fluid is hypovolemic, receptors shrink and ADH is secreted to retain water.

Plasma
1. False—Plasma is composed of serum and plasma proteins.
2. True
3. True
4. True
5. True
6. False—More plasma proteins are found in the intravascular compartment.
7. False—Each end of the capillary bed has a different pressure gradient.
8. True
9. True
10. False—At the venous end, the blood pressure is lower than the osmotic pressure.

Blood-Forming Organs
1. True
2. True
3. True

4. False—Kupffer's cells filter and destroy bacteria.
5. True
6. True

Normal Red Blood Cell Production, Function and Destruction
1. False—Bone marrow is a soft tissue.
2. False—Bone marrow is found in long bones and in spaces between the trabeculae of cancellous bone.
3. True
4. False—Yellow bone marrow is mostly fat cells.
5. True
6. True
7. False—Erythrocytes are mature red blood cells.
8. True
9. True
10. False—The outer membrane covering of an erythrocyte is permeable to water, chloride, hydrogen and bicarbonate ions. It is semipermeable to sodium and potassium.
11. True
12. True
13. True
14. False—Cell division occurs in all of the maturational stages.
15. False—Stem cells form hemocytoblasts
16. True
17. True
18. True
19. False—Vitamin B_{12} is stored in the liver.
20. True
21. True
22. True
23. False—Four heme molecules combine with globin to form hemoglobin.
24. False—The normal range for hemoglobin in the female is 14 to 18 gm/100 ml of blood.
25. True
26. True
27. False—Excess iron is stored in the liver as ferritin.

Normal White Blood Cell Production and Function
1. False—Neutrophils, eosinophils and basophils are known as granulocytes.
2. False—Neutrophils are formed in the bone marrow.
3. True
4. True
5. True
6. False—Lymphocytes
7. False—*T* cells
8. False—Plasma cells are responsible for specific antibodies. *B* cells = humoral immunity.

The Inflammatory Process
1. False—Pain, heat, redness, swelling and loss of function

2. True
3. False—Leukocytosis occurs in the inflammatory process.
4. True
5. False—Neutrophils and macrophages engulf, and lysosomal enzymes digest, the bacteria.

Immunity
1. False—T cells
2. True
3. False—Macrophages are attracted to the area.
4. False—It invades the cell membrane of the antigen.
5. True
6. True
7. False—IgM
8. True
9. True
10. True
11. False—This is a cytolytic immune response. An example is transfusion reaction.
12. True
13. True
14. True

Blood Groups
1. False—AB = universal recipient
2. True
3. True
4. True
5. False—AB has no plasma antibodies.
6. True
7. True
8. True
9. True

Hemostasis
1. True
2. True
3. True
4. False—By prothrombin activator and calcium
5. False—Thrombin converts fibrinogen to fibrin.
6. False—Vitamin K is necessary for formation of prothrombin.
7. False—Calcium
8. True
9. False—Heparin prevents clotting.
10. True

Assessment of the Hematopoietic System
1. True
2. True
3. True
4. False—Hepatomegaly is evaluated by percussion.

5. False—Sternal tenderness is an indicator of a hematopoietic problem.
6. True
7. False—Vital signs may be normal.
8. True
9. True
10. True
11. False—Infection is usually found on the skin, in the throat or in the respiratory and urinary tracts.
12. True
13. True
14. False—Hematocrit is decreased in anemia and hemorrhage.
15. False—A decrease in mean corpuscular hemoglobin concentration indicates hypochromic anemia.
16. False—Reticulocytes decrease in conditions suppressing bone marrow production.
17. False—Hemoconcentration causes an increase in the platelet count.
18. True
19. True
20. False—The normal partial thromboplastin time is 20 to 45 seconds.

Pathological States and Nursing Management
1. True
2. True
3. True
4. True
5. False—Hemoglobinopathy is a hereditary defect.
6. True
7. False—Aplastic anemia may be due to chemical toxins and radiation, and in some cases the etiology is unknown.
8. False—Clinical presentation varies, as do laboratory results.
9. True
10. True
11. True
12. False—Leukemia may involve the kidneys, nervous system, bone and skin.
13. True
14. True
15. True
16. True
17. True
18. False—Elevated BUN and decreased clotting factors may be indicative of leukemia.
19. True
20. False—Chronic lymphocytic leukemia rarely occurs before 40.
21. True
22. False—All nodes may be involved.
23. True
24. True
25. True
26. True
27. True

28. True
29. True
30. True
31. True
32. True
33. True
34. False—DIC is characterized by free thrombin and aggregation of platelets.
35. True
36. False—Purpura of the chest and abdomen is the first sign of DIC.
37. True
38. False—The prothrombin time is normal in hemophilia.
39. True
40. True
41. True
42. True
43. True
44. False—Sickle cell disease may cause the blood's pH to be acidotic.
45. True
46. True
47. False—Sickle cell disease is seen in children under two years of age.
48. False—Hemolytic crisis is a rapid decrease in the hematocrit level.
49. True
50. True
51. True

Care Common to Hematopoietic Problems
1. True
2. False—Red blood cells are administered to increase erythrocytes.
3. True
4. True
5. False—Parenteral medications should be given intravenously.
6. False—Platelets are not included.
7. True
8. True

PASS ANSWER SHEET

1. a
2. b
3. a
4. c
5. c
6. a
7. d
8. b
9. a
10. d
11. c
12. b
13. a
14. c
15. d
16. d
17. d
18. c
19. b
20. c
21. d
22. c
23. a
24. b
25. d
26. a
27. c
28. a
29. d
30. d
31. b
32. a
33. c
34. d
35. b
36. a
37. b
38. a
39. d
40. c
41. a
42. c
43. b
44. d
45. b
46. c
47. c
48. d
49. b
50. d
51. a
52. c
53. d
54. b
55. a
56. c
57. a
58. c
59. b
60. c
61. d
62. a
63. a
64. d
65. c
66. b
67. b
68. a
69. c
70. b

SURVEY SUMMARY
HEMATOPOIETIC SYSTEM

I. **The Hematopoietic System: Overview**
   A. Blood is a sticky substance that carries oxygen and nutrients; helps maintain electrolyte balance; assists in heat regulation; and serves as a defense against infection.
   B. *Blood-forming* organs consist of the:
      1. Bone marrow
      2. Liver
      3. Spleen
      4. Lymph nodes
      5. Thymus
   C. *Blood-circulating* organs consist of the:
      1. Heart
      2. Blood vessels

II. **Anatomy and Physiology**
   A. *Blood*
      1. The *components* of blood are *solid* substances consisting of erythrocytes, leukocytes and platelets, and a *fluid* substance, plasma.
      2. The *color* of blood is dependent upon the oxygen saturation level of the hemoglobin.
      3. *Specific gravity* ranges between 1.048 and 1.066.
      4. The *blood buffer system* is composed of:
         a. Carbonic acids
         b. Carbonates
         c. Bicarbonates
         d. Proteins
         e. Phosphates
      5. The *functions* of blood are to:
         a. Transport oxygen and nutrients to the cells
         b. Maintain fluid and electrolyte balance
         c. Aid in temperature regulation
         d. Aid in the defense against infection
      6. *Blood volume* is normally 5 to 6 liters.
         a. Forty percent of the blood is found in the venous system.
         b. Blood volume is controlled by ADH secreted by the posterior pituitary.
   B. *Plasma*
      1. The *components* of plasma are serum and plasma proteins, which are albumin, serum, globulins, fibrinogen, plasminogen and prothrombin.
      2. The *functions* of plasma are to carry food, antibiotics, hormones, vitamins and minerals to the cells, and to remove waste products from the cells.
      3. *Volume control* is maintained by osmotic pressure.
   C. *Blood-forming organs*
      1. *Bone marrow* is the soft tissue of the bone.
         a. Yellow marrow is predominantly fat cells.
         b. Red marrow is concerned with *hematopoiesis.*

2. The *liver* has hematologic functions.
   a. It synthesizes clotting factors.
   b. Kupffer's cells filter out bacteria.
   c. Bile pigments are excreted.
3. The *spleen* acts as a reservoir for RBCs, and contains lymphoid elements.

D. **Normal red blood cell production, function and destruction**
   1. *Bone marrow*
      a. It is found in both long bones and cancellous bone.
      b. Marrow is of two types:
         1. *Red* marrow is concerned with red blood cell production.
         2. *Yellow* marrow is mainly fat cells.
   2. *Erythrocytes* are mature red cells.
      a. They are formed by the process of *erythropoiesis.*
      b. Their cellular structure includes an outer membrane and *stroma.*
      c. Red blood cell development begins with *primordial stem* cells.
      d. Stem cells form hemocytoblasts.
      e. Hemocytoblasts form *basophil erythroblasts.*
      f. *Diapedesis* is the process by which the mature cell, the erythrocyte, moves through the capillary membrane into the blood stream.
      g. *Cyanocobalamin* (vitamin B_{12}) is stored in the liver and released for RBC maturation.
   3. *Hemoglobin* is the functional unit of the erythrocyte.
      a. Normal hemoglobin is 12 to 16 gm/100 ml in the female, and 14 to 18 gm/100 ml in the male.
      b. Oxygen combines with hemoglobin to form oxyhemoglobin.
   4. A lowered oxygen tension stimulates the release of erythropoietin.
   5. *Hemolysis* is the destruction of RBCs.
      a. The normal RBC life span is 120 days.
      b. Bilirubin is the end product of the heme molecule.
      c. Red cells can be destroyed other than physiologically.
      d. Excessive destruction of RBCs results in a jaundiced condition.

E. **Normal white blood cell production and function**
   1. There are five major types of *leukocytes:*
      a. Neutrophils
      b. Eosinophils
      c. Basophils
      d. Monocytes
      e. Lymphocytes
   2. *Neutrophils, eosinophils* and *basophils* are formed in the blood marrow.
   3. *Lymphocytes* and *monocytes* are produced in the lymphoid tissues of the spleen, thymus and lymph nodes.
   4. Each plays a role in protecting the body by either the process of *phagocytosis* or *immune body formation.*
   5. *Lymphocytes* differentiate into *T* and *B* cells.
      a. *T* cells provide tissue immunity.
      b. *B* cells provide humoral immunity.

6. **Plasma cells** are differentiated successors of lymphocytes that produce specific antibodies.

F. **Inflammatory process**
   1. The **signs** and **symptoms** of inflammation include:
      a. Pain
      b. Heat
      c. Erythema
      d. Swelling
      e. Loss of function
   2. The **inflammatory process** includes the release of histamine, vascular dilatation, increased capillary permeability and exudation of fluid into the interstitial spaces.
   3. The body's response is **phagocytic.**

G. **Immunity** is the ability of the body to defend itself against foreign organisms or toxins.
   1. **Cellular immunity** is important in foreign tissue grafts, autoimmune processes, cancer and some allergies. *T* cells are involved in cellular immunity.
   2. The **complement system** potentiates the phagocytic action.
   3. **Humoral immunity** is due to circulating antibodies as a result of differentiated *B* cells.
      a. There are five classes of immunoglobulins:
         1. IgG
         2. IgA
         3. IgM
         4. IgD
         5. IgE
      b. Allergies result from an immunoglobulin deficit.
   4. Alterations in immunologic response include **hypersensitivity,** which can be induced by a genetic predisposition coupled with an external factor or by prior sensitization. It may be immediate or delayed.

H. The **blood groups** are divided into two systems: ABO and Rh.
   1. The ABO system is composed of O, A, B and AB, and is based on the presence or absence of antibodies and antigens in the blood.
   2. **Agglutination** is a tool for cross-matching blood.
   3. The Rh factor can be either positive or negative.
      a. Transfusion of Rh positive blood to an Rh positive patient can result in hemotysis.
      b. The **Coombs test** is used to determine the presence of Rh antibodies in an Rh negative patient.

I. **Hemostasis** involves **vasoconstriction, coagulation** and **clot contraction.**
   1. Arterioles and capillaries constrict, aided by serotonin. Platelets aggregate.
   2. **Coagulation** is initiated by either the **intrinsic** or **extrinsic** pathway.
      a. **Prothrombin** is converted to **thrombin.**
      b. **Thrombin** converts **fibrinogen** to **fibrin.**
      c. **Fibrin threads** make a network of RBCs and plasma.
   3. The **clot** is a meshwork of fibrin threads and begins to retract soon after formation.

4. *Factor III* removes thrombin from the blood, blocking thrombin's effect on fibrinogen.

III. **Physical Assessment of the Hematopoietic System should include:**
   A. *Assessment of history*
      1. Family
      2. Medical
      3. Medications
   B. General Signs and Symptoms
      1. Level of consciousness
      2. Fatigue
      3. Weakness
      4. Weight loss
      5. Fever
      6. Malaise
   C. Specific Signs and Symptoms
      1. Involvement of skin
      2. Visual disturbances
      3. Gastrointestinal disturbances
      4. Skeletal impairment
      5. Cardiorespiratory changes
      6. Genitourinary problems
   D. Physical examination
      1. Inspection
      2. Palpation
      3. Percussion
      4. Auscultation

IV. **Hematopoietic Nursing Assessment includes evaluating:**
   A. For *level* of *consciousness*
   B. Subjective and objective findings
   C. Laboratory and radiologic studies:
      1. Blood
      2. Urine
      3. X-ray
      4. Radionuclide scan
      5. Lymphangiography
   D. Vital signs

V. **Pathological States and Nursing Management**
   A. *Anemia*
      1. Types
         a. Aplastic
         b. Hemolytic
      2. The patient may present with:
         a. Pallor
         b. Cyanosis
         c. Tachycardia
         d. Vertigo
         e. Tenderness

3. Bone marrow is the best diagnostic aid.
4. Nursing care includes:
   a. Watch for infection.
   b. Maintain fluid and electrolyte balance.
   c. Watch for bleeding.
   d. Reverse isolation.
   e. Provide meticulous skin and mouth care.
   f. Conserve energy.

B. **Leukemia**
   1. Leukemia is a neoplastic disease with disorderly proliferation of white blood cells.
   2. The patient presents with:
      a. Hepatomegaly
      b. Splenomegaly
      c. Fatigue
      d. Bone pain
      e. Fever
   3. Diagnostic data includes blood and bone analysis.
   4. Nursing care includes:
      a. Provide patient education.
      b. Observe for and prevent infection.
      c. Monitor WBC.
      d. Prevent complications.

C. **Lymphomas** are divided into Hodgkin's disease and non-Hodgkin's disease.
   1. Hodgkin's disease is a histocytic lymphoma, beginning with painless enlargement of lymph nodes.
   2. Diagnostic data is made by excision of a node and pathological examination for presence of Sternberg-Reed cells.
   3. Nursing care includes developing a realistic approach to the illness.
      a. Provide patient education.
      b. Provide emotional support.
      c. Prevent complications.
      d. Provide meticulous skin and mouth care during radiotherapy.
   4. Non-Hodgkin's disease
      a. The clinical picture similar to Hodgkin's disease.
      b. Diagnostic data are similar to Hodgkin's disease.
      c. Nursing care is the same as for Hodgkin's disease.

D. **Polycythemia**
   1. Polycythemia is caused by an overabundance in the production of RBCs.
   2. The patient may present with:
      a. Bleeding
      b. Headache
      c. Pruritis
      d. Dyspnea
   3. Red blood cell count is the best diagnostic aid.
   4. Nursing care includes:
      a. Perform phlebotomy.
      b. Administer drugs.

c. Monitor diet.
d. Provide emotional support.
e. Prevent infection.

E. *Anaphylaxis*
1. Anaphylaxis is a severe hypersensitivity occurring shortly after the introduction of the antigenic agent.
2. The patient may present with:
   a. Dyspnea
   b. Cyanosis
   c. Convulsions
   d. Hives
   e. Respiratory distress
3. Diagnostic data are by physical findings.
4. Nursing care includes:
   a. Perform basic life support.
   b. Perform advanced life support.

F. *Disseminated Intravascular Coagulation*
1. DIC is a complication as a result of a severe injury or trauma.
2. The patient may present with:
   a. Hemorrhage
   b. Purpura
3. Laboratory studies are the best diagnostic aid.
   a. Thrombocytopenin
   b. Prolonged PT, and PIT
4. Nursing care includes:
   a. Maintain an adequate airway and circulation.
   b. Monitor vital signs.
   c. Maintain fluid and electrolyte balance.
   d. Prevent complications.
   e. Prevent hemorrhaging.

G. *Hemophilia*
1. Hemophilia is a hereditary coagulation disease.
2. The male patient may present with:
   a. Hemoptysis
   b. Melena
   c. Epistaxis
   d. Hematuria
3. Serum assay for factors VIII and IX is the best diagnostic aid.
4. Nursing care includes:
   a. Prevent bleeding.
   b. Prevent deformities.
   c. Maintain fluid and electrolyte balance.
   d. Provide emotional support.

H. *Sickle cell disease*
1. Sickle cell disease is a congenital hemolytic anemia.
2. The patient may present with:
   a. Pain in joints and abdomen.
   b. Swelling of hands and feet.
   c. Mitral stenosis.

3. The definitive diagnosis is made by laboratory studies.
   a. Sickle cell prep
   b. Sickledex
4. Nursing care includes:
   a. Maintain adequate hydration.
   b. Maintain fluid and electrolyte balance.
   c. Prevent deformities.
   d. Prevent infection.

I. *Multiple myeloma*
1. Multiple myeloma is a plasma cell dyscrasia.
2. The patient may present with:
   a. Weakness
   b. Skeletal pain
   c. Hemorrhage
   d. Renal failure
   e. Lethargy
   f. Weight loss
3. Laboratory studies are the best diagnostic aid.
   a. Elevated ESR
   b. Hypercalcemia
   c. Elevated creatinine
4. Nursing care includes:
   a. Maintain fluid and electrolyte balance.
   b. Control pain.
   c. Maintain mobilization.

VI. **Care Common to Hematopoietic Problems**
   A. Reduced erythrocytes, observe for:
      1. Fatigue
      2. Weakness
      3. Hypotension
   B. Reduced white blood cells, observe for:
      1. Infection
      2. Fever
      3. Pulmonary infiltrates
      4. Chest pain
   C. Decreased platelet function, observe for:
      1. Hemorrhage
      2. CNA
      3. Ulcerations
   D. Administration of blood
      1. Reactions
      2. Complications

CHAPTER TEN
HOW TO PREPARE FOR
and
TAKE AN EXAMINATION

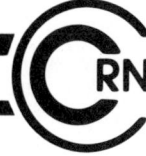

HOW TO PREPARE FOR AND TAKE AN EXAMINATION

WHY TAKE THE EXAMINATION?

The CCRN examination measures the minimum critical care nursing competency designated by nursing standards and guidelines. Subjects tested include anatomy, physiology, pathophysiology and nursing care. The CCRN examination not only reflects your core knowledge, but also that of others practicing in the critical care nursing field. Testing becomes a tool with which to measure competency and maintain minimum standards within critical care nursing. A growing number of hospitals require certification for employment in the critical care department. Salary scales are also linked to the successful completion of the certification process.

THE CCRN EXAMINATION

The four-hour examination comprises 250 multiple choice questions. Subject areas include the cardiovascular, pulmonary, renal, metabolic, hematopoietic and gastrointestinal systems, and the psychosocial aspects of critical care nursing. The number of test items for each subject area appears to be evenly distributed. Each examination contains some experimental questions that will be used on future tests. These questions are not counted in your score.

Dress comfortably and layer your clothing. It is easy to remove or put on a jacket or sweater, depending on temperature changes.

Carefully read all instructions for testing needs, such as pencils, admission tickets, identification and a watch. Organize all materials the night before the examination. If possible, plan your route to avoid heavy traffic.

Arrive early enough on the examination day to park, locate the site and refresh yourself before testing begins. Leave all review books and outlines at home. Reviewing just prior to the examination will only heighten your anxiety level.

When the testing site opens, find a seat, prepare your materials and relax. Once the examination begins, work as rapidly and carefully as possible. You probably will not be able to correctly answer all the questions. All questions count equally toward your score. Use this knowledge to your advantage. Progress at a consistent rate. Do not spend an unreasonable amount of time on one difficult question; return to it later. You have approximately one minute for each question. You must complete 60 questions per hour to finish within the time limits. Check the time and maintain a steady pace.

PHYSICAL CHANGES RELATED TO THE STRESS OF TEST-TAKING

Testing is a measure of competency. Therefore, the words *test* or *examination* cause both physical and emotional changes in the individual to be tested. The emotions evoked often result in *stress* and *anxiety*.

The body reacts to stress and anxiety with defense or coping mechanisms. Physiologically, the general adaptation system (also called fight or flight) becomes dominant, with the sympathetic nervous system overriding the parasympathetic division. Norepinephrine is secreted, causing blood pressure to increase. Epinephrine is secreted and the central nervous system is activated, resulting in increased cardiac output, increased oxygen exchange and dilated pupils, which enhances vision. The release of ACTH contributes to higher energy levels.

The physiological responses to stress and anxiety may have a positive or negative effect, depending on an individual's ability to harness stress levels. In moderate amounts, stress and anxiety can increase concentration and mobilize energy, thereby benefiting the test-taker. However, high levels of stress can cripple the test-taker by increasing anxiety levels and decreasing concentration. Energy is not productively harnessed, and energy reserves are depleted. Therefore, the test-taker must be aware of individual tolerance levels in order to put the body's general adaptation system to efficient use. This awareness begins by properly preparing for an examination.

EXAMINATION PREPARATION

To successfully take an examination, you must organize your efforts.

Begin studying early so that your normal work and sleep habits are not interrupted. Normal, unhurried schedules help lessen anxiety and stress. Develop a written timetable that includes all of the material to be covered, daily study times, self-testing and a review of unmastered material.

More specifically, review the contents of CRITICAL CARE REVIEW FOR NURSES to formulate an overall picture. Decide what areas will require additional study. Read the summary outlines *daily*. Use them to place concepts and facts in perspective, then study a specific part of the outline in depth.

Maintain an established study routine that includes scheduled breaks for both exercise and nourishment. Stand and stretch for five minutes every hour.

The day before the examination should be used for review and relaxation. If you have used your study time wisely, you know the material; and if not, it is too late. Eat well, relax and get a good night's sleep.

Begin the examination day with a well-balanced meal. Studying on the morning of the examination will only increase anxiety and tend to make you question your knowledge base.

Upon your arrival at the examination site, do not panic. Do not allow yourself to be drawn into the pre-examination paranoia of frenzied colleagues. Remember the confidence you have developed from the past study periods.

Be sure to carefully read the directions. Skipping or misreading important directions could cost you points. Quickly skim the test and plan your time accordingly. Ask yourself: How many questions are there? How much time can I spend on each question? Check the time, set your watch on the desk top and begin the test.

Read or skim each question. Eyeball key terms or important words and phrases. If possible, supply the correct answer before reading the choices. Select the correct answer, but do not mark the answer sheet. Now actively read the question. Underline or mark key words and phrases. Ask yourself what the test item wants and mark the best answer.

If you cannot answer a question, remain calm. Take a deep breath and use common sense. Since you will not be penalized for guessing, guess. Enhance your chances by eliminating the answers that you know are incorrect. Do not spend too much time on difficult questions. You may want to skip difficult questions and come back to them later. But at least make a guess before finishing the examination.

After completing the test, return to the first question and review your answers. Think very carefully before changing an answer. Your first response is usually the best or correct response. Check the answer sheet for stray marks, incorrect placement of answers and blanks.

Do not second-guess yourself or participate in test postmortems. Forget it until the results arrive.

KEY CONCEPT:
- Provide ample review time
- Assess the test situation
- Survey the answer sheet
- Stay calm and wait for the results

CHAPTER ELEVEN
PRACTICE EXAMINATION

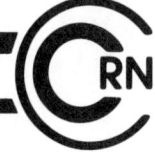

PRACTICE EXAMINATION

This practice examination contains 250 questions. It is similar in format to the actual exam, and is designed to give you practical experience before you actually take the AACN examination.

You should take this exam under simulated testing conditions. Upon completion, immediately identify the content areas requiring additional study, and refer to the appropriate sections in the text. When you feel that you have mastered these content areas, take this practice examination again.

It might be advantageous to wait several days before retaking the examination. Repeating the practice examination several days before the certifying examination is also recommended.

Answers to the practice examination questions are on page 667.

1. Anxiety is
    a. common among critically ill patients.
    b. always a result of threat from environment.
    c. always maladaptive.
    d. all of the above

2. The action of vasopressin is to
    a. increase portal venous pressure by constricting the splanchnic vein.
    b. decrease portal venous pressure by constricting the splanchnic vein.
    c. increase portal venous pressure by dilating the splanchnic vein.
    d. decrease portal venous pressure by dilating the splanchnic vein.

3. The three cranial nerves responsible for eye movement are the
    a. trochlear, accessory and optic nerves.
    b. oculomotor, trochlear and abducens nerves.
    c. optic, oculomotor and trochlear nerves.
    d. optic, trigeminal and facial nerves.

4. Diabetes insipidus is characterized by:
    (1) dilute urine up to 15 to 29 liters per day
    (2) increased ADH level as a causative factor
    (3) a negative history of diabetes mellitus or renal disease
    a. 1, 2, 3
    b. 1, 3
    c. 1
    d. 2, 3

5. The pathology of gastric ulcers seems to be
    a. an increased acid-pepsin secretion.
    b. a breakdown in the defense barrier of the mucosa.
    c. an increased amount of fundic cells.
    d. a decreased amount of Brunner's cells.

6. A lesion affecting the right optic tracts will result in
    a. left homonymous hemianopsia.
    b. bitemporal hemianopsia.
    c. right homonymous hemianopsia.
    d. right monocular blindness.

7. The four functions of the kidney are:
   (1) fluid balance
   (2) electrolyte balance
   (3) acid-base balance
   (4) metabolic waste excretion
   (5) regulation of salt intake
   (6) regulation of intra-arterial temperature
   a. 1, 3, 4, 5
   b. 2, 3, 4, 5
   c. 3, 4, 5, 6
   d. 1, 2, 3, 4

8. Increased levels of PEEP in a hemodynamically unstable patient may
   a. decrease cardiac output
   b. increase preload.
   c. decrease blood pressure.
   d. all of the above

9. The patient with a duodenal ulcer typically has an increased secretion of acid and pepsin caused by a(n)
   a. increase in the amount of parietal cells in the gastric mucosa.
   b. increase in the amount of acid secreted by the parietal cells.
   c. decreased amount of stimulation needed by the parietal cells to secrete acid.
   d. all of the above

10. An allergy is due to a deficit of
    a. immunoglobins.
    b. antigens.
    c. B cells.
    d. T cells.

11. Nursing care for the patient with a Sengstaken-Blakemore tube includes
    a. continuous nasogastric suction.
    b. intermittent inflation and deflation of the gastric balloon.
    c. maintenance of correct inflation pressures in the gastric and esophageal balloons with traction applied to the tube to prevent descent into the stomach.
    d. continuous iced saline lavage.

12. The cause of acute tubular necrosis is
    a. gangrene of the kidney.
    b. total absence of urine output.
    c. fluid overload.
    d. reduced renal perfusion.

13. The most significant symptom of peptic ulcer disease is
    a. gastrointestinal bleeding.
    b. abdominal cramping.
    c. episodic abdominal pain.
    d. nausea and vomiting.

14. Mr. Jones, a successful banker, enters the coronary care unit with acute myocardial infarction. He does not stay in bed or use his light to ask for help. The nurse should recognize that he feels threatened because of
    a. loss of job.
    b. loss of self-respect.
    c. isolation from family.
    d. his dependency.

15. Three ways in which the kidney influences acid-base balance are:
    (1) reabsorption of bicarbonate
    (2) acidification of phosphate salts
    (3) secretion of ammonia
    (4) maintenance of urine pH at 5.5 to 6.5
    a. 1, 2, 3, 4
    b. 1, 3, 4
    c. 1, 2, 4
    d. 1, 2, 3

16. A patient's perception of his illness may be altered by
    a. past experiences.
    b. family experiences.
    c. no experience.
    d. all of the above

17. Blood grouping is based on
    a. agglutination of recipient cells by donor cells.
    b. agglutination of donor cells by recipient serum.
    c. agglutination of donor cells by recipient cells.
    d. agglutination of recipient cells by donor serum.

18. To allay the apprehension of the critically ill patient, you should
    a. always assign the same nurse to care for the patient when possible.
    b. assign different nurses to care for the patient.
    c. inform the patient this is your first day in the unit.
    d. answer the patient's question with a question.

19. Homeostasis is
    a. equilibrium between physiological and emotional changes.
    b. equilibrium between physiological and environmental changes.
    c. none of the above
    d. a and b

20. The recommended procedure for the infusion of a vasopressin drip is to
    a. start the infusion at 0.6 units per minute and titrate the dosage to stop the bleeding.
    b. start the infusion at 0.3 units per minute and observe for 30 minutes; if bleeding continues, titrate the dose to a maximum of 0.8 units per minute every 30 minutes.
    c. start the infusion at 0.8 units per minute for two hours; if bleeding continues, notify the physician.
    d. start infusion at 0.1 unit per minute and observe for two hours; if bleeding continues, notify the physician.

21. Depression is an indicator that
    a. the patient is denying his problem.
    b. the patient has a personal grudge with the physicians and nurses.
    c. the patient has begun to realize his problems.
    d. the patient has not realized his problem.

22. The body's inability to recognize self from nonself is the definition of
    a. Arthus phenomenon.
    b. allergy.
    c. autoimmune disease.
    d. anaphylaxis.

23. The function of the loop of Henle is:
    (1) reabsorption of sodium
    (2) reabsorption of water
    (3) reabsorption of H^+ ion
    (4) reabsorption of chloride
    a. 1, 2
    b. 1, 2, 3, 4
    c. 1, 4
    d. 3, 4

24. Which of the following is true concerning production of cerebrospinal fluid?
    a. 150 cc per day are produced and there are approximately 500 cc in the system at any time.
    b. Cerebrospinal fluid is produced by the arachnoid granules and reabsorbed by the choroid plexus.
    c. At any given time, there is approximately four times as much cerebrospinal fluid in the ventricles as in the lumbar subarachnoid space.
    d. 500 cc per day are produced and there are approximately 150 cc in the system at any time.

25. Mr. Jones has been in the critical care unit for three days. He is on hourly vital signs and neurological checks. He is beginning to show behavioral changes. You suspect this may be due to
    a. sensory overload.
    b. sensory deprivation.
    c. sleep deprivation.
    d. all of the above

26. An example of a localized phagocytosis with hemorrhagic necrosis is
    a. the Arthus phenomenon.
    b. an allergy.
    c. anaphylaxis.
    d. cytotropic reaction.

27. The spinal nerves exit in such a manner that there are
    a. 8 cervical, 13 thoracic and 6 lumbar nerves.
    b. 6 cervical, 11 thoracic and 4 lumbar nerves.
    c. 8 cervical, 12 thoracic and 5 lumbar nerves.
    d. 6 cervical, 13 thoracic and 5 lumbar nerves.

28. The most important factor in alleviating a patient's anxiety is
    a. the nurse who provides limited information concerning hospitalization.
    b. the nurse who provides factual information.
    c. the nurse who provides explanations which are brief and factual.
    d. having the physician visit daily.

29. All of the following may be factors in ulcer formation, *except*
    a. increased autonomic stimulation.
    b. endogenous and/or exogenous cortisones.
    c. glucocorticoids.
    d. an increased number of Brunner's glands.

30. The Cushing triad is
    a. decreased blood pressure, increased heart rate and pupillary changes.
    b. increased pulse pressure, decreased heart rate and respiratory irregularities.
    c. decreased pulse pressure, decreased heart rate and respiratory irregularities.
    d. increased pulse pressure, increased heart rate and Cheyne-Stokes respirations.

31. Impairment of the right cranial nerve XII will result in
    a. the tongue deviating to the right.
    b. the tongue deviating to the left.
    c. an inability to move the tongue from the midline.
    d. an inability to move the neck to the right.

32. The formation of an acute stress ulcer
    a. has the same pathology as peptic ulcers.
    b. involves the deep musculature of the stomach.
    c. is thought to be caused by ischemia.
    d. occurs mostly in neurosurgical patients.

33. At what age does a child develop a concept of body image?
    a. 6 to 8 months
    b. one year
    c. 14 to 18 months
    d. over 2 years

34. Severe generalized vasodilation with hypotension and third spacing of fluids is:
    a. autoimmunity.
    b. immune reaction.
    c. anaphylactic shock.
    d. Arthus phenomenon.

35. The four most common abnormal blood chemistry findings in renal failure are
    a. Na,↑↑K,↑BUN and ↓creatine.
    b. Na,↓↓K,↓BUN and ↑creatine
    c. Na,↓↑K,↑BUN and ↑creatine
    d. Na,↑↑K,↑BUN and ↑creatine

36. The cristi galli and cribriform plate are parts of the
    a. sphenoid bone.
    b. sella turcica.
    c. petrous ridges.
    d. ethmoid bone.

37. In Maslow's hierarchy of needs, which of the following statements are not correct?
    (1) Physiological needs are our basic needs and can be obtained with a paycheck.
    (2) It is important to meet each level of need.
    (3) Needs are always fully achieved.
    (4) Meeting one's physiological needs is not important.
    a. 1, 3, 4
    b. 2, 3, 4
    c. 1, 2, 4
    d. 1, 2, 3

38. Myasthenic crisis may be differentiated from cholinergic crisis by which of the following tests?
    a. measurement of vital capacity
    b. small doses of edrophonium chloride
    c. asking the patient to smile, raise the eyebrows and show the teeth
    d. arterial blood gases

39. Treatment for hyperkalemia includes:
    (1) increasing K intake
    (2) insulin, glucose and sodium bicarbonate I.V.
    (3) hemodialysis or peritoneal dialysis
    (4) kayexalate resin exchange by mouth or rectally
    a. 1, 2, 3
    b. 1, 2, 4
    c. 1, 3, 4
    d. 2, 3, 4

40. The chemical released in a hypersensitive response is
    a. histamine.
    b. serotonin.
    c. bradykinin.
    d. none of the above

41. A patient informs you that he is going to die and starts to cry. His diagnosis is terminal cancer. As a nurse, you should
    a. inform him that is is wrong.
    b. tell him not to think about dying.
    c. hold his hand.
    d. leave him alone.

42. The treatment for diabetes insipidus includes:
    (1) replacing water loss, preventing dehydration, preventing hypovolemic shock
    (2) replacing water loss with vasopressin therapy
    (3) replacing water loss with isotonic saline or protein solutions
    (4) correcting intracranial condition
     a. 1, 2, 3, 4
     b. 1, 2, 3
     c. 3, 4
     d. 1, 2, 4

43. Oliguria is defined as a urine output of less than
     a. 400 to 500 cc per day.
     b. 600 to 700 cc per day.
     c. 700 to 800 cc per day.
     d. 800 to 900 cc per day.

44. Characteristics of the adrenocorticotropic hormone include:
    (1) It is secreted by the anterior pituitary.
    (2) The target organ is the adrenal medulla.
    (3) It stimulates the adrenal cortex to increase its secretion of mineral corticoids and glucocorticoids.
    (4) It decreases production level in the presence of Addison's disease.
     a. 1, 2
     b. 3, 4
     c. 2, 3
     d. 1, 3, 4

45. All three ego states, adult, parent and child, exist in all people. These states are referred to as
     a. concepts of the superego, ego and id.
     b. psychological realities.
     c. Maslow's hierarchy of needs.
     d. none of the above

46. The patient with frontal lobe dysfunction may exhibit the following signs and symptoms:
     a. speech and sensation dysfunction
     b. vision and motor movement impairment
     c. motor and mentation impairment
     d. memory loss and mentation impairment

47. The first line of treatment for the patient with gastrointestinal bleeding is
     a. to find the source of bleeding.
     b. to correct electrolyte imbalance.
     c. to prevent and treat shock.
     d. to perform selective angiography.

48. Erythroblastosis fetalis
     a. results from a sensitized antigen-antibody reaction.
     b. does not occur with the first pregnancy.
     c. causes hemolysis of red blood cells.
     d. all of the above

49. Signs and symptoms of renal insufficiency include
    a. anemia.
    b. extracellular edema and anemia.
    c. metabolic acidosis and anemia.
    d. hyperkalemia and metabolic acidosis.

50. The most frequently associated findings in acute pancreatitis are:
    a. steroids and biliary tract disease.
    b. trauma and steroids.
    c. alcohol and biliary tract disease.
    d. alcohol and dyazide diuretics.

51. The effect of too much parathyroid hormone can be manifested by
    a. demineralization of bones.
    b. decreased renal phosphate excretion.
    c. hypocalcemia.
    d. a and b

52. Postrenal failure is caused by
    a. obstruction in ureters and strictures of the urethera.
    b. transfusion reaction.
    c. acute tubular necrosis.
    d. renal artery thrombosis.

53. Associated symptoms of acute pancreatitis include all of the following *except*
    a. severe pain over the entire abdomen with radiation to the back
    b. nausea and vomiting
    c. abdominal distention
    d. febrile state above 102° F

54. The hypothalamus is instrumental in the metabolic system by
    a. producing oxytocin and antidiuretic hormone, and storing the hormones in the posterior pituitary.
    b. monitoring hormone levels in the body.
    c. controlling hormone secretion in the pituitary gland.
    d. all of the above

55. The patient with acute pancreatitis will usually have the following lab data *except:*
    a. elevated serum amylase
    b. elevated direct bilirubin
    c. elevated calcium
    d. decreased serum albumin

56. The single most important indicator of neurologic status is
    a. pupillary response.
    b. motor ability.
    c. level of consciousness.
    d. respiratory pattern.

57. Critical care patients feel more secure with
    a. nurses in constant attendance.
    b. technical equipment.
    c. monitoring alarms.
    d. physician visits.

58. The Circle of Willis is composed of
    a. internal carotids, posterior cerebral and basilar arteries.
    b. posterior and anterior communicating, posterior and anterior cerebral and middle cerebral arteries.
    c. posterior and anterior communicating, posterior and anterior cerebral and middle meningeal arteries.
    d. posterior and anterior cerebral, posterior and anterior meningeal and basilar arteries.

59. These are five stages to death and dying. A terminal patient may experience
    a. all the stages.
    b. none of the stages.
    c. going back and forth between stages.
    d. all of the above

60. The thyroid gland
    a. is controlled mainly by ACTH.
    b. secretes thyroxin and calcitonin.
    c. secretes thyrotropic hormone.
    d. has three lobes and is one of the smaller glands of the metabolic system.

61. The pathology of acute pancreatitis includes
    a. blockage of the flow of the pancreatic enzymes, stagnation in the ducts and acini, activation of the enzymes, and digestion of the pancreas.
    b. free flow of the pancreatic enzymes, overabundance of trypsinogen, activation of enzymes, and digestion of the pancreas.
    c. blockage of the pancreatic flow, overabundance of trypsin inhibitor, and complete inactivation of the enzymes.
    d. blockage of the pancreatic flow, overabundance of bile salts, and complete inactivation of the enzymes.

62. Denial can have a beneficial effect in illness. It allows the patient the opportunity to
    a. learn coping mechanisms.
    b. continue life as before.
    c. visit with family without a devastating effect.
    d. express anger.

63. Which best describes the circulation of cerebrospinal fluid?
    a. lateral ventricles to foramen of Monro to third ventricle to fourth ventricle to foramina of Luschka and Magendie
    b. lateral ventricles to foramen of Magendie to third ventricle to fourth ventricle to foramina of Luschka and Monro
    c. third ventricle to foramen of Magendie to lateral ventricles to fourth ventricle to foramina of Luschka and Monro
    d. lateral ventricles to foramen of Luschka to third ventricle to fourth ventricle to foramina of Magendie and Monro

64. The muscles involved in respiration are the
    a. diaphragm.
    b. intercostals.
    c. sternocleidomastoids.
    d. a and b

65. Osmosis is
    a. the movement of water across a semipermeable membrane from lesser to greater concentration of particles.
    b. the movement of particles across a semipermeable membrane from area of greater to lesser concentration of particles.
    c. movement of water across a permeable membrane.
    d. movement of particles across a semipermeable membrane from less concentration to greater concentration.

66. The ego states include the adult, the parent and the child. Which of the following statements is true concerning the ego states?
    a. Everyone has all three stages.
    b. When anger dominates, the adult is in command.
    c. One's goal should be to do away with the parent and child states.
    d. Most people only experience two of the three stages.

67. The goal(s) of therapy for the patient with acute pancreatitis is (are)
    a. to keep the pancreas at rest.
    b. to maintain adequate circulating blood volume.
    c. to alleviate pain.
    d. all of the above

68. A 54-year-old woman presents in the emergency department complaining of a severe headache. Photophobia and nuchal rigidity are noted on physical examination. Her temperature is 101°F orally. History is unremarkable except for a severe otitis media several weeks ago. She stopped taking the medication once she felt better. The most likely diagnosis is
    a. Guillain-Barre.
    b. subarachnoid hemorrhage.
    c. sinusitis with recurrent otitis media.
    d. meningitis.

69. It is not uncommon for the elderly to develop delusions, illusions and hallucinations, especially if they live alone. This may be due to
    a. sensory overload.
    b. sensory deprivation.
    c. sensory stimulation.
    d. sensory override.

70. When a patient experiences denial of an illness, this may indicate
    a. an increase in anxiety.
    b. failure to accept the situation.
    c. a personality disorder.
    d. an abnormal state requiring psychotherapy.

71. When obtaining a history from the patient with a gastrointestinal disorder, the nurse should elicit a history of
    a. previous gastrointestinal disorders.
    b. abdominal pain.
    c. heartburn.
    d. all of the above

72. The major complication following jugular insertion is
    a. air embolism
    b. pneumothorax.
    c. infection.
    d. bleeding.

73. In the intensive care unit, the patient is frequently deprived of an adequate sleep cycle. This interruption interferes with proper rest. The patient should have a sleep cycle of at least
    a. 2 hours.
    b. 3 hours.
    c. 4 hours.
    d. 5 hours.

74. Which of the following factors can lower the glomerular filtration rate?
    a. lowered renal blood flow
    b. increased cardiac output
    c. decreased cardiac output
    d. hypovolemia
    e. a, c, d

75. Potential complications of peptic ulcer disease are
    a. perforation, bleeding and pyloric obstruction.
    b. peritonitis, ileus and bleeding.
    c. ileus, liver failure and intestinal obstruction.
    d. sepsis, ascites and ileus.

76. The basic mechanism of coagulation is
    a. thrombin to fibrinogen.
    b. conversion of prothrombin to thrombin.
    c. thromboplastin to fibrinogen.
    d. fibrin to fibrinogen.

77. Aggressive sexual behavior is
    a. more common in males over 30 years of age.
    b. more common in males over 45 years of age.
    c. usually brought on by the action demonstrated by the nurse.
    d. more common in males over 60 years of age.

78. Diffusion is the movement of
    a. water from an area of greater concentration to an area of lesser concentration across a semipermeable membrane.
    b. particles from an area of lesser concentration to an area of greater concentration across a semipermeable membrane.
    c. solids across a permeable membrane from smaller concentration to larger concentration.
    d. particles across a semipermeable membrane from area of greater concentration to area of lesser concentration of particles.

79. Which factor listed below is not one of the causes of adult respiratory distress syndrome?
    a. shock: septic or hypovolemic
    b. pneumonia
    c. pulmonary embolism
    d. prolonged cardiopulmonary bypass

80. A patient was admitted to the recovery room following a cholecystectomy. The initial blood pressure of 140/80 dropped to 70/50. The patient's skin became cyanotic and clammy. The pulse was rapid and weak. The patient had been taking prednisone by mouth on a daily basis for ten years for arthritis. The patient is exhibiting
    a. acute adrenal crisis.
    b. insulin shock.
    c. hyperosmolar coma.
    d. diabetes insipidus.

81. Vitamin K is required for the formation of
    a. thromboplastin.
    b. fibrin.
    c. prothrombin.
    d. thrombin.

82. Decreased FRC accompanies the following pathological condition:
    a. emphysema
    b. pulmonary embolus
    c. adult respiratory distress syndrome
    d. pulmonary edema

83. The normal ratio of BUN to creatinine is
    a. 20:1.
    b. 1:10.
    c. 10:1.
    d. 1:20.

84. Hyperosmolar coma is manifested by
    a. dehydration/dry skin and seizures.
    b. enhanced sensorium.
    c. dehydration, clammy skin and seizures.
    d. Kussmaul breathing.

85. A 62-year-old man presents in the emergency department with right hemiparesis with the arm weaker than the leg, and a right facial droop. He is alert and appears oriented. He is able to follow commands involving his left side, but has expressive aphasia. The most likely cause of the problem is
    a. right internal carotid occlusion.
    b. left middle cerebral artery infarct.
    c. right anterior communicating artery infarct.
    d. ruptured cerebral aneurysm.

86. In an inferior wall myocardial infarction, the nurse should observe for
    a. changes in V_1 and V_2.
    b. changes in II, III and aVF.
    c. reciprocal changes in leads I and aVL, and some precordial leads.
    d. b and c

87. The product(s) of protein metabolism is (are):
    a. blood urea nitrogen
    b. creatinine
    c. uric acid
    d. amino acids
    e. a, b, c

88. Diabetic ketoacidosis presents with an elevation of blood sugar. Further pathophysiology of the disease is evidenced by
    a. blood glucose levels 50 to 70 mg.
    b. fatty acid mobilization and utilization.
    c. serum calcium levels of 8 mg/L.
    d. ketone bodies that cause a decrease in hydrogen ions and an increase in bicarbonate ions.

89. The diabetic who increases exercise will need
    a. less insulin.
    b. more insulin.
    c. longer-acting insulin.
    d. an additional dose of regular insulin.

90. Prevention of tracheal necrosis in the intubated patient is best accomplished by
    a. periodic cuff deflation for 5 minutes every hour.
    b. use of low-pressure cuffed tubes with minimal occlusive volume.
    c. careful positioning of the head and support of the tube to prevent pulling.
    d. use of high-pressure cuffed tubes.

91. Platelets are fragments of the precursor
    a. reticulocytes.
    b. hemocytoblasts.
    c. megakaryocytes.
    d. mast cells.

92. A patient enters the hospital with a diagnosis of end stage renal disease. He tells the nurse that he will be fine as soon as he is dialyzed. This patient is using the coping mechanism known as
   a. denial.
   b. projection.
   c. rationalization.
   d. depression.

93. The type of pressure used to remove excess water by ultrafiltration in the dialysis patient is
   a. osmotic.
   b. blood.
   c. hydrostatic.
   d. pneumatic.

94. After several days, the patient tells you that he cannot wait for the numbness in his arms and legs to go away so that he can get up and move around. An appropriate response would be:
   a. "These things take a long time."
   b. "Have you discussed this with your doctor? Maybe we should mention it today."
   c. "Don't worry, you'll be your old self in no time at all."
   d. "What makes you think you will ever walk again?"

95. Heparin is constantly circulated by
   a. stem cells.
   b. factor VIII.
   c. megakaryocytes.
   d. basophilic mast cells.

96. In thyrotoxicosis, treatment can be accomplished by
   a. subtotal thyroidectomy.
   b. propylthiouracil 50 mg orally every 8 hours or Tapazole 5 to 10 mg every 8 hours and Lugol's solution 15 to 30 drops per day.
   c. radioactive iodine I131 treatments.
   d. all of the above

97. Bowel sounds will be absent in the following disease states, except
   a. peritonitis.
   b. ileus.
   c. gangrene.
   d. cirrhosis.

98. In the intubated patient, three bypass functions of upper airway anatomy to consider are
   a. filtration, humidification and temperature control.
   b. olfaction, filtration and temperature control.
   c. distribution of gas, olfaction and humidification.
   d. oxygen and carbon dioxide equilibration, filtration and distribution of gas.

99. A patient is admitted to the intensive care unit with crushing chest pain. He verbalizes to the nurse his fear of dying. To relieve his anxiety, the nurse should
    a. orient the patient and his family to the unit, including routine, equipment and policies.
    b. send the family home to provide rest for the patient.
    c. sedate the patient.
    d. none of the above

100. Hereditary hemolytic anemias with unstable red cell membranes leading to destruction are
    a. thalassemia and sickle cell.
    b. spherocytosis and glucose-6-phosphate dehydrogenase.
    c. aplastic and thalassemia.
    d. sprue and aplastic.

101. The patient comes into the physician's office with complaints of nervousness, insomnia, fatigue, palpitations, diarrhea and heat intolerance. This patient exhibits, on examination, a fine hand tremor, palpable thyroid and exophthalmos. Diagnostic studies show a PBI of 8 mg/100 ml serum and an elevated BMR. EKG shows atrial fibrillation with a heart rate of 120 beats per minute. This is a classic presentation of
    a. myxedema.
    b. Addison's disease.
    c. Grave's disease.
    d. hypoglycemia.

102. Indications for endoscopic evaluation include
    a. upper gastrointestinal bleeding.
    b. evaluation of peptic ulcer disease.
    c. detection of perforations.
    d. a and b

103. Arterial blood gases of pH 7.55, PO_2 100, pCO_2 25, HCO_3 23, BE -1 are indicative of
    a. metabolic acidosis.
    b. metabolic alkalosis.
    c. respiratory acidosis.
    d. respiratory alkalosis.

104. A 21-year-old man is admitted to the emergency department following a motorcycle accident. He is awake and alert and in no apparent respiratory distress. Vital signs are blood pressure 98/60, pulse 102, respirations 26. His extremities are flaccid, with no sensation below the shoulders. Radiographs reveal a dislocation fracture of C7. The emergency department nurse should
    a. prepare for immediate intubation since cervical injuries result in impaired respirations.
    b. prep the patient for surgery, because immediate reduction of the fracture will reverse the neurological deficit.
    c. anticipate placement of Gardner-Wells tongs to reduce the fracture with traction.
    d. contact the patient's family and inform them of his accident and resultant permanent paralysis.

105. A patient is admitted to the intensive care unit following an automobile accident. According to Maslow's hierarchy of needs, the patient at this point has
    a. self-esteem needs.
    b. physiological needs.
    c. social needs.
    d. safety and security needs.

106. Hereditary anemia with a defective hemoglobin molecule found predominately in blacks is
    a. sprue.
    b. thalassemia.
    c. spherocytosis.
    d. sickle cell.

107. Pernicious anemia results in
    a. demyelination of dorsal and lateral columns and peripheral nerves.
    b. cardiomegaly.
    c. angina.
    d. jaundice.

108. In peritoneal dialysis the catheter is inserted
    a. within the peritoneal cavity.
    b. between the peritoneal cavity and the peritoneal space.
    c. above the membrane.
    d. below the membrane.

109. Artificial kidney systems, both peritoneal and hemodialysis, are designed to
    a. remove waste products of protein metabolism.
    b. maintain homeostatic concentration of serum electrolytes.
    c. compensate for metabolic acidosis and restore the body buffer system.
    d. remove water.
    e. all of the above

110. Respiratory acidosis is caused by
    a. hypoventilation.
    b. hyperventilation.
    c. gain of nonvolatile acid.
    d. loss of nonvolatile acid.

111. Glucagon is
    a. produced in the alpha and beta cells of the islets of Langerhans.
    b. responsible for increasing the concentration of blood sugar and is produced in the islets of Langerhans by the alpha cells.
    c. stimulated by high blood-sugar concentration.
    d. responsible for decreasing blood-sugar concentration.

112. A nurse can check a patient's visual field by
    a. asking him to read the newspaper.
    b. testing for color identification.
    c. moving an object toward his eyes and observing for movement.
    d. observing to see which areas of his meal tray he appears to ignore.

113. The typical paralysis in Guillain-Barre is
    a. descending.
    b. ascending.
    c. more pronounced on one side of the body.
    d. more pronounced distally than proximally.

114. Chronic renal patients are usually anemic with hematocrits as low as 16 percent to 18 percent, with the average approximately 25 percent. This may be due to
    a. anorexia.
    b. blood loss during dialysis.
    c. decreased production of erythropoietin.
    d. not taking iron supplements.
    e. b and c

115. Mr. Roberts is admitted to the intensive care unit with a concussion. He is unconscious at the present time. Nursing actions include
    a. telling the family to be quiet in order for the patient to rest.
    b. not allowing the family to visit.
    c. providing continuous external stimulation.
    d. providing brief explanations of care while at the bedside.

116. Diagnostic studies in hyperosmolar coma show
    a. moderate urine acetone and normal BUN.
    b. blood sugar greater than 1,000 mg/dl and normal or low blood pH.
    c. low blood pH and high BUN.
    d. normal BUN and low blood sugar.

117. The lower lobes are best auscultated over the
    a. midaxillary area.
    b. sternum.
    c. lower back posteriorly.
    d. lower anterior chest.

118. A patient with a right facial droop involving the entire face has a lesion located in the
    a. right facial nerve.
    b. left motor cortex.
    c. left trigeminal nerve.
    d. right trigeminal nerve.

119. Fluid is lost from the body through
    a. skin and lungs.
    b. lungs, urine and feces.
    c. skin and urine.
    d. skin, lungs, urine and feces.

120. Bone marrow dysfunction can be caused by
    a. isoniazid (INH).
    b. gentamycin.
    c. chloramphenicol.
    d. all of the above

121. An 18-year-old woman with a history of diabetes mellitus is seen in the emergency department with a diagnosis of hypoglycemic reaction. Hypoglycemic reaction is characterized by:
    (1) flushed dry skin and tachycardia
    (2) blurred vision and personality changes
    (3) headache and dilated pupils
    (4) hunger
    a. 2, 3, 4
    b. 1, 3
    c. 3, 4
    d. all of the above

122. Negative nitrogen balance occurs if
    a. the consumed nitrogen is equivalent to the amount excreted.
    b. the consumed nitrogen is greater than the amount excreted.
    c. the consumed nitrogen is less than the amount excreted.
    d. none of the above

123. In a true or absolute shunt, the V/O is
    a. .25.
    b. .50.
    c. .75.
    d. 0.

124. Adrenal crisis may be precipitated by:
    (1) trauma, infection, surgery
    (2) adrenal hemorrhage associated with anticoagulant therapy
    (3) sodium waste with depletion of plasma volume
    (4) hypoglycemia
    a. 2, 4
    b. 2, 3
    c. 1, 2, 3
    d. all of the above

125. A lesion along a given dermatome, which causes unilateral sensory loss, probably is located
    a. in the parietal lobe.
    b. along the peripheral nerve at its entry point into the spinal cord.
    c. along the ipsilateral thoracic cord below the level of T4.
    d. in the right frontal lobe.

126. Blood enters the glomerulus via the
    a. afferent arteriole.
    b. efferent arteriole.
    c. proximal tubule.
    d. loop of Henle.

127. Enteral hyperalimentation is indicated when the patient
    a. has a functioning gastrointestinal tract.
    b. is unable to swallow.
    c. is debilitated.
    d. all of the above

128. A patient in the critical care unit tells the nurse that she is cute and extends an invitation to take her to dinner. He is exhibiting behavior known as
    a. paranoid.
    b. depressive reactive.
    c. sexually aggressive.
    d. normal sexual.

129. From the time a patient is admitted to the critical care unit the nurse should be preparing the patient for
    a. recovery.
    b. transfer.
    c. discharge.
    d. none of the above

130. Reticulocytosis is seen in
    a. agranulocytosis.
    b. polycythemia.
    c. sickle cell anemia.
    d. spherocytosis.

131. The phrase "less than 0.20 second" best refers to which of the following?
    a. abnormal P-R interval
    b. normal QRS interval
    c. normal Q-T interval
    d. normal P-R interval

132. Fistulization of the trachea post intubation frequently occurs in the
    a. carina.
    b. posterior trachea.
    c. larynx.
    d. cricoid cartilage.

133. Blast cells are commonly seen in
    a. polycythemia.
    b. aplastic anemia.
    c. thalassemia.
    d. leukemia.

134. The innermost covering of the kidney is loosely attached to the
    a. perirenal fat.
    b. renal cortex.
    c. adipose tissue.
    d. renal fascia.

135. A patient has no pupillary reaction to light in the left eye. There is reaction to light in both eyes when the light is shined in the right eye. The lesion is located in the
    a. 2nd cranial nerve-left side.
    b. 2nd cranial nerve-right side.
    c. 3rd cranial nerve-left side.
    d. 3rd cranial nerve-right side.

136. Mrs. Smith is very depressed about the admission of her husband to the intensive care unit. After every visit, Mr. Smith requires pain medication. You suspect the wife may be causing Mr. Smith's pain. You should
    a. ask her not to visit.
    b. carefully monitor her visits.
    c. suggest she visit her clergy for counseling.
    d. spend a few minutes with her; tell her it is normal to feel depressed; and let her know she is upsetting her husband.

137. According to Elizabeth Kübler-Ross's five stages of death and dying, a patient may
    a. not progress through all the stages.
    b. progress through some of the stages, slip back to denial and start over.
    c. not go through the stages systematically.
    d. never go through any of the stages.

138. Disorderly proliferation of white blood cells is
    a. leukemia.
    b. anemia.
    c. thalassemia.
    d. agranulocytosis.

139. When observing a seizure, the nurse should record the following information:
    a. duration, aura, time of last meal, deviation of head or eyes, and pupillary size and reaction.
    b. duration, aura, focal onset and spread, the names and titles of others observing the seizure, and the postictal state
    c. duration, aura, focal onset and spread, pupil size and reaction, deviation of head or eyes, and postictal state
    d. duration, aura, focal onset and spread, temperature of the room, pupil size and reaction, deviation of head or eyes, and postictal state

140. Nephrotic syndrome is chiefly characterized by
    a. proteinuria.
    b. oliguria.
    c. an elevated serum creatinine and BUN.
    d. hematuria.

141. Symptoms of adrenal crisis are
    a. edema, nervousness, weight gain and hyperpigmentation.
    b. hypotension, dehydration, hyperpigmentation and lethargy.
    c. hypotension, polyuria, dehydration and weight loss.
    d. hypotension, dehydration, polyuria and hypopigmentation.

142. Normal pH of arterial blood gases is
    a. 7.40.
    b. 7.30.
    c. 7.50.
    d. 7.20.

143. Acute and chronic leukemia are differentiated by
    a. rate of growth.
    b. number of cells present.
    c. predominance of immature or mature cells.
    d. response to treatment.

144. Vomiting may cause the following electrolyte disturbances, except
    a. alkalosis.
    b. hypokalemia.
    c. hyponatremia.
    d. hypercalcemia.

145. Diabetic ketoacidosis may be precipitated by:
    (1) unusual exercise
    (2) too little food ingestion
    (3) infections of respiratory or urinary tracts
    (4) surgery or trauma
    a. 1, 4
    b. 2, 3
    c. 3, 4
    d. all of the above

146. Colicky abdominal pain associated with borborygmi is indicative of
    a. peritonitis.
    b. intestinal obstruction.
    c. appendicitis.
    d. cholecystitis.

147. The "physiological pacemaker of the heart" is a term used to describe the
    a. AV node.
    b. SA node.
    c. bundle of His.
    d. bundle of Kent.

148. Blastic crisis converts
    a. chronic myelogenous leukemia to acute myelogenous leukemia.
    b. chronic lymphocytic leukemia to acute lymphocytic leukemia.
    c. acute myelogenous leukemia to myelogenous leukemia.
    d. a and b

149. Airway resistance is the
    a. amount of pressure needed to create a given change in volume.
    b. relationship between pressure and airflow in the lung airways.
    c. relationship between capillary hydrostatic pressure and colloidal osmotic pressure.
    d. process by which gas molecules pass from an area of higher to lower partial pressure.

150. The generalized edema associated with nephrotic syndrome is the result of
    a. fluid overload.
    b. a decreased glomerular filtration rate.
    c. pump failure.
    d. fluid shift secondary to hypoalbuminemia.

151. In teaching the patient with Addison's disease, the nurse should instruct the patient to:
    (1) conserve energy level
    (2) eat foods high in potassium and low in sodium
    (3) avoid infection
    (4) eat foods high in sodium and low in potassium
    a. 3, 4
    b. 1, 2, 3
    c. 2, 3
    d. 1, 3, 4

152. The hematuria and proteinuria of acute glomerulonephritis is due to
    a. deposits of the antigen-antibody complex on the endothelial cells.
    b. interstitial fibrosis.
    c. the escape of blood and protein through the porous glomerular capillary.
    d. sclerosis of the arterioles and atrophy of the glomeruli.

153. Palpation of the abdomen is useful in evaluating the patient's condition, except for
    a. differentiating pain.
    b. detecting masses.
    c. verifying organomegaly.
    d. determining presence of dilated veins.

154. A 32-year-old male is admitted to the critical care unit following an automobile accident. He is awake and alert, but was unconscious for several minutes following the accident. Physical examination is unremarkable except for a right linear temporal-parietal skull fracture. The nurse will be performing hourly assessment and observing for
    a. the development of an epidural hematoma.
    b. the development of seizures within the first 24 hours.
    c. the development of cerebrospinal fluid leakage from his ears.
    d. the development of adrenal crisis.

155. The most common leukemia to attack children is
    a. CLL.
    b. ALL.
    c. AML.
    d. CML.

156. Parathormone is secreted by the parathyroid gland and
    (1) is stimulated by a high calcium level in the extracellular fluid.
    (2) increases reabsorption of bone salts.
    (3) increases phosphate excretion in the kidneys.
    (4) is stimulated by a low calcium level in the extracellular fluid.
    a. 1, 2, 3
    b. 2, 3
    c. 3, 4
    d. 2, 3, 4

157. The primary cause of hypoxemia is
    a. decreased minute ventilation.
    b. V/O abnormality.
    c. acid-base imbalance.
    d. increased PCWP.

158. Uncontrollable hypertension secondary to renal failure is due to the increase in
    a. serum renin levels and tubular reabsorption of sodium.
    b. renal blood flow.
    c. tubular reabsorption of sodium only.
    d. serum renin level and a decrease in tubular reabsorption of sodium.

159. A sucking chest wound may produce an extreme medical emergency known as
    a. bleeding.
    b. tension pneumothorax.
    c. shock.
    d. respiratory failure.

160. Total parenteral nutrition should be initiated when the patient has
    a. a poorly functioning gastrointestinal tract.
    b. an extremely high caloric requirement.
    c. anorexia.
    d. a and b

161. Manifestations of the somatotropin hormone include:
    (1) a decreased secretion in children which causes acromegaly
    (2) a decreased secretion in adults which causes panhypopituitarism
    (3) a secretion known as the growth hormone
    (4) an overproduction that may cause acromegaly in the adult
    a. 3, 4
    b. 2, 3, 4
    c. 1, 2
    d. 2, 3

162. Complications associated with total parenteral nutrition include
    a. sepsis.
    b. catheter insertion dysfunction.
    c. metabolic disorders.
    d. all of the above

163. The artery that carries unoxygenated blood is the
    a. aorta.
    b. radial.
    c. pulmonary.
    d. brachial.

164. The ventricular rate is 30 to 40 beats per minute, rhythm is regular, P-P interval is regular, P-R interval is not constant, atrial rate is 70. You are most likely looking at an EKG strip of
    a. idioventricular rhythm.
    b. complete heart block.
    c. Mobitz I.
    d. Mobitz II.

165. The heart rate is 150 to 300 uncoordinated beats per minute. Rhythm is very irregular; P waves may be present, but are unrecognizable; no P-R interval; QRS complexes are absent. Multiple ectopic pacemaker sites produce waves of varying amplitude and shapes. The EKG strip is most likely
    a. idioventricular rhythm.
    b. atrial fibrillation.
    c. ventricular fibrillation.
    d. dying heart.

166. Deficiency of pulmonary surfactant frequently results in a pathological condition referred to as
    a. asthma.
    b. pneumonia.
    c. pleurisy.
    d. atelectasis.

167. Cranial radiation may be used to reduce central nervous system involvement in
    a. acute myelogenous leukemia.
    b. chronic lymphoblastic leukemia.
    c. acute lymphoblastic leukemia.
    d. chronic myelogenous leukemia.

168. A nephron is composed of the following:
    a. Bowman's capsule, afferent and efferent arterioles
    b. renal pyramid, calyx, glomerulus
    c. glomerulus, proximal tubule, loop of Henle, distal tubule, collecting tubule
    d. a and b

169. Distended jugular veins in an upright position are an indication of
    a. low blood pressure.
    b. left heart failure.
    c. right heart failure.
    d. intra-septal rupture.

170. The Philadelphia chromosome is present in 80 percent of
    a. ALL.
    b. AML.
    c. CML.
    d. CLL.

171. To obtain cardiac output, which of the following equations should be used?
    a. CO = SV + HR
    b. CO = SV times HR
    c. CO = SV minus HR
    d. CO = SV + HR minus BP

172. With regard to blood pressure, cardiac tamponade would clinically manifest in which of the following ways?
    a. increased systolic; decreased diastolic
    b. increased diastolic; increased systolic
    c. decreased diastolic; decreased systolic
    d. increased diastolic; decreased systolic

173. Lymphoma involving both sides of the diaphragm, but excluding the spleen is classified as
    a. stage III.
    b. stage I.
    c. stage II.
    d. stage IV.

174. Metabolic acidosis may be caused by all of the following, *except*
    a. anaerobic metabolism.
    b. renal failure.
    c. salicylate poisoning.
    d. diuretic therapy.

175. The most common treatment of flail chest is
    a. chest tubes.
    b. surgical stabilization of the fractured ribs.
    c. splint dressings.
    d. intubation and mechanical ventilation.

176. Total body radiation for leukemia may be used
    a. prior to bone marrow transplant.
    b. as an alternative to chemotherapy CLL.
    c. CML.
    d. a and b

177. Gastric secretion is stimulated by
    a. pepsinogen, hydrochloric acid and intrinsic factor.
    b. pepsin, H2 receptor blockers and pepsinogen.
    c. histamine, hydrochloric acid and mucus.
    d. gastric, acetylcholine and histamine.

178. Treatment for the patient in hyperosmolar coma includes:
    (1) establishing a patient airway, maintaining adequate ventilation, and inserting a levine tube
    (2) correcting metabolic acidosis with bicarbonate
    (3) correcting fluid balance and dehydration
    (4) providing emotional and psychological support to the patient and family members
    a. 2, 3
    b. 1, 2, 3
    c. 1, 3, 4
    d. all of the above

179. Facial nerve lower motor neuron paralysis is best described as
    a. dysarthria, dysphagia and postural hypotension.
    b. dysarthria, dysphagia and diplopia.
    c. ipsilateral inability to close an eye, control mouth or move lips.
    d. ipsilateral inability to open an eye, move tongue or move lips.

180. Coombs' test is to determine
    a. mast cells.
    b. effectiveness of RhoGAM.
    c. sensitivity.
    d. presence of IgH antibodies in a RH negative person.

181. The most effective chemotherapeutic agent for lymphocytic lymphoma is
    a. vincristine.
    b. methotrexate.
    c. bisulfate.
    d. cytosine arabinoside.

182. The liver contributes to digestion by
    a. secreting proteolytic enzymes.
    b. secreting bile salts.
    c. gluconeogenesis.
    d. all of the above

183. Complications associated with subtotal thyroidectomy include:
    (1) decreased serum calcium
    (2) thyroid storm
    (3) respiratory distress due to bleeding and edema
    (4) hoarseness
    a. 3, 4
    b. 1, 2
    c. 1, 2, 3
    d. all of the above

184. The pharmocologic treatment of choice for rate-dependent PVCs would be which of the following?
    a. lidocaine 50 to 100 grams intravenously
    b. lidocaine 1 to 2 mg in 500 cc of dextrose in water
    c. atropine 0.5 grams intravenous push times 2
    d. atropine 0.5 mg intravenous push times 2

185. Which of the following diseases would increase PCWP?
    a. pulmonary edema
    b. adult respiratory distress syndrome
    c. spontaneous pneumothorax
    d. asthma

186. The dead space volume in a person weighing approximately 150 pounds would be
    a. 125 cc.
    b. 150 cc.
    c. 175 cc.
    d. 200 cc.

187. The immunoglobulins that respond first to an invasion of a foreign substance are
    a. IgA.
    b. IgG.
    c. IgM.
    d. IgE.

188. Complications associated with diabetes ketoacidosis include:
    (1) coma and death
    (2) hypokalemia
    (3) shock
    (4) seizures
    a. 1, 2
    b. 1, 2, 3
    c. 3, 4
    d. all of the above

189. Which of the following statements is true concerning psychomotor seizures?
    a. The patient has complete recall of the event.
    b. The seizure begins in one extremity and gradually spreads.
    c. During the course of the seizure the patient retains motor function.
    d. The patient is incontinent and unconscious.

190. The function(s) of the gallbladder is (are)
    a. to connect the common hepatic duct with the pancreatic duct.
    b. to store and concentrate bile.
    c. to store and concentrate triglycerides and amino acids.
    d. to connect the common bile duct with the pancreatic duct.

191. The coronary arteries fill during
    a. atrial contraction.
    b. systole.
    c. formation of the P wave.
    d. diastole.

192. The immunoglobulin responsible for anaphylactic reaction is
    a. IgD.
    b. IgE.
    c. IgA.
    d. IgM.

193. Venous flow of blood in the liver consists of
    a. portal vein, liver sinusoids, ventral vein, hepatic vein, inferior vena cava.
    b. portal vein, hepatic vein, liver sinusoids, inferior mesenteric, inferior vena cava.
    c. hepatic vein, liver sinusoids, inferior vena cava.
    d. hepatic vein, liver sinusoids, central vein, inferior vena cava.

194. The function of the pancreas is:
    (1) an exocrine and endocrine gland
    (2) to produce insulin
    (3) effected by levels of ACTH
    a. 2
    b. 2, 3
    c. 1, 3
    d. all of the above

195. Suctioning or deep coughing may clear the lung fields of
    a. wheezes.
    b. rales.
    c. rhonchi.
    d. pleural rub.

196. Which of the following cardiac dysrhythmias is not usually seen with hyperkalemia?
    a. tall, peaked T waves
    b. S-T segment depression
    c. atrial fibrillation
    d. widened QRS

197. Which of the following is a physiological volatile acid?
    a. lactic acid
    b. pyruvic acid
    c. carbon dioxide
    d. carbonic acid

198. Diagnostic studies of a patient in diabetic coma reveal:
    (1) serum blood glucose levels 300 to 800 mg percent or higher
    (2) ketonemia and ketonuria
    (3) metabolic acidosis
    (4) hemoconcentration and an elevated BUN
    a. 1, 3
    b. 1, 2, 3
    c. 1, 4
    d. all of the above

199. Which of these statements is *not* true regarding the intrinsic factor?
    a. Intrinsic factor is secreted by parietal cells.
    b. Intrinsic factor is a mucoprotein.
    c. Intrinsic factor binds to vitamin B12.
    d. Intrinsic factor aids in the digestion of vitamin B12.

200. In progressive renal failure, when workload is shifted to the remaining functioning nephrons, which of the following compensatory events takes place?
    (1) hypertrophy of the working nephrons
    (2) an increase in the GFR through the functioning nephrons
    (3) an increase in the solute load
    (4) an increase in tubular reabsorption
    a. 1, 3
    b. 1, 2, 3
    c. 3
    d. all of the above

201. Pulmonary emphysema is frequently complicated by
    a. left ventricular failure.
    b. cor pulmonale.
    c. premature ventricular contractions.
    d. pulmonary emboli.

202. The patient arrives in the emergency department with a diagnosis of diabetic coma. Which of the following physical signs are seen?
    (1) diaphoresis, pale appearance, sinus tachycardia, muscle twitching and unresponsiveness
    (2) deep, rapid respirations
    (3) unresponsive; dry, warm skin; flushed face; sinus tachycardia
    (4) acetone breath
    a. 3, 4
    b. 1, 2, 4
    c. 2, 3, 4
    d. all of the above

203. A patient's wife tells you about her episodes of blurred vision in the right eye several times a day. She describes it as "a veil covering my eye." As a nurse you would respond by
    a. telling her she has probably had a small stroke in her vision center and suggesting that she see a doctor immediately.
    b. advising her to see a doctor since it may be a warning sign of impending stroke.
    c. suggesting she mention it to her doctor at her next annual physical.
    d. telling her it is only eye fatigue and recommending that she see opthalmologist.

204. Functions of the liver include:
    a. vitamin storage
    b. mineral storage
    c. metabolism of protein, carbohydrate and fat
    d. all of the above

205. The primary treatment of DIC is
    a. Amicar.
    b. heparin.
    c. transfusion.
    d. antibiotics.

206. In the diuretic stages of acute renal failure, the high urine volume is **due to**
    (1) the decreased blood urea concentration.
    (2) osmotic diuresis secondary to an increased blood urea concentration.
    (3) the impaired ability of the tubules to conserve water and salt.
    (4) the uneven distribution of blood flow throughout the kidney.
    a. 1, 3
    b. 2, 3
    c. 1, 3, 4
    d. 3, 4

207. The secretion of epinephrine and norepinephrine is regulated by the autonomic nervous system. This secretion may be
    a. stimulated by fear or anger.
    b. secreted by the medulla of the adrenal gland.
    c. synonymous with catecholamines.
    d. all of the above

208. The ability to recognize an object by touch is called
    a. aphasia.
    b. apraxia.
    c. agnosia.
    d. agraphia.

209. The coronary circulation has a rather unique ability to compensate for blocked or damaged vessels, helping the heart to mend itself. This feature is called
    a. unilateral circulation.
    b. bilateral circulation.
    c. collateral circulation.
    d. trilateral circulation.

210. Hypovolemia in anaphylactic shock is the result of
    a. third-spacing of fluids.
    b. hemorrhage.
    c. inappropriate ADH.
    d. diuresis.

211. Right to left shunt effect in adult respiratory distress syndrome is primarily due to
    a. collapsed alveolar units.
    b. blocked pulmonary capillaries.
    c. ventricular septal defect.
    d. increased interstitial fluid.

212. Manifestations of aldosterone deficiency can be seen as:
    (1) hypovolemia, hypotension and increased sodium absorption
    (2) decreased cardiac size, decreased cardiac output and decreased renal flow
    (3) weight gain, hypotension and elevated BUN
    (4) hypovolemia, hypotension and increased sodium excretion
    a. 1, 2, 4
    b. 1, 2, 3
    c. 1, 3
    d. 2, 4

213. Which of the following symptoms usually is indicative of bilateral mechanical obstruction involving the renal arteries?
    a. oliguria
    b. anuria
    c. proteinuria
    d. hematuria

214. Anaerobic metabolism may result in
    a. metabolic alkalosis.
    b. metabolic acidosis.
    c. respiratory alkalosis.
    d. respiratory acidosis.

215. A lesion of the left hemisphere in Broca's area results in a deficit of
    a. verbal comprehension.
    b. written comprehension.
    c. verbal expression.
    d. written expression.

216. Replacement of platelets and fibrin in DIC would usually be by infusion of
    a. whole blood.
    b. packed cells.
    c. cryoprecipitate.
    d. albumin.

217. A pathological state that causes fine, moist rales is
    a. mucous in the large bronchi and trachea.
    b. irritation of the pleura.
    c. bronchospasm.
    d. pulmonary edema.

218. Prerenal failure associated with cardiac failure is the direct result of
    a. obstruction of the renal vessels.
    b. decreased cardiac output and decreased renal perfusion.
    c. fluid overload leading to glomerular solute overload.
    d. an increased retention of sodium.

219. Treatment of the patient in diabetic coma includes:
    (1) establishing a patent airway and maintaining adequate ventilation
    (2) correcting fluid balance
    (3) monitoring blood glucose and arterial blood gases
    (4) correcting electrolyte imbalance
    a. 1, 2, 4
    b. 1, 2
    c. 1, 3
    d. all of the above

220. The oculomotor nerve is responsible for all of the following, except
    a. elevating the eyelid.
    b. lateral eye movement.
    c. pupillary constriction to light.
    d. medial eye movement.

221. The greatest danger in immunosuppressed diseases is
    a. hemorrhage.
    b. infection.
    c. allergic reaction.
    d. none of the above

222. Renal failure that is the result of injury or necrosis to the renal parenchyma is classified as
    a. chronic.
    b. postrenal.
    c. intrinsic.
    d. acute.

223. In Addison's disease, the patient may exhibit the following symptoms:
    (1) weight loss and anorexia
    (2) hypotension and weakness
    (3) impaired tolerance to stress
    (4) hyperpigmentation of skin
    a. 1, 2, 4
    b. 2, 3
    c. 1, 2, 3
    d. all of the above

224. A patient presents with a unilateral loss of all sensory modalities in a single extremity. The lesion is most likely located in the
    a. ipsilateral sensory strip of the parietal lobe.
    b. peripheral nerve or its entry point into the spinal cord.
    c. cervical spinal cord.
    d. contralateral sensory strip of the parietal lobe.

225. Normal pulmonary hydrostatic pressure is:
    a. 3 mm/Hg.
    b. 5 mm/Hg.
    c. 8 mmg.
    d. 10 mm/Hg.

226. Electrical cardioversion may be dangerous in the presence of which of the following drugs?
   a. Lasix
   b. Digitalis
   c. Valium
   d. morphine sulfate

227. The most common cause of cardiogenic shock is
   a. failure of the heart.
   b. failure of the lungs.
   c. failure of the brain.
   d. failure of the kidney.

228. A precipitating factor of adult respiratory distress syndrome which may increase mortality is
   a. drug ingestion and overdose.
   b. septic shock.
   c. hypovolemic shock.
   d. trauma.

229. Neurons in the peripheral nervous system
   a. have myelin but no neurilemma.
   b. are incapable of Wallerian degeneration.
   c. have myelin and neurilemma but lack nodes of Ranvier.
   d. are capable of regeneration.

230. The characteristic symptoms of Parkinson's disease are
   a. tremor, muscle rigidity and athetosis.
   b. tremor, muscle atrophy and akinesia.
   c. tremor, muscle wasting and athetosis.
   d. tremor, muscle rigidity and akinesia.

231. Stimulation of the parasympathetic nervous system affects the heart rate by
   a. increasing the heart rate.
   b. increasing contractility.
   c. decreasing the heart rate.
   d. There is no effect on the heart rate.

232. The adrenal glands are located above each kidney and
   (1) consist of a medulla and cortex
   (2) are stimulated by ACTH and the sympathetic nervous system
   (3) are called upon in stress situations
   (4) are not necessary for life
   a. 1, 4
   b. 1, 2
   c. 1, 3
   d. 1, 2, 3

233. The patient presents his complaints as anorexia, apathy, intolerance to cold and loss of libido. These symptoms are usually early signs of:
   (1) Addison's disease
   (2) Grave's disease
   (3) myxedema
   (4) diabetes mellitus
   a. 2, 4
   b. 2, 3, 4
   c. 2
   d. 3

234. The most prevalent cause of COPD in the United States is
   a. air pollution.
   b. asthma.
   c. smoking.
   d. occupational hazards.

235. The elevated serum ammonia level seen in patients with hepatic failure may be caused by
   a. malnutrition and excessive alcohol consumption.
   b. lack of detoxification by the liver.
   c. portal-systemic shunting.
   d. b and c

236. Ventricular systole best refers to which of the following?
   a. relaxation
   b. contraction
   c. filling
   d. pressure

237. The pain associated with an acute myocardial infarction can best be described as
   a. pressure lasting longer than 20 minutes, accompanied by fear of death.
   b. pressure lasting less than 20 minutes, relieved with nitroglycerine.
   c. relievable with nitroglycerine, rest and oxygen; and accompanied by fear of death.
   d. nonradiating pain that is low in intensity and accompanied by fear of death.

238. There are two major classifications for angina. The predictable angina is referred to as
   a. postinfarction.
   b. unstable.
   c. stable.
   d. preinfarction.

239. Bronchial breath sounds heard over the periphery of the lungs may be indicative of
   a. pulmonary edema.
   b. pulmonary embolus.
   c. consolidation.
   d. bronchospasm.

240. The most important of the glucocorticoids is cortisol. Its functions include:
    (1) decreasing glucose utilization in body cells
    (2) blocking the inflammatory process
    (3) increasing blood glucose concentration
    (4) decreasing blood glucose concentration
    a. 1, 2
    b. 1, 3
    c. 1, 2, 3
    d. 1, 2, 4

241. Of the following pathological states, which is due to mechanical failure of the heart?
    a. arteriosclerosis
    b. congestive heart failure
    c. angina
    d. myocardial infarction

242. In the presence of ventricular fibrillation, ineffective countershock attempts might be caused by
    a. presence of metabolic acidosis.
    b. ventricular irritability.
    c. inadequate oxygenation.
    d. all of the above

243. Asystole represents the lack of electrical and mechanical activity in the heart. The initial treatment should consist of
    a. cardiopulmonary resuscitation.
    b. fibrillation.
    c. calcium chloride.
    d. sodium bicarbonate.

244. Esophageal varices are formed by
    a. dilatation of the small veins in the esophageal submucosal plexus at the portal-systemic anastamotic site in the lower third of the esophagus.
    b. dilatation of the esophageal branch of the left gastric artery due to portal hypertension.
    c. dilatation of the azygos veins due to portal hypertension.
    d. dilatation of the esophageal vein due to portal hypertension.

245. The process by which a gas molecule passes from an area of higher to lower partial pressure is called
    a. perfusion.
    b. osmosis.
    c. diffusion.
    d. internal respiration.

246. In chronic renal failure there is a(n)
    a. decrease in the GFR, decrease in ionizable calcium, and a rise in serum phosphate.
    b. increase in the GFR, decrease in ionizable calcium, and a decrease in serum phosphate.
    c. decrease in the GFR, ionizable calcium and serum phosphate.
    d. increase in the GFR and ionizable calcium, and a decrease in serum phosphate.

247. Which cartilage in the trachea forms the only complete ring and makes cuffed endotracheal tubes unnecessary in a child under six years of age?
    a. arytenoid
    b. cricoid
    c. thyroid
    d. adenoid

248. The circumflex artery branches from the
    a. right coronary artery.
    b. left coronary artery.
    c. pulmonary artery.
    d. aorta.

249. A patient is most likely to rupture a necrotic area post myocardial infarction
    a. within the first two hours.
    b. within 24 hours.
    c. within the first week.
    d. after the second week.

250. On a standard 12-lead EKG, a Q wave is prominent in leads II, III, and aVF. Where is the area of the infarct?
    a. posterior
    b. anterior
    c. inferior
    d. septal

PRACTICE EXAMINATION ANSWERS

1. a	51. a	101. c	151. d	201. b
2. b	52. a	102. d	152. c	202. c
3. c	53. d	103. d	153. d	203. b
4. a	54. d	104. c	154. a	204. d
5. b	55. c	105. b	155. b	205. b
6. a	56. c	106. d	156. c	206. b
7. d	57. b	107. a	157. b	207. d
8. d	58. b	108. c	158. c	208. c
9. d	59. c	109. d	159. b	209. c
10. a	60. b	110. a	160. d	210. a
11. c	61. a	111. b	161. b	211. a
12. d	62. a	112. d	162. d	212. a
13. c	63. a	113. b	163. c	213. b
14. d	64. d	114. e	164. b	214. b
15. d	65. a	115. d	165. c	215. c
16. d	66. a	116. b	166. d	216. c
17. b	67. d	117. c	167. c	217. d
18. a	68. d	118. a	168. c	218. b
19. b	69. b	119. d	169. c	219. d
20. b	70. b	120. c	170. c	220. b
21. c	71. d	121. a	171. b	221. b
22. c	72. a	122. c	172. d	222. c
23. b	73. b	123. d	173. a	223. d
24. d	74. e	124. d	174. d	224. d
25. d	75. a	125. b	175. d	225. b
26. a	76. b	126. a	176. d	226. b
27. c	77. a	127. d	177. d	227. a
28. c	78. d	128. c	178. d	228. b
29. d	79. c	129. b	179. c	229. d
30. b	80. a	130. b	180. d	230. d
31. a	81. c	131. d	181. a	231. c
32. c	82. c	132. b	182. b	232. d
33. b	83. c	133. d	183. d	233. d
34. c	84. a	134. d	184. d	234. c
35. d	85. b	135. a	185. a	235. d
36. a	86. d	136. d	186. c	236. b
37. a	87. e	137. b	187. c	237. a
38. b	88. b	138. a	188. d	238. c
39. d	89. a	139. c	189. c	239. c
40. a	90. b	140. a	190. b	240. b
41. c	91. c	141. b	191. d	241. b
42. d	92. a	142. a	192. b	242. d
43. a	93. c	143. c	193. a	243. a
44. d	94. b	144. d	194. d	244. a
45. b	95. d	145. d	195. c	245. c
46. c	96. d	146. b	196. c	246. a
47. c	97. d	147. b	197. c	247. b
48. a	98. a	148. a	198. d	248. b
49. d	99. a	149. b	199. d	249. c
50. a	100. b	150. d	200. d	250. c

BIBLIOGRAPHY
PSYCHO-SOCIAL SYSTEM
CHAPTER 2

Benolierl, J.Q. and S. Vande Velde. As the patient views the intensive care unit and the coronary care unit. Heart Lung 260-264, 1975.

Berne, E. Transactional analysis in psychotherapy. New York: Grove Press, 1961.

Cassem, N.H. and T.P. Hackett. Stress on the nurse and therapist in the intensive care unit and the coronary care unit. Heart Lung 4:252-58, 1975.

Davidson, D. and J. Groccin. A humanistic approach to counseling in critical care. Critical Care Nurse, Jul./Aug., 1981.

Eisendrath, S.J. and J. Dunkel. Psychological issues in intensive care unit staff. Heart Lung 8:751-58, 1979.

Gardner, D. and N. Stewart. Staff involvement with families of patients in critical care units. Heart Lung 7:105-10, 1978.

Harris, T.A. I'm OK, you're OK. New York: Avon Books, 1973.

Helton, M.C., et al. The correlation between sleep deprivation and the intensive care unit syndrome. Heart Lung 9:464-68, 1980.

Jillings, C.R. Nursing intervention with the family of the critically ill patient. Critical Care Nurse, Sep./Oct., 1981.

Kubler-Ross, E. On death and dying. New York: MacMillan, 1969.

Scalzi, C. Nursing management of behavioral responses following acute myocardial infarction. Heart Lung 2:62-68, 1973.

Sekelin, A. Sleep deprivation and biological rhythms in critical care units. Critical Care Nurse, May/Jun., 1981.

NERVOUS SYSTEM
CHAPTER 3

Bannister, R. Brain's clinical neurology. Edinburgh: Oxford University Press, 1978.

Bates, B. A guide to physical examination. Philadelphia: J.B. Lippincott Co., 1979.

Clusid, J. Correlative neuroanatomy and functional neurology. Los Altos: Lange Medical Publications, 1979.

Conway, B.L. Carini and Owens neurological and neurosurgical nursing. St. Louis: C.V. Mosby Co., 1978.

Core curriculum. Chicago: AANN, 1977.

Plum, F. and J. B. Posner. Diagnosis of stupor and coma. Philadelphia: F.A. Davis Co., 1980.

Simpson, J. and K. Mayer. Clinical evaluation of the nervous system. Boston: Little, Brown and Co., 1973.

Taylor, J. and S. Ballenger. Neurological dysfunctions and nursing interventions. New York: McGraw Hill, 1980.

PULMONARY SYSTEM
CHAPTER 4

Advanced cardiac life support, Part 4. Emerg. Med. 12:107-10+, Aug. 15, 1980.

Anderson, C.L., et al. Physiological significance of sternomastoid muscle contraction in chronic obstructive pulmonary disease. Resp. Care 25:937-39, Sep., 1980.

Anthony, C. and N. Kalthoff. Textbook of anatomy and physiology. St. Louis: C.V. Mosby Co., 1971.

Brigham, K.L., et al. The pulmonary circulation. Resp. Care 25:264-66+, Feb., 1980.

Brown, H.V., et al. Evaluation of an oxygen concentrator in patients with COPD. Resp. Ther. 8:55-57, Sep./Oct., 1978.

Bubis, M.J., et al. Differences between slow and fast vital capacities in patients with obstructive disease. Chest 77:626-31, May, 1980.

Burki, N.K. Resting ventilatory pattern, mouth occlusion pressure, and the effects of aminophylline in asthma and chronic airway obstruction. Chest 76:629-35, Dec., 1979.

Cardin, S. Acid-base balance in the patient with respiratory disease. *Symposium on fluid, electrolyte, and acid balance.* Nurs. Clin. North Am. 15:593-601, Sep., 1980.

Chernick, R., et al. Respiration in health and disease. Philadelphia: W.B. Saunders Co., 1972.

Chusid, E.L. Diagnostic procedures in bronchopulmonary diseases. Hosp. Pract. 16:99-108, Jun., 1981.

CPR and emergency cardiac care: new standards and guidelines. Basic life support in adults, Part 2. Emerg. Med. 12:49+, Aug., 1980.

Felson, B. The chest roentgenologic workup—what and why? Conventional methods. Resp. Care 25:955-59, Sep., 1980.

Grossback-Landis, L. Successful weaning of ventilator-dependent patients. Top. Clin. Nurs. 2:45-68, Oct., 1980.

Guyton, A. Textbook of medical physiology. Philadelphia: W.B. Saunders Co., 1976.

Hall, J.P., et al. Adult respiratory medical emergencies. *Symposium on emergency nursing.* Nurs. CLin. North Am. 16:75-84, Mar., 1981.

Hudak, C. M., et al. Critical care nursing. Philadelphia: J.B. Lippincott Co., 1977.

Jayamanne, D.S., et al. Flow-volume curve contour in COPD: correlation with pulmonary mechanics. Chest 77:749-57, Jun., 1980.

Kosanke, C.W., Jr., et al. Expiratory reserve volume: an understressed indicator of respiratory impairment. CVP 8:61-62, Aug./Sep., 1980.

Lavin, M.J., et al. Lung contusion—a chimera. Resp. Care 25:242-46, Feb., 1980.

Lippmann, M., et al. Pulmonary embolism in the patient with chronic obstructive pulmonary disease. Chest 79:39-42, Jan., 1981.

Luce, J.M., et al. Intermittent mandatory ventilation. Chest 79:678-85, Jun., 1981.

Massaro, D. Clinical implications of the effect of breathing pattern on the lung. Resp. Care 25:377-78+, Mar., 1980.

Mathews, J.J. Chronic obstructive pulmonary disease. Top. Emerg. Med. 2:13-24, Jul., 1980.

McCarthy, D.S. Chronic obstructive pulmonary disease following obstructive pulmonary fibrosis. Chest 77:473-77, Apr., 1980.

Meador, B. Why COPD can end in heart failure—and what you can do about it. RN 43:64-66+, May, 1980.

Millar, S. Methods in critical care. Philadelphia: W.B. Saunders Co., 1980.

Morrison, M.L., et al. Respiratory intensive care nursing. Boston: Little, Brown and Co., 1979.

Netter, F.H. Respiratory System. New Jersey: CIBA, 1979.

Perdue, P. Urgent priorities in severe trauma. Life-threatening respiratory injuries, Part 1. RN 44:26-33, Apr., 1981.

Prior, John A., et al. Physical diagnosis. St. Louis: C.V. Mosby Co., 1973.

Ramsdell, J.W., et al. Determination of bronchodilation in the clinical pulmonary function laboratory: role of changes in static lung volumes. Chest 76:622-28, Dec., 1979.

Rokosky, J.S. Symposium on respiratory care. Assessment of the individual with altered respiratory function. Nurs. Clin. North Am. 16:195-209, Jun., 1981.

Rosenfeld, M., et al. Manual of medical therapeutics. Boston: Little, Brown and Co., 1973.

Sibbald, W.J., et al. Alveolo-capillary permeability in human septic ARDS: effect of high-dose corticosteroid therapy. Chest 79:133-42, Feb., 1981.

Spragg, R.G. Adult respiratory distress syndrome. Hosp. Med. 15:31-33+, Mar., 1979.

Stroud, S. Shock lung—adult respiratory distress syndrome—on the rise. Crit. Care. Update 7:25-26+, Jan., 1980.

Thorn, G., et al. Harrison's principles of internal medicine. New York: McGraw-Hill, 1977.

Viji, D., et al. A simplified concept of complete physiological monitoring of the critically ill patient. Heart Lung 10:75-82, Jan./Feb., 1981.

West, J. Respiratory physiology. Baltimore: Williams and Wilkins, 1978.

White, R.D. Airway management: esophageal obturator airway, endotracheal intubation, and cricothyrotomy. EMT J. 4:31-36, Mar., 1980.

Worthington, L. Hypoxemia. RN 43:48-53+, May, 1980.

Wyka, K. Techniques for the detection of small airways disease. Resp. Ther. 10:50-52, Jan./Feb., 1980.

Yancey, W., et al. Unrecognized tracheal intubation: a complication of the esophageal obturator airway. ANN Emerg. Med. 9:18-20, Jan., 1980.

CARDIOVASCULAR SYSTEM

CHAPTER 5

A blow to the heart—blunt chest trauma. Emerg. Med. 12:59-60, Sep. 15, 1980.

Advanced cardiac life support. American Heart Assoc., 1977.

Alspach, J.A. Electrical axis: how to recognize deviations on the ECG and interpret them. Am. J. Nurs. 79:1976-83, Nov., 1979.

Athayde, M.P. Interpreting normal electrocardiograms. AORN J. 33:1267-77, Jun., 1981.

Bates, B. A guide to physical examination. Philadelphia: J.B. Lippincott Co., 1974.

Bennett, B.R. EKG changes following penetration trauma to the heart. EMT J. 5:202-5, Jun., 1981.

Borg, N. Care curriculum for critical care nursing, ed. 2. Philadelphia: W.B. Saunders, 1981.

Botvinick, E.H. Nuclear cardiology, myocardial infarction, avid and blood-pool scintigraphy, Part 2. CVP 9:41-42+, Jun./Jul., 1981.

Crampton, R. High- versus low-energy defibrillation in cardiac arrest. Top. Emerg. Med. 3:69-78, Jul., 1981.

Crumlish, C.M. Cardiogenic shock: catch it early! Nursing (Horsham) 11:34-41, Aug., 1981.

Daily, E.K. and J.S. Schroeder. Techniques in bedside hemodynamic monitoring, ed. 2. St. Louis: C.V. Mosby Co., 1981.

Danzi, D.F., et al. Ventricular septal defect following blunt chest trauma—case report. ANN Emerg. Med. 150-54, Mar., 1980.

Dubb, A., et al. A study in left bundle branch aberration. Heart Lung 9:144-45, Jan./Feb., 1980.

Edwards Laboratories. Hemodynamic training manual. Division of American Hospital Supply Corp., 1979.

Ehsani, A.A., et al. Noninvasive assessment of changes in left ventricular function induced by graded isometric exercise in healthy subjects (research med.). Chest 80:51-55, Jul., 1981.

Eisenberg, M.S., et al. Out-of-hospital cardiac arrest: a review of major studies and a proposed uniform reporting system. Am. J. Public Health 70:236-40, Mar., 1980.

Franciosa, J.A. Nitroglycerin and nitrates in congestive heart failure. Heart Lung 9:873-82, Sep./Oct., 1980.

Gaines, H.P. The multi-problem patient...diabetes...congestive heart failure. J. Pract. Nurs. 30:13-16+, Feb., 1980.

Gibson, J.A. Arterial line placement, monitoring, and maintenance. NITA 4:140-41, Mar./Apr., 1981.

Giles, T.D. Principles of vasodilator therapy for left ventricular congestive heart failure. Heart Lung 9:271-76, Mar./Apr., 1980.

Gould, L., et al. Usefulness of the electrocardiogram and vectorcardiogram in left bundle branch block and myocardial infarction. Chest 77:208-10, Feb., 1980.

Green, E.D., et al. Cardiac concussion following soft-ball blow to the chest—case report. ANN Emerg. Med. 9:155-57, Mar., 1980.

Hayward, R. Reading the electrocardiogram. Chest Heart Stroke J. 3:54-61, #5, 1979.

Houser, S.R. Cardiac electrophysiology: cellular events that underlie the ECG. CVP 8:44-47+, Apr./May, 1980.

Hummeloard, A.B., et al. Calcium and calcium slow channel blockers: an overview. CCQ 4:17-28, Sep., 1981.

Jones, R.H., et al. Radionuclide angiocardiography. Appl. Radiol. 8:188-94+, Nov./Dec., 1979.

Julihn, M. Cardiac tamponade. Emergency 13:18+, Jun., 1981.

Karliner, J.S. and G. Gregoratos. Coronary care. New York: Churchill Livingston, 1981.

Marguard, C.L., et al. A case of Prinzmetal's angina with right bundle branch block. Heart Lung 9:531-33, May/Jun., 1980.

Marriott, H.J.L. AV block: an overdue overhaul. Emerg. Med. 30:1384-87+, Mar., 1981.

McCarthy, E. Hemodynamic effects and clinical assessment of dysrhythmias. CCQ 4:9-15, Sep., 1981.

McEvoy, M. Functional heart murmurs. Nurse Pract. 6:34+, Mar./Apr., 1981.

Meislin, H.W. The esophageal obturator airway: a study of respiratory effectiveness. ANN Emerg. Med. 9:54-59, Feb., 1980.

Nowak, R.M., et al. Bretylium tosylate as initial treatment for cardiopulmonary arrest: randomized comparison with placebo (research med.). ANN Emerg. Med. 10:404-7, Aug., 1981.

Panteleo, N., et al. The noninvasive evaluation of ventricular function by performance of equilibrium radionuclide ventriculography. CCQ 4:55-65, 1981.

Papenhausen, J.L. Data-based criteria for cardiovascular nursing intervention. CCQ 4:1-7, Sep., 1981.

Roberts, A. Systems and signs: the cardiovascular system. Part 69 of Systems of life. Nurs. Times 76: center pages, Sep., 1980.

Roffman, J.A., et al. Ventricular conduction defects: significance and prognosis. Heart Lung 9:111-21, Jan./Feb., 1980.

Seager, S.B. Cardiac enzymes in the evaluation of chest pain. ANN Emerg. Med. 9:346-49, Jul., 1980.

Shively, M. The physiologic principles of intraortic balloon counterpulsation. CCQ 4:83—8, Sep., 1981.

Sokolow, M. and M.B. McIlroy. Clinical cardiology, ed. 2. Los Altos: Lange Medical Publications, 1979.

Sprung, C.L., et al. Ventricular arrhythmias during Swan-Ganz catheterization of the critically ill. Chest 79:413-15, Apr., 1981.

Wilson, R.F. Critical care manual, Vol. 1. The Upjohn Co., 1976.

RENAL SYSTEM
CHAPTER 6

American Association of Critical Care Nursing. Core curriculum for critical care nursing. Philadelphia: W.B. Saunders Co., 1981.

Anderson, R.J., T. Berl, et al. Clinical disorders of water metabolism. Kidney Int. 10:117, 1976.

Aronoff, G. Antimicrobial therapy in patients with impaired renal function. Dialysis Transplant 1, 8:14, 1979.

Christopherson, L.K. and T.A. Gonde. Patterns of grief: end-stage renal failure and kidney transplantation. J. Thanato 3:49-57, 1975.

Drutz, D. Altered cell-mediated immunity and its relationship to infection susceptibility in patients with uremia. Dialysis Transplant 4, 8:320, 1979.

Fischbach, F. A manual of laboratory diagnostic tests. Philadelphia: J.B. Lippincott Co., 1980.

Friedman, E.A. Strategy in renal failure. New York: John Wiley & Sons, 1978.

Gambertoglio, J. Pharmacokinetic principles and renal disease. Dialysis Transplant 1, 8:8, 1979.

Gibson, T. Dialyzability of common therapeutic agents. Dialysis Transplant 1, 8:24, 1979.

Gulyassy, P. Abnormal drug binding in uremia. Dialysis Transplant 1, 8:19, 1979.

Guyton, A.C. Textbook of medical physiology. Philadelphia: W.B. Saunders Co., 1981.

Hall, R., et al. Attitudes toward illness as a predictor of adjustment of chronic hemodialysis. Dialysis Transplant 2, 8:138, 1979.

Hariprasad, M. and R. Eisinger. Experience with a one-bed acute hemodialysis unit. Dialysis Transplant 6, 8:596, 1979.

Hekelman, F.P. and C.A. Ostendarp. Nephrology nursing perspectives of care. New York: McGraw-Hill, 1979.

Kossoris, P. Family therapy: an adjunct to hemodialysis and transplantation. Am. J. Nurs. 70:1730, 1970.

Kroah, J. An exploratory study of the strategies that renal nurses use in response to emotional reaction and behaviors of hemodialysis patients. Image 5:16, 1972.

Leaf, A. and R. Cotran. Renal pathophysiology. New York: Oxford University Press, 1976.

Merrill, R.H. Review of vascular access. Dialysis Transplant 6, 9:22-28, 1977.

Rose, B. Clinical physiology of acid-base and electrolyte disorders. New York: McGraw-Hill, 1977.

Schrier, R.W. Renal and electrolyte disorders. 304-5. Boston: Little, Brown and Co., 1976.

Schroeder, J. and E. Daily. Techniques in bedside hemodynamic monitoring. St. Louis: C.V. Mosby Co., 1976.

Stark, J. Renal failure: imbalances inevitable. *In* Monitoring fluid and electrolytes precisely. Philadelphia: Nursing Skills Books, 1978.

Stark, J. BUN/creatinine—your keys to kidney function. Nursing 80 5, 10:33, 1980.

Strout, V., C. Lee and C.A. Schapen. Fluid and electrolytes. Philadelphia: F.A. Davis Co., 1977.

Teschan, P. Neurologic aspects of renal disease. Dialysis Transplant 6, 8:646, 1979.

Ulrich, B. Nephrology nurse: teaching the teachers to teach. Dialysis Transplant 7, 8:744, 1979.

Valtin, H. Renal dysfunction: mechanisms involved in fluid and solute imbalance. Boston: Little, Brown and Co., 1979.

Villazon, A., J. Portos and A. Sierra. Polyuric syndromes in the critically ill patient. Crit. Care Med. 4:25, 1976.

Weiner, M., Pepper et al. Clinical pharmacology and therapeutics in nursing. New York: McGraw-Hill, 1979.

Widmann, F. Clinical interpretation of laboratory tests. Philadelphia: F.A. Davis Co., 1973.

Zschoche, D. Comprehensive review of critical care. St. Louis: C.V. Mosby Co., 1976.

ENDOCRINE SYSTEM

CHAPTER 7

American Association of Critical Care Nursing. Core curriculum for critical care nursing. Philadelphia: W.B. Saunders Co., 1981.

Beeson, P.B., W. McDermott and J.B. Wyngaarden. Textbook of medicine. Philadelphia: W.B. Saunders Co., 1979.

Bolinger, R.E. Hypoglycemia. Crit. Care Q. 3:99, 1980.

Bondy, P.K. and L.E. Rosenburg. Duncan's diseases of metabolism: endocrinology. Philadelphia: W.B. Saunders Co., 1974.

Brunner, L.S. and D.S. Suddarth. Textbook of medical-surgical nursing. Philadelphia: J.B. Lippincott Co., 1980.

Brunner, L.S. and D.S. Suddarth. The Lippincott manual of nursing practice. Philadelphia: J.B. Lippincott Co., 1978.

Cataland, S. Hypoglycemia: a spectrum of problems. Heart Lung 7:455, 1978.

Cryer, P.E. Diagnostic endocrinology. New York: Oxford University Press, 1979.

Fairchild, R.S. Diabetes insipidus: a review. Crit. Care Q. 3:111, 1980.

Fischbach, Frances. A manual of laboratory diagnostic tests. Philadelphia: J.B. Lippincott Co., 1980.

Forsham, P.H. Abnormalities of the adrenal cortex. Clin. Symp. 15:35, 1976.

Guyton, A.C. Textbook of medical physiology. Philadelphia: W.B. Saunders Co., 1981.

Hamburger, S.C. and D.R. Rush. Syndrome of inappropriate secretion of antidiuretic hormone. Crit. Care Q. 3:119, 1980.

Hellman, R. The evaluation and management of hyperthyroid crises. Crit. Care Q. 3:77, 1980.

Kubo, W.M. and M.M. Grant. The syndrome of inappropriate secretion of antidiuretic hormone. Heart Lung 7:469, 1978.

Kyner, J.L. Diabetic ketoacidosis. Crit. Care Q. 3:65, 1980.

Luckmann, J. and K.C. Sorenson. Medical-surgical nursing: a psychophysiologic approach. Philadelphia: W.B. Saunders Co., 1980.

Rodman, M. and D. Smith. Clinical pharmacology in nursing. Philadelphia, J.B. Lippincott Co., 1979.

Schimke, N.R. Adrenal insufficiency. Crit. Care Q. 3:19, 1980.

Skillman, T.G. Diabetic ketoacidosis. Heart Lung 7:594, 1978.

Sneid, D.S. Hyperosmolar hyperglycemic nonketotic coma. Crit. Care Q. 3:29, 1980.

Something to sniff at. Emerg. Med. 8:92, 1976.

Thorn, G., R. Adams et al. Harrison's principles of internal medicine. New York: McGraw-Hill, 1977.

Tzagournis, M. Acute adrenal insufficiency. Heart Lung 7:603, 1978.

Urbanic, R.C. and E.L. Mazzaferri. Thyrotoxic crisis and myxedema coma. Heart Lung 7:435, 1978.

Weiner, M., Pepper et al. Clinical pharmacology and therapeutics in nursing. New York: McGraw-Hill, 1979.

Williams, R.H. Textbook of endocrinology. Philadelphia: W.B. Saunders Co., 1974.

GASTROINTESTINAL SYSTEM

CHAPTER 8

AMA drug evaluations, ed. 4. Chicago: American Medical Association, 1980.

Bates, B. A guide to physical examination, ed. 2. Philadelphia: J.B. Lippincott, Co., 1979.

Beeson, P.B. and W. McDermott. Textbook of medicine, ed. 14. Philadelphia: W.B. Saunders Co., 1975.

Condon, R.E. and L.M. Nyhus. Manual of surgical therapeutics, ed. 4. Boston: Little, Brown and Co., 1978.

Conn, H.F. and R.B. Conn. Current diagnosis. Philadelphia: W.B. Saunders Co., 1974.

Cooperman, A.M., Ed. The surgical clinics of North America: symposium on peptic ulcer disease, 56, No. 6. Philadelphia: W.B. Saunders Co., Dec., 1976.

Copenhauer, W.M., et al. Baily's textbook of histology, ed. 17. Baltimore: Williams and Wilkins, 1978.

Delp, M.H. and R.T. Manning. Major's physical diagnosis, ed. 8. Philadelphia: W. B. Saunders Co., 1975.

Freitag, J.J. and L.W. Miuer. Manual of medical therapeutics, ed. 23. Boston: Little, Brown and Co., 1980.

Freston, J.W., Ed. Clinics in gastroenterology: GI pharmacology and current therapy, 8, No. 1. London: W.B. Saunders Co., Jan., 1979.

Gilman, A.G., et al. Goodman and Gilman's the pharmacological basis of therapeutics, ed. 6. New York: MacMillan, 1980.

Given, B.A. and S.J. Simmons. Gastroenterology in clinical nursing, ed. 3. St. Louis: C.V. Mosby Co., 1979.

Guyton, A.C. Textbook of medical physiology, ed. 6. Philadelphia: W.B. Saunders Co., 1981.

Hollinshead, W.H. Textbook of anatomy, ed. 3. Hagerstown: Harper and Row, 1974.

Kaminski, M.V., et al. Intravenous hyperalimentation in modern hospital practice. Tuckahoe: USV Pharmaceutical Corp., 1977.

Mountcastle, V.B. Medical physiology, 2, ed. 14. St. Louis: C.V. Mosby Co., 1980.

Mullen, J.L., Ed. The surgical clinics of North America: surgical nutrition, 61, No. 3. Philadelphia: W.B. Saunders Co., Jun., 1981.

Netter, F.H.   The CIBA collection of medical illustrations: digestive system, Part III, liver, biliary tract and pancreas, 3.   New Jersey: CIBA Pharmaceuticals, 1975.

Netter, F.H.   The CIBA collection of medical illustrations: digestive system, Part I, upper digestive tract, 3.   New Jersey: CIBA Pharmaceuticals, 1975.

Netter, F.H.   The CIBA collection of medical illustrations: digestive system, Part II, lower digestive tract, 3.   New Jersey: CIBA Pharmaceuticals, 1975.

Robbins, S.L., et al.   Basic pathology, ed. 3.   Philadelphia: W.B. Saunders Co., 1981.

Sabiston, D.C.   Davis-Christopher textbook of surgery, ed. 11.   Philadelphia: W.B. Saunders Co., 1977.

Sisson, J.A.   The bare facts of general pathology, ed. 3.   Philadelphia: J.B. Lippincott Co., 1979.

Snell, R.S.   Clinical anatomy for medical students.   Boston: Little, Brown and Co., 1973.

Torsoli, A., Ed.   Clinics in gastroenterology: gastrointestinal emergencies, 10, No. 1.   London: W.B. Saunders Co., Jan., 1981.

Warwick, R. and P.L. Williams.   Gray's anatomy, ed. 35 British.   Philadelphia: W.B. Saunders Co., 1973.

HEMATOPOIETIC SYSTEM
CHAPTER 9

Battezzati, M.   The lymphatic system, rev. ed.   New York: John Wiley and Sons, 1972.

Behnke, H.   Guidelines for comprehensive nursing care in cancer.   New York: Springer Publishing Co., 1973.

Beland, I. and J. Passos.   Clinical nursing—pathophysiology and psychosocial approaches.   New York: MacMillan, 1975.

Beutler, E.   Hemolytic anemia in disorders of red cell metabolism.   New York: Plenum Medical Book Co., 1978.

Biggs, R.   Human blood coagulation, hemostasis, and thrombosis. Blackwell Scientific Publications, ed. 2.   Philadelphia: J.B. Lippincott, 1976.

Bouchard, R. and N.F. Owens.   Nursing care of the cancer patient.   St. Louis: C.V. Mosby Co., 1976.

Brinkhouse, K.M., R.W. Shermer and F.K. Mostofi.   The platelet.   Baltimore: Williams and Wilkins, 1971.

Brunner and Suddorth.   Textbook of medical-surgical nursing, ed. 4.   Philadelphia: J.B. Lippincott Co., 1980.

DeGruchy, G.   Clinical hematology in medical practice, ed. 4.   London: Blackwell Scientific Publications, 1978.

Germain, C.   The cancer unit: an ethnography.   Wakefield, Mass.: Nursing Resources, Inc., 1979.

Gung, F. and A. Baikie.   Leukemia.   New York: Grune and Stratton, 1974.

Katz, A.   Hemophilia.   Springfield: Charles C. Thomas, 1970.

Kinney, M.R.   AACN's clinical reference for critical-care nursing.   New York: McGraw-Hill, 1981.

Lacher, M.   Hodgkin's disease.   New York: John Wiley and Sons, 1976.

Leavell, B.S. and O.A. Thorup.   Fundamentals of clinical hematology, ed. 4.   Philadelphia: W.B. Saunders Co., 1976.

Lichtman, M.A.   Hematology for practitioners.   Boston: Little, Brown and Co., 1978.

Petz, L.D. and G. Garritty.   Acquired immune hemolytic anemias.   New York: Churchill Livingston, 1980.

Platt, W.R.   Hematology, ed. 2.   Philadelphia: J.B. Lippincott, 1979.

Race, R.R. and R. Sanger. Blood groups in man, ed. 6. Philadelphia: J.B. Lippincott, 1970.

Roberts, S.L. Behavioral concepts and the critically ill patient. Englewood Cliffs, New Jersey: Prentice Hall, Inc., 1976.

Schleicher, E.M. Bone marrow morphology and mechanics of biopsy. Springfield, Illinois: Charles C. Thomas, 1973.

Smith, D.W. and C.P. Germain. Care of the adult patient, ed. 4. Philadelphia: J.B. Lippincott, 1975.

Tiffany, R. Oncology for nurses and health care professionals, Vol. 1. Boston: George Allen and Unwin, 1978.

Williams, W.J., E. Beutler and R.W. Rundles. Hematology, ed. 2. New York: McGraw-Hill, 1977.

INDEX

Abdomen,
   auscultation, 508-09
   examination, 506-511
      in assessment of shock, 307
   palpation, 509
   percussion, 509
   physical assessment, 506-510

Abducens nerve, 74, 75

Absorption,
   in capillary dynamics, 145-48
   in small intestines, 495-96

Acetylcholine,
   in myoneural junction, 58
   as neurotransmitter, 58
   in regulation of peripheral
      regulation, 241

Acid-base balance, 143-158
   buffer system, 149
   in carbon dioxide, 377-79
   chemical buffers, 149
   function, 149
   in homeostasis, 143
   regulation of, 143-45
   renal, 399

Acid secretions of stomach, 491

Acidosis,
   causes, 153
   electrolyte imbalance, 152
   Henderson-Hasselbalch equation, 150-51
   metabolic, 153
      in renal disease, 153, 379
      signs & symptoms, 153
   respiratory, 153
      signs & symptoms, 153

Acinar cells, 432

Acoustic nerve, 75

Acromegaly, 434

Actin in sarcoplasm, 237

Action potential, 247-48
   refractory period, 248

Active transport,
   in small intestines, 494

Addiction, 25-26

Adrenal androgens, 433

Adrenal arteriography, 442

Adrenal cortex, 433
   adrenal androgens of, 433, 442
   glucocorticoids of, 433, 442
   mineralocorticoids of, 433, 444

Adrenal crisis, 450-51

Adrenal glands, 433
   location of, 433

Adrenal medulla, 433, 442

Adrenocorticotropic hormone (ACTH), 435

Afferent fibers of central
   nervous system, 68

Afterload, 258

Aggressive sexual behavior, 24-25

Airway,
   maintenance of, 183
   obstruction of, 182
   resistance, 145
   suctioning, 141-42

Aldosterone, 375

Alimentary tract (*see* Gastrointestinal)

Alkalosis,
   electrolyte imbalance, 155
   metabolic, 155
      signs & symptoms, 155
   renal, 379
   respiratory, 154
      signs & symptoms, 154

Alveolar ventilation, 142

Alveoli, 148
   adult respiratory distress, 168
   collapse, 148

Anaphylactic reactions, 590

Androgens, adrenal, 433

Anemia, 259
   aplastic, 582
   hemolytic, 585
   hypoxia, 259
   leukemia, 585-86
   treatment in renal failure, 350

Anemic hypoxia, 259

Angina, 298

Angiography,
   pulmonary, 164

Angiotensin,
   in fluid balance, 375
   production of, 375

Angle of Louis, 159

Anion gap, 154

Anterior pituitary gland, 433-440

Antibody(ies),
   in immune defense
      mechanisms, 573

Anticoagulants,
 in balloon pumping, 321
Antidiuretic hormone (ADH), 432
 in autonomic nervous system, 432
 blood level of, in osmosis
  in kidneys, 564
 in regulation of body water, 349
 in regulation of osmolality
  of body fluids, 349-360
 in urine concentration, 349
Antigens, 576
Antrum,
 of stomach, 488
Anxiety, 29
 in family of critical-care patient, 29
 guides for nursing action related
  to, 29-30
 management of, 29-30
 in psychosociodynamics of sick
  role, 19-30
Aorta,
 palpation of, 261-63
Aortic bodies, 251
Aortic ejection clicks, 266
Aortic valve,
 murmur, 267
Apex cardiography, 269
Apex of heart, 236
Aplastic anemia, 582-83
 assessment, 582
 nursing care, 582
 pathophysiology, 582
 treatment, 583
Appearance (see Assessment)
Aqueduct of Sylvius, 67
ARDS, 168
Arrest,
 block, 284
 sinus, 285
Arrhythmias,
 assessment—myocardial
  infarction, 299
 atrial pacing, 312
 pulmonary artery pressure
  monitoring, 321
 sinus, 283-85
Arterial waveforms, 323-24
Arteriosclerosis (see Atherosclerosis)
Arteriovenous fistula for
 hemodialysis, 395
Arteriovenous shunt for
 hemodialysis, 395

Artery(ies),
 colon, 501
 esophagus, 501
 gallbladder, 501
 kidneys, 368
 liver, 501
 pulmonary, 303
 small intestines, 501
 stomach, 501
Arthus's phenomena, 575
Assessment,
 cardiovascular, 260-67
 endocrine, 441-42
 gastrointestinal, 440-44
 hematopoietic, 578-581
 nervous, 73-79
 pulmonary, 158-166
 renal, 480-84
Asthmaticus, status, 172-73
 clinical presentation, 173
 nursing care, 173
 pathophysiology, 172
Atelectasis, 149
Atherosclerosis, 297
Atria,
 anatomy, 238
 conduction, 239
Atrial contraction,
 premature, 285-86
Atrial fibrillation, 288
Atrial flutter, 288
Atrial tachycardia, 286
Atrioventricular (AV) node, 238-39
Atrioventricular valves, 239
Atropine sulfate, 283
Auscultation,
 of abdomen, 508
 of heart, 262-63
 of lung, 163-64
Autoimmune diseases, 575
Automaticity,
 heart rate, 241
Autonomic nervous system,
 anatomy of, 70
 cardiac regulation, 249
 physiology of, 70-71
Autoregulation,
 coronary blood flow, 250-51
 peripheral circulation, 251
 renal blood flow, 368
 stroke volume, 254
Axis, 275

Axons, 55

B cell, 574

B cell immune response, 574

Bainbridge reflex, 256

Balloon, intra-aortic, 321-22

Baroreceptors,
  in regulation of arterial pressure, 143
  in regulation of peripheral pressure, 143
  in shock, 305

Bicarbonate ions,
  concentration in body fluids, 147-49

Bile,
  function, 503
  metabolism, 503
  regulation, 503

Bile canaliculi, 503

Bile pigments, 503

Bile salts, 503

Biliary tract disease, 523

Bilirubin, 581

Blood,
  cells, 563
    red, 568
    white, 570
  color, 563
  composition & characteristics, 563-64
  distribution of, 563-66
  groups, 576-77
  hydrogen ion concentration, 563
  loss of, 565
  osmotic pressure, 565
  oxyhemoglobin, 569
  pH, 563
  plasma, 563-64
  specific gravity, 563
  tests on, 580
  viscosity of, 563
  volume, 563-64

Blood count in hematopoietic disorders, 580

Blood gases, arterial, 148-49

Blood pressure,
  assessment of shock, 305
  regulation, 393

Blood urea nitrogen, 383

Blood vessels,
  anatomy, 245
  diameter in hemodynamics, 245, 250-51
  renal, control mechanisms, 373-74

Body fluid, buffer system in acid-base, 149

Body of stomach, 488

Bone marrow,
  blood cell production, 566-67
  erythrocyte production, 568
  specimen of, in assessment, 581

Bones,
  growth, 434
  organ, 566

Bowman's capsule, 367

Bradycardia, sinus, 283
  drug therapy, 283

Brain,
  anatomy, 51-62
  blood flow, 63-64
  circulation, 63-64
  increased intracranial pressure, 95-96
  metabolism, 60-61
  monitoring, 96
  ventricular system, 66-67

Brain stem,
  divisions, 59-60
  functions, 61-62

Breath sounds, auscultation, 163

Bronchi, 136

Bronchial breath sounds, 163

Bronchitis,
  chronic, 170

Bronchophony, 163

Bronchovesicular breath sounds, 163

Bruit in monitoring AV fistula, 396

Brunner's glands, 494

Buffer system, 149

Bundle-branch block,
  left, 279-280
  right, 278-79

Cable in EKG monitor, 271-74

Calcitonin,
  deficiency of, 437
  functions of, 437
  regulation, 437

Calcium,
  deficiency of,
    effects of kidney, 375
    effects of/on parathormone on/of, 375, 437
  regulation, 437

Canaliculi, bile, 503

Cannula, hemodialysis, 394-95

Capillary anatomy, 245

Carbohydrates,
  absorption small intestines, 496
  in total parenteral nutrition, 528-29

Carbon dioxide,
  effects of, on ventilation, 147

Cardia of stomach, 488

Cardiac cycle, 252-53

Cardiac index, 253

Cardiac output, 135
  control of, 253
  definition of, 253
  factors influencing, 253-55
  measurement, 254-55
  thermal dilution, 255

Cardiac pacemaker, 308

Cardiac patient,
  differential diagnosis, 267-297
  evaluation, 267-297
  monitoring techniques, 267-297
    angiographic, 296-97
    echocardiographic, 268
    electrophysiologic, 246

Cardiac pump (*see also* Heart), 235-36

Cardiac tamponade,
  nursing care, 180
  pathophysiology, 180

Cardiogenic pulmonary edema, 301

Cardiogenic shock,
  assessment, 305
  intra-aortic balloon pumping, 321

Cardiovascular system, 235-322
  action potential, 248
  anatomy, 235-242
  assessment, 260-297
  cardiac pump, 235-38
  circulation, 243-46
  electrical conduction, 241-42
  electrocardiography, 267
  electrophysiology, 246
  evaluation of, 260-68
  hemodynamics, 321
  pathophysiology, 297-315
  physiology, 246-48
  pulmonary circulation, 235
  surgery, 316
  vector cardiography, 269

Carotid arteries, 262

Carotid bodies, 250

Catecholamines, 439
  in shock, 305

Catheters,
  cardiac catheterization, 295
  peritoneal dialysis, 394
  Swan-Ganz, 295
  total parenteral nutrition, 529

Cauda equina, 67

Cecum of colon, 497-98

Cell bodies of neurons, 55

Cell-mediated immunity, 573
  T cell, 573

Central nervous system,
  anatomy, 61-69
    brain, 61-66
    cranial nerves, 69-75
    spinal cord & spinal nerves, 67
  physiology,
    motor testing, 76
    reflex activities, 59-60
    sensory, 76
  support,
    cerebral circulation, 63-63
    cerebrospinal fluid, 67
    meninges, 52
    skull, 51-53
    ventricles, 66-67
    vertebral column, 53-54

Central venous pressure, 257

Cerebellum,
  anatomy, 60
  motor integration, 60-61

Cerebral aneurysm, 81-82

Cerebral circulation, 63-64

Cerebral hemispheres, 61

Cerebral vascular accident, 79-81

Cerebrospinal fluid, 67

Chemoreceptors, 250
  in blood gases, 250
  in peripheral regulation, 143

Chest physiotherapy, 192

Chest trauma, 176-180

Cheyne-Stokes respiration, 78

Chief cells, 432, 491

Chloride, 147, 376

Cholecystokinin, 493

Choroid plexus, 66

Chronic obstructive pulmonary disease (COPD), 170-72

Chymotrypsin, 523

Cimetidine, 49

Circle of Willis, 63

Circulation,
    cerebral, 63-64
    coronary, 243
    hemodynamics, 251-55
    portal, 501
    liver, 505-6

Cirrhosis, 512
    hepatic failure, 515
    portal hypertension, 514

Clubbing of nails, 162

Coagulation, intravascular disseminated, 591-92

Coagulation factor(s), 577-78
    I, fibrinogen, 577
    II, prothrombin, 577
    III, tissue thromboplastin, 577
    V, proaccelerin, 577
    VII, proconvertin, 577
    VIII, antihemophilic factor, 592
    X, Stuart factor, 577
    XI, plasma thromboplastin antecedent, 577
    XII, Hageman factor, 577

Colon (see Intestines)

Color,
    of blood (see Assessment), 563

Coma,
    hyperosmolar hyperglycemic nonketotic, 449

Compliance,
    pulmonary, 144
    ventilatory, 144

Computer, cardiac output, 253

Computerized axial tomography (CAT), 78

Conduction, electrical, 241-42
    blood supply, 244

Congestive heart failure, 301

Consciousness,
    assessment, 441

Continuous positive airway pressure (CPAP), 192

Contractility, myocardial, 258

Contractions,
    atrial, premature, 285
    junctional, premature, 289
    muscular (see Seizures)

Convulsions (see Seizures)

Coronary circulation, 243

Cor pulmonale in emphysema, 170

Cortex,
    adrenal, 433, 438

Cortical nephrons, 366-67

Corticospinal motor tracts, 68

Corticosteroids, 438

Cortisol, 438

Cranial nerves, 74-75

Creatine phosphokinase (CPK), 267

Creatinine, 383

Cricothyrotomy, 185

Crisis, 27

Critical care,
    problems, 27
    psychosocial basis, 19-30

Cushing's reflex, 251

Cyanosis (see Assessment)

Death, 30-31

Decerebrate, 77

Decorticate, 77

Defense mechanism, 22-23

Dehydration, 397

Dehydrogenase deficiency, 583

Dendrites, 55

Denial, 23

Depression, 24

Dermatomes, 76

Diabetes insipidus, 444-46

Diabetes mellitus, 447

Diabetic ketoacidosis, 447-49

Dialysis, 393-95

Diastolic murmurs, 266

Diazepam, 93, 190

Diencephalon, 61

Diffusion, 145-46

Disseminated intravascular coagulation, 591-92

Diuretic phase of acute renal failure, 385

Diuretics, 384

Dopamine, 308

Dura mater, 52

Dying, 30-31

Dysuria, 381

Echocardiography, 268

Edrophonium chloride, 89

Effector T cells, 573
Efferent fibers of central nervous system, 68
Egophony, 163
Einthoven's triangle, 271
Ejection clicks, 265
Ejection murmurs, 265
Electrical conduction (*see* Conduction)
Electrocardiography, 269-295
Electrodes, leads, 271-73
Electrolyte balance, 398
Electrolytes,
    balance, kidneys, 375-77
    EKG changes, 282
    loss, small intestines, 495
    total parenteral nutrition, 529
Electrophysiology, cardiac, 246-49
Emotional impact, complicating ventilatory assistance, 194
Emphysema,
    critical care, 170
    diagnostic data, 171
    nursing care, 171
    pathophysiology, 170
Endocrine system, 431-451
    adrenal crisis, 450-51
    assessment, 441-43
    pancreas, 432
    thyroid crisis, 446
Endotracheal intubation, 184-85
Enzymes,
    cardiac, 267
    in digestion of proteins, 496
    intestine, in digestion of carbohydrates, 496
    pancreatic, 428, 504
Epidural technique for intracranial pressure, 96
Epinephrine,
    in regulation of systemic pressure, 251
    secretion of adrenal medulla, 437
Erythrocytes, 568-69
    regulation, 568
Erythropoiesis, 568
Esophogeal obturator airway, 184
Esophageal varices, 517-520
Esophagus, 485-87
    traumatic injuries, 182

Facial nerve (VII), 75
Family of critical care patient, 29
Fat(s), absorption by small intestines, 496
Feedback, negative, of pituitary, 432
Fibrinogen, 563
Fibrinogen-activating factor, 572
Fick technique, 254
Filtration, glomerular, 369
First-degree heart block, 29
Fistulas, AV, hemodialysis, 393
Flail, chest, 176
Fluids,
    in adrenal crisis, 450-53
    balance of, in homeostasis, 397
    in diabetic ketoacidosis, 447-48
    in hyperosmolar hyperglycemic nonketotic coma, 449
    intake and output, 453
    in intestinal obstruction, 529-531
    intravenous, TPN, 529
    osmolality, 392
    regulation, 392
Follicle-stimulating hormone (FSH), 435
Foramen magnum, of skull, 52
Foramen of Monro, 66
Frequency, urinary, 381
Fundus, stomach, 488

Gallbladder, 502
Gallop rhythm, 265
Gastric analysis, 511
Gastric glands, 488
Gastric phase, 491
Gastrin,
    function, 491
    gastric motility, 491
    regulation, 491-92
Gastritis, 520-22
Gastroesophageal sphincter, 487
Gastrointestinal system, 485-542
    anatomy, 485-506
    blood supply, 491
    disorders, 512-527
    nervous intervention, 501
    nutrition, 528
    pancreatitis, 522-23
Genitourinary system (*see* Renal)

Glands,
  acinar, in pancreas, 432
  adrenal, 433
  Brunner's, 494
  gastric, 491
  parathyroid, 432
  pituitary, 432
  thyroid, 432, 433, 437

Glial cells, 56

Glomerular filtration, 370

Glomerular filtration rate, 369

Glomerulus, 367

Glossopharyngeal nerve (IX), 75

Glucose,
  hyperosmolar hyperglycemic nonketotic coma, 449
  in TPN, 529
  intravenous, for hypoglycemia, 449

Glucose 6-phosphate, 583

Glutamic-oxaloacetic transaminase (SGOT), 267

Growth hormone, 434

Guillain-Barre syndrome,
  nursing care, 84
  pathophysiology, 83

Head,
  closed head injury, 84-86
  increased intracranial pressure, 95
  management, 86

Health history (see Assessment)

Heart,
  apex, 235
  atria, 238
  auscultation, 263-67
  base, 235
  circulation, 243
  cycle, 252-53
  examination, 261-67
  inspection, 261
  murmurs, 265-66
  myocardial infarction, 301
  nervous control, 249
  palpation, 262
  percussion, 262
  shock, 429
  sounds, 263-67
    extra, diastolic and systolic, 264-65
    first, 263
    fourth, 265
    normal, 263
    second, 263
    third, 265
  valves, 238
  ventricles, 238

Heart block, 290

Hematomas,
  epidural, 85
  intracranial, 85
  subdural, 85

Hematopoiesis, 563

Hematopoietic system, 563-597
  assessment, 578-582
  pathological states, 582-594

Hemiblocks, 258

Hemodialysis, 393

Hemodynamic monitoring, 321

Hemoglobin, 569
  oxygen-carrying capacity of, 559
  in oxygen transport, 559
  saturation, 559
  studies, 580

Hemolysis, 563

Hemolytic anemia, 582-85
  nursing care, 585
  pathology, 582

Hemolytic crisis, 593

Hemophilia B, 592

Hemophilia C, 592

Hemopneumothorax, 176

Hemorrhage,
  esophageal varices, 517
  peptic ulcer disease, 520

Hemorrhagic shock, 385

Hemostasis, 577

Hemothorax, 175

Henderson-Hasselbalch equation, 150-55

Henle's loops, 371

Heparin, 578, 394

Hepatic failure, 515

Hepatojugular reflex, 261

Hering-Breuer expiratory reflex, 143

His, bundle of, 280

History (see Assessment)

Hodgkin's disease, 587

Hormones,
  adrenocorticotropic, 434
  antidiuretic, 432
  follicle-stimulating, 435
  growth, 434
  luteinizing, 435
  melanocyte-stimulating, 436
  parathyroid, 437-38
  thyroid, 437

Humidification, 192

Humoral immunity, 573

Hydroxybutyrate dehydrogenase, 267

Hyperalimentation,
 enteral, 529
 parenteral, 529-530
 peripheral, 531

Hyperglycemia,
 complicating TPN, 529

Hyperkalemia, 152
 signs & symptoms, 152

Hyperosmolar hyperglycemic nonketotic coma, 449

Hypertension in renal disease, 392

Hypertensive crisis, 305

Hypoglossal nerve (XII), 75

Hypoglycemia, 449-450
 in TPN, 529

Hypoparathyroidism, 447

Hypovolemia (see Shock)

Hypoxia, 259

IgA, 574

IgE, 574

Immune response, 574

Immunity,
 acquired, 573
 cell mediated, 573-74
 humoral, 574

Immunoglobin, 574

Indicator dilution technique in measurement of cardiac output, 254

Infarction, myocardial, 533

Inflammatory response, 573-74

Inspection (see Assessment)

Insulin (see Pancreas)

Intermittent mandatory
 ventilation, 191
 weaning, 191

Intermittent positive pressure breathing, 192

Interstitial cell-stimulating hormone, 435-36

Intestines (see Colon),
 large, 493-99
  anatomy, 498
  motility, 498
  secretion & absorption, 498
 small, 493-97
  absorption, 496-97
  anatomy, 493
  motility, 494
  secretions, 497

Intra-aortic balloon pump, 321

Intracranial pressure, 95-97
 increased, 95
 monitoring, 96
 pathophysiology, 95

Intravenous fluids in parenteral alimentation, 529

Intubation, endotracheal, 134

Ions, bicarbonate, 147

Ischemia, myocardial, 321

Islets of Langerhans, 432

Isoenzymes, 268

Junctional contraction, premature, 289

Junctional rhythm, 289

Junctional tachycardia, 290

Juxtaglomerular cells, 368

Kidney(s),
 acid-base balance, 377-79
 ammonia generation, 379
 anatomy, 365
 blood flow, 368
 blood pressure regulation, 373
 calcium regulation, 375
 chloride regulation, 376
 complications, 400
 concentration of urine, 372
 electrolyte regulation, 375-77, 383
 failure, acute renal, 384
 failure, chronic renal, 388
 glomerular filtration, 369
 glomerulonephritis, 389-390
 pathological states, 384
 physiology, 369-371
 pyelonephritis, 388-89
 radiologic studies, 383
 tubules, 368

Kubler-Ross, 30-31

Kupffer cells, 566

Kussmaul's respirations, 448

Laboratory studies,
 cardiovascular, 297
 endocrine, 442
 gastrointestinal, 510
 hematopoietic, 580-82
 nervous, 78
 pulmonary, 163-64
 renal, 382

Lactate dehydrogenase (LDH), 267
Langerhans, islets of, 432
Left bundle-branch block, 279-280
Left ventricular filling pressure, 256
Leukemia, 585
Liver, 503
   cirrhosis, 512
   palpation, 509
   percussion, 509
Loops of Henle, 371
Louis, angle of, 159
Lungs,
   assessment, 159
   auscultation, 158-163
   palpation, 162
   pathological states, 170
   pathophysiology, 137-38
   percussion, 162
Luteinizing hormone (LH), 435

Lymphocytes, 570-75
Lymphomas, 587-88

Magnesium, 376
Maslow's Hierarchy, 19-20
Mechanical ventilation, 187-192
Medulla, adrenal, 433
Melanocyte-stimulating hormone, 436
Melanocytes, 436
Meninges, 52
Meningitis, 82-83
Mental attitudes, 20-21
Metabolic acidosis, 157
Metabolic alkalosis, 157
Mineralocorticoids, 438
Mitral valve, 241
Monitoring,
   intracranial pressure, 96
   pulmonary capillary wedge, 257-58
   waveforms, 324
Monro, foramen of, 66
Motility,
   gastric, 491
   small intestines, 491
Mouth, 486-87
Mucosa,
   esophageal, 488
   gastrointestinal, 488

Multiple myeloma, 594
Murmurs,
   diastolic, 266
   heart, 266
Myasthenia gravis, 89-91
Myelin sheath, 55
Myocardial infarction, 299
Myofibrils, 237
Myosin in sarcoplasm, 237

Nails (*see* Assessment)
Nasopharynx, 487
Nephron, 367
Nephrotic syndrome, 367
Nerve,
   abducens (VI), 75
   acoustic (VIII), 75
   cranial, anatomy, 74-75
   facial (VII), 75
   glossopharyngeal (IX), 75
   hypoglossal (XII), 75
   oculomotor (III), 73
   olfactory (I), 73
   optic (II), 73
   spinal accessory (XI), 75
   trigeminal (V), 75
   trochlear (IV), 75
   vagus (X), 75
Nervous system, 51-97
   anatomical divisions, 51
   anatomy, 51-54
   autonomic, 70-72
   brain, 61-66
   cerebral blood flow, 63
   cerebral metabolism, 60
   cranial nerves, 71-75
   parasympathetic, 70
   sympathetic, 70
   spinal cord, 67
Neuroglial cells, 56, 60
Neurologic states, 79-92
   increased intracranial pressure, 95-97
   nursing care, 95-97
   seizures, 91
Neurological assessment, 73-79
   examination, 76
Neurological status in endocrine disorders, 453
Neurons, 55-56
   impulse transmission, 56-57
Neutrophil, 570

Nitroprusside, 308

Norepinephrine, 251, 431

Nosocomial infection, 194

Nutrition,
   gastrointestinal disorders, 528-531
   parenteral, 529-531
   renal, 399

Oculomotor nerve (III), 73

Olfactory nerve (I), 73

Oliguria, 385

Oliguric phase of acute renal failure, 385

Optic nerve (II), 73

Oropharynx, 493

Osmolality, 372

Osmolarity, 372

Osmoreceptors, 251

Overhydration, 397

Oxygen,
   partial pressure, 145-46
   therapy, 192
   transport, 146-47

Oxygen equipment, 193-94

Oxyhemoglobin dissociation curve, 146

Pacemakers, 308-315

Pacing, 312

Pain, 28, 298, 299

Pancreas, 431, 432, 438

Pancreatitis, 522

Parasympathetic nervous system, 249

Parathormone (PTH), 431-32, 437-38

Parenteral hyperalimentation, 529

Parenteral nutrition, total, 529

Paroxysmal atrial tachycardia, 286
   with block, 287

Pepsinogen, 491

Peptic ulcer, 520-22

Pericarditis, 303

Peritoneal dialysis, 394

Peyer's patches, 494

pH, 149, 151, 157, 377, 379

Phagocytosis, 570

Phenobarbital,
   in status epilepticus, 93

Phenytoin, 92

Phosphate, 375

Physical assessment (*see* Assessment)

Physiotherapy, chest, 192

Pia mater, 53

Pituitary gland, 431-32

Plasma, 565

Plasma cells, 565

Plasma proteins, 565

Platelets, 563

Pleural friction rubs, 163

Pneumothorax, 178-79

Polycythemia, 589

Polydipsia, 444, 447

Polyuria, 444, 447

Portal hypertension, 517

Portal vein, 505

Positive end-expiratory pressure, 189

Potassium, 375

Preload, 256

Premature atrial contractions, 285
   with block, 286

Premature junctional contractions, 289

Premature ventricular contractions, 292

Pressoreceptors, 250

Prolactin, 436

Proteins,
   absorption, small intestines, 496

Psychological hazards, 19-31

Psychosocial nursing, 19-31

Pulmonary arterial pressure, 295

Pulmonary artery wedge pressure, 295
   measurement of, 323-24

Pulmonary capillary wedge pressure, 240, 295
   monitoring of, 257, 258

Pulmonary edema, 301

Pulmonary embolism,
  clinical features of, 174
  diagnosis of, 175
  nursing care, 175
  pathophysiology, 174

Pulmonary embolus, 174

Pulmonary system, 135-194
  diffusion of respiratory
    gases in, 149-158
  effects of kidney disease on, 149-158
  transportation of respiratory
    gases in, 146

Pulse, 262-63

Pulse pressure, 263

Pulsus alternans, 263

Pulsus paradoxus, 263

Pumps (see Heart)

Pupil(s),
  assessment of, 77

Pupillary reflexes, 77

Purkinje system, impulse
  transmission through, 241

Pylorus of stomach, 490

Q wave, 269

QS complex, 270

R wave, 270

Rales, 163

Red blood cells (see Erythrocytes)

Regurgitant murmurs, 263

Renal anatomy, 365

Renal assessment, 381

Renal insufficiency, 392

Renal physiology, 368-377

Renal system (see also Kidney(s)),
  365-417

Renin-angiotensin, 374, 433

Respiration (see Pulmonary system)

Respiratory,
  acidosis, 157
  alkalosis, 157
  anatomy, 138-142
  distress syndrome (RDS), 168-69
  failure, 166
  muscles, 143

Respiratory gases,
  diffusion of, 145
  transportation of, 146-47

Respiratory system,
  in acid-base balance regulation, 149
  disorders of, 149-158

Rh system, 576

Rhonchi, 163

Rhythm of heart (see Heart)

Right bundle-branch block, 278-79

Rigidity,
  decerebrate, assessment of
    comatose patient, 77
  decorticate, assessment of
    comatose patient, 77

Salts, bile, 503

Sarcolemma, 236

Scans, lung, 164

Second degree heart block, 291

Secretory IgA, 574

Seizures, 91-92
  generalized, 91
  grand mal, 91
  petit mal, 91

Semilunar valves, 241

Sensory deprivation, 27, 28

Sensory overload, 27, 28

Shock, 305-7

Sickle cell anemia, 583

Sinus, coronary, 243

Sinus arrest, 285

Sinus arrhythmia, 284

Sinus block, 284

Sinus bradycardia, 283

Sinus rhythm, normal, 283

Sinus tachycardia, 283

Skull, 51

Spherocytosis, 583

Spinal accessory nerve (XI),
  assessment, 75

Spinal cord,
  anatomy of, 67
  injuries, 86-88
  nursing care, 88
  shock, 86-87

Spleen, 567

S-T segment, 269

Status asthmaticus, 172-73

Status epilepticus, 92-93

Stomach,
    acid, 491-92
    gross anatomy of, 488
    motility of, 490
    secretions of, 490-92

Stress, 21-22

Stroke, 79

Stroke volume, 254

Suctioning,
    as adjunct to ventilation, 190
    of airway in patient on continuous assisted ventilation, 190

Suicide, 25-26

Supraventricular arrhythmias, 290

Swan-Ganz catheter, 295

Sylvius, aqueduct of, 66

Sympathetic nervous system, 70
    in control of heart rate, 249

Synaptic cleft in nerve impulse conduction for muscular contraction, 58

Systolic murmurs, 266

T cell subsets in immune response, 573

T wave, 269-270

Tachycardias (see also Arrhythmias),
    atria, paroxysmal, 287
    sinus, 283
    ventricular, 294

Tensilon for myasthenia gravis, 89

Tension pneumothorax, 176

Tetanus, 90-91

Thalassemia, 583

Thermodilution in measurement of cardiac output, 255

Third degree heart block, 292

Thoracic cage,
    inspection of, 159-160

Thyrocalcitonin, 437

Thyroid crises, 446

Thyroid gland, 432
    assessment of, 442
    location of, 432

Thyroid-stimulating hormone (TSH), 434

Thyrotoxic crises, 446

Thyroxine (T_4), 437

Tidal volume, 141

Tissue(s),
    and blood, gas exchange between, 141-157
    injury to, DIC, 591
    metabolic demands of, in internal respiration, 27, 157

Trachea, 135-36

Tracheal rupture, 181

Tracheostomy, 185
    emergency, indications for, 185, 186

Transmission of nerve impulses, 56

Tricuspid valve, 241

Trigeminal nerve (V), 75

Trochear nerve (IV), 75

Uremic syndrome, 401

Urinalysis in endocrine disorders, 442

Vagal stimulation, cardiac effects of, 249

Valsalva's maneuver, 277

Valve,
    aortic, 241
    cardiac, 241
    mitral, 241
    tricuspid, 241

Vascular anatomy, 243

Vascular access for hemodialysis, 396

Vasopressin, 251, 341

Vectorcardiography, 269

Veins, coronary, 243

Ventilation, 141-42
    adjuncts to, in advanced life support, 193
    intermittent mandatory, 191
    perfusion ratio, abnormalities, 148

Ventilators, mechanical 187-89

Ventilatory assistance emotional, impact complicating, 194

Ventricles, cardiac, 238-241
    afterload, 258
    anatomy, 308-311
    contractility, 241

Ventricular contractions, premature, 292

Ventricular fibrillation, 294

Ventricular tachycardia, 293

Vertebral column, 54

Vitamins,
   absorption by small intestine, 495
   B_{12}, 495
   D, 495
   production of, in colon, 499

Voice sounds, auscultation of, 163

Volume-cycled ventilators, 187-89

Weaning, 191

Wenckebach heart block, 291

White blood cells, 570-71

Willis, circle of, 63